The Road to Modern Surgery

Saleh Abbas • David Watters

The Road to Modern Surgery

A Historical Journey Through Surgical Landmarks

Springer

Saleh Abbas
Department of Surgery
University Hospital Geelong
Deakin University
Geelong, VIC, Australia

David Watters
Department of Surgery
University Hospital Geelong
Deakin University
Geelong, VIC, Australia

ISBN 978-981-96-4336-3 ISBN 978-981-96-4337-0 (eBook)
https://doi.org/10.1007/978-981-96-4337-0

This Springer imprint is published by the registered company Springer Nature Singapore Pte Ltd.
The registered company address is: 152 Beach Road, #21-01/04 Gateway East, Singapore 189721, Singapore

Preface

Surgery, in its essence, represents humanity's enduring quest to heal the body and alleviate suffering. It is both a science and an art, emerging as a profession in which the frontiers of knowledge are combined with increasing technical precision. Over millennia, surgery has evolved from a crude practice shaped by desperate necessity, often laced with superstition, to become a sophisticated discipline guided by evidence, reason, and technological innovation.

The Road to Modern Surgery traces this extraordinary journey from the ancient civilizations of Babylon to the dazzling advances of the present era. It has been written to document the successes and failures of the past, in the hope of informing our future. Current surgical practice reflects both the ingenuity and misconceptions of its pioneers, but also the courage and resilience of those who placed their trust in it, even when surgery was a last resort, performed with rudimentary tools, and based on a limited understanding of anatomy and pathophysiology, without the ability to adequately relieve pain.

We wrote this book so that those living in the twenty-first century might understand how today's surgical principles and practices have emerged. We wish to take the reader on a journey from the ancient civilizations of the Sumerians, Babylonians, Egyptians, and Greeks, through the Middle Ages (fifth to fourteenth centuries), and then on to the Renaissance (fifteenth to sixteenth centuries), Enlightenment (seventeenth to eighteenth centuries), and Modern Era. En route we have highlighted major milestones, acknowledging that medical knowledge and surgical practice often went backwards as well as forwards, as from age to age, essential knowledge might be forgotten and then later [re-] "discovered." There were dark periods when religious leaders and power brokers were more inclined to suppress science, so delaying, in some cases for centuries, medical advancement.

We have also sought to address some of the topics often only scantily covered by other medical and surgical historians. These include the role of the Arab physicians, surgeons, and scholars through the Middle Ages. We honour them as innovators in their own right, but also as custodians of knowledge that was at risk of being lost to the world following the collapse of the Roman Empire (476 CE). Another issue we have addressed is the omission of the role of women physicians and surgeons. So we have documented their struggle to be recognized, respected, remembered, and recompensed for their contributions along a bumpy journey toward gender equity in medicine and surgery.

The ethics of surgical practice have changed little through the millennia. Hippocrates (fourth century BC) is famous for the oath that bears his name and promotes ethical practice. But long before Hippocrates, was the seventeenth-century BCE Babylonian Code of Hammurabi, in which we discover that the ancients had similar views to ourselves as to what is expected of ethical medical practice. In the early eleventh-century CE, Ibn Sina (Avicenna), whose Canon of Medicine became a cornerstone of medical education, made significant contributions to surgical ethics and postoperative care. Even in the Middle Ages, there were hospitals in cities such as Baghdad, Cairo, and Damascus functioning as centers of medical excellence, hosting scholars from diverse backgrounds. Islamic medical texts emphasized the importance of patient welfare, meticulous cleanliness, and the ethical responsibilities of surgeons in similar vein to today. Guy de Chauliac's text, *Chirugia Magna*, which guided European surgical practice from the fourteenth to nineteenth century, promoted similar ethical standards to those of his predecessors and of what is expected of surgical professionalism today.

The pioneers of asepsis, anaesthesia, and countless procedures were not necessarily those whose gave their names to the current eponymous term, nor those who are normally credited with a discovery or development. *The Road to Modern Surgery* has tried to faithfully cover some of the rivalry, and race to be "first," in some cases unwitting, and where credit for a discovery has generally been given to those working in high-ranking institutions or with the ability to ensure their paper was published in English.

Yet despite those who sought the glory of primacy, surgical progress has always been a collective endeavor. It has been shaped by diverse cultures, enriched by the rise and fall of empires, and now, increasingly, by global collaboration. The twentieth and twenty-first centuries have witnessed an explosion of progress, propelling surgery into realms that would have been inconceivable to earlier generations. From the advent of minimally invasive techniques to the use of robotic systems, modern surgery is defined by its precision and adaptability. Advances in imaging, with today's MRI and CT scans, intensive care units, and interventional radiology, allow surgeons and other proceduralists to navigate the human body with unprecedented accuracy. Meanwhile, breakthroughs in genetics and biotechnology hold the promise of personalized surgical interventions tailored to an individual's unique biology. As this book is published we are witnessing the early application of Virtual Reality, 3D printing and Artifical Intelligence (AI) to many fields of medicine.

The Road to Modern Surgery is not merely a historical account; it is also a celebration of the human spirit. The story of surgery is, in many ways, a story of humanity itself—a testament to our resilience, creativity, and compassion. It pays tribute not only to the pioneers whose contributions—big and small—have shaped the field but also to the patients who endured unimaginable pain in the hope of a better future. Each chapter and section of this book highlights a pivotal period or topic in surgical history, illustrating the gradual, often arduous, and sometimes disputed, path toward progress.

Whether you are a medical professional, a history enthusiast, or simply a curious reader, we invite you to journey with us on *The Road to Modern Surgery*.

Geelong, VIC, Australia Saleh Abbas
Geelong, VIC, Australia David Watters

Contents

Chapter 1
The Executive Summary

Or a Brief History of How Things Came to Be

1.1 Introduction

> *The charm of history and its enigmatic lesson consist in the fact that, from age to age, nothing changes and yet everything is completely different.* Aldous Huxley

This book is written to highlight the advances in surgery from antiquity to the present day. We will take you on an epic journey highlighting human spirit and ingenuity spanning the millennia. This account is not intended to be a comprehensive review of all events but instead covers key milestones, each of which represents progress towards the state of surgery today. With every major advance there were failures, false starts and disasters impacting the lives of who were not healed, their suffering was not relieved, or whose lives were not saved (Fig. 1.1).

Surgery has always been performed in an effort to relieve pain and suffering, correct deformity, or treat disease. There has been clear documentation of operative procedures from the earliest pictorial and written accounts of human history. In ancient Egypt, India and China there were skilled surgeons over the pre-Christian millenia. It is likely that much medical and surgical knowledge was forgotten and had to be re-learned over the centuries, as civilizations and empires rose and later declined. This was certainly true of all that was known by Greco-Roman doctors and surgeons when the Roman Empire collapsed. The Arab world then acted a repository and library of medical knowledge for some 600 years before Europe emerged from its dark ages into a Renaissance in the fourteenth century.

S. Abbas, D. Watters, *The Road to Modern Surgery*,
https://doi.org/10.1007/978-981-96-4337-0_1

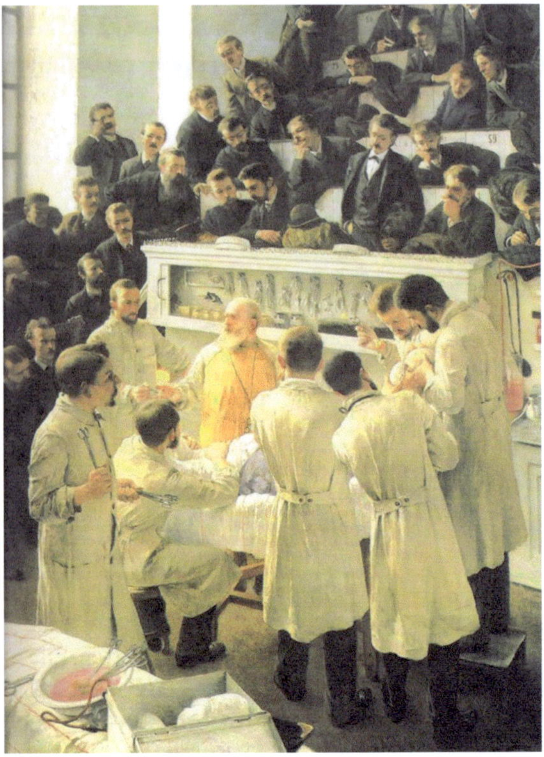

Fig. 1.1 Theodore Billroth demonstrating a surgical operation in 1890. Painting by Franz Seligman 1890. Belvedere, Wien, Austria. (Photo by author, DW)

1.1.1 The Surgical Profession

During the last millennia, and all around the world, the surgical profession emerged from the guild of barbers, at a time when its skill was acquired, not in universities, but through apprenticeship, knowledge, and techniques being handed down from master to student, similar to anyone learning a trade. Without anaesthesia, surgery was, until the mid-nineteenth century, reserved for the desperate and the dying.

For centuries, the barber surgeons enjoyed a lower social standing than those who practiced "physic," the physicians, who were typically university-educated and held more prestigious positions in society. In many cases, surgeons were barred from practicing in hospitals and other medical institutions, so were relegated to working in shops, on a battlefield, whilst some, less sought after, travelled around offering their limited skills at a market place stall or fairground.

It wasn't until the mid-nineteenth century, with the advent of new surgical techniques made possible by the development of anaesthesia and antiseptic practices, that surgery began to gain more respect and prestige as a medical specialty. At this time all doctors were being trained in Universities or Medical Colleges. All doctors undertook training in basic surgery and all surgeons were required to undertake a licenciate or graduate in medicine prior to undertaking surgical training. This led to the establishment of surgical schools and the development of surgical residencies, which helped to elevate the status of surgeons within the medical profession.

Today, all surgeons are doctors, and all doctors undergo some surgical education. However, although many doctors perform some surgery, to acquire specialist registration with a Medical Council or Board and be licensed to use the title "surgeon," many years of surgical education and training are now required after graduating from medical school. However, the delivery of optimal surgical care now also depends on a multidisciplinary team involving nurses, anesthetists, theater technicians, and allied health professionals as well as surgeons.

The increase of human life expectancy by almost 30 years over the last century is indeed a profound but recent development in human history. This extended lifespan can be attributed to several factors, particularly advances in living standards, education, public health, and medicine. Improved living standards, including better nutrition and sanitation, have played the major role particularly as a result of access to clean water, improved hygiene, and better housing. The increased access to good healthcare has also contributed to the improvement of health outcomes and longevity.

1.1.2 The Role of Surgery Within the Health System

A surgical service not only treats disease, usually in hospitals, but represents a vital part of the health system because many surgical conditions need surgery as part of their primary care (eg injuries), but also when there is need for an essential, rescue procedure such as a cesarean section for the 10–15% of pregnancies and deliveries that develop complications or are high risk and prone to do so. Timely surgery saves lives, limbs, and prevents organ dysfunction or failure. When surgery is needed, there usually isn't another option. Modern health systems cannot function effectively without the delivery of both planned and emergency surgical care. Where these are under-resourced, there cannot be good health for all, nor equitous access. Across the world it is estimated that more than five billion of the world's eight billion people do not have safe, timely or affordable access to surgical care. Most of those people live in low- and middle-income countries.

Surgical advances have also made a significant impact; for example those resulting in the cure of cancer, repair of damaged heart valves, coronary artery revascularization, muscle and tendon transfers to restore function and transplantation of vital organs. In the second half of the twentieth century cancers that previously presented too late for cure from surgery such as breast, esophageal and rectal cancer have become amenable to higher disease-free survival as a result of adjuvant and neoadjuvant chemoradiotherapy. Public health screening programs have also resulted in more cancers being diagnosed and treated early, such as breast, cervical, prostate, and colorectal cancers.

The best surgical outcomes are achieved today through the input and coordination of multidisciplinary teams involving perioperative nurses, allied health in supporting and engaging the patient in their own preparation, treatment, and recovery.

There are many opportunities to improve a patient's preparation for major surgery, as well as an expectation that the techniques of surgery and anaesthesia will continue to advance.

Today, the delivery of best surgical care involves bundles of care aimed at enhancing recovery after surgery (ERAS). These include better preparation before surgery, providing best care whilst undergoing surgery and anesthesia, including monitoring for and managing any deterioration or complications promptly. High risk, comorbid patients undergoing major surgery need and deserve a higher level of monitoring and postoperative support, often in an intensive care unit. It is also essential to promote safe and effective recovery through appropriate support of the patient's return to independent function with early mobilization, eating, avoidance of hospital acquired infection, and prevention of thromboembolism. In addition to the surgeon and anaesthetist, those involved may include nursing staff, physiotherapists, pharmacists, intensive care physicians, dieticians, occupational therapists, and social workers. Best care involves a whole team of healthcare professionals while the effectiveness of individual perioperative teams depends on their ability to communicate, collaborate, and be well coordinated.

1.2 An Executive Summary of the History of Surgery

While surgery is often seen as a lifesaving and miraculous practice today, its history is marked by gruesome, and sometimes barbaric, practices that required a few thousands of years of development to enable them to be delivered safely.

The earliest surgical procedures can be traced back to ancient times, where trepanation—the practice of drilling holes in the skull to relieve pressure—was performed by the Egyptians, Incas, Melanesians, and other ancient cultures. However, these procedures were often done without anaesthesia or antiseptics, resulting in a high rate of infection and death. Nonetheless, some of the documented successes attest to the skill, sound clinical judgment and professionalism of the ancients. These accounts are found in Chinese, Indian, Persian, Greek, Roman and Arab literature, and are in no way limited to the documented history of surgery in Europe.

1.2.1 The Code of Hammurabi

The practice of surgery demands professionalism and a high standard of ethics, so the potential for harm has meant that it has been regulated since the earliest of times. The Code of Hammurabi, written in ancient Babylon around 1750 BCE, is one of the oldest known legal codes. It contained over 280 laws covering a wide range of topics, including commerce, property, marriage, and criminal law but one section was devoted specifically to medical practice.

These regulations cover rules governing medical malpractice and compensation for its victims. For example, if a surgeon caused the death of a patient, the surgeon's hands would be cut off. However, if a patient died during surgery as a result of their own actions, such as not following the surgeon's instructions, then the surgeon was not held responsible. The Code of Hammurabi also established fees for medical services and set out guidelines for the treatment of patients. Surgeons were required to provide medical care to all patients, regardless of their ability to pay, and were expected to provide a certain standard of care and attention to their patients.

1.2.2 The Ancient Egyptians

Ancient Egyptian surgeons were skilled in a range of surgical techniques, including the immobilisation of fractures, the excision of tumours, and the suturing of wounds using linen thread. There is also evidence that the practice of mummification played a significant role in the development of surgical skills in ancient Egypt.

Mummification was a complex process that involved the removal of internal organs and the preservation of the body using a variety of techniques. A knowledge of anatomy derived from mummification informed ancient Egyptian surgeons as to human structure and function, enabling them to diagnose and treat many conditions. For example, they were able to successfully perform trepanation (drilling a hole in the skull), based on their knowledge of the anatomy of the scalp, skull, brain, and its coverings.

In addition to their anatomical knowledge, ancient Egyptian surgeons also developed a range of tools and techniques to perform surgery, including scalpels, forceps, and cautery. They also used natural substances like honey and plants as antiseptics and painkillers.

1.2.3 The Greeks

Hippocrates (460–377 BCE) of Cos was someone who based his medical practice and writing on observation and experience of clinical cases and their outcomes. He likely also inherited considerable knowledge from the Egyptians. He provided many original descriptions of disease as well as progressing the understanding of human anatomy. Nonetheless his concept of health and disease still centred around a balance in "the four bodily humours": Black bile from the gallbladder (melancholic), yellow bile from the spleen (choleric), phlegma from the brain and lungs, and blood from the liver (sanguine).

He advocated for high standards of professionalism in medical practitioners and, indeed, the Hippocratic oath, or a modification thereof, is still the basis of professional codes of conduct today.

Although Alexander the Great (356–323 BCE) reached northern India, there is no evidence of the works of Sushruta, who was performing quite advanced reconstructive surgery including rhinoplasties in 600 BCE. His texts (Sushruta Samhita), written in Sanskrit, were translated into Arabic during the Middle Ages, his surgical procedures did not reach Europe until the Renaissance.

In Alexandria, Herophilus (330–250 BCE) and Erisistratus (335–280 BCE) advanced the knowledge of anatomy in third century BCE.

Agnodice, a female doctor, also trained in Alexandria but returned to practice in Athens where she became a controversial but popular figure. She was initially forced to practice as a man, but after this she was wrongly accused and her gender was discovered through a court case, the law was changed to allow women to practice medicine as well. Later, Julius Caesar (100-44 BC) permitted women doctors not only to practice in Rome, but they were granted the right to be Roman citizens.

1.2.4 The Romans

For some centuries it was Greek doctors who practiced medicine and surgery in Rome, as the Romans thought medicine was beneath them. Early in the Christian Era these attitudes changed.

Celsus (25 BC–50 CE), probably an encyclopedist and writer, rather than a doctor, compiled an influential book, *De Medecina*, which consisted of 8 volumes two of which are devoted to surgery. The surgical procedures described have much similarity to the procedures performed today, and well in advance of the standards in Europe over the next millenium.

Galen (129-216 CE) who became personal physician to Roman Emperor Marcus Aurelius in 168 AD, studied medicine in Greece and traveled throughout the Mediterranean world, where he gained a reputation as a skilled surgeon and physician. He wrote extensively on anatomy, physiology, and medical practices, and his works remained influential in the field of medicine for centuries after his death.

One of Galen's most significant contributions to surgery was his development of the technique of ligature, which involved tying off blood vessels to control bleeding during surgery. He also performed surgeries to treat conditions such as cataracts, tumours, and injuries to the head and brain.

As was common in his day, Galen experimented on animals to inform his medical research and surgical practice. His work included the dissection of animals such as monkeys, pigs, sheep, goats, among others. He believed that by studying the anatomy and physiology of these animals, he could gain a better understanding of the human body, so enabling him to develop new surgical techniques and medical treatments.

Though Galen's work was influential in the development of medicine, many of his ideas and practices would later be shown to be based on misconceptions and erroneous beliefs. Nonetheless, his works were widely disseminated and studied in medical schools for centuries, and his ideas became entrenched in medical dogma even until the fourteenth century.

For example, Galen erroneously believed in the concept of the four Hippocratean humours, which held that the body was composed of four fluids—blood, phlegm, yellow bile, and black bile—and that good health depended on the balance of these fluids!

Galen's work on the anatomy of the human body was also flawed, as he was limited by the available methods of observation and dissection at the time. As his descriptions of human anatomy were largely based on animal dissections, his descriptions of the structure and function of organs such as the heart and brain were limited.

Galen's works also mention a number of female practitioners, mainly from Greece, who made significant contributions to medical treatment in the second century CE, particularly in gynaecology.

1.2.5 Europe and the Middle Ages (Sixth to Fourteenth Centuries)

The separation of medicine and surgery from magic and religion was a gradual process that occurred over several centuries, from the ancient world and continuing through the medieval period and into the Fourteenth and Fifteenth centuries.

During the European medieval period, medicine and surgery were heavily influenced by religious beliefs and practices. Many of the physicians and surgeons of the time were monks, nuns or members of various religious orders, with the available medical knowledge often written and stored in their libraries and their skills passed down through apprenticeship within those orders.

However, there were still some significant advances made in the understanding and practice of medicine and surgery during the medieval period. Following the fall of Rome, the Islamic world became the repository of medical knowledge and made further contributions, including the development of hospitals and some use of anesthesic techniques to ameliorate the pain of surgery.

Between the eleventh and thirteenth centuries, the first Universities and medical schools were founded in Europe, so in the early days these schools often relied upon sourcing some of their teaching from the Islamic world and/or the religious orders.

1.2.6 Guy de Chauliac (1298–1368)

Guy de Chauliac was a prominent French surgeon who wrote the *Chirurgia Magna* [the Great Surgery] in the fourteenth century. This was a comprehensive text that covered a wide range of topics in seven volumes. These included anatomy (Treatise 1), swellings (Treatise 2) wound care (Treatise 3), ulcers (Treatise 4), fractures (Treatise 5) and described surgical instruments, and surgical procedures in relation to the conditions covered. It was one of the most influential surgical texts of the late

Middle Ages and was widely read and studied by surgeons and physicians throughout Europe until the nineteenth century. De Chauliac was known for his innovative surgical techniques and placed an emphasis on the importance of cleanliness and hygiene in surgical practice.

However, generally during the Middle-Ages, physicians and surgeons had a limited understanding of much of the internal structure of human body. Also, the role of microorganisms in causing infections had not been discovered. As a result, they were unable to prevent or treat infections, Surgeons often performed operations in unsanitary conditions, their instruments were not properly sterilized even if clean, so many patients suffered or died from infectious complications of surgery.

1.2.7 The Renaissance Period (Fifteenth to Seventeenth Centuries)

The Renaissance was a period of significant intellectual and cultural growth in Europe from the fifteenth to the seventeenth century. A collective scientific conscience emerged that challenged long-held Galenic or magical beliefs and revolutionised many fields of study, including maths, physics, chemistry, biology, anatomy, human physiology, philosophy, and religion. During this period, surgery was transformed from a crude and often deadly practice into a more effective medical discipline based on scientific knowledge.

The fall of Constantinople (Istanbul) in 1453 to Sultan Mehmed II resulted in the collapse of the Eastern Roman (Byzantine) empire. This provoked a period of anti-Muslim sentiment and mistrust between Christian Europe and Islam. On the Iberian peninsula, the Moors were progressively defeated throughout the late 1400s, with the fall of Granada in 1492.

In 1517, the Reformation under Martin Luther led to the splitting of the Christian church into catholic and protestant and a lessening of the grip of the church over science and its advancement. One of the key characteristics of the Renaissance was a greater emphasis on humanism, which placed the individual at the center of the universe and promoted the importance of human reason and observation. This approach to philosophy and science led to significant advancements in many fields of study, but required a separation of science from religious dogma, and was made all the more possible by the reformation providing an alternative Christian religion to Roman Catholicism.

The introduction of the wooden printing press in Europe by the German, Johannes Gutenberg (c1400–1468) was to fast-track the spread of anatomical, medical, and surgical knowledge in the fifteenth century. However it should be noted that wooden (China) and metal (Korea) printing presses had already been used in the Far East for centuries, perhaps from the ninth century.

One of the most important developments during the Renaissance period was an expansion of anatomical knowledge, which allowed surgeons to perform more precise surgical procedures. Cadaveric dissection was illegal in the islamic world, which had limited the Islamic physicians' and surgeons' ability to advance medical knowledge during the medieval period. With the church's permission in 1315, dissection was restored to the field of medicine by Mondino de Luzzi (1270–1326) in Bologna. He published *Anatomia corporis humani* in Latin the following year (1316), though it could not be printed until the European development of printing in 1478.

Further work by Italian anatomists such as Andreas Vesalius (1514–1564) laid the foundation for modern surgical techniques and established the critical importance of dissection in medical education. Vesalius' illustrations of the human body were incredibly detailed and largely accurate. He is credited with revolutionising the profession's knowledge of anatomy, bringing it to a new level of understanding and detail. In addition there was collaboration between anatomists and artists, so that Vesalius' work also inspired better approaches to medical education and teaching. Rather than relying solely on textbooks and lectures, medical students began to use Vesalius's illustrations to gain a more hands-on understanding of human anatomy. This led to the establishment of anatomy labs, where students could practice dissection and gain practical experience. Vesalius' work also inspired other anatomists and physicians to make new discoveries and advancements in surgery. Many European universities and medical schools began to allow human dissections to take place and their medical students were required to attend dissections during their training.

1.2.8 Andreas Vesalius (1514–1564)

Andreas Vesalius was a Renaissance-era physician and anatomist who played a significant role in challenging the long-held ideas of Galen and advancing our understanding of human anatomy.

In 1543, Vesalius published his landmark work "*De Humani Corporis Fabrica*" ("On the Fabric of the Human Body"), which included detailed illustrations of human anatomy based on his own dissections of cadavers. His work challenged many of the assumptions made by Galen and other ancient authorities and represents a critical period of progress in medicine and surgery. He helped break the Galen-based tradition which had persisted during the Middle Ages, partly as a result of human dissections being then prohibited by both the Islamic and Catholic religions. His contributions to anatomy paved the way for many important medical discoveries and advancements in the centuries that followed.

1.2.9 William Harvey (1578–1657)

The next major step forward medicine was to add to this growing anatomical knowledge an understanding of physiology. William Harvey, an English physician with a doctorate from the then leading European University of Padua, is credited with describing the body's full circulation for the first time. His *Exercitatio Anatomica de Motu Cordis et Sanguinis in Animalibus* was first published in Latin in 1628, and then in 1653, in English (*Anatomical Exercise on the Motion of the Heart and Blood in Animals*). An understanding of the heart and circulatory system saw the emergence of physiology from an anatomical foundation to connect human structure and function.

Better surgical tools and techniques also contributed to some growth of surgery during the Renaissance. Rediscovery of the use of ligatures to control bleeding, the metal scalpel, and the use of surgical sutures all contributed to more effective surgery during this period. Thus surgery was able to achieve more than the rather limited, and often ineffective or dangerous, bloodletting, amputation, and trephination procedures of earlier periods.

1.2.10 The Barber Surgeons

During the early Renaissance, surgery was considered a lower form of medicine and was often looked down upon by physicians who had been trained in universities. These physicians were primarily trained in Galen's ideas, but were often unaware of their limitations when applied to human patients. As a result, surgery was often left to the barbers, who were skilled in cutting hair, wielding a razor and performing some limited procedures such as bloodletting and amputations. However, in the absence of anaesthesia, analgesia and asepsis, their procedures were generally crude, swift and barbaric, so surgery was not considered such a respectable profession. Today's red-and-white-striped barber poles have their origins in the medieval practice of barber-surgeons. Then it was common for barbers and surgeons to be members of the same profession—the barber pole outside their shop with its red and white stripes representing the blood and bandages used in surgical procedures.

As scientific knowledge advanced during the Renaissance, surgery began to be seen as a more sophisticated and essential aspect of medicine. Better surgical techniques were developed, so physicians began to recognise the importance of surgical intervention in the treatment of a wider range of medical conditions.

1.2.11 Ambrose Paré (1510–1590)

Ambroise Paré was a French barber-surgeon who made several important contributions to the field of surgery during the Renaissance period. One of his most significant innovations was the use of ligatures to control bleeding during surgical procedures. At the time, the prevailing method for controlling bleeding was to use a hot iron or cauterise the wound, which was often painful and ineffective. However, in 1536, while treating soldiers wounded in battle, Paré ran out of the hot oil used for cauterisation and instead used silk threads to tie off the blood vessels and stop the bleeding. This technique, known as ligation, proved to be much more effective and less painful than cauterisation. Paré also introduced other important surgical techniques, such as improving the design of artificial limbs and developing better, less painful methods for treating gunshot wounds.

1.2.12 The Eighteenth Century

During the 1700s, body snatching was a common practice among individuals who sought to sell cadavers to anatomists and medical schools. This was due to the high demand for cadavers for dissection and medical research, but a limited supply of legally available bodies. At the time, the only legal way to obtain a cadaver for dissection was obtaining the bodies of executed criminals. However, the number of executions was relatively low, and the bodies of executed criminals were not always made available for dissection. This led to a shortage of cadavers for medical research and education.

Body snatchers would typically target recently buried corpses, digging them up at night and then selling them to medical schools or individual anatomists. This practice was illegal and highly controversial, as it involved the desecration of graves and the violation of families' wishes for the proper burial of their loved ones.

Body snatching eventually led to the passage of legislation in many countries, such as the Anatomy Act of 1832 in the UK, which permitted the legal donation of bodies for medical research and education. This reduced the demand for illegally obtained cadavers and helped to reduce the criminal practice of body snatching.

1.2.13 John Hunter (1728–1793)

John Hunter was a significant figure in the history of medicine and surgery and is deservedly credited with being one of the founders of scientific surgery. He was born in Scotland in 1728, from where he moved to London to pursue a career in medicine in 1748. He never studied at any University, as was common practice for a surgeon of his day. He was instead trained at the Chelsea hospital by the famous London surgeon, William Cheselden (1688–1752). Hunter initially worked in his brother's school of anatomy until appointed master of anatomy at Surgeon's Hall in 1753. He practiced as a surgeon at St George's hospital and eventually became surgeon to King George III in 1776, the year the American States declared their independence. Hunter was known for his rigorous approach to scientific investigation and experimentation, which he applied to the study of anatomy, physiology, and surgery. He believed that a thorough understanding of the human body was essential for successful surgery, and emphasized the importance of careful observation, experimentation, and analysis in the science of medicine [1].

Hunter undoubtedly obtained many of his specimens from bodysnatchers which enabled him to amass a remarkable collection to inform his teaching and research. One of his most significant contributions to the field of surgery was the development of new surgical techniques based on his scientific investigations. He also studied comparative anatomy and conducted experiments on animals to inform the development of surgical procedures. After his death, his collection of anatomical specimens was purchased by the British government for the Royal College of Surgeons whose museum is now called the Hunterian museum. The reputation of surgery was very much better at the end of Hunter's life than it had been earlier in the eighteenth century.

1.3 The Nineteenth Century

1.3.1 Surgical Infection, Puerperal Sepsis, and Micro-organisms

> *A man laid on the operating table of one of our hospitals is exposed to more chance of death than the English soldier on the field at Waterloo.* Sir James Simpson, 1869 [1]

In the early nineteenth century, doctors did not know about the role of microorganisms in causing infections and, as a result, they did not take the necessary measures to prevent the spread of disease. This is in spite of De Chauliac's and others' earlier advocacy for cleanliness. There were high rates of infection and procedure-related death, with surgeons and attendants unaware that their bare hands transmitted infection between cases, and nowhere more so than the maternity ward.

Although micro-organisms had not yet been discovered and their connection to disease would await Louis Pasteur's later work on germ theory, there were still strong advocates in the eighteenth and early nineteenth centuries for cleanliness. Their work, based on observation and protocol, was rewarded by lowering maternal mortality without being able to provide the scientific evidence as to what was causing puerperal sepsis, nor how doctors, whose overcoats were often smeared with blood, pus, and other bodily matters, were responsible for transmitting it.

The high incidence of nosocomial puerperal sepsis during the mid-nineteenth century prompted Harvard's Oliver Wendell Holmes (1809–94) in 1843, to pen a classic essay on *The Contagiousness of Puerperal Fever* with rules for the obstetrician to mitigate this risk including handwashing, changes of clothing and avoidance of autopsies when managing obstetric cases [2, 3].

On the other side of the Atlantic, Hungarian Ignác Semmelweis (1818–65)—never one for conducting laboratory research or showing respect to colleagues with whom he disagreed—reduced the Maternal Mortality in Vienna's *Allgemeine Krankenhaus* in 1847 from 16% to 2% by enforcing handwashing with *chlorina liquida* in the obstetrics ward [3, 4]. There were also other pioneers in the first half of the nineteenth century who advocated for hand hygiene including Semmelweis's own students Routh (1848), Weiger (1848) and Skoda (1849). Another brave advocate was Thomas Watson in London (1842), These pioneers and champions suffered ridicule, professional isolation and, in Semmelweis' case, non-renewal of contract [3, 4]. Semmelweis was forced to return to his native Hungary and so that the women of Budapest became the beneficiaries of his hand hygiene practice where, as in Vienna, his protocols greatly reduced death rate from puerperal sepsis [3].

1.3.2 Louis Pasteur (1822–1895)

Louis Pasteur was responsible for "germ theory." His first discovery was made through study of fermentation. His paper on spontaneous generation described *"les corpuscles organises dans l'atmosphere"* may have been meant to apply to wine but would have far wider implications ever after. Pasteur's later work studied other infections such as fowl cholera before he successfully introduced vaccination for rabies (which has a long latent period) post exposure.

With the discovery of germs or microbes, surgeons began to understand the importance of sterilisation in preventing infections. They developed new methods of sterilization, such as the use of heat and chemical disinfectants, then began to implement more rigorous protocols for cleaning and sterilising surgical instruments and equipment. This helped to significantly reduce the risk of infections during surgical procedures, and allowed for more complex and extensive surgeries to be performed with greater safety and success [3].

1.3.3 Vaccination

The potential value of exposing healthy people to pathogens in order to render them immune to disease was practiced for centuries prior to the first successful vaccine utilizing cow pox being introduced by Dr. Edward Jenner in 1796. This advance, whilst not specifically surgical, was founded on earlier observations of the efficacy of inoculation in China (1549), and Turkey (1721), that cowpox infection protected against smallpox (1774). Then in the 1800s Louis Pasteur made further progress, developing the first laboratory produced vaccine against cholera in fowls, before successfully preventing rabies through post-exposure vaccination. The further development of vaccines in the twentieth century resulted in significant reductions in deaths from infectious diseases.

1.3.4 Joseph Lister (1817–1912)

The discovery of asepsis in surgery is a crucial milestone in the history of medicine, and it is widely attributed to the work of Joseph Lister and others in the 1860s (Fig. 1.2). At the time, surgical procedures were often carried out in unsanitary conditions, and infections were a major cause of patient mortality. For example, the mortality from amputations in Paris between 1836 and 1850 was 66%. Lister, having served under Syme in Edinburgh (1853–60), was appointed Professor of Surgery at Glasgow Medical school and Glasgow Royal Infirmary. There he reported that 16 of 35 amputations performed died between 1864 and 1866. He still believed that infections were caused by some *influence of the atmosphere* but correctly surmised that by disinfecting/sterilising surgical instruments, wounds, and even the air in the operating room, he could prevent infections and improve patient outcomes.

Lister, on the advice of Thomas Anderson, the Professor of Chemistry in Glasgow, began using carbolic acid (phenol), as an antiseptic during surgical

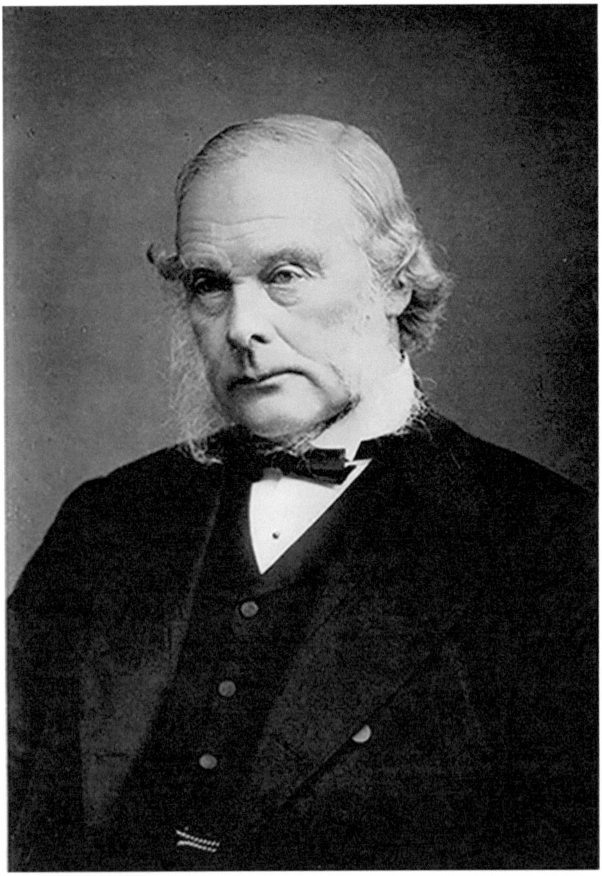

Fig. 1.2 Joseph Lister, 1st Baron Lister (1827–1912) surgeon Wellcome M0006745. Portrait of The Right Honourable Joseph Lister, 1st Baron Lister, British surgeon. (This image is published with open access under the Creative Commons Attribution license, CC. https://commons.wikimedia.org/wiki/File:Joseph_Lister,_1st_Baron_Lister_(1827_-_1912)_surgeon_Wellcome_V0027875ER.jpg#/media/File:Joseph_Lister,_1st_Baron_Lister_(1827_-_1912)_surgeon_Wellcome_L0034558.jpg)

procedures. He soaked his surgical instruments in carbolic acid solution and sprayed the air in the operating room with the solution to kill germs. He also used the solution to clean wounds before and after surgery. His first case series involved 12 compound fractures (8 of whom survived), before extending his techniques to amputations, of which 34 of 40 survived between the years of 1867–1869.

Lister's use of antiseptic techniques in surgery was initially met with resistance and skepticism from his peers, but his success rate in preventing infections and improving patient outcomes soon became widely recognized across Europe and in North America. His methods eventually became widely adopted in the medical community, and by the early 1900s, aseptic techniques had become standard practice in surgery. The carbolic that Lister originally used is not only toxic to the microbes but also to the wounds so later aseptic solutions were discovered that caused less tissue damage [5].

The nineteenth century was a time of great advances. There were also many eponymous names added to conditions and procedures. Surgical practice was very general, covering most parts of the body. Many doctors and surgeons had their names attached to early descriptions of conditions in multiple specialties. There was very little subspecialization until the twentieth century.

1.3.5 Anaesthesia

Anaesthesia, which is used to reduce or eliminate pain during surgery, was not available before the mid-nineteenth century. Instead, patients were often held down or given alcohol or other substances to dull the pain during surgery. It was only during the nineteenth century that the true development of anaesthesia, with inhalational ether took place. The first successful use of anaesthesia in surgery is often credited to an American dentist named William Morton in Boston, who used ether as an anesthetic during a tooth extraction in 1846. There were others that gave ether before Morton, but given his demonstration had occurred at the Massachusetts General Hospital in Boston, and that he had the personality and bravado seize the primacy he is usually credited with its discovery. Morton's contribution was followed by the introduction of chloroform as an anesthetic by James Simpson, an Edinburgh obstetrician, in 1847, who popularized its use. However he was also not the first to use it. These advances in anaesthesia spread rapidly around the world with operations being performed even in Tasmania, Australia within a few months.

1.3.6 Maternal Mortality

In the nineteenth century, even in Europe, the maternal mortality rate (MMR) was 500–1000 deaths per 100,000 live births. Today, although rates persist in the 100's in low-middle income countries, in many high income countries the MMR may be single figures. Cesarean section was practised in many ancient cultures including Hindu, Egyptian, Grecian, and Roman but mostly when the mother had died and to save the infant. The first well documented survival of both mother and baby comes from Switzerland in 1500 when Jakob Nufer, a pig gelder, operated on his wife after a prolonged labour. Skilled birth attendants and the ability to access a safe, timely Caesarean section is another factor that has reduced maternal and neonatal mortality for those experiencing obstructed labour.

1.3.7 The Twentieth Century

The discovery of X-rays in 1895, allowing the introduction of imaging at the start of the twentieth century was a major advance. Throughout the century there were developments in ultrasound and imaging, including the second half of the century, Computerised Tomography, Magnetic Resonance Imaging, and Positron emission scanning (PET). These have enabled doctors and surgeons to visualize internal structures of the body in great detail, without the need for invasive procedures. This has allowed for more accurate diagnosis of conditions and injuries, more precise planning of surgical procedures as well as better recognition and management of complications.

World War I saw a number of key advances in surgery around resuscitation of the injured soldier, the management of haemorrhagic shock, and the ability to provide blood transfusion. At the start of the war, femoral shaft fractures were poorly treated and carried a 50–70% mortality. Once the Thomas splint was introduced to facilitate transport of the soldier with a fractured thigh, in association with better resuscitation and wound management, the mortality fell. The earlier operative management of abdominal and chest wounds closer to the front also improved survival rates of trunk injuries during the war.

After the war, cancer treatment had more options with radiotherapy units being established in France, Poland, and then throughout Europe and North America. Chemotherapeutic agents were not introduced until the second half of the century.

Operations that were dangerous and offered only as a last resort in the nineteenth century began to be able to be performed safely over the first half of the twentieth century. These include resections of rectal carcinoma, pituitary adenoma, the pancreatic head, duodenum, and pneumonectomy. The ability to give thyroid extract and then the commercial synthesis of thyroxine made thyroidectomy safer.

The specialties of plastic surgery and neurosurgery were developed early in the century, then spurred on by the need to manage the terrible facial and head injuries of WWI. Thoracic surgeons in the first half of the twentieth century treated tuberculosis until the introduction of streptomycin and other anti-tuberculous drugs after WWII. Between the wars, general surgeons still practiced gynecology, managed fractures, and would perform a prostatectomy.

Antibiotics contributed significantly to the prevention and treatment of infection. The first anti-bacterial agent to be introduced was prontosil, a sulphonamide, developed by Gerhard Domagk (1895–1964) in 1935. Penicillin was discovered in 1928, trialled early in World War II, then manufactured for use by the Allied troops in 1943. The introduction of streptomycin and other anti-tuberculous drugs after WWII resulted in surgery for pulmonary tuberculosis becoming almost never needed. The role of surgery for extrapulmonary tuberculosis in many parts of the world soon became limited to making a diagnosis. A wide-range of antibiotics have been discovered or developed but with their advent the prevalence of antibiotic resistance has grown and protocols for antibiotic use and stewardship have had to be designed.

After WWII in the 1950s and 1960s, cardiothoracic surgery and vascular surgery began to develop as specialties in response to the increasing incidence cardiac and peripheral vascular diseases. The 1960s and 1970s saw the introduction of transplant surgery, multimodality treatment of cancer, and the development of oncology as a medical specialty. Since the 1970s and 1980s, the development of microsurgical vascular anastomosis has allowed a variety of free flaps to be used for reconstruction of tissue defects from injury and cancer resection. For example, free flaps were first performed in Sweden for breast cancer reconstruction in the 1970s.

From the late 1950s, the formation of the Association for Osteosynthesis (AO) in Switzerland led to huge improvements in the instrumentation and treatment of fractures, allowing accurate reduction and internal fixation. The introduction of safe and effective joint arthroplasties needed by the ageing populations of high-income countries led to a huge increase in joint replacements, now the commonest planned orthopedic procedure. Also, towards the end of the twentieth century, orthopedic surgeons began to sub-specialise in hip, knee, shoulder, foot and ankle, and spinal surgery. In the late twentieth century, specialist oro-maxillo-facial surgeons who were accustomed to enter the profession from a dental background began to first obtain both medical and dental degrees prior to their specialist training.

General surgeons based in the cities of high- income countries also began limiting their scope of practice through sub-specialization in colorectal, upper gastrointestinal, hepatobiliary, breast, endocrine, trauma, or burns surgery.

From the 1980s, minimally invasive surgery emerged from the domain of surgeons practicing urology or gynecology into abdominal and thoracic surgery. The advent of laparoscopic cholecystectomy led to much of planned and some emergency general abdominal surgery being performed laparoscopically by early in the twenty-first century. The introduction of robotic surgery resulted in robotic prostatectomy replacing laparoscopic and open radical prostatectomy for prostatic cancer. Robotic procedures are progressively being introduced for glossectomy (base of tongue cancers), hysterectomy, colorectal surgery, and thoracic surgery. These allow the surgeon to operate from a console whilst an assistant is at the operating table.

1.3.8 Women and Surgery

The history of surgery until the nineteenth century was largely, but not exclusively, written by men about men. Although European Universities, particularly in Italy, admitted women in the twelfth to fifteenth centuries, women were progressively excluded from the profession of medicine and surgery from the fourteenth to eighteenth centuries. A licence, or at least permission, was granted to some wives and/or widows of surgeons, the latter being allowed to continue to run their late husband's practice, including operating on what they had been trained to do, and particularly in Europe. It was an intense struggle for women to enter medical schools, to be trained as doctors and later, as surgeons, though the pioneers started to make headway in the second half of the nineteenth century. Yet still, the medical women of many countries including the United States and Great Britain even had to found their own hospitals to provide positions for their gender to gain clinical experience and later to practice. During the First World War (1914–1918), many military forces would not enlist women on grounds of their gender. This led to Women Doctor volunteers setting up hospitals serving frontline troops on the Eastern Front in France, Serbia, and Russia, or being allowed to work as Civilian/Contract doctors on home shores. Later the twentieth century saw women doctors being able to specialize, finally allowed to progress their careers in medicine and finally, the first female Professors or Heads of Department appointed. The twenty-first century saw the first female Presidents of Surgical Colleges, but also increasing awareness of, and progress towards reducing, discrimination, bullying, and sexual harassment in surgery. The profession also woke up to the need to provide better opportunities and career progression for women in the profession, the need to champion pay parity, and the right to flexible working hours. As a result, the surgical profession will be better and broader in its representation in the twenty-first century and beyond.

1.4 Conclusion

Surgery is, and has become, a proud profession through the ages. We use the word proud in its best sense, and emphasize that surgeons should not be arrogant, or self-righteous, but be proud of what they can offer to their patients, while empathic towards their needs and suffering. This introduction has rapidly summarised some of the major milestones of surgical history. It is necessarily brief with the chapters to follow providing more detail of the development of surgery and the surgical profession over the millennia. It is only by understanding how today's surgical practices, and even today's dogma, have come into being, that we can appreciate why contemporaneous surgical practice is what it is.

The journey to where we have reached today has not been straightforward. Nor should the perioperative care of today be seen as our point of arrival. Surgeons, anesthetists, and their perioperative colleagues must continue to improve the care they provide to their patients and the community. The opportunities lie before, during, and after the procedure because the preparation/optimization and recovery/rehabilitation phases are as important as the operation itself. The principles of care include showing empathy, not doing harm, not exploiting a patient's vulnerability, choosing an operation that offers an outcome that the patient wants, and managing expectations as to what surgery can realistically achieve. These principles remain as true today as when the medical profession had no knowledge of microbes, when pain relief was limited, when there was no hormone replacement, when we couldn't internally fix a fracture, yet there was suffering to be relieved. They were true for those who wrote the Code of Hammurabi in ancient Babylon (1792–1750 BCE), true in the day of Hippocrates (460–367 BCE) compiling his oath, true when Guy de Chauliac wrote Chirugia Magna in the fourteenth century CE, just as they are true today and expressed in many medical or surgical codes of conduct. Surgery is a proud profession but that pride should only be based on sound professional behaviour and striving to deliver the best outcomes of care for our patients and communities.

References

1. Simpson J. Our existing system of hospitalisation, its effect on the results of surgical operations. Edinb Med J. 1869;14:816–30.
2. De Costa CM. The contagiousness of childbed fever: a short history of puerperal sepsis and its treatment. Med J Aust. 2002;177:668–71.
3. Carter KC, Tate GS. The earliest-known account of Semmelweis's initiation of disinfection at Vienna's Allgemeines Krankenhaus. Bull Hist Med. 1991;65:252–7.
4. Nuland SB. The enigma of Semmelweis – an interpretation. J Hist Med Allied Sci. 1979;34:255–72.
5. Lister J. The antiseptic principle in the practise of surgery. BMJ. 1867;ii:246–8.

Chapter 2
Surgery in Antiquity

How the Ancient World Laid the Foundations

2.1 Surgery in the Sumerian Civilization (Sixth to Fifth Millennia BCE)

The Sumerians, who lived in ancient Mesopotamia in what is now southern Iraq, clearly had some understanding of medicine and utilised limited surgical techniques. Their civilization emerged during the early Bronze Age between the sixth and fifth millennia BCE. Later Sumerian texts dating back to around 2000 BCE contain descriptions of various medical treatments and surgical procedures, including the use of knives, forceps, and other instruments. The Mesopotamian medical practice of the Akkadians had two types of practitioners: the ashipu (sorcerer) and asu (physician). The Gods were honoured in both kinds of healers – Gula, the Sumerian Goddess of healing (Fig. 2.1) – was the patron of doctors and her temples were places of healing; Ninazu, Lord of Physicians, and Ningishzida, his son, are credited with being the originators of the medical caduceus emblem, the double-edged snake (Fig. 2.2). A description of the surgeon's knife (naglabu) used at the time represents an interesting first description of the relationship between the barbers and surgeons.

One of the first known surgical procedures recorded in Sumerian clay tablets is the treatment of skull fractures that required the repositioning of the bone fragment via a trephine. The Sumerians also record treatments for broken bones, other injuries, and tumors. They also described the use of analgesics, hypnotics, and antibiotics [1].

Although there are no accurate records, the earliest example of cranial surgery dates back to around 6000 years in Turkey in the form of trephining of the skull. The indications for the procedure then are unknown, but may have had have nothing to

---

This chapter covers the ancient world from the Sumerians, Babylonians, Egyptians, Greeks, to the Byzantine era.

S. Abbas, D. Watters, *The Road to Modern Surgery*,
https://doi.org/10.1007/978-981-96-4337-0_2

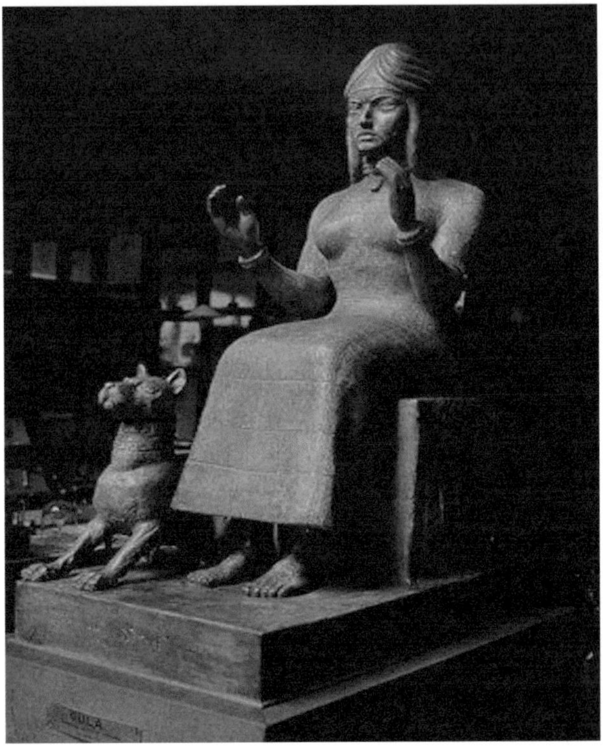

Fig. 2.1 Legend: Gula (Ninkarrak), the Sumerian Goddess of healing, is the divine patron of doctors, healing arts, and medicine. She is referred to as Lady of healing, the Great physician in various Sumerian documents from 2047 to 1750 BCE. (This image is published with open access. Wellcome Collection, CC. https://wellcomecollection.org/works/ebd8vd44/images?id=fk46ra38)

do with an injury. The skulls that have been collected suggest that some patients survived whilst others did not.

Nancy Demand of Indiana University wrote: "Most of the information available to modern scholars is derived from cuneiform tablets. Unfortunately, while an abundance of cuneiform tablets have survived from ancient Mesopotamia, relatively few describe medical practice. Many of the tablets that do mention medical practices have survived from the library of Asshurbanipal, the last great king of Assyria. This was housed in the king's palace at Nineveh, and when the palace was burned by invaders, around 20,000 clay tablets were baked (and thereby preserved) by the great fire [2].

Flint and bronze surgical instruments were among the articles found in the grave of Sumerian Queen Shubad of Ur (c 2600 BCE).

In the early 1920s, some translations from the 660 medical tablets from the library of Asshurbanipal were published by Campbell Thompson. Other medical texts have been published more recently. For example, Franz Kocher has published a series of volumes called *Die Babylonishch-Assyrische Medizin*. The first four are based on 420 tablets found from sites other than Assurbanipal's library, including the library of a medical practitioner (an asipu) from Neo-Assyrian Assur, as well as Middle Assyrian and Middle Babylonian texts.

Sumerian clay tablets from around 2000 BCE contain detailed descriptions of various medical treatments and surgical procedures, along with corresponding incantations and rituals to be performed by priests. The texts often include the use of magic words and symbols, believed to have healing powers. The texts also contain some information about the diagnosis of diseases [1, 3].

Castration of captives was also common practice for captives who could then be employed as eunuchs at the royal court. The procedure was associated with high mortality rates [3–5].

In 1849, Lord Austin Henry Layard excavated the vast majority of the clay tablets that we now associate with Assyrian times [1, 2]. This occurred about four thousand years after their original creation. There are now thousands of tablets and approximately 800 complete medical texts attributable to the Assyrian and Babylonian era [5].

The responsibilities of the surgeon were, interestingly, somewhat similar to those of surgeons now. Surgeons were responsible for evaluation of ailments that were considered mechanical in nature. Ophthalmologic surgeries are noted as being done as early as 3500 BC. Other Assyrian surgical procedures were directed at the management of bowel obstruction, with descriptions of "opening the bowels" to let impacted contents spew documented in these texts. It is unclear whether these were enterotomies or early stomas. Other treatments appear to be orogastric lavage, massage with ointments and oils, and the provision of enemas. Keeping patients *nil per os* (NPO) was also described. Sesame seed oil was used to dress wounds as an antiseptic [6].

Another task within the surgeon's scope of practice was incision and drainage of abscesses. One tablet describes a procedure in which the surgeon performs what appears to be a thoracotomy to drain an empyema (pus in the pleural cavity around the lungs) [7].

Cesarean sections were also described. In 1960, a tablet was translated describing a boy being extracted from the womb of his mother. There is little information about the indications, and it is assumed that most were carried out on slave women for economic purposes. Cesarean sections were, as a practice, avoided for free women due to high risk of maternal death [8].

2.2 Surgery During the Babylonian Period

The Babylonians lived in ancient Mesopotamia in what is now Iraq. Their civilization predates the Sumerians, and like the Sumerians, the Babylonians developed an understanding of medicine and performed some surgical procedures. Babylonian clay tablets from around 2000 BCE contain descriptions of procedures such as amputations, setting of fractures and reduction of dislocations, and the treatment of head wounds. They also described treatments for tumors and abscesses [9, 10].

2.2.1 *Esagil-kin-apli (Eleventh Century BCE)*

Esagil-kin-apli was the chief scholar of the Babylonian king, Adad-apia-iddina (1067–1046 BCE). He wrote a medical textbook that is often referred to as the "*Hippocratic Corpus of Babylon*" which covered diagnosis, prognosis, and therapy for a wide variety of diseases. Some of the surgical instruments used by Babylonian doctors were similar to those used by the Sumerians, such as knives and forceps, but they also developed new instruments such as the "swallow's beak" (which was probably a type of probe), and the "hooked instrument" (which was probably used for pulling out tumors or other growths [9].

The Babylonians also had a strong belief in supernatural causes of illness and injury, similar to the Sumerians, and they believed that certain rituals, incantations, and offerings could drive away evil spirits and placate the gods.

2.2.2 *Urlugalidine (2300 BCE)*

One of the earliest surgeons in Babylonia was probably a man by the name of Urlugalidine (2300 B.C.), whose "logo" was two knives intertwined. Today his stamp can be seen at the Louvre in Paris. The services of this type of surgeon included branding slaves on the forehead or hand, barber duties, and dental extractions. These barber duties provide further evidence of long historical relationship between barbers and surgeons [9].

2.2.3 *Circumcision in Babylonian Civilization*

Circumcision was also a common practice in ancient Mesopotamia, including among the Babylonians. The procedure provided a rite of passage into adulthood, was commonly performed on young boys, and dates as far back as the eighth century BCE. It was seen as a way of honoring the gods and performed as part of religious and cultural rituals. Although Babylonian medical texts reference the practice, it is not clear if the indications were medical.

2.2.4 *Surgical Tools in Ancient Mesopotamia*

The ancient Mesopotamians, including the Sumerians and Babylonians, developed a variety of surgical tools and instruments. They had non-specific instruments which were derived from household equipment and included various types of sieve. These were made from reeds or rushes and had different sizes and were of different sizes of mesh. Sieves were certainly used to concoct medical prescriptions. Mortars and pestles were made of stone or of wood. They were hand-operated, used to crush seeds and cereals to grind them into fine granules just as in a modern kitchen [9–11].

Some examples of surgical tools used in ancient Mesopotamia include:

Knives and scalpels: These were used for making incisions and performing amputations. There were variety of knives of different shapes and sizes for various surgical procedures including household instruments.

- Forceps: For grasping and manipulating tissues and similar to the forceps used today.
- Hooks: For pulling out tumors or other growths.
- Probes: For examining wounds and other injuries.
- Drills: For drilling holes in bones, possibly for the treatment of fractures or other injuries.
- Needles: For stitching wounds and other surgical procedures.
- Scissors and knives were sharpened on a grindstone, the blade to be sharpened may have been of metal, stone, flint, or obsidian.
- The thorns from a tree or plants were used by the surgeon for wound suturing, which indicates that wound suturing was known in antiquity.
- The hollow stalk of a reed was used as a pipette. Pipettes may also have been made of lead or tubes of copper or bronze.
- A tube small enough in diameter to be suitable for insertion into the urethra or external auditory meatus, or for the instillation of eye drops.
- Barber razors were used as knives, usually made from copper.
- A blunt, club-shaped instrument was used in obstetrics. It was made from different metals, and its use for extraction of the fetus suggests that it may have been some form of primitive scoop.
- Threads were known to ancient Mesopotamians, who were capable of manufacturing the sapiiru net of fine, thin mesh.
- Bandages were used for a variety of problems including treatment of fractures. They were made from woven materials from wool or horse hair.

Nonspecific instruments which were derived from household included the razor, bandages and sapiiru (thread) mentioned above.

A blunt, club-shaped instrument used in obstetrics was made from different metals, was for extraction of the fetus formed some type of primitive scoop.

Several drugs were added to dressings and bandages before their application to the patient, and were replaced when necessary [11–14].

2.2.5 Anatomy and Dissection

The Mesopotamian surgeons had a good understanding of surface (external) anatomy. Their knowledge of internal anatomy was limited and was based on the dissection of animals, not humans as their laws forbade dissection [12–14].

2.2.6 *Analgesia*

In no text relating to operations is there any mention of anaesthesia, despite the ancient Mesopotamians having considerable knowledge of pharmacy, relying mainly on plants, though some chemical substances were also used. It is probable that wine was given to patients before surgery. Frankincense was used for analgesia. The bark and leaves of willow (sarbatu) contain salicylates, and they were taken internally for the relief of pain. Stronger analgesic and narcotic drugs were, however, available and were given to the patient orally. These drugs have a long history of use in Mesopotamia, certainly from early in the second millennium BCE. Mandrake was often prescribed alone and could be combined with other drugs. Henbane is widely distributed in the eastern Mediterranean region and was certainly used in medical prescriptions. Hemp was used as for pain relief and as an intoxicant, while the opium poppy was widely available and used for pain control [11, 12, 15].

2.2.7 *Law and Medicine in Ancient Mesopotamia: The Code of Hammurabi (1792–1750 BCE) [13, 14]*

Law and medicine were closely intertwined in ancient Mesopotamia. The Sumerians and Babylonians, who lived in what is now southern Iraq, had a sophisticated understanding of law and medicine, and their legal and medical texts contain detailed descriptions of various treatments and procedures.

Doctors were required to follow certain rules and codes of conduct. Medical texts from this period contain legal codes governing the practice of medicine, including rules for the qualifications and training of doctors.

Doctors were also held liable for any mistakes or negligence in their practice, and patients or their families could bring a legal case against a doctor if they felt they had been wronged. There were also penalties for unqualified persons who practiced medicine. In the case of malpractice, the law required the doctor to pay compensation to the patient or the patient's family for any harm caused.

One of the most famous Babylonian law code was the "Code of Hammurabi" which had a section related to the profession of medicine, it contains several laws that regulated the profession and set standards for the qualifications and conduct of physicians.

Hammurabi, the king of Babylon who reigned from 1792 to 1750 B.C., is known for creating the Code of Hammurabi, which is considered to be the oldest existing set of laws known for its portrayal of retributive justice and praised for its thoroughness and fairness this book contains 282 legal precedents with clear procedures and consequences. Prior to being etched into the eight-foot-high black diorite stone, most of the laws had already been established. Hammurabi codified them into a fixed and standardized set of laws.

215. *If a physician make a large incision with an operating knife and cure it, or if he open a tumor (over the eye) with an operating knife, and saves the eye, he shall receive ten shekels in money.*

216. *If the patient be a freed man, he receives five shekels.*
217. *If he be the slave of some one, his owner shall give the physician two shekels.*
218. *If a physician make a large incision with the operating knife, and kill him, or open a tumor with the operating knife, and cut out the eye, his hands shall be cut off.*
219. *If a physician make a large incision in the slave of a freed man, and kill him, he shall replace the slave with another slave.*
220. *If he had opened a tumor with the operating knife, and put out his eye, he shall pay half his value.*
221. *If a physician heal the broken bone or diseased soft part of a man, the patient shall pay the physician five shekels in money.*
222. *If he were a freed man he shall pay three shekels.*
223. *If he were a slave his owner shall pay the physician two shekels.*
224. *If a veterinary surgeon perform a serious operation on an ass or an ox, and cure it, the owner shall pay the surgeon one-sixth of a shekel as a fee.*
225. *If he perform a serious operation on an ass or ox, and kill it, he shall pay the owner one-fourth of its value.*
226. *If a barber, without the knowledge of his master, cut the sign of a slave on a slave not to be sold, the hands of this barber shall be cut off.*
227. *If any one deceive a barber, and have him mark a slave not for sale with the sign of a slave, he shall be put to death, and buried in his house. The barber shall swear: "I did not mark him wittingly," and shall be guiltless.*

Source: The Code of Hammurabi—Translated by L. W. King.

The oldest imagery of the caduceus is rooted in Mesopotamia with the Sumerian god of healing Ningishzida; his symbol, a staff with two snakes intertwined around it, dates back to 4000 BC to 3000 BC (Fig. 2.2).

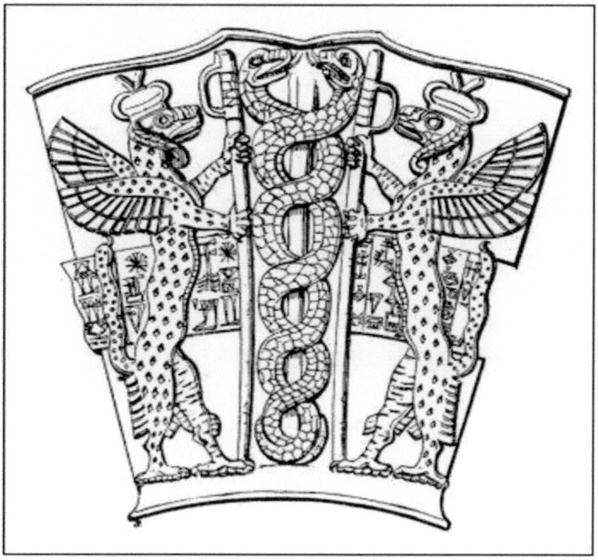

Fig. 2.2 Entwined snakes of Mesopotamia. Black plaster cast. (This image is published with open access under the Creative Commons Attribution license, CC. https://en.wikipedia.org/wiki/Snakes_in_mythology#/media/File:Ningizzida.jpg)

2.3 Surgery in Ancient Egypt

Ancient Egyptians had considerable knowledge of medicine and surgical techniques. They performed a wide range of surgical procedures, including those related to trauma, tumours, and other injuries and illnesses. Knowledge of Ancient Egyptian medicine primarily derives from a dozen important medical papyri dating from ca 1550 BCE (Edwin Smith Papyrus) to 300 BCE (Brooklyn Snake Papyrus), these documents were written in hieratic, a cursive form of hieroglyphics. The Ebers Papyrus provides the best knowledge about anatomy and physiology in the ancient Egyptian times.

The Egyptian conception of the human body was as a network of interconnected channels and was likened to the branches of the Nile, with the heart as the center of the human body – the central engine of all the bodily functions. From the heart proceeded various channels, conveying not only the blood, but also air (reaching the heart from the nose and lungs), tears, saliva, mucus, sperm, urine, nutriment, and faeces, as well as harmful substances conceived to be the agents of pain and illness.

Ancient Egyptian surgical instruments have been found in tombs and include knives, forceps, needles, and probes. They also used catheters, pessaries, and surgical illumination during their procedures. The Ebers Papyrus, one of the oldest medical texts in the world dating back to around 1550 BCE, contains detailed descriptions of surgical procedures, including the treatment of wounds, fractures, dislocations, tumors, and abscesses (Fig. 2.3).

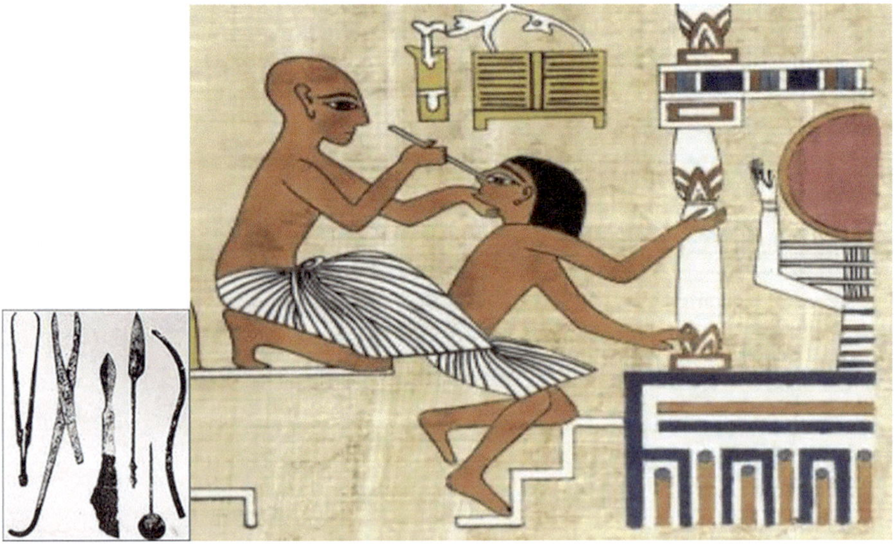

Fig. 2.3 Ancient Egypt Medical tools1. A collection of ancient Egyptian medical knives, cupping cups, spatula, and forceps. Dated to about 4000 B.C. (This image is published with open access under the Creative Commons Attribution license, CC. https://commons.wikimedia.org/w/index.php?search=ancient+Egyptian+medical+knives%2C+cupping+cups%2C+spatula%2C+and+forceps&title=Special:MediaSearch&go=Go&type=image)

Ancient Egyptian doctors also performed a wide range of obstetric and gynecological procedures, including the use of instruments for the treatment of uterine prolapse, and the delivery of babies by cesarean section. Some of the texts reveal that these procedures were used for saving the lives of both mother and child, but also to save the life of the mother in case of fetal death [16].

Their surgical practices and procedures were also deeply rooted in superstition and the belief in supernatural causes of illness and injury.

Egyptians also examined the dead body to ascertain the cause of death. Clean wounds were treated by stitching and adhesive bandages. Other wounds were treated by trimming (debriding) the edges and suturing and treating them with honey and herbs, possibly as antiseptics.

Ancient Egyptian doctors also had a knowledge of cataract surgery with different types of surgical instruments used to remove the cataract, including a needle-like instrument used to puncture the eye and scoop out the cloudy lens.

Ancient Egyptian medical texts, such as the Ebers Papyrus, dating back to around 1550 BCE, describe the surgical procedures used to treat cataracts. The texts describe the use of different types of surgical instruments, including a needle-like instrument used to puncture the eye and scoop out the cloudy lens [17, 18].

The Edwin Smith papyrus (1600 BCE) documents 48 injuries involving the cranium, chest, neck, upper limbs and spine.

Merit Ptah may be the first female medical practitioner to be mentioned in history, living around 2700 BCE, (Fig. 2.4). The surviving texts do not describe any surgical procedures. Medicines were applied to affected body parts or swallowed. There is a description of a vaginovesical fistula with incontinence of urine "in an irksome place." [16, 17].

The texts also describe the use of a tool called the "couching" technique in which a small metal or bronze rod was used to push the cataract to the bottom of the eye, allowing the patient to see again. This method was considered to be less invasive than the removal of the lens, and it has been suggested that the technique was likely to have been used to treat patients with early stages of cataracts. After the operation, patients were prescribed to use eye drops made of honey, and other medicinal plants, to prevent infections and to speed up the healing process (Fig. 2.5).

It is worth noting that these surgical procedures were performed without the use of anesthesia and surgical sterilization as we know today, which could have led to serious complications and infections. The texts also indicate that some patients suffered from partial or complete blindness after the operation.

The Egyptians had a good understanding of orthopaedic conditions and injuries, and developed a range of surgical techniques to treat them.

The Ebers Papyrus describes the surgical procedures used to treat fractures, dislocations, and spinal injuries. The texts describe the use of different types of surgical instruments, including splints, slings, and traction devices, to immobilize the affected limb and promote healing. They also describe the techniques of reduction and fixation of the fractures using wooden splints, metal pins, and wires [17].

With regards spinal injuries, they developed methods of traction to straighten the spine and also surgical procedures to reduce spinal fractures and dislocations.

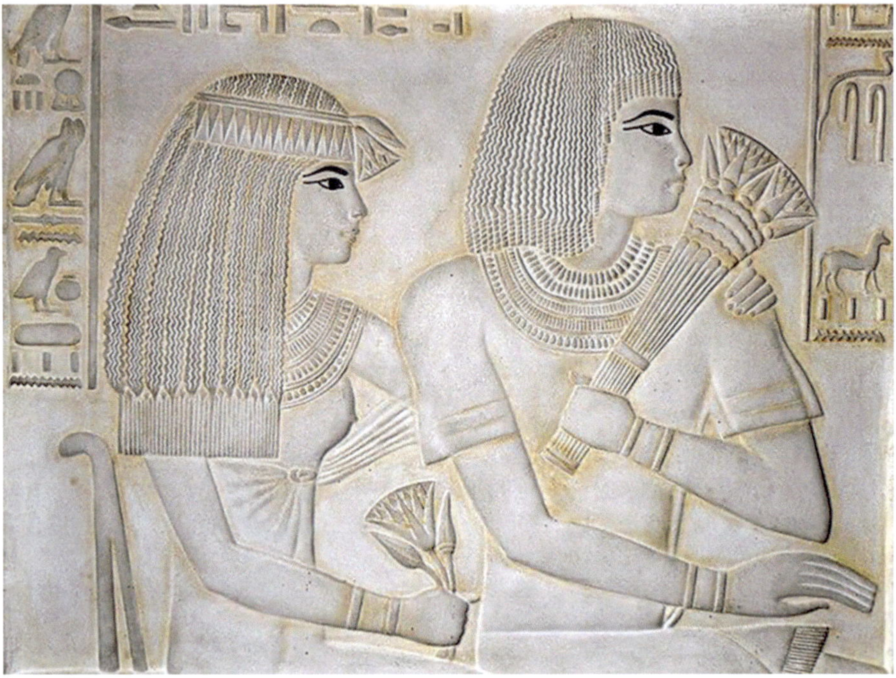

Fig. 2.4 Merit Ptah: A copy from TT55 tomb, stored; vezir Ramose during the reign of Amenhotep III and Akhenatenre. (By Stzeman; Creative Commons Attribution-Share AlikeCC. https://en.wikipedia.org/wiki/Ramose_(TT55)#/media/File:Vezir_Ramose_and_spouse_Merit-Ptah.jpg)

Patients were given herbal medicine to alleviate pain and promote healing. They also used rudimentary physiotherapy to help patients to regain the function of the affected limb.

The Ebers Papyrus, dating back to around 1550 BCE, also describes surgical procedures used to treat urologic conditions such as bladder stones and tumours of the urinary tract. The texts contain detailed descriptions of surgical procedures and instruments to remove bladder stones and tumors, and even to relieve urinary incontinence [17, 18].

They also described their management of the male reproductive system and treated conditions such as hydrocele, hernias, and phimosis including incision, excision, and suturing to repair or remove the pathological tissue.

Ancient Egyptians had a surprisingly sophisticated understanding of the cardiovascular system.

Although Egyptians had a surprisingly sophisticated understanding of the cardiovascular system, as mentioned above, with the heart as the centre, there is no clear evidence that they had a good understanding of vascular conditions nor developed any surgical techniques to treat them.

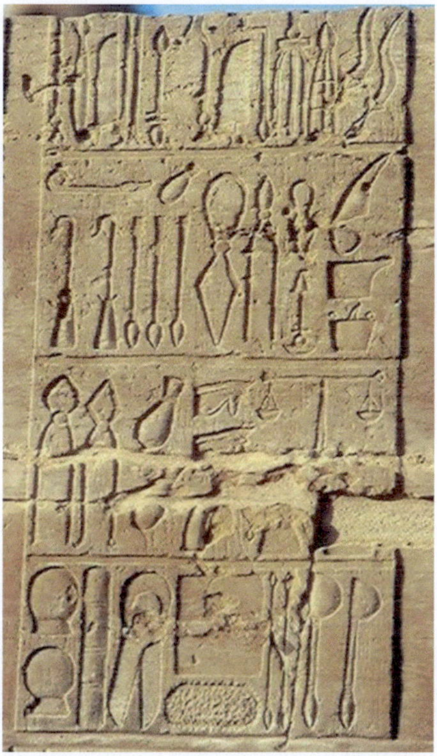

Fig. 2.5 Photo of medical aid kit, ancient Egypt. (This image is published with open access under the Creative Commons Attribution license, CC, https://wellcomecollection.org/works/m6p4u3jf/images?id=a6xnjw53)

Their knowledge of the circulatory system, was limited to the heart pumping blood throughout the body. They mainly dealt with traumatic injuries or conditions that could be treated by external means such as compression. They did describe varicose veins and arterial aneurysm. They also described treating that with heated knife to reduce the bleeding [19].

The Greek King, Philip of Macedon, was succeeded by his son Alexander the Great in 336 BCE. Following his victorious conquest of the Persians in Asia Minor, Alexander easily extended his rule to Egypt. The source of further surgical advancement then shifted to Greece from Egypt. In the year B.C. 332, Alexander the Great founded Alexandria, which rapidly grew into the most magnificent and prosperous city in the known world under the rule of the Ptolemies. Around 300 B.C., the renowned School of Alexandria was established, with Aristotle, Alexander's former teacher, as its Master. The school remained significant until the time of Hypatia, who tragically met a cruel fate in 415 CE. The school persisted until 640 CE when Alexandria was conquered by the Arabs [20, 21].

Following the tragic demise of Cleopatra in 30 BCE, the Ptolemaic dynasty came to an end, and Egypt was annexed as a Roman province. Consequently, Alexandria's significance declined, and as Rome emerged as the hub of civilization [19, 22].

Although the Edwin Smith papyrus (dating from 1600 BCE) contains case scenarios and recommended treatment (or no treatment) for 48 injuries with six that relate to the spine. The spinal and head injuries are further discussed in the section on neurosurgery. In brief, the papyrus attests to the skills of Egyptian doctors, but it is likely that these skills were lost for a millennia until they began to be rediscovered by the Greeks such as the historian, Herodotus (484–425 BCE), and Hippocrates (460–377 BCE) [21, 22].

Whilst the Ebers papyrus also describes aneurysms (probably false aneurysms and mycotic aneurysms), and varicose veins (serpentine windings), surgery was wisely discouraged on the grounds of being potentially fatal. There are descriptions of later descriptions of how to ligate and excise varicosities in Egypt around 237 BCE but these belong to the Greek era and the school of Medicine in Alexandria.

2.4 Surgery in Ancient India and the Work of Sushruta (600 BCE)

> *A person who possesses courage and presence of mind, a hand free from perspiration, tremorless grip of sharp and good instruments and who carries his operations to the success and advantage of his patient who has entrusted his life to the surgeon. The surgeon should respect this absolute surrender....* Sushruta Samhita

In ancient India, surgery was known as *Shalya Tantra* with *Shalya* representing a broken arrow or sharp part of a weapon and *Tantra* representing maneuver. Ayurveda (the Science of Life), the fifth Indian Veda, lays the foundation for the classical medical system of India, including a compendium of medical science, the *Charak Samhita*, and the work of medical practitioners, such as Acharya Agnivesh around 800 BCE. This was the standard Ayurveda textbook for some 2000 years [23, 24].

2.4.1 Sushruta

Sushruta (meaning renowned) was a specialist in cosmetic, reconstructive and dental surgery around 600 BCE (Fig. 2.6). He lived in Kashi (today Varanasi or Banaras) on the banks of the Ganga in North East India. His *Samhita* covers cesarean, cataract, prostheses, fractures, urinary stones, reconstructive procedures, and the pre and postoperative management of these conditions. Surgery and the conditions it manages were described under eight different sections representing Chedya (excision), Lekhya (Scarification), Vedhya (Puncturing), Esya (Exploration), Ahrya (extraction), Vasraya (evacuation), and Sviya (Suturing). The *Sushruta Samhita,* written in Sanskrit, described 60 types of upkarma for treating wounds, 120 surgical instruments, and 300 surgical procedures. There was a holistic approach to health and wellbeing that included balanced humours, good nutrition, elimination of wastes, and contentment.

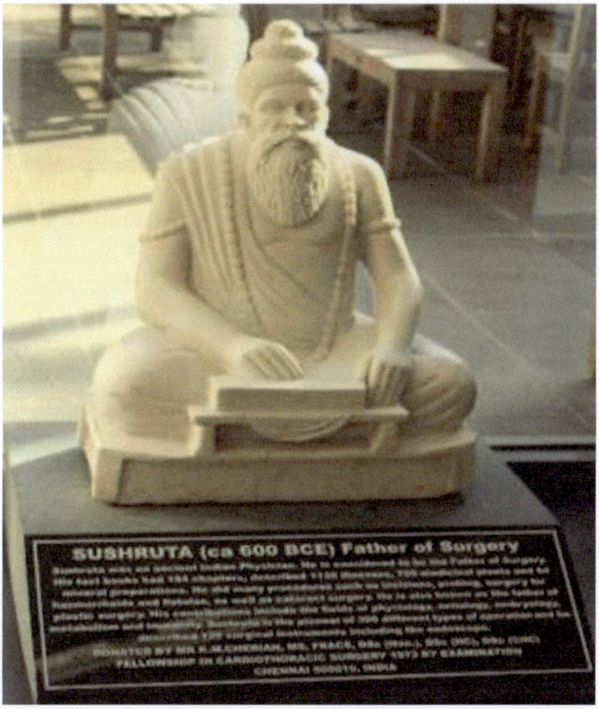

Fig. 2.6 Statue of Sushruta at the Royal Australasian College of the Surgeons, Melbourne. (Photo: the author, DW)

Blunt and penetrating injuries are classified with reconstructive procedures described including those for the nose and ears. The management of fractures and dislocations is described. Trainees had to study for years and practice surgical techniques on models made of fruit (e.g., watermelons or cucumber) or wood [25].

The *Sushruta Samhita* also has a complete and detailed section on anatomy (*Sarira Sthana*) which includes embryology and a system of dissection of the human body. Sushruta recognized that surgery is founded on anatomy and despite Hindu law forbidding the desecration of a body aged two years or older after death. Somehow it was possible to obtain bodies, perhaps many being under two years which might be why the Samhita described the human skeleton as having 300 bones (also counting epiphyses).

The cadaver was prepared by being wrapped in grass, flax, or bark, placed in a cage and suspended in a slow flowing river allowing it to decompose for seven days and then dissected. *"Anyone desirous of acquiring a thorough knowledge of anatomy should prepare a dead body and carefully observe it by dissecting it and examining its different parts."*

> *Surgery has the superior advantage of producing instantaneous effects by means of surgical instruments and appliances and hence is the highest in value of all medical tantras. It is the eternal source of infinite piety, imports fame, and opens the gates of heaven to its votaries. It prolongs the duration of human existence on earth and helps humans in successfully completing missions and wearing a decent competence in life.* [26].

2.4.2 *Sushruta's Legacy*

Sushruta's methods of rhinoplasty and other reconstructive procedures were passed down through the centuries from Guru (master) to Sisya (pupil) and undoubtedly modified through the ages. The "Indian method" became known to the Arab world when the Caliph Mansur (714–775 CE) ordered the *Samhita* to be translated from Sanskrit into Arabic. A further translation was made by Ibn Abi Usaybia (1203–1269). The Arabic translations of the *Sushruta Samhita* were later translated into Latin to form a foundation for European medical knowledge as Europe emerged from the "Dark Ages."

In 1793, two British surgeons working in India, James Findlay and Thomas Crusoe, saw an Indian surgeon perform a rhinoplasty for someone whose nose had been amputated a year earlier as a punishment for his driving a bullock for the British Army during the Mysore war of 1792. An illustrated and detailed account was published in the *Gentleman's magazine of London*. London surgeon, Joseph Constantine Carpue (1764–1846), successfully carried out two rhinoplasties based on the Indian approach using a forehead flap in September 1814 and January 1815. His publication in 1816 highlighted its superiority over the Italian approach described by Gaspare Tagliacozzi (1545–1599) describing the methods of the Scicilian Branca and Vianeo families from the 1400's. These were modifications of the original procedures described in the *Sushruta Samhita* [26, 27].

2.5 Surgery in Ancient Greece

The Greeks laid many of the foundations of philosophy, mathematics, and medicine that guide our practice today. They probably rediscovered what was known earlier, as well as deriving their principles de novo. Alexander the Great (356–323 BCE), who had been tutored by Aristotle (384–322 BCE), acceded to the throne at the age of 20 in 336 BCE. He was to be undefeated in battle and established one of the largest empires in human history. It extended north into the Balkans, Eastwards into Anatolia in today's Turkiye, across Asia Minor and Persia to North-Western India, then South to the Syria and Egypt, establishing the Greek City of Alexandria that was to become a center for learning, hosting a library. Alexander's empire had the opportunity to benefit from the knowledge of the countries he conquered; these included those already discussed - Persia, Assyria, Egypt, and India. However, well before the short reign of Alexander, ancient Greece was already renowned for its medical knowledge and expertise. The foundation of Hippocratic medicine (see below) relied on evidence based knowledge, as physicians of that time were expected to provide comprehensive and detailed medical histories to support their practice [28, 29].

Medical remedies were sourced from nature, including seawater, honey, vinegar, and powdered medicinal plants. Homer's *Iliad* (c eighth century BCE) provides descriptions of injuries and amputations that were representative of real-life care of wounds incurred through warfare.

The worship of Asklepios, or the Latin equivalent, Jesculapius, dates back to a time before the destruction of Troy, approximately around 1200 BCE. Homer's accounts suggest that Esculapius and his sons were involved in surgical practices, resembling modern army surgeons. During the mythical or fictional siege of Troy, Podalirius and Machaon were actively engaged in performing various procedures, including the extraction of barbed arrows through incisions and controlling bleeding from wounds [30, 31].

Lay physicians' guilds, known as Asclepiadse, were established and played a more significant role in the development of Greek medicine. These guilds were instrumental in shaping the course of Grecian medicine. There were also specialized practitioners known as lithotomists who focused exclusively on performing lithotomy procedures for bladder stones.

2.5.1 *Hippocrates (460–377 BCE)*

The Greek physician Hippocrates of Cos is often called the "father of medicine." He described the natural causes of many diseases, differentiating them from a "punishment of God." Hippocrates largely relied upon clinical observation to make a diagnosis, rather than mythology or superstition.

Born in 460 BCE on the island of Cos, Hippocrates the Second was the son of the Asclepiad Heraclides and proudly asserted his lineage, claiming to be the seventeenth descendant of Hippocrates the Great. He lived during an extraordinary era of intellectual growth, surrounded by renowned figures like Pericles, the Athenian statesman, Socrates, the philosopher, Herodotus, the historian, and Phidias, the greatest sculptor of ancient Greece. Hippocrates the Second holds the distinction of being the first to document his medical expertise in writing. His writings have been preserved as a valuable record of the surgical practices that were executed with remarkable precision and skill during his time [30].

For example, he described breast cancer and established the medicine as a scholarly discipline, distinguishing it from philosophy. He was the first known chest surgeon, describing the removal of breast cancer, abscesses, and placement of chest drains and dealing with varicose veins (Fig. 2.7).

Hippocrates may have been one of the first after the Egyptians to describe the treatment of varicose veins (varix = grape), as well as their association with ulceration and that they could be treated by compression bandaging, still an effective treatment today [28, 32].

Hippocrates' view of pathophysiology was that human health and disease were related to the imbalance of "the four bodily humours": *Black bile* from the gallbladder (melancholic), *yellow bile* from the spleen (choleric), *phlegma* from the brain and lungs, and *blood* from the liver (sanguine).

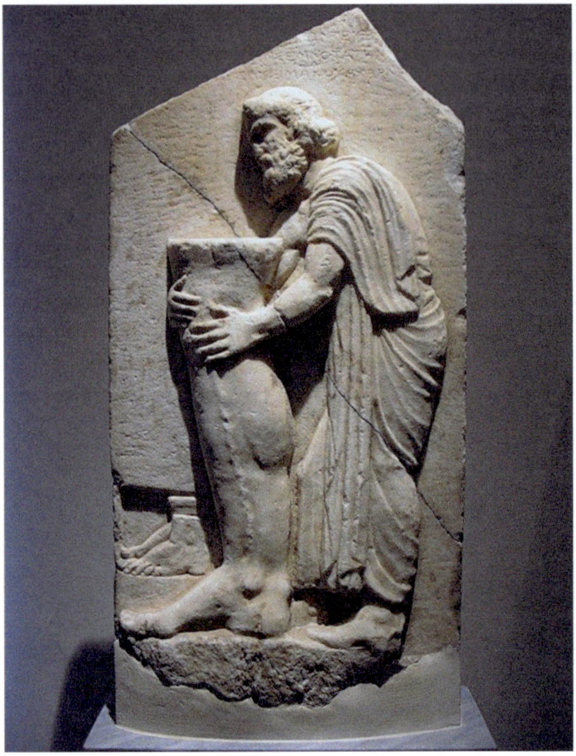

Fig. 2.7 Tablet found at the base of the Acropolis in Athens—earliest known illustration of varicose veins. (This image is published with open access under the Creative Commons Attribution license, CC. https://commons.wikimedia.org/w/index.php?search=varicose+veins+Greece&title=Special:MediaSearch&go=Go&type=image)

2.5.2 The Hippocratic Oath

"The Hippocratic Oath" was written by Hippocrates and is still taken today by many doctors. The oath addresses ethical issues of practice that even a doctor today must embrace: to treat patients the best of one's ability, to preserve patient confidentiality, to teach the next generation of physicians, and to avoid any lethal injection. The oath also promises to leave surgery to those to whom the craft of surgery belongs.

However, it has often been re-worded to be rendered more applicable to what is regarded as current practice of the day. For example, the original oath honours the Gods of healing, promises to look after the siblings of one's teacher as one's own, and agrees not induce an abortion. The translation below was made by Michael Norton of the National Library of Medicine (US) in 2002.

> *I swear by Apollo the physician, and Asclepius, and Hygieia and Panacea and all the gods and goddesses as my witnesses, that, according to my ability and judgement, I will keep this Oath and this contract:*
>
> *To hold him who taught me this art equally dear to me as my parents, to be a partner in life with him, and to fulfill his needs when required; to look upon his offspring as equals to my own siblings, and to teach them this art, if they shall wish to learn it, without fee or contract; and that by the set rules, lectures, and every other mode of instruction, I will*

impart a knowledge of the art to my own sons, and those of my teachers, and to students bound by this contract and having sworn this Oath to the law of medicine, but to no others.

I will use those dietary regimens which will benefit my patients according to my greatest ability and judgement, and I will do no harm or injustice to them.

I will not give a lethal drug to anyone if I am asked, nor will I advise such a plan; and similarly I will not give a woman a pessary to cause an abortion.

In purity and according to divine law will I carry out my life and my art.

I will not use the knife, even upon those suffering from stones, but I will leave this to those who are trained in this craft.

Into whatever homes I go, I will enter them for the benefit of the sick, avoiding any voluntary act of impropriety or corruption, including the seduction of women or men, whether they are free men or slaves.

Whatever I see or hear in the lives of my patients, whether in connection with my professional practice or not, which ought not to be spoken of outside, I will keep secret, as considering all such things to be private.

So long as I maintain this Oath faithfully and without corruption, may it be granted to me to partake of life fully and the practice of my art, gaining the respect of all men for all time. However, should I transgress this Oath and violate it, may the opposite be my fate.

2.5.3 Surgical Instruments in Ancient Greece

Greek surgical instruments have been found in archaeological excavations and include knives, forceps, needles, and probes. Greek surgical texts, such as the writings of Hippocrates, contain detailed descriptions of surgical conditions, procedures, and the use of surgical instruments. For example, the treatment of wounds, fractures, dislocations, tumors, and abscesses. The ancient Greeks, as did the civilizations before them, treated bladder and kidney stones, gynecological conditions and performed ophthalmic procedures.

2.5.4 Herophilus and Erisistratus in Alexandria

It was at Alexandria, at the beginning of the third century BC that cadaveric dissection was performed by two Greek doctors, Herophilus and Erasistratus 304–250 BCE). Herophilus (335–280 BCE) worked in Anatolia (part of Turkey today), Athens and Alexandria. He undertook cadaveric dissections so made a number of anatomical contributions including on the brain, cerebellum, and cranial nerves. He described the superior saggital sinus and the duodenum. Erasistratus, also originated from Anatolia and was the younger colleague of Herophilus. Among other anatomical contributions he described the heart valves (naming them triscuspid and sigmoid) and also recognized that nerves originated from the brain [33].

2.5.5 *Agnodice (Fourth Century BCE)*

Gaius Julius Hyginus, a Roman author wrote in *Fabulae* of how women were forbidden from practice in ancient Athens but Agnodice was able to study medicine in Alexandria under Herophilus. She returned to practice in Athens disguised as a man, and treated women as "an obstetrix." She became very popular but was accused of seduction. She was forced to reveal her gender to the jury during her trial which led to her acquittal. The case resulted in the law against the practice of female physicians being revoked. Greek women were then able to practice medicine and continued to do so during the Roman period.

Most medical practitioners over the next millennium based their practice on Hippocrates' teachings, and later from the second century CE, those of Galen—whose underlying philosophy of health and disease remained mistakenly trying to restore the imbalance of the four bodily humors.

2.6 Surgery During the Roman Empire (280 BCE–476 CE)

A series of wars were fought between the Greek kingdoms and Rome in the period 280 BC, leading to the final conquest of the Ptolemic kingdom and Alexandria in 30 BC. However, the Roman Empire had already extended to Anatolia (modern day Turkey) and Asia Minor by the middle of the second century BC.

The majority of "Greek" physicians originated from what was the ancient Greek empire, but not from modern day Greece but rather from Anatolia or Asia Minor, part of Turkey today. Examples were Herophilus, Soranus, Aeretaeus, and Galen from Ephesus, Cappadocia, and Pergamon. In Ancient Rome, the physicians all originated from what were formerly Greek kingdoms.

This was because, for a considerable period, the upper-class Romans viewed the practice of medicine as disreputable. However, this perception changed significantly due to the achievements of Asclepiades (128–56 BCE). After studying in Alexandria, he settled in Rome and formed friendships with prominent figures like Cicero and other distinguished individuals of his era. Asclepiades gained renown as the first surgeon to perform tracheotomy. His success helped to diminish the prejudice against medical practitioners in Roman society.

Thereafter, the most skilled surgeons were enlisted in the army, and many of them received their education from renowned medical schools in Alexandria, Egypt, or schools in proximity to Athens, Greece. Some even pursued specialized training at schools dedicated to training gladiators to prepare for their roles as surgeons in the Roman legions. These highly trained surgeons played a vital role in military hospitals, where they performed a variety of surgical procedures, albeit these were limited when inside body cavities. They had a variety of surgical instruments enabling them to operate on virtually every part of the body [28, 31, 34, 35].

2.6.1 Roman Surgical Operations and Provision of Anesthesia/Sedation

In an optimal scenario, four specialists participated in each surgical procedure. The *medicus chirurgus* took charge of conducting the surgical interventions to repair injuries. Assisting during and after surgery, the *chirurgus nutrix* (surgical nurse) ensured a clean and hygienic environment for the operations and helped in patient care post-surgery. The *medicus ordinarius*, a medical doctor skilled in anaesthesia, administered the anaesthesia. Lastly, the *miles medicus* (hospital orderly) attended to supplementary tasks not directly associated with the surgical procedure [36, 37].

In ancient Rome, anaesthetists employed the dissociative (sedation) method of anesthesia, combining sedatives with strong analgesics and local anesthetics. This approach induced catalepsy, amnesia, and analgesia in the patient. The preferred analgesic was powdered opium, which was mixed with wine. However, opium had to be imported from the East through the Silk Road, so was scarce. In such cases, the anesthetist would use powdered mandrake (*Mandragora officinarium*) in a draft of wine, which was locally grown in Italy. Additionally, the sedative powdered corn poppy (*Papaver rhoeas*) was added to the wine.

For local anaesthesia during surgery, a mixture of memphitic stone and henbane seeds (*Hyoscyamus niger*) was ground up and applied to the areas about to undergo surgery. Once these agents were administered to the patient, he or she would enter a state of twilight sleep, and the surgeon would proceed with the operation, aiming to conduct it as swiftly as possible. Postoperative care held significant importance in Roman medicine, with hemorrhagic shock and infections being frequent concerns. To replenish blood levels, a legionnaire would be provided with foods abundant in heme iron and non-heme iron. Roman physicians lacked knowledge about the specific relationship between heme and non-heme iron in treating anemia. Instead, their understanding of which foods could effectively restore a soldier's strength after blood loss was based on observation from generations of trial and error, but with documented findings of their effectiveness. In the realm of postoperative care, antiseptics like vinegar and honey played a crucial role in managing wounds to minimize infections. Additionally, addressing the impact of inflammation and fever were vital aspects of the postoperative care process. Tumeric, imported from India or China, was used to control inflammation, but when not available the locally grown rosemary was used [38–40].

Roman surgical instruments have been found in archaeological excavations and include knives, forceps, needles, and probes. These include those recovered from Pompeii which was destroyed by lava flow and pumice from Mt. Vesuvius in 79 CE. Roman surgical texts, such as the *Corpus Hippocraticum* and *De Medicina* by Celsus, contain detailed descriptions of surgical procedures and the use of surgical instruments.

Julius Caesar (100–44 BCE), who was not born by cesarean section as his mother survived him, passed legislation that allowed women physicians to become Roman citizens. As Roman law forbade Romans from practicing medicine, this was delegated to foreigners, including women, and mainly the Greeks most of whom came from Anatolia.

2.6.2 *Aulus Celsus (25 BCE–50 CE)*

The Roman nobleman and encyclopedist, Aulus Cornelius Celsus, wrote an encyclopedia, *De Artibus*, with an eight volume medical compendium, *De Medicina* [42, 43]. Two volumes are devoted to surgery, VII and VIII. Celsus may not have been a doctor or a surgeon but rather an archivist who collected and compiled the knowledge of the first century of the Christian era in Latin. After the fall of Rome, his work was lost until 1443, when rediscovered, and was the first medical text to be printed in Europe with the advent of the printing press in 1478.

The repair of an umbilical hernia is described with reduction, excision of the sac and closure of the fascial defect. The Roman surgeons certainly had a curved needle with an eyelet for suturing. For soft tissue abscesses the treatment was incision(s), and drainage, sufficient to "afford the necessary relief" and "that the deepest part of the cavity gets a vent." After drainage honey was infused into the wound to clean it. Scalpels were often used to incision and those recovered from the house of the surgeon at Pompeii were similar to the scalpels of today but the handle and blade were one single instrument (Fig. 2.8).

Other operations included extraction of a missile, probing and laying open an anal fistula and even performing a laparotomy for an abdominal stab wound.

> *The larger intestine can be sutured, not with any certain assurance, but because a doubtful hope is preferable to certain despair, for occasionally it heals up. The if either intestine is livid or pallid or black, in which case there is necessarily no sensation, all medical aid is in vain....*

And for uninjured intestine herniating through a stab wound:

> *The patient is to be laid on his back with his hips raised; and if the wound is too narrow for the intestines to be replaced, it is to be cut until sufficiently wide. If the intestines have already become too dry, they are to be bathed in water.*

The text goes on to describe a closure of all layers of the abdominal defect after returning the bowel and/or omentum to the peritoneal cavity.

Celsus described dermatologic conditions, surgical procedures, and cancer, using the word cancer for crab in Latin, because he recognized the dilated tortuous veins surrounding a breast cancer and their similar appearance to the legs of crabs.

De Medicina is considered one of the most important surviving ancient medical and surgical texts. Although the first century CE original work did not survive, it was paraphrased in the ninth century AD by a Byzantine scholar, and this version and is still available [28, 31, 34, 35].

Roman doctors carried out basic plastic surgery, such as repairing cleft lips, and surgical procedures related on the eyes and ears. "*De Medicina*" has detailed

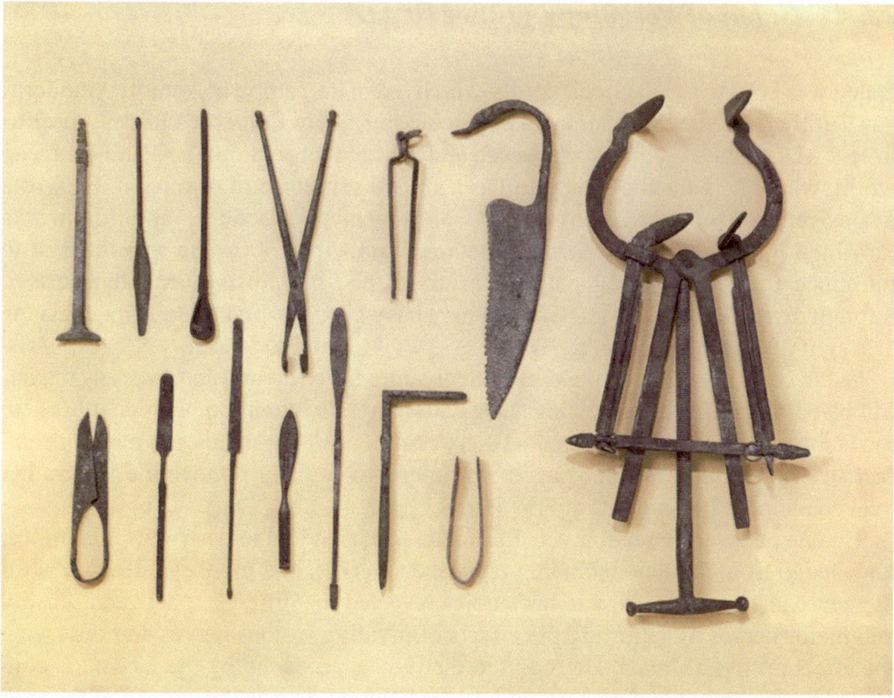

Fig. 2.8 Surgical instruments from the Roman era. (This image is published with open access under the Creative Commons Attribution license, CC. https://upload.wikimedia.org/wikipedia/commons/2/2b/Graeco-Roman_surgical_instruments._Wellcome_L0012385.jpg)

descriptions of surgical procedures and instruments used to treat (couch or remove) cataracts and urologic conditions such as bladder stones, tumors of the urinary tract, as well as hydrocoeles, hernias, and phimosis [39–41]. To remove urinary (bladder or urethral calculus (stone), either the finger or a tool called the crotchet was employed. The credit for this technique is attributed to Ammonius of Alexandria, also known as "Lithotomos," who lived around B.C. 230 BCE [35, 36].

2.6.3 Soranus of Ephesus and Aeraetus of Cappadocia

Soranus of Ephesus (98–138 CE) wrote a textbook on Obstetrics and Gynecology for female students of his day.

> *...knowledge of anatomy of the hidden organs should match that of the organs that can be seen.*

Aeraetus of Cappadocia (Second Century CE) described trigeminal neuralgia. He wrote about the whole range of medical conditions and was also the first to give an account of diabetes and coeliac disease.

2.6.4 Galen of Pergamon (129–210 AD)

Galen was born to a rich Greek family who lived in Pergamon in Anatolia (modern-day Turkiye). He became personal physician to Roman Emperor Marcus Aurelius in 168 AD, studied medicine in Greece and traveled throughout the Mediterranean world, where he gained a reputation as a skilled surgeon and physician. He wrote extensively on anatomy, physiology, and medical practices, and his works remained influential in the field of medicine until the 1500s. He was the first to introduce the idea of prognosis, as prior to this, prognosis was often derived through divination and mysticism. He may have been the first to describe melaena as a sign of impending death.

Galen certainly adopted the use of the ligature for tying off blood vessels to control bleeding during surgery. This was almost certainly common practice in Roman medicine by this time. Galen treated a cataract in a similar manner to modern cataract surgery, using a needle shaped instrument to actually remove the lens rather than couching it (pushing it into the inferior eye).

Human cadaver dissection was forbidden so Galen had to derive his anatomical knowledge from animals including pigs, sheep, goats, and monkeys. He described the neuroanatomy of pigs, and his studies revealed the difference between sensory and motor nerves by reporting the effects of dividing various nerves and observing the effect on live animals. He reported that voice, produced by the larynx, is controlled by the brain via the recurrent laryngeal nerve. As was the custom of the ages he was a proponent of venesection and bloodletting for various ailments.

His ideas about physiology were reproductions of the philosophy of Plato and Aristotle. Galen hypothesized that the human body has three systems: the brain and nerves for sensation; the heart and arteries for life-giving energy; and the liver and veins, responsible for nutrition and growth. He thought the liver was the blood producing organ, and that air mixing with blood in the heart via small holes between the left and right side rather than within the lungs [37, 38].

Galen's written works and theories had a profound influence on Byzantine and Arab medicine after the fall of Rome. In the ninth century Greek manuscripts began to be collected and translated by Arabs, and about 850 CE Hunayn bin Ishaq, a physician at the court of Baghdad, prepared a list of 129 works of Galen that were translated to Arabic. Medicine in the Arab world thus became heavily based upon the work of Galen.

The legacy of Galen persisted until the Renaissance, until in 1543, Andreas Vesalius showed that Galen's anatomy of the body was more animal, and his concepts included many errors. Galen's notions of physiology lasted until the English physician William Harvey explained the circulation of the blood.

He served as the personal physician to several emperors, and wrote on anatomy, physiology, pathology, and philosophy. Galen used catgut for suturing, and understood that pneuma (air) was essential for life [42–44].

He continued to espouse the theory of the four humours, and mistakenly believed pus (for example in an abscess) should not be removed by surgery (unlike those surgeons documented by Celsus). His anatomical drawings, based on monkey and pig dissections, remained uncontested until the Renaissance period, when an updated understanding of anatomy based on human dissection was published [42, 43].

Although the profession of medicine was largely dominated by male doctors, Galen, in his writings, also made mention of a number of renowned female physicians of his day including Origenia, who had remedies for hemoptysis and diarrhea; Eurgerasia, who treated nephritis; Margareta, an army surgeon; also Favilla, Samithra, and Xanita are mentioned [44].

2.6.4.1 Aspasia (Fourth Century CE)

Aspasia was an influential female physician and gynecologist in the fourth century CE. She practiced abortions only when the life of the woman was in danger, and was skilled in version of the fetus, procedures on the vulva and uterine hemorrhoids. She was well regarded and cited by later surgeons, Aetius of Amida (d 575 CE) and Paul of Aegina (ca 625–690 CE), who both referred to her work and procedures with admiration [44].

2.6.4.2 The Fall of the Roman Empire (476 CE)

Throughout the previous eight centuries, Greek and Roman physicians had advanced the scientific medical-surgical knowledge in Europe, North Africa, and the Middle-East. The development would now stall for a while. Arabian scholars became the guardians of earlier Greeko-Roman medical knowledge and continued to advance that knowledge within their own sphere of influence [28, 34].

2.7 Ancient China, Its Early Dynasties to the Mongol Empire

2.7.1 Bian Que (407–310 BCE)

The legendary, Bian Que, (Fig. 2.9), may have used hemp and wine to induce anaesthesia. He wrote an account called the *Yellow Emperor's Cannon of 81 difficult issues*. He is also reported to have advocated for the four-step diagnoses of *"Looking (at their tongues and their outside appearances), Listening (to their voice and breathing patterns), Inquiring (about their symptoms), and Taking (their pulse)."*

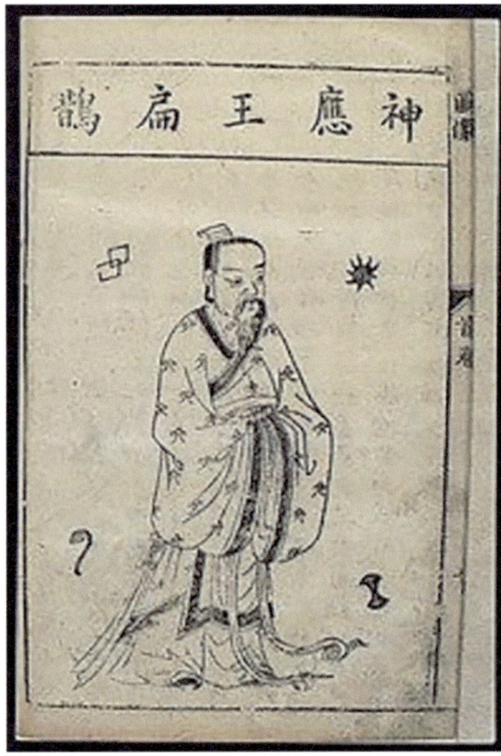

Fig. 2.9 Bian Que's Yellow Emperor's Cannon of 81 Difficult Issues. (This image is published with open access under the Creative Commons Attribution license, CC. https://commons.wikimedia.org/w/index.php?search=Bian+Que's+Yellow+Emperor&title=Special:MediaSearch&go=Go&type=image)

2.7.2 Hua Tuo (c140–c208 CE)

Hua Tuo was a Chinese surgeon also renowned for the use of hemp and wine (mafeisan) to provide a form of anaesthesia to his patients. He performed laparotomies, excised pathological tissue, parts of viscera (partial splenectomy), and may even have performed intestinal anastomoses. He also practiced acupuncture (as was then normal in China) and developed a series of physiotherapy exercises based on five animals, in which the patient imitated the movement of the tiger, deer, bear, ape, and bird. Unfortunately, he met an untimely end at the hand of the king of Wei Cao Cao, who executed him for suggesting he be trephined, and this despite Cao Cao's own wife advocating for the procedure to be performed. His medical treatise, *Qingnang shu* (Book of the Blue Bag), was burned at the time of his death. Cao Cao later regretted putting him to death as there was no one to save his son who soon afterwards fell ill and died.

2.7.3 *Sun Simiao (d 682 CE)*

Sun Simiao was an early Tang dynasty (618–907 AD) Chinese medicine author who wrote two well-regarded texts with prescriptions on Emergency measures. The first was *Essential Formulas for Emergencies [Worth] a Thousand Pieces/Catty of Gold* (5300 recipes) and the second was a supplement with a further 2000 recipes. He also wrote a text on the *Absolute Sincerity of Great Physicians*, [sometimes called the Chinese Hippocratic Oath], which Chinese medical education still endorses today.

> *A Great Physician should not pay attention to status, wealth or age; neither should he question whether the particular person is attractive or unattractive, whether he is an enemy or friend, whether he is a Chinese or a foreigner, or finally, whether he is uneducated or educated. He should meet everyone on equal grounds. He should always act as if he were thinking of his close relatives.*

2.7.4 *Couching*

Couching (*jin pi shu*), not a particularly successful procedure for treating a cataract; it aims to push the lens down into the lower eye chamber, and was first introduced to Chinese surgery during the West Han dynasty (206 BC–9 AD) via the Silk Road. The technique, combined with acupuncture, spread throughout China during the Tang dynasty (607–907 AD). Maharshi Sushruta, an ancient Indian surgeon, had first described the procedure around 600 BCE. The technique has been superseded by much more successful techniques today, first involving extraction of the opaque lens and, later, introduction of a prosthetic intra-ocular lens (IOL) by British ophthalmologist, Sir Harold Ridley, in 1949.

2.7.5 *Human Cadaveric Dissection*

The first recorded anatomical human dissection occurred in China in 13 CE during the Han dynasty (201 BCE - 220 CE). There were also illustrations of anatomical dissections of the internal organs which were published in 1113 CE during the Song dynasty (960–1279 CE) but then reproduced with little further modification for centuries. They were updated to modern standards when Western Medical missionaries arrived in China during the nineteenth century.

2.7.6 *Pax Mongolica (1250–1350 CE)*

Although it had a violent inception, established by Genghis Khan (1162–1227), the dominance of the Mongols across Asia and the Middle East led to a period of stability lasting a century, known as the Pax Mongolica. The impact of this era on the trajectory of medical and surgical advancements in Asia, the Levant, and Western Europe was significant. For more than a century, the Pax Mongolica made trade, cultural interaction, and science collaboration possible throughout Eurasia. This was possible because of the Silk Road's unification, which led to significant and historic contact between Europe and China for the first time.

This early form of global interconnectedness involving the exchange of goods and innovations introduced significant advances to various regions, including the Mongols and their neighboring societies. These regions included Europe and the Middle East, where the Pax Mongolica facilitated the introduction of gunpowder, paper manufacturing, systems of exchange and banking through bills of exchange, and insights into anatomy and pharmaceutical practices.

The Mongol Khans actively fostered the expansion and sharing of medical expertise across their empire. They established hospitals, inspired by the Persian model. Teams of physicians were dispatched from various corners of the empire to serve in these hospitals. Prominent Mongol leaders sought medical assistance from a diverse array of practitioners, including those from Chinese, Indian, Uighur, Arabic, and Nestorian backgrounds. Abundant evidence supports the notion of medical interchange and collaboration among these different schools of thought.

Especially pertinent is the transfer of groundbreaking anatomical insights obtained through human cadaver dissections from Yuan China to Europe. A pivotal figure during this period was Rashid al-Din (1247–1313), a Persian Jew who embraced Islam in his mid-thirties. He emerged as a renowned physician, and crucial chronicler of the Mongol era. Notably, he established an academic institution called the Rabi Rashidi in Tabriz. This establishment featured a research-focused hospital, a medical school, a paper production facility, and an extensive library containing an impressive collection of over 60,000 books.

Rabi Rashidi printed the first known manuscript on Chinese surgery and medicine in 1313. It was called *Tansūqnāma-i Īlkhān dar funūn-i 'ulūm-i Khatā'ī* (Treasure Book of the Ilkhans on the Branches of the Chinese Sciences). Within its content, there are comprehensive discussions, including numerous anatomical illustrations. These illustrations were based on the cadaveric dissections that were conducted on around fifty rebels executed in China's Guangxi Province in the year 1045 CE. Chinese and Persian medical practitioners collaborated to translate and compile these texts into both Persian and Arabic. The origins of these remarkable illustrations trace back to an original manuscript discovered in 1931 within the Süleymaniye Library in Istanbul, bearing the date 1313. It is proposed that the *Tansūqnāma* potentially played a role in rekindling European curiosity in the field of anatomy and the practice of cadaveric dissection.

The Rabi Rashidi establishment also served as a venue for the renowned Persian physician and anatomist, Mansur ibn Ilyas. Mansur's predecessors undertook journeys to Eastern oriental countries and authored manuscripts that integrated Eastern medical knowledge. However, the most significant contribution from Mansur is his work titled *Tashrih-i Mansuri* (Mansur's Anatomy), which stands as the world's earliest color atlas of human anatomy. This remarkable work was published in 1386.

"Mansur's Anatomy" drew extensively from the writings of prominent Arabic scholars such as Avicenna and Rhazes. These scholars, in their own right, were influenced by the writings of Galen and Hippocrates.

Mansur's atlas offers an astonishingly precise account of the anatomy and physiology of the optic nerves, their interconnections, and the distinctive cruciform optic chiasm. Furthermore, it introduced an innovative approach to anatomical education. Notably, it included the first-ever depiction of a pregnant uterus within the context of the circulatory system. The atlas's distinctiveness also arises from its use of numerous color images.

In this manner, Mansour's works were absorbed into the libraries and lecture rooms of the newly founded European University medical institutions during the fourteenth century. Mansur's contribution to the instruction of anatomy was significant, with a long-lasting impact on successive generations of anatomy students. Western historians have often overlooked the influence of the Pax Mongolica during the twelfth to fifteenth centuries, focusing rather on the revival of Greco-Roman medical texts in Europe through interactions with Byzantium and the Arabic realms, which then spanned from southern Spain to Palestine.

More contemporary sources, however, have brought attention to several events that occurred within the framework of the Pax Mongolica, which challenge the oversimplified paradigm. During this period of prosperity, the standing of "modern" Islamic medicine experienced a noticeable ascent in Europe. By the year 1467, an intriguing shift was observable: over half of Ferrari's library at Pavia University were either Arabic or Persian books. His 1471 textbook featured a remarkable 3000 citations from Avicenna, in contrast to 1000 from Galen and a mere 140 from Hippocrates. Furthermore, the university initiated weekly lectures specifically dedicated to the teachings of Rhazes.

In the twelfth to thirteenth centuries, Universities in Europe began conferring advanced degrees in medicine, similar to the systems already used in Eastern academies. This shift ushered in a more permissive, if not completely secular, University system.

Due to their martial lifestyle, the Mongols had acquired extensive experience in handling traumatic injuries. The treatment of fractures and dislocations was entrusted to *Bariachi*, skilled bonesetters who operated independently from physicians. Chinese surgeons who were brought under Mongol rule began specializing in orthopaedics. Among them, Wei Yilin gained prominence for his contributions. He authored a manual on fracture reduction techniques, introduced rudimentary anaesthesia utilizing opium, and pioneered the suspension method for joint reduction. Interestingly, this suspension technique did not emerge in Western medical practice until its independent development in 1927 by Dr. G. Davis.

The Mongols provided the means by which European and Islamic medical knowledge was included in medieval Beijing. In 1263, they set up the "Medical Bureau of the Capital." This institution was aimed at spreading Western medicine in China. The Imperial library in Beijing had Chinese translations of Western medical classics, including Avicenna's Canon of Medicine. This work later became a standard teaching text in Europe from the fourteenth to eighteenth centuries.

The first Archbishop of Beijing, John of Montecorvino, had a diary. In it, he wrote that the Great Khan Temür employed a Lombard surgeon. This insight offers an interesting perspective on the intersection of medical knowledge and cultural exchange during this period.

2.7.7 Ming Dynasty (1368–1662)

The Ming Dynasty followed the Mongol-led Yuan dynasty.

2.7.7.1 Tan Yunxian (1461–1554)

Tan Yunxian was a female physician treating women during the Ming Dynasty. Her grandmother was the daughter of a physician and she learned from her grandmother. Women were not able to learn from masters, they had to learn through family training and this training was often directed at assisting the males in the family with supporting work. They were not able to set up their own clinics but practiced in the country amongst family and acquaintances. Women in Ming China could not consult male doctors about certain "female" conditions. Tan Yunxian completed a book *Sayings of the Female Doctor* but was not able to publish it until her son ordered the plates to be cut on his behalf.

Wang Ji (1463–1539) was a contemporary male physician who published an early medical casebook.

2.7.7.2 An Early Smallpox Vaccination (1549)

Wan Quan (1495–1585), also known as *Wan Mizhai*, was a pediatrician who was the third in his family to practice medicine. Wan was the first individual to have written about variolation, an early smallpox vaccination in a treatise *Douzhen Xinfa*, published in 1549, well before Edward Jenner's (1749–1823) introduction of the vaccine in Britain and Europe.

2.8 Guy de Chauliac (1300–1368)

Guy de Chauliac (Fig. 2.10) was born to a poor family in the final years of the thirteenth century and was to become the pre-eminent surgeon not only of his day, but he also exerted a dominant influence over surgical thinking until the late 1500s. His book, *Chirugia Magna*, was first written in Latin in 1363, but as a mark of its popularity was then translated and transcribed into many European languages [45, 46]. Before providing more biographical detail, it is important to understand the

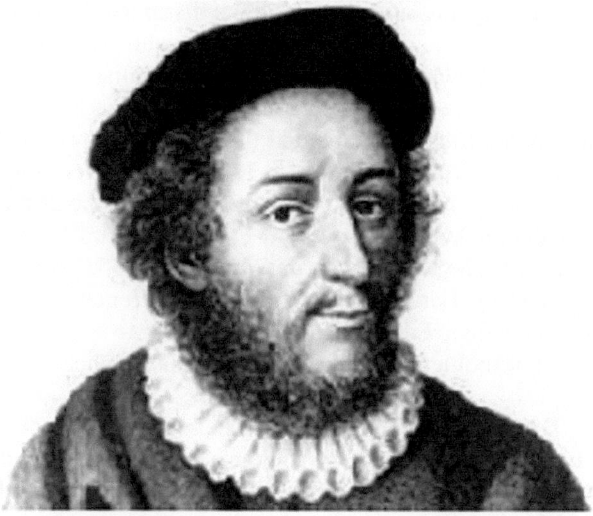

Fig. 2.10 Guy de Chauliac. Stipple engraving by A. Tardieu Wellcome. (This image is published with open access under the Creative Commons Attribution license, CC. https://commons.wikimedia.org/w/index.php?search=guy+de+chauliac&title=Special:MediaSearch&go=Go&type=image)

political landscape of Europe in the fourteenth century, as it was recovering from its Dark Ages.

In the early fourteenth century, Europe developed global trade with China, Japan, and India. Venice and Genoa, the major Italian cities, were fierce rivals vying for control of shipping commerce between Africa, the Middle East, and Eurasia. The Mongolian empire extended close to the Black Sea, with trade focused on the port of Caffa (Feodosiya) under Genoa's protection. This trade route facilitated the entry of the Black Death into Caffa and its subsequent spread to Genoa. In 1347–1348, the Black Death struck Europe, causing the death of approximately one third of its 75 million population [46–48].

In the thirteenth and fourteenth centuries, the Mongols held dominion over the most extensive landmass in human history, with their influence extending to the Black Sea. The Mongols sacked Baghdad in 1258 and subsequently posed threats to Syria in 1271 and 1281, though they were repelled. A peace treaty between the Mamluks and Mongols was eventually signed in 1323. After the Norman invasion of England led by William the Conqueror in 1066, a period of English-Norman/French collaboration ensued. English and French leaders assembled armies and, with the approval of the Pope, embarked on Crusades to the Middle East (the Holy Land) with the aim of capturing and retaining Jerusalem. Intermittent conflicts on the frontiers between regions under Muslim and Christian control persisted during the Middle Ages until the 1600s. During this period in Europe, the Christian Byzantine Empire faced challenges from the Muslim Turks, and the Iberian peninsula witnessed prolonged conflict. These events were of great significance, especially considering the dominant influence of leading Arab physicians on medical understanding at that time [48, 49].

The ongoing wars and conflicts disrupted the usual international collaboration between physicians from both sides, who were primarily focused on advancing medical knowledge. Before Guy de Chauliac's birth, the Mamluks, led by Emir Baibars, were determined to expel Christian armies from the Middle East. The Mamluk Sultanate emerged as the dominant power in the region, ruling over Egypt and Syria from 1250 to 1517. They achieved significant victories, capturing Antioch in 1268 and Tripoli in 1289. During the prime years of Guy de Chauliac's practice in Avignon, Southern France, Edward III (r1327–1377) was the King of England. The Hundred Years War (1337–1453) between England and France was sparked by Edward III's claim to the French throne. After the deaths of three French Kings, Edward III was not chosen to succeed as the French nobility argued that his mother, Isabella, could not have inherited the throne, so neither could he [49].

Guy de Chauliac, born into a humble family, received an ecclesiastical scholarship to study medicine in Toulouse and later in Montpellier, France. He pursued a fellowship in anatomy at Bologna under Nicola Bertuccio, who had been a student of Mondino de Luzzi. The significance of a thorough understanding of anatomy in medicine had recently been incorporated into the medical curriculum at Bologna during the previous decades. He took a further fellowship in Paris, the leading European center for surgery at the time. In 1325, he earned his Master's degree in medicine from the University of Montpellier, the highest academic honor for a doctor at that time. He was a physician who specialized in surgery, not a Barber Surgeon. He also took Holy Orders (prior to medical education), which included a vow of celibacy, so he never married. He initially practiced in Lyon, but later became the physician to three Popes based in Avignon: Clement VI (1342–1352), Innocent VI (1352–1362), and Urban V (Pope 1362–1370) [49–51].

Despite the fear of infection, Guy cared for patients, including Pope Clement VI who was surrounded by fires. Both the pope and Guy survived, but Guy himself later contracted the plague with an axillary bubo. His famous book *Chirugia Magna* (La Grande Chirugie) was written in medieval Latin in 1363, long before the invention of printing. It circulated as a manuscript before being printed in 1478 and later translated into French, There were 70 editions in the different languages which remained in circulation for centuries. Chirugia Magna remained the most influential surgical text for the next 200 years, from the late fourteenth century until Paré (1510–1590). In his work, Guy de Chauliac drew from the leading medical writers who preceded him, spanning from Hippocrates and Galen to the prominent Egyptian, Persian, and Arabian physicians of the eleventh to thirteenth centuries. He made a total of 3299 references to the works of others, including 120 quotes from Hippocrates, 890 from Galen, 661 from Avicenna, 173 from Albucasis, 161 from Rhazes, and 149 from Haly Abbas [46, 47, 49].

During the thirteenth century in Italy, inhalational anesthesia using opium and mandragora was already being administered, a practice that had been introduced in the twelfth century. The ability to provide some form of anesthesia enabled him to perform a wide variety of operations. Guy de Chauliac's advice on wound management acknowledged the healing power of nature and emphasized the importance of removing foreign bodies before closing the wound edges using sutures. He also emphasized the need for hemostasis, including the value of ligating bleeding arteries. In Guy de Chauliac's time, surgical practice saw advancements in antiseptic surgery, with the use of strong wine (spirits of wine) to cleanse wounds and serve as a dressing, often mixed with oil. He emphasized the importance of absolute cleanliness for the surgeon. In cases of infection, he recommended warm red oil fomentations with added egg albumen for wound treatment [49, 50].

Guy de Chauliac's surgical expertise extended beyond wounds, ulcers, and bleeding to include procedures involving the skull, thorax, and abdomen. He provided a thorough account of trephination and had some experience with brain injuries and brain tissue loss, noting cases of patient recovery. He also described thoracic drainage techniques for fluid release. Moreover, he recommended opening penetrating abdominal wounds to suture the perforated intestines, using a special needle he had invented for this purpose. He also advised suspension and traction for femoral fractures, centuries before the Thomas splint. Guy de Chauliac was aware of his limitations and advised against attempting to remove kidney stones, suggesting that bladder stones should be left to the expertise of travelling lithotomists. He cautioned about the risks of abscesses when cutting for bladder stones, stating, "if other complications occur, may the Lord help you." Additionally, he provided descriptions of catheterization techniques and methods for removing urethral stones [49, 50].

Guy de Chauliac explored various conservative measures for hernia treatment, including the use of a truss, which he even designed himself. During his time, several surgical approaches were described, such as excision of the testicle and using cautery, arsenic, or gold thread to strengthen the weakened tissue responsible for hernias. Guy wrote separate monographs on hernia and cataract treatment.

In his preface on professional requirements for all surgeons, Guy de Chauliac identified four essential characteristics of a skilled and competent surgeon. An English version of these qualities is as follows: "First he should be learned; second, he should be expert; third he must be ingenious; and fourth, he should be able to adapt himself. It is required for the first, that the surgeon should know not only the principles of surgery, but also those of medicine in theory and practice; for the second, that he should have seen others operate; for the third, that he should be ingenious, of good judgement, and memory to recognize conditions; and for the fourth, that he be adaptable and able to accommodate himself to the circumstances."

Guy de Chauliac was ahead of his time in recognizing the significance of non-technical competencies in surgery. He emphasized the importance of professionalism, respecting the autonomy and needs of the patient, effective communication, showing respect to colleagues, and avoiding recklessness or exploitation. These qualities were crucial for providing compassionate and ethical medical care [49–51]. His fame and influence stemmed from his exceptional skill in assimilating and incorporating the teachings of his predecessors. He relied on meticulous clinical observations and was not afraid to scrutinize the outcomes of his treatments. Moreover, his unwavering commitment to professionalism placed the needs of his patients above all else, solidifying his reputation as a renowned surgeon.

References

1. Adamson PB. Medical History. 1991;35:428–35.
2. The Asclepion, Prof. Nancy Demand, Indiana University – Bloomington.
3. Barber KE. Hospitals and treatment facilities in the ancient world. In: Schlager N, Lauer J, editors. Science and its times, vol. 1. Detroit: Gale; 2001. p. 131–4.
4. Jastrow M. The medicine of the Babylonians and Assyrians. Proc R Soc Med. 1914;7(109–176):2.
5. Layard AH. Nineveh and its remains. 1st ed. The Lyons Press; 2001.
6. Legrain L. The Boudoir of Queen Shubad. Mus J. 1929;XX(3–4):210–45. Accessed August 30, 2023. https://www.penn.museum/sites/journal/9246/
7. Pastena JA. Women in surgery: an ancient tradition. Arch Surg. 1993;128:622–6.
8. Breasted JH. The Edwin Smith surgical papyrus. 1991.
9. Retief FP, Cilliers L. Mesopotamian medicine. S Afr Med J. 2007;97(1):27–30.
10. Pearn J. Hammurabi's code: a primary datum in the conjoined professions of medicine and law. Med Leg J. 2016;84(3):125–31. https://doi.org/10.1177/0025817216646038. Epub 2016 May 5. PMID: 27151189.
11. Stiefel M, Shaner A, Schaefer SD. The Edwin Smith Papyrus: the birth of analytical thinking in medicine and otolaryngology. Laryngoscope. 2006;116(2):182–8. https://doi.org/10.1097/01.mlg.0000191461.08542.a3. PMID: 16467701.
12. Kinnier Wilson JV. Childbirth and congenital disorders. In: Brothwell D, Sandison AT, editors. Diseases inantiquity. Springfield, Il: Charles C. Thomas; 1967. p. 203–6, on p. 203.
13. Kramer SN. History begins at Sumer. Philadelphia: University of Pennsylvania Press; 1981.
14. Salem SI. Medicine in Ancient Mesopotamia. In: Selin H, editor. Encyclopaedia of the history of science, technology, and medicine in Non-Western cultures. Dordrecht: Springer; 2016.
15. White AJ, Herbeck J, Scurlock JA, Mayberry J. Ancient surgeons: a characterization of Mesopotamian surgical practices. Am J Surg. 2022;224(Issue 2):790–3.
16. Ritner RK. The cardiovascular system in ancient Egyptian thought. J Near East Stud. 2006;65:99–109.
17. The cardiovascular system in ancient Egyptian thought. J Near East Stud. 2006;65:99–109.
18. Boisaubin EV. Cardiology in ancient Egypt. Tex Heart Inst J. 1988;15:80–5.
19. Ascaso FJ, Lizana J, Cristóbal JA. J Cataract Refract Surg. 2009;35(3):607–8. https://doi.org/10.1016/j.jcrs.2008.11.052.
20. Feldman RP, Goodrich JT. The Edwin Smith surgical papyrus. Childs Nerv Syst. 1999;15:281–4.
21. Lifshutz J, Colohan A. A brief history of therapy for traumatic spinal cord injury. Neurosurg Focus. 2004;16:E5.
22. van Middendorp JJ, Sanchez GM, Burridge AL. The Edwin Smith papyrus: a clinical reappraisal of the oldest known document on spinal injuries. Eur Spine J. 2010;19:1815–23.
23. Singh V. Editorial. Sushruta: the father of surgery. Natl J Maxillofac Surg. 2017;8:1–2.
24. Samhita S. https://archive.org/details/SushrutaSamhita_201701 (free download).
25. Dave T, Habte A, Vora V, Sheikh MQ, Sanker V, Gopal SV. Sushruta: the Father of Indian Surgical History. Plast Reconstr Surg Glob Open. 2024;12(4):e5715. https://doi.org/10.1097/GOX.0000000000005715. PMID: 38596573; PMCID: PMC11000756.
26. Loukas M, Lanteri A, Ferrauiola J, Tubbs RS, Maharaja G, Shoja MM, Yadav A, Rao VC. Anatomy in ancient India: a focus on the Susruta Samhita. J Anat. 2010;217(6):646–50. https://doi.org/10.1111/j.1469-7580.2010.01294.x. Epub 2010 Sep 30. PMID: 20887391; PMCID: PMC3039177.
27. Bhattacharya S. Sushruta – the very first anatomist of the world. Ind J Surg. 2022;84:901–4.
28. Campbell B. The Oxford handbook of warfare in the classical world. Oxford University Press; 2013.
29. Tipton C. Sports medicine: a century of progress. J Nutr. 1997;127(5):878S–85S.
30. Mac Auley D. A history of physical activity, health and medicine. J R Soc Med. 1994;87:32.
31. Potter DS. A companion to the Roman empire. Wiley-Blackwell; 2009.

32. Ombrellino M, Kabnick LS. Varicose vein surgery. Semin Intervent Radiol. 2005;22(3):185–94. https://doi.org/10.1055/s-2005-921951. PMID: 21326692; PMCID: PMC3036286.
33. Ghosh SK. Human cadaveric dissection: a historical account from ancient Greece to the modern era. Anat Cell Biol. 2015;48(3):153–69. https://doi.org/10.5115/acb.2015.48.3.153. Epub 2015 Sep 22. PMID: 26417475; PMCID: PMC4582158.
34. Hornblower S. The Oxford classical dictionary. Oxford University Press; 2012.
35. Richard AG. Mil Hist. 2011;28:36–41.
36. Scarborough J. Roman Medicine. Ithaca, New York: Cornell University Press; 1969. p. 70–5.
37. Vegetius FR. De Rei Militaris. Liverpool: Liverpool University Press 1.6, 8.28; 1993.
38. Dioscorides. Opium is a powerful analgesic containing morphine, codeine and thebaine. In: De Medica Materia, 4.64.3.
39. Dioscorides. Mandrake is a less potent analgesic containing scopolamine, hyoscyamine and atropine. In: De Medica Materia, 4.75.3.
40. Discorides. 1.104 Willowbark contains salicylic acid, an anti-febrile. In: De Medica Materia.
41. Fitz-Henry J. The ASA classification and peri-operative risk. Ann R Coll Surg Engl. 2011;93:185–7.
42. Köckerling F, Köckerling D, Lomas C. Cornelius Celsus--ancient encyclopedist, surgeon-scientist, or master of surgery? Langenbecks Arch Surg. 2013;398(4):609–16. https://doi.org/10.1007/s00423-013-1050-0. Epub 2013 Jan 24. PMID: 23344725; PMCID: PMC3627856.
43. Celsus CA. (c30 AD) De Medecina (on medicine) Book VII. Loeb Classical Library Edition; 1935.
44. Gregory T, Markos S. Aspasia and Cleopatra Metrodora, two majestic female physician – surgeons in the early byzantine era. J Univ Surg. 2016;4:3.
45. Watters DAK. Guy de Chauliac. ANZ J Surg. 2013;83:730–4. https://doi.org/10.1111/ans.12349.
46. Wheelis M. Biological warfare at the 1346 Siege of Caffa. Emerg Infect Dis. 2002;8:971–5.
47. Mellick SA. The Montpellier school and the Guy de Chauliac. ANZ J Surg. 1999;69:297–301.
48. Wallner B. The Middle English translation of Guy de Chauliac's anatomy. Lunds Universitets Arsskrift. Lund: CWK Gleerup; 1964.
49. Murphy GH. The surgery of Guy de Chauliac. Can Med Assoc J. 1951;65:68.
50. Thevenet A. Guy de Chauliac (1300–1370): the 'Father of Surgery'. Ann Vasc Surg. 1993;7:208–12.
51. Royal Australasian College of Surgeons. Continuing professional development program, 10th edn. Melbourne: Royal Australasian College of Surgeons, 2012.

Chapter 3
Surgery in Medieval Arab and Islamic Times

The Islamic World Comes to the Rescue of Medical and Surgical Knowledge

God has not caused a single disease to descend upon men without providing a remedy.

Prophet Mohammed

3.1 Islam's Contribution to Medicine and Surgery in Medieval Times

A new chapter begins as the spread of Islamic power in Asia resulted in the preservation and transmission of the scientific knowledge of the Greeks. With the death of Mohammed in A.D. 632 CE, his religious beliefs spread, establishing a vast empire surpassing Alexander's. In 637 CE, the Arabs captured Jerusalem, and in 640 CE, after a 14-month siege, Alexandria suffered the same fate. The Arab and Islamic surgical tradition has a long history, dating back to the seventh century CE. During the Islamic Golden Age (eighth–thirteenth century CE), Arab and Muslim surgeons were known for their advanced surgical skills and the development of new surgical techniques and tools.

The Arabians elevated the status of the medical profession from a menial occupation to that of one of the esteemed learned professions. They were the pioneers in incorporating systematically arranged illustrations into their medical writings and introduced their efficient system of numbering, which largely replaced the cumbersome Roman numerals. Additionally, they advanced the science of chemistry as applied to medicine and significantly enhanced the art of dispensing through the use of elegant preparations like rose and orange water. The Arabians were instrumental in the introduction of the concept of the legal regulation of qualifying examinations for admission to the medical profession. Although they were not the originators of the idea of establishing hospitals, they were responsible for the establishment of a considerable number of these institutions.

This chapter covers the Islamic and Arab world's contribution during the seventh to fourteenth centuries.

S. Abbas, D. Watters, *The Road to Modern Surgery*,
https://doi.org/10.1007/978-981-96-4337-0_3

Muslim physicians were strong proponents of bathing, particularly for treating fevers and utilizing steam baths. Their methods for managing smallpox and measles still hold considerable merit today. Practicing medicine legally necessitated passing an examination and obtaining a state diploma [1–3].

At the time of the birth of Islam, there was a known physician in Mecca called Hareth Ibn Kelda, but few details are available about him and the practice of medicine in that era. During the seventh century, the old world Empires (Romans and Persians had collapsed), as the Arab domain expanded and encompassed the former previous empires of Persia, Greece, and Rome, the emerging Islamic empire inherited and embraced various scholarly disciplines, including those of medicine and pharmacology. Acknowledging the significance of these disciplines, Islamic leaders facilitated the translation of works from diverse languages, especially Greek, into Arabic. This enabled the ongoing research and study in these fields to continue and flourish in the centuries ahead. The translations of Greek scholarly works into Arabic played a crucial role in the subsequent translations into Latin. Later, this, in turn, facilitated the return of Greek knowledge to the scientists and scholars of the European Renaissance, thereby paving the way for its widespread dissemination and influence during that era. In Baghdad during the eighth century, Islamic scholars and physicians translated medical works from various regions, including those of the Roman physician Galen, but also texts from Persian and Indian medical traditions.

Muslim scholars and physicians made significant contributions to the advancement of medical knowledge and practice. Alongside the translation of important works, they introduced novel fields of research and clinical care. These included gynecology, embryology, and a special emphasis on the well-being of mothers and children. Recognizing the crucial role of women as the mothers of future generations, medieval Muslims prioritized their healthcare to ensure the flourishing of the Arab empire.

Furthermore, early Arab scholars played a vital role in the understanding, treatment, and prevention of diseases such as smallpox and measles. In contrast to the prevailing superstitions and strict Catholic doctrines that hindered progress in European medicine, which saw disease as a punishment of God, Islamic scholars and physicians pushed the boundaries of medical knowledge, as they understood that disease is another of humanity's problems that needs to be solved [2, 3].

They were pioneers in incorporating surgery as a distinct discipline within the broader field of medicine. The enduring impact of Islamic hospitals can be observed in the structure of modern hospitals. These early healthcare facilities served as a concrete legacy, as they established a blueprint for the organization and operation of hospitals in the next millennium until today. Notably, these hospitals embraced a progressive approach by implementing open admission policies, welcoming patients from diverse economic backgrounds, irrespective of their gender, religion, or ethnicity. The administration of these hospitals was efficiently managed by a sizeable administrative staff, and the patients were allocated to gender-specific wards based on their medical conditions [3].

Moreover, the early Islamic hospitals were pioneers in the concept of having pharmacies on-site, recognizing the importance of readily available medications within the healthcare setting. Additionally, they prioritized education and training by offering programs for students to gain practical experience under the guidance of experienced physicians. They improved the operation of lithotomy and methods to reduce joint dislocations. They knew how to ligate the arteries and veins four centuries before Ambrose Paré. They used hooks for the extraction of nasal polyps. The seton for anal fistula was their invention. Ibn Zuhr (943–1008 CE) was the first to re-describe the operation of tracheotomy since the Roman Asclepiades. They proposed the use of concoctions of narcotic plants like darnel, also known as *Lolium Temulentum*, to induce complete loss of consciousness and sensation before performing surgeries. Moreover, they seemed to have an awareness of the consequences of microbial infection, although the actual cause was not yet understood [1–3].

Islamic medical texts, such as Ibn Sina's (also known as Avicenna, 980–1037 CE) *Canon of Medicine*, Al-Razi's *Libor Almartsoris*, and Al-Zahrawi's *Kitab al Tasrif*, played a central role in medical education across European universities for many centuries.

The Arab and Islamic surgical tradition has a long history, dating back to the seventh century CE. During the Islamic Golden Age (eighth–thirteenth century CE), Arab and Muslim surgeons were known for their advanced surgical skills and the development of new surgical techniques and tools.

Islamic surgical texts, such as the works of the Persian physician Al-Zahrawi (936–1013 CE) and the Persian-Arab physician Avicenna, contain detailed descriptions of surgical procedures and the use of surgical instruments. These texts also include information on surgical techniques, wound healing, and the use of anaesthesia. Under the leadership of physician-vizier Ali ibn Isa Al-Kahal (fl.1010) (a famous ophthalmologist), a team of doctors was organized to offer medical care to the sick, with certain physicians making daily visits to prisons. Furthermore, there was a notably compassionate approach to caring for the mentally ill [3, 4]. They developed many surgical tools and instruments that were not known in the West before the Islamic Golden age, such as surgical scissors, forceps, scalpels, and various types instruments for cataract surgery.

According to S P Scott: "*Five centuries after the Moorish physicians of Spain had treated disease by the rational principles of medicine, surgery, and hygiene, Europe still adhered to the archaic conceptions of barbaric ignorance; to the belief that all illness was a manifestation of divine displeasure; to the possession by evil spirits; to the delusive expedients of priestly artifice,—the exhibition of relics, the muttering of texts, the performance of exorcism.*" [5].

They translated, synthesized, and expanded upon the works of renowned ancient physicians and scientists, such as Hippocrates, Galen, and Dioscorides. Through the translation movement and the establishment of renowned centers of learning, such as the "House of Wisdom" in Baghdad, knowledge from diverse cultures was preserved, synthesized, and further developed.

One of the most influential figures in Arab and Islamic surgery was Al-Zahrawi (also known as Albucasis), who was active during the tenth century. His comprehensive medical encyclopedia, "*Al-Tasrif*," contained a dedicated treatise on surgery that covered a wide range of topics and surgical procedures. Arab and Islamic surgeons made significant advancements in various surgical fields. They performed complex operations, including neurosurgery, orthopedic surgery, plastic surgery, and ophthalmic surgery. Techniques for cataract removal, lithotomy (stone extraction), amputations, and even early forms of rhinoplasty (nose reconstruction) were developed.

The use of anaesthesia during surgery was also recognized in Arab and Islamic medicine. Distraction techniques, pressure point methods, and the use of opium and alcohol were employed to alleviate pain during surgical procedures. Arab pharmacies underwent government supervision to ensure the purity and quality of medications, employing verified scales for accurate measurements and proper labeling [5, 6].

Arab and Islamic surgeons made contributions to the understanding of anatomy as well. They conducted some human dissections when permitted, studied the skeletal system, and provided a number of detailed anatomical descriptions. Ibn al-Nafis, a thirteenth-century Arab physician, challenged the prevailing belief of Galenic anatomy and made important observations on the circulatory system, including the pulmonary circulation [5, 6].

Surgical knowledge was disseminated through medical schools, hospitals, and academic centers across the Arab and Islamic world. These institutions provided an environment for the exchange of knowledge and the training of aspiring surgeons. Many renowned medical scholars emerged from these institutions, and their writings and teachings influenced generations of medical practitioners [2, 4, 5].

In the ninth century, the renowned Islamic physician Al Razi played a significant role in overseeing the "Audidi Hospital" in Baghdad, which boasted a staff of around two dozen doctors. The expansion of medical facilities continued, and by the year 1000, Baghdad had five public hospitals. Similar institutions were established in Cairo, Aleppo, Damascus, and Al-Andalus. These early Islamic medical centers closely resembled present-day hospitals, as they featured specialized wards for different diseases, outpatient clinics, postoperative areas for surgical patients, and on-site pharmacies. Additionally, they served as educational hubs, providing training programs for aspiring doctors [6, 7].

Islamic hospitals were at the forefront of introducing antiseptic practices for wound cleaning, utilizing substances like alcohol, vinegar, and rose-water. Their emphasis on cleanliness was strikingly different from the prevailing lack of sanitation and hygiene in Christian territories during that era. Although William Harvey is commonly attributed with the discovery of blood circulation in 1616, the concept of pulmonary circulation was already elucidated by the Arabic physician Ibn Al-Nafis three centuries earlier. Although Al-Nafis's understanding was not entirely comprehensive, he recognized that the heart consists of two halves and that blood traverses the lungs when moving from one side of the heart to the other. Additionally, he grasped the concept that the heart is supplied with nutrients through capillaries [6, 7].

Some examples of surgical tools used in the Islamic Arab civilization include:

- Scalpels: These were used for cutting and dissecting tissue. They came in various shapes and sizes, and some had a curved blade for cutting in tight spaces.

- Forceps: These were used for grasping and holding objects, such as tissues during surgery. They came in various sizes and shapes, and some had a curved or angled jaw to fit in tight spaces.
- Needles: These were used for suturing and stitching wounds. They were made of bronze and had a sharp point on one end and a hole on the other end for threading.
- Hooks: These were used for grasping and manipulating tissue during surgery. They came in various shapes and sizes, and some had a curved or angled tip for reaching into tight spaces.
- Drills: These were used for drilling into bone. They were made of bronze or iron and had a sharp, pointed tip.
- Probes: These were used for exploring wounds and examining internal organs. They were made of metal and had a sharp, pointed tip.
- Cataract surgical instruments: They were also used for cataract surgery, as well as other ophthalmological procedures.
- Scissors: They were known in the Arab and Islamic civilization for its diversity of designs and uses, for example, Abulcasis has described several types of surgical scissors, such as curved scissors, which are still used in modern surgery today [2, 4, 6, 8].

Hygiene and preventive measures held significant importance in Islamic medicine. Islamic pathology emphasized that numerous disorders were caused by overburdening the digestive organs. The Qur'an and Muslim traditions strongly advocated for abstemious and moderate lifestyles, drawing inspiration from the disciplined and temperate habits observed in desert living.

Muslims also embraced various healing techniques, including cautery, as demonstrated by al-Zahrawi in the following examples. He acknowledges the widespread belief that cautery marks the end of medicine, referred to as "al-kayy akhir al-tibb." However, he clarifies that this saying is indeed true, but not in the manner that it is commonly interpreted.

The Arabians remained faithful to their responsibility until the sack of Baghdad by the Mongols in 1258. After the conquest of Cordova by Ferdinand III of Castile in 1236 and the capture of Baghdad, the progress of surgery among the Arabians essentially came to a halt. Despite this significant event, their influence continued to extend until the seventeenth century [2, 7, 8]. Through their writings and the translation of their works into Latin.

3.2 Significant Islamic Physicians and Surgeons

3.2.1 Ali Ibn Abbas (930–994)

Ali Ibn Abbas Al-Majusi (Haly Abbas) was a Persian physician to the patron of medicine, Adhud al-Dawlah (Governor of Baghdad). He was in Shiraz, before he went to Baghdad, and later built the famous Adhudi Hospital in Baghdad. He was born in the city of Shiraz, Iran, and is best known for his significant contributions to the field of medicine through his influential work, *Kitab al-Maliki* (The Royal Book). Also he wrote *Liber Regius*, an extensive medical encyclopedia that encompasses various medical disciplines, including surgery, pharmacology, and internal medicine. It is one of the most comprehensive medical works of the medieval era and has had a lasting impact on medical knowledge [10, 11].

Haly Abbas' work includes detailed descriptions of various diseases, their symptoms, and methods of treatment. He also introduced new surgical techniques and provided insights into pharmaceutical preparations and their uses. The Arabic manuscript was organized into 20 discourses with numerous chapters. The initial ten discourses focus on medical theory, while the subsequent ten delve into medical practice. The nineteenth discourse, comprising 110 chapters, is solely dedicated to the subject of surgery. The *Liber Regius* contains the earliest mention of a capillary circulation. This section, found in the chapter discussing Animal Virtues or Vital Functions, primarily addresses the opposing movements of expansion and contraction, which form diastole and systole in the heart and arteries, as well as the respiratory actions of inspiration and expiration.

At the end of the chapter he puts emphasis on the importance of the training a physician. His medical knowledge and achievements earned him respect and recognition not only in the Islamic world but also in Europe, where his works were translated and studied by many subsequent scholars and physicians. Stephen of Antioch's translation of the *Liber Regalis* is found in numerous manuscripts and two early editions were printed at Venice in 1492 and at Lyons in 1523 [5, 9, 11] (Fig. 3.1).

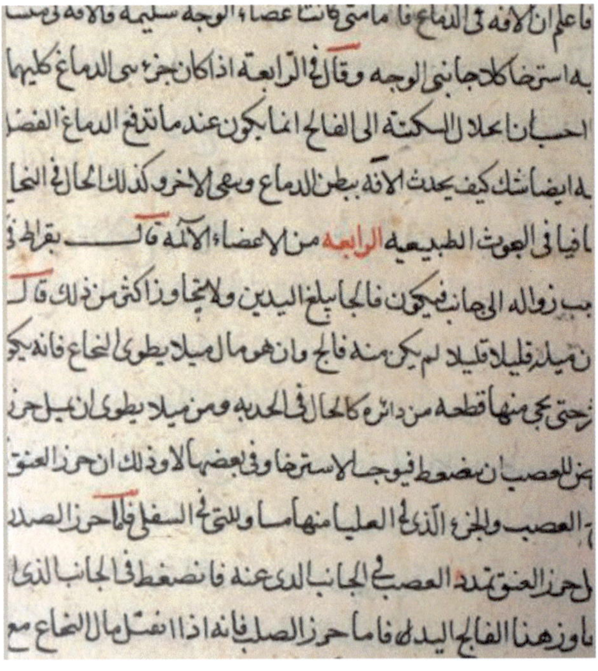

Fig. 3.1 Text from the *Tastif* (Al/Zahrawi). https://upload.wikimedia.org/wikipedia/commons/d/dc/Zahrawi1.png

3.2.2 *Abu al-Qasim al-Zahrawi (936–1013); "the father of modern surgery"*

Abu al-Qasim al-Zahrawi (936–1013) was a prominent Arab Muslim physician and surgeon who lived in the tenth century CE in Spain. He is widely considered to be one of the greatest surgeons of the medieval Islamic world. He achieved considerable renown as a physician and authored a significant compendium of existing medical knowledge called *Tasrif*, Figure [1], also known as *Liber Servitoris* in Latin. This extensive work encompasses thirty volumes. The last volume is the most important in that it deals with all aspects of surgery. This was the pioneering textbook of surgery that included illustrations of the instruments employed, marking the first-ever publication of its kind. With the assistance of drawings, he elaborately described the utilization of these instruments and the intricacies of surgical procedures. The book achieved such immense popularity that it became the established standard textbook of surgery in prominent universities across Christian Europe and was widely read. Al-Zahrawi emphasized the crucial importance of possessing knowledge of anatomy and physiology before engaging in any surgical procedures.

> *Before practicing surgery, he [the surgeon] should gain knowledge of anatomy and the function of organs so that he will understand their shape, connections and borders. He should be familiar with nerves, muscles, bones, arteries and veins. Not understanding the structure and function of the body can lead to an error that may lead to the patient's demise. I have seen someone incise into a swelling in the neck thinking it was an abscess, when it was an aneurysm, and the patient dying on the spot.*

Certain surgical procedures detailed by him are still performed today following the very methods he described almost a millennium ago. These include operations on varicose veins, the treatment of skull fractures, dental extractions, and the use of forceps for delivering a deceased fetus, to name just a few examples. The scientific and rational approaches initiated by Muslims in the Eastern lands were further refined in the medical institutions of Muslim Spain [5, 7].

3.2.3 *Avicenna or ibn Sina (980–1037)*

Avicenna, also known as ibn Sina, (Fig. 3.2) was a Persian Muslim physician, scientist, and philosopher who lived in the tenth and eleventh centuries CE. He was the author of many important works, including the Canon of medicine, which is considered one of the most famous and influential books in the history of medicine.

In his Canon of Medicine, Avicenna described the symptoms, causes, and treatment of a wide range of diseases and conditions. He provided detailed descriptions of surgical procedures, including those related to ophthalmology, orthopedics, urology, and gynecology. He also described the use of surgical instruments and techniques, including surgical procedures for cataracts, hernias, and tumors.

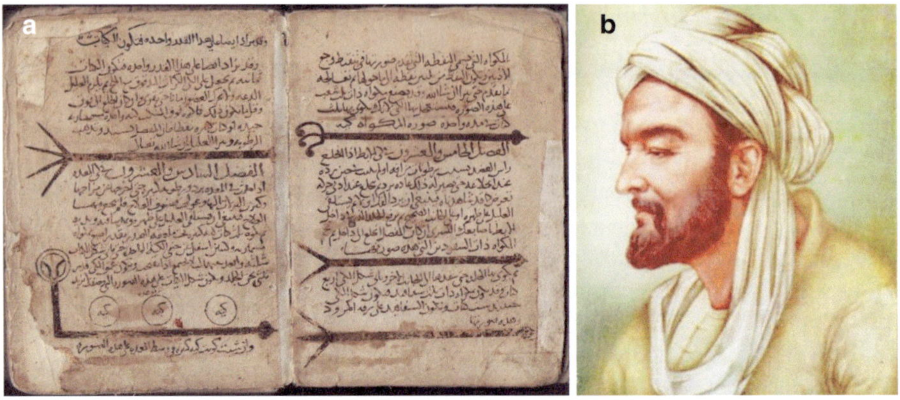

Fig. 3.2 (**a**) (Canon of Medicine). (**b**) Ibn Sina

Avicenna's canon of medicine was widely read and used in Europe and the Islamic world for several centuries. It was translated into Latin in the twelfth century and played an important role in the development of European medicine during the Renaissance period.

Islamic medicine acknowledged the infectious nature of certain diseases, such as leprosy, smallpox, and sexually transmitted infections. Avicenna also wrote about tuberculosis and the spread of contagious diseases how contagious diseases spread as well as the importance of implementing quarantine measures [2, 9, 10].

3.2.4 Ibn Al-Haytham (965–1040 AD)

Ibn Al-Haytham (also known as Alhazen) was an Arab Muslim scientist, mathematician, and philosopher who lived in the eleventh century CE. He is considered one of the greatest scientists of the Islamic Golden Age, particularly in the fields of optics, astronomy, and mathematics.

His book *Kitab al-Manadhir* (Book of Optics) was a groundbreaking work in the field of optics, focusing on the study of light, vision, and optics rather than surgical procedures.

The treatment of the eye disease received more attention from the Muslim practitioners than any other branch of medicine. From its inception, ophthalmology and eye surgery were subjects of particular interest, and regarded by many as having been of high caliber, exhibiting a remarkable skill for their time. One contributing factor to their progress may have been both the prevalence of eye diseases among the population and the willingness of those affected to undergo assessment and treatment. Cataracts were classified into nine distinct types which were managed through procedures like couching and puncture. Their needles came in various shapes, including round and triangular, and some were hollow, made from glass [1, 3, 5].

3.2.5 *Ali Ibn Issa (d1010)*

Also known as (Jesu haly) (d.1010) from Baghdad. His *Tadkiratul-Kahhaleen* (Notebook of the Oculist) is the second oldest complete Arabic text that survives, focusing on the study of the eyes and based on both earlier texts and personal experiences. The book is divided into three sections, the first dedicated to anatomy, the second to external eye diseases, and the third to internal eye diseases not apparent upon inspection. Surgery was included in the third part, which covered general ophthalmological medicine. In this segment, he provided descriptions of the effects of 143 different drugs [1, 3, 10].

3.2.6 *Ibn Albitar (1197–1248)*

Ibn Al-Bitar (also spelled Albitar) was an Arab Muslim physician and surgeon who lived in the thirteenth century CE. He is known for his surgical treatise, *Al-Tashrih al-Qanuni fi al-Tadbir wa al-Tadbeer* (The Canon of medicine in treatment and management) which was written in 1203 and was widely read and used in the Islamic world and Europe.

The *Al-Tashrih al-Qanuni* was a surgical encyclopedia that contains detailed descriptions of surgical procedures and the use of surgical instruments. It covers a wide range of surgical procedures, including those related to ophthalmology, urology, and gynecology. It also includes information on surgical techniques, wound healing, and the use of anaesthesia, as well as descriptions of surgical instruments and their uses [8, 9]. The text was translated into Latin in the thirteenth century, which helped to spread his surgical teachings in Europe. Europe woke up intellectually from its dark ages and the Renaissance dawned [5, 8, 9].

3.2.7 *Ibn Al-Nafis (1213–1288)*

Ibn al-Nafis, also known as Ala al-Din Abu al-Hasan al-Dimashqi, was an Arab physician, scientist, and polymath who lived during the thirteenth century. He was born in Damascus, Syria, and was a pioneer in anatomy. His writings emphasized the importance of evidence-based medicine, meticulous observation, and the integration of theoretical knowledge with practical experience.

He challenged the prevailing Galenic anatomical concepts, though it is not clear whether or how Ibn al-Nafis conducted human dissections and still conformed to the religious restrictions of his day. However he certainly provided valuable descriptions of the structure and function of the human body, including the circulatory system and the heart, possibly largely based on animal dissections. Al-Nafis certainly advocated for the practice of dissection as a means to understand anatomy and physiology. However, he also publicly noted that he personally refrained from performing dissections due to his devout adherence to Islamic beliefs. Nonetheless, in his extensive medical encyclopedia, Al-Nafis achieved detailed observations on various anatomical structures, including the brain, nervous system, bone structure, and gall bladder, among others. Regrettably, only a limited number of Al-Nafis' writings were translated into Latin, resulting in a significant delay in Europeans benefitting from his anatomical descriptions.

In his major work, *"Al-Shamil fi al-Tibb"* (The Comprehensive Book on Medicine), Ibn al-Nafis described the human circulatory system in detail. He proposed a revolutionary theory that challenged the prevailing belief of the time, namely the concept of the cardiac "pulmonary circulation." According to Ibn al-Nafis, blood flows from the right ventricle of the heart to the lungs, where it undergoes oxygenation, and then returns to the left ventricle of the heart. This concept of pulmonary circulation was proposed centuries long before its rediscovery by William Harvey in the seventeenth century.

Ibn al-Nafis's works were highly regarded during his time and beyond. His writings on anatomy and physiology were influential, while his theories sparked discussions and further exploration in the medical community. His works were widely studied and referenced by subsequent scholars, both in the Arab and Islamic world, but only belatedly in Europe.

In addition to his contributions to medicine, Ibn al-Nafis was also recognized for his intellectual pursuits in other fields, such as philosophy, theology, and literature [4, 5, 9, 10].

3.2.8 Ibn al-Quff (1233–1286)

Ibn al-Quff, born in Karak (Jordan) in 1233 and passing away in Damascus in 1286, was a multifaceted scholar engaged in various fields, including medicine, physiology, natural sciences, and philosophy. After relocating to Damascus, Ibn al-Quff's family settled in the Syrian capital. He pursued a diverse range of studies, including metaphysics, philosophy, medicine, natural sciences, and mathematics. Subsequently, he was appointed as an army physician-surgeon at the citadel of Ajiun in Jordan, where he served for several years. Even with his demanding duties as a physician-surgeon for the Mamluk army, Ibn al-Quff managed to be a highly productive writer. One of his primary works is a comprehensive medical compendium known as *Kitab jami' al-gharad fi hifd al-Sihha wadaf al-marad* and a treatise on surgery, *Kitab al-umda fi sinaat al-jiraha* (The Pillar of Surgery). The second of these writings is split into two sections, theory and practice, each comprising ten chapters. The initial part commences with a detailed anatomical introduction, followed by discussions on pathology and a classification of diseases.

In Kitab al-umda, Ibn al-Quff elucidated the crucial link between the arteries and veins, emphasizing the flow of life-sustaining blood and pneuma from the former to the latter. Notably, he refers to the capillaries, making this reference almost four centuries before Malpighi's work, which had benefited from the utilization of the microscope. Additionally, Ibn al-Quff provided explanations regarding the role of cardiac valves, their quantity, and the direction of their opening and closing. He also advocated for the unification of weights and measures utilized in pharmacy and medicine across all Arab territories. In addition to his other works, Ibn al-Quff composed a comprehensive commentary on Hippocrates' Aphorisms, titled *Kitab al-usul fi sharb al-fusul*, which still exists. Moreover, he wrote commentaries on Ibn Sina's *Qanun* and *Kitab al-isharat*; however, regrettably, these commentaries are no longer extant.

In his work *Jami al-Gharad*, Ibn al-Quff delves into various subjects such as embryology, child growth, diet, drug therapy, health preservation, presenting innovative approaches and ideas. For instance, he theorized about the origin of the embryo and the stages it undergoes in its development, particularly noting the formation of a foam-like cluster after the sixth day of fertilization and the early development of the embryo after the twelfth day. He also discussed how the head distinctly emerges as separate from the shoulders, and emphasized that the brain is the first major organ to form during this process [3, 4, 7, 10].

3.3 Medical Institutions and Hospitals

The hospital was a remarkable accomplishment of medieval Islamic society. While the connection between the design and establishment of Islamic hospitals and the earlier poor and sick relief facilities provided by certain Christian monasteries has not been fully explored, it is evident that the medieval Islamic hospital was a more intricate institution, offering a broader spectrum of services. The earliest recorded hospital founded under Islamic rule emerged in the ninth century in Baghdad, most likely constructed by the Vizier serving Caliph Harun al-Rashid. Limited information is available concerning the specifics of this establishment. The most significant hospital in Baghdad (372H) was established in 982 CE by the ruler `Adud al-Dawlah. At its inception, the hospital boasted a staff of 25 doctors, encompassing oculists, surgeons, and bonesetters.

According to S. P Scott "*In the polished capitals of Damascus and Cairo numbers of splendidly appointed medical institutions—colleges, hospitals, dispensaries, laboratories—arose*." The hospital provided free services from distinguished doctors and had advanced hygienic measures. It was spacious, well-equipped, and had a thorough ventilation system. Fountains were present throughout the facility and each disease had its own dedicated ward with competent specialists. Patients with mental illness were treated like any other patient, with their own attendants and recreational activities. Entertainment options were available for patients with insomnia and those in recovery.

A millennium ago, the concept behind hospitals in the Muslim world was to offer a comprehensive array of services, catering to treatments, recuperation, shelter, and retirement needs. These hospitals cared for individuals from all walks of life, regardless of their wealth or status, as Muslims believed in their moral duty to provide healthcare to the ill, irrespective of their background [5].

The funding for these hospitals primarily came from charitable religious endowments known as "Waqf," although some hospitals also received financial support from the State treasury for their maintenance. Thanks to this funding, the hospitals rapidly evolved into prominent scientific institutions and an essential component of city life.

The most well-known structured hospital was constructed in Cairo during the period of 872–874 CE. The hospital, otherwise referred to as the Ahmad ibn Tulun Hospital, offered complimentary medical care to all individuals seeking treatment. The hospital boasted two bathhouses, separate for men and women, a well-stocked library, and a dedicated psychiatric wing, showcasing its advanced nature. Upon admission, patients entrusted their regular attire and valuables to the hospital authorities for safekeeping, while they were provided with special ward clothes and assigned to their respective beds [5, 7, 11].

3.3.1 Al-Qayrawan Hospital

The Al-Qayrawan hospital (Fig. 3.3) of the ninth century was an advanced institution, featuring well-organized halls that included waiting rooms for visitors. The hospital employed female nurses from Sudan, provided a mosque for patients to pray and study, and had regular physicians along with teams of Fuqaha al-Badan, a group of scholars who practiced medicine and offered services such as bloodletting, bone setting, and cauterization. Additionally, the hospital had a special ward for lepers known as Dar al-Judhama, constructed nearby, at a time when leprosy was widely regarded as an untreatable sign of evil elsewhere. The hospital received funding from the state treasury and generous contributions from individuals to enhance its income, ensuring the provision of the best possible care [10, 11].

3.3.2 Al-Mansuri Hospital, Cairo

In the thirteenth century, Cairo housed three hospitals, with the most renowned being the Al-Mansuri Hospital. During a military campaign in Syria, Al-Mansur Qalawun, who would later become the thirteenth-century ruler of Egypt, fell ill with renal colic. The care he received at the Nuri Hospital in Damascus was exceptional,

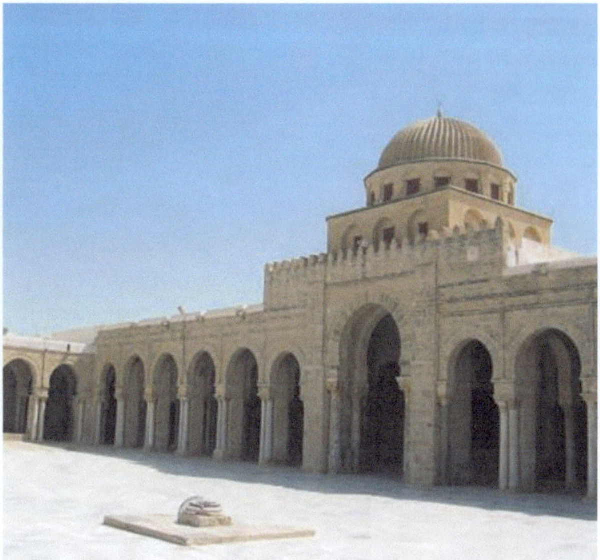

Fig. 3.3 Al/Qayrawa hospital. https://en.wikipedia.org/wiki/Kairouan#/media/File:Montage_ville_de_Kairouan.png

prompting him to promise the establishment of a similar institution once he became the ruler. Staying true to his word, he built the Al-Mansuri Hospital in Cairo, stating… "I hereby devote these waqfs for the benefit of my equals and my inferiors, for the soldier and the prince, the large and the small, the free and the slave, for men and women."

The Al-Mansuri Hospital Fig. 3.4, constructed in 1284, boasted four entrances, each featuring a fountain at its center. The Mamluk sultan Qalawun ensured that the hospital was adequately staffed with physicians and equipped with all the necessary resources to care for the sick. Male and female attendants were appointed to cater to patients, who were accommodated in separate wards. The hospital beds were equipped with comfortable mattresses, and specialized areas were well-maintained. Continuous running water was available throughout the hospital premises. In a designated section of the building, the physician-in-chief was provided with a room for teaching and lecturing purposes. There were no limitations on the number of patients who could be treated, and the in-house dispensary supplied medications for patients to take home [5, 10, 11].

3.3.3 Al-Nuri Hospital in Damascus

The new one [the Nuri Hospital] is the most frequented and largest of the two [hospitals in Damascus], and its daily budget is about 15 dinar. The overseer is responsible for maintaining registers that list the patients' names and expenses for necessary medications, food, and other items. Each morning, physicians come to examine the patients and prescribe beneficial treatments and meals tailored to their needs… Ibn Jubayr, twelfth century traveller [4, 5, 11].

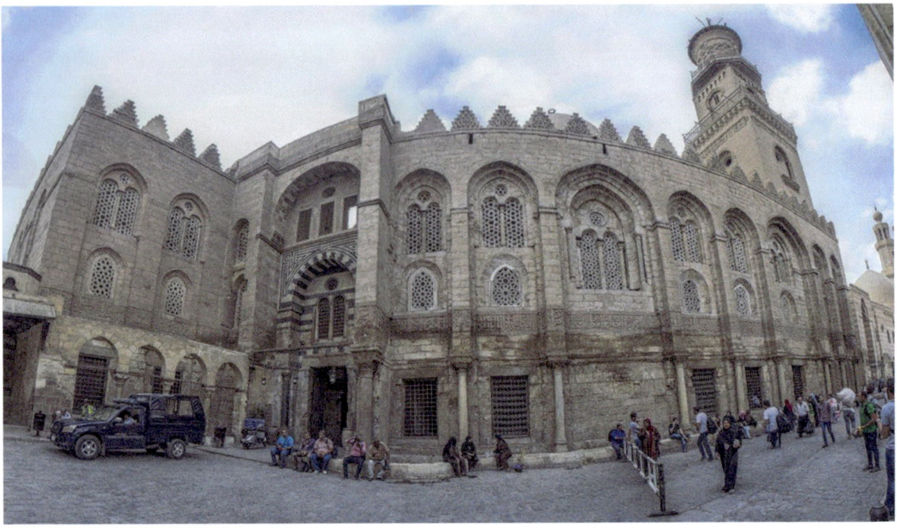

Fig. 3.4 Sultan Al-Mansor Complex (Wikipedia). https://en.wikipedia.org/wiki/Qalawun_complex#/media/File:Cairo,_madrasa_del_sultano_qalaun,_04.JPG

Eight centuries ago, teaching hospitals formed the cornerstone of medical education, much like they do in contemporary times. These institutions provided both practical and theoretical lessons to medical students.

Teaching sessions occurred in group settings and through one-on-one interactions, mirroring the methods used today. Lectures took place in a spacious hall within the hospital, where a reading from a medical manuscript was conducted by the "reading-out physician." Following the reading, the chief physician or surgeon engaged the students in question-and-answer sessions. Numerous students studied under renowned physicians, and owing to the abundant availability of paper in the Muslim world, manuscripts inscribed with the phrase "for personal own use" have been preserved. Conversely, these same texts were scarce and seldom owned by students in Europe [2, 4, 10].

Bedside teaching, an integral part of medical training involved groups of students accompanying the attending physician or surgeon on their ward rounds. More advanced students had the opportunity to observe the doctor as they obtained patient histories, conducted examinations, and prescribed medications in the outpatient department of the hospital.

One of these esteemed medical schools was situated within the Al-Nuri hospital in Damascus. Nur al-Din ibn Zangi (1118–1174), the twelfth-century ruler, established the hospital under the guidance of the physician Abu al-Majid al-Bahili. The hospital was aptly named after Nur al-Din ibn Zangi, and he ensured it was well-provisioned with food and medication. Additionally, he made a generous contribution of numerous medical books, which were carefully housed in a dedicated hall [2, 4, 10].

3.4 Summary of Medieval Islamic Contributions to Modern Surgery

The surgical advances of the Islamic world during the medieval period had a significant impact on the development of modern surgery. Islamic surgeons of the medieval period were known for their advanced surgical skills, the development of new surgical techniques and tools, and their contributions to the field of surgical hygiene. These contributions were influenced by the Islamic Golden Age (eighth–thirteenth century CE) where scientific and medical knowledge flourished.

Islamic surgeons made many important contributions to the field of surgery, including the following:

- Development of new surgical instruments: Islamic surgeons developed many surgical tools and instruments that were not known in the West before the Islamic Golden Age. These included surgical scissors, forceps, scalpels, and various types of cataract surgery instruments.
- Introduction of anesthesia: Islamic surgeons were among the first to use anesthesia, such as opium and mandrake, to reduce pain during surgical procedures.
- Importance of surgical hygiene: Islamic surgeons placed a strong emphasis on surgical hygiene, including the use of antiseptic agents and the use of dressing on wounds to promote healing and prevent infections.
- Advancements in surgical techniques: Islamic surgeons made advancements in surgical techniques in fields such as ophthalmology, orthopedics, urology, and gynecology. They also were known for the development of new surgical procedures, such as cataract surgery, rhinoplasty, and surgical management of tumors.

These contributions were transmitted to Europe through translations of Islamic surgical texts and through interactions between European and Islamic surgeons. The surgical knowledge and techniques developed in the Islamic world played an important role in the development of European surgery during the Renaissance period and in the modern era [10, 11].

Guy de Chauliac's Churiugia Magna cited the Arab literature many times. Indeed surgical techniques and the use of sedation were possibly better in the thirteenth and fourteenth centuries than they were in 200 years later when the lessons Arab texts had been forgotten.

References

1. Durant W. The age of faith. New York: Simon and Shuster; 1950. p. 245–6.
2. Campbell D. Arabian medicine and its influence on the middle ages. Amsterdam: Philo Press; 1926.
3. Montgomery Watt W. The influence of Islam on medieval Europe. Edinburgh; 1972. p. 65; C. Hillenbrand, The Crusades, Islamic Perspectives, Edinburgh University Press, 1999.

4. Montgomery Watt W. The influence of Islam on medieval Europe, op. cit., p. 65. See also: Medieval Sourcebook: Usmah Ibn Munqidh (1095–1188): Autobiography, excerpts on the Franks.
5. Scott SP. History of the Moorish Empire, Philadelphia: The Lippiuncot Company, 3 vols.; vol. 3.
6. Lewis. The surgery of Albucasis. Islamic Cult. 1999;73:21.
7. Savage Smith E. Medicine. In: Rashed R, editor. Encyclopedia of the history of Arabic science, vol. 3. London: Routledge; 1996.
8. Wensinck J. A handbook of early Mohammedan tradition, alphabetically arranged. Leiden: Brill; 1920.
9. Haddad FS, Syyed IB. Medicine and medical education in Islamic history. In: Athar S, editor. Islamic perspectives. p. 45–56.
10. Meyerhof M. Science and medicine. In: The legacy of Islam. Sir Thomas Arnold and Alfred Guillaume. Oxford: The Clarendon Press; 1931.
11. Whipple A. The role of the Nestorians and Muslims in the history of medicine, op. cit., p 41.

Chapter 4
The History of Anatomy

How We Learned About the Body's Structure

4.1 History of Anatomy

An understanding of the structure of the human body is essential to medicine and surgery. However, where culture, religion, and taboo forbade human cadaveric dissection, the anatomically curious had to rely on dissecting animals on the assumption that their comparative anatomy is similar. Those practicing the art of surgery would have also developed a limited anatomical understanding of the structures they operated on, as well as what they observed exposed in the traumatic wounds of their patients. However, most of the surgery was superficial and external, rather than within body cavities.

4.1.1 The Ancient Egyptians

The ancient Egyptians mummified the bodies of their Pharaohs, their families, and other rich noblemen. The process of mummification began around 2600 BCE during the fourth and fifth dynasties and continued until Roman times. It involved removal (usually via an incision in the left side of the abdomen) and preservation of the internal organs with only the heart being left in situ, as it was regarded as the center of a person's being. The other organs were preserved in canopic jars and either stored in the tomb separately or replaced embalmed in the body. The removal of the organs gave Egyptians a reasonable understanding of the anatomy of the body's major organs, but without much understanding of their functions. The body was then dried using natron, a type of salt, to extract the moisture, and then embalmed with strips of linen [1]. The mummified corpse was ready for burial about 70 days after death.

The anatomy section covers the thirteenth to eighteenth centuries and deserves to be a chapter in its own right.

S. Abbas, D. Watters, *The Road to Modern Surgery*,
https://doi.org/10.1007/978-981-96-4337-0_4

4.1.1.1 Anatomical Knowledge of the Greeks

The writings of Homer (eighth century BCE) already indicate some anatomical knowledge. Hippocrates (c400 BCE) had a reasonably accurate knowledge of the skeleton, but could not differentiate between arteries and veins, nor did he recognize that what he termed "nerves" were actually ligaments or tendons. Aristotle (330 BCE) derived his knowledge of anatomy from the dissection of animals, particularly the pig. He had an accurate understanding of the aorta and its branches as well as describing a number of parts of the intestine. One of his contemporaries, Praxagolas of Cos, recognized the difference between the arteries and veins but thought arteries were air vessels due to the presence of air post mortem [2].

It was at Alexandria, at the beginning of the third century BCE that cadaveric dissection was performed by two Greek philosophers, Herophilus and Erasistratus. Erasistratus described the heart valves (naming them triscuspid and sigmoid) and also recognized that nerves originated from the brain. Herophilus described the superior saggital sinus and the duodenum [2]. However, by the time of Galen (second century CE), the Romans had reverted to only allowing physicians to dissect animals, so he had to derive his anatomical knowledge of organs based on dissections of monkeys and pigs. Galen's knowledge of the skeleton was sound, of muscles incomplete, yet much greater than previously described, and he recognized that arteries contain blood not air. Galen's understanding of the vascular system was nonetheless very limited, but his knowledge of the brain was more detailed, including descriptions of the falx, ventricles, and choroid plexus.

4.1.2 Arabic Knowledge of Anatomy

The Arabs through the Middle Ages were not able to publicly dissect as this was forbidden and therefore there was little progress made during this period. The writings of some Arab scholars such as Ibn al-Nafis (1210–88) suggest that some human dissection may have been carried out during the Middle Ages regardless of its legality. This led them to an understanding of the cardiopulmonary circulation centuries before William Harvey (1578–1657) (see Chap. 3). Ibn al-Nafis recognised that blood flows from the right ventricle of the heart to the lungs, where it undergoes oxygenation, and then returns to the left ventricle of the heart. Also, in *Kitab al-umda*, Ibn al-Quff (1233–1286) recognised the crucial link between the arteries and veins, emphasising the flow of life-sustaining blood and pneuma from the former to the latter. He also identified capillaries almost four centuries before Malpighi's work, which was to benefit from the utilisation of the microscope. Nevertheless, the development of a sound and more complete understanding of human anatomy only began when permission for cadaveric dissection was reintroduced in Western Europe during the Renaissance from the fourteenth century.

4.1.3 *Anatomical Education in Italian Universities of the Twelfth to Fifteenth Century*

During the tenth and eleventh centuries Salermo emerged as a European center for medicine. In the twelfth century formal regulations for the education and examination of physicians were instituted including anatomy. However in 1231, the Holy Roman Emperor, Frederick II (1194–1250), decreed that all medical students should attend at least one human dissection and that a human body should be dissected at least once every 5 years [2].

During the thirteenth century other Universities were being founded and introducing medical studies, particularly those at Bolongna (Italy) Montpellier (France), and Paris (France). By the end of the century Henry de Mondeville in Montpellier was conducting anatomical demonstrations, while William de Saliceto in Bologna was performing post mortems to determine the cause of death. These demonstrations became popular with students from all over Europe.

4.1.3.1 Cadaver Dissections

In 1315, Mondino de Luzzi (1270–1326) performed the first public dissection on an executed criminal with the blessing of the church. De Luzzi then published an anatomical textbook *Anatomia Corporis Humani* in 1316.

Bolgna continued in this tradition with Nicola Bertruccius (d 1347). Some private dissections also went on in houses where a member of faculty taught a small group of students. However, the cadavers dissected were usually acquired illegally from graves [2].

> *My master Bertruccius conducted the dissection very often after the following manner: the dead body having been placed upon a bench, he used to make four lessons on it. In the first the nutritional portions were treated, because they are so likely to become putrefied. In the second he demonstrated the spiritual members; in the third the animate members; in the forth, the extremities. (Roth, 1896, cited by Walsh)*

These late medieval anatomists still held to the Galenic concepts of medicine, even as they advanced their knowledge of anatomy and surgery. To some extent the demonstrations in anatomy followed a prescribed text (read by the anatomist or lector) involving a commentator (ostensor) highlighting to the audience what was being described, while the sector, a barber surgeon, undertook the dissection. These dissections were not performed to advance knowledge but to illustrate knowledge.

Guy de Chauliac (1300–1368), surgeon to three Popes in Avignon, actively promoted the value and necessity of cadaveric dissection in his day and through his writings which were to influence European surgery for centuries. Guy de Chauliac had specifically gone to Bologna following his Masters degree in Montpellier to study anatomy from Bertruccius.

During the middle of the fourteenth century, the Universities of Perugia, Padua, and Florence made it mandatory for medical students to attend at least one dissection during their studies.

4.1.3.2 Andreas Vesalius (1514–1564)

Andreas Vesalius was a Renaissance-era physician and anatomist who played a significant role in challenging the long-held ideas of Galen and advancing our understanding of human anatomy. In 1543, Vesalius published his landmark work *De Humani Corporis Fabrica* (On the Fabric of the Human Body), which included detailed illustrations of human anatomy based on his own dissections of cadavers. His work challenged many of the anatomical assumptions made by Galen and other ancient authorities which had held sway through the Middle Ages and the anatomists of the early Renaissance in the fourteenth and fifteenth centuries [2].

Vesalius had started his career by dissecting small animals. He became critical of those who accepted Galen's work without performing their own dissections. His conclusions led to a fierce dispute with his superior Jacques du Bois (or Sylvius), who was a convinced Galenist. Somewhat incredibly, du Bois' explanation to the differences between some structures as described by Vesalius that were different from Galen was that humanity must have changed between the centuries (Figs. 4.1, 4.2, and 4.3).

4.1.4 Anatomical Education in France

Henri de Mondeville (1260–1320), who wrote *La Chirugie,* was Professor of Anatomy from 1301 to 1304 in Montpellier. He performed the first unauthorized human dissection in 1315, the same year that de Luzzi performed an authorized one in Bologna. De Mondeville, with a Masters from Montpellier, had originally learned to dissect whilst undertaking postgraduate study in Bologna (under Borgogni). He

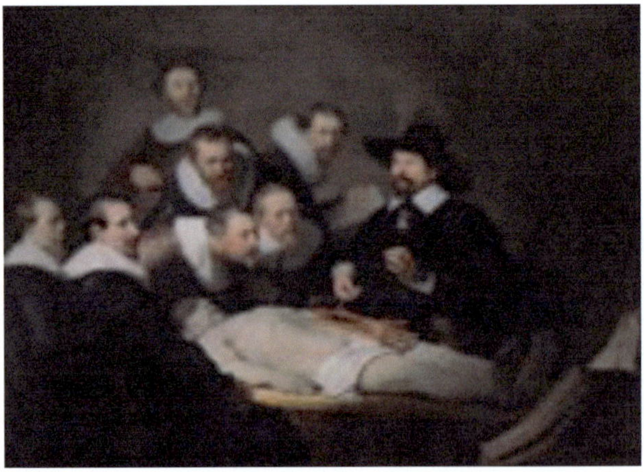

Fig. 4.1 Oil painting by Rembrandt van Rijn entitled The Anatomy Lesson of Dr. Nicolaes Tulp (c. 1632 CE), demonstrating an educational. (This image is published with open access under the Creative Commons Attribution license. CC. https://en.wikipedia.org/wiki/The_Anatomy_Lesson_of_Dr._Nicolaes_Tulp#/media/File:Rembrandt_-_The_Anatomy_Lesson_of_Dr_Nicolaes_Tulp.jpg)

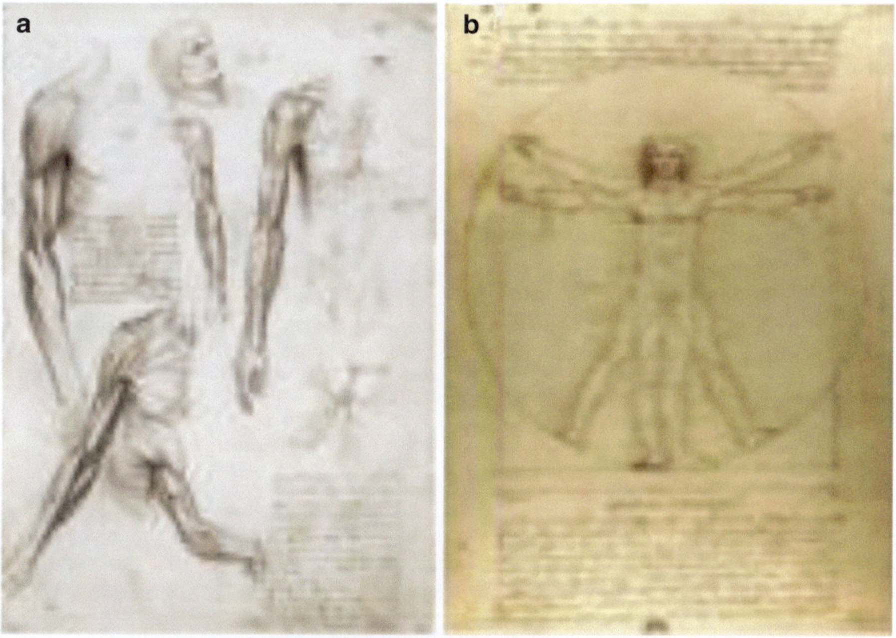

Fig. 4.2 Sketches by Leonardo da Vinci entitled (**a**) A Dead or Moribund Man in Bust Length (c. 1487 CE), detailing the muscles of the arm and the veins of the arm and trunk, and (**b**) The Vitruvian Man (c. 1490 CE), showing the proportions of the human body. (This image is published with open access under the Creative Commons Attribution license. CC. https://upload.wikimedia.org/wikipedia/commons/4/4d/A_Dead_or_Moribund_Man_in_Bust_Length.jpg)

was one of the first surgeons to show that pus was not necessary for wound healing and that wounds if cleaned could be sutured, thus breaking on this point with Galenic tradition. He was appointed surgeon to Kings Philip the Fair (d 1314) and Louis X (d 1316) but much preferred his academic activities to Royal duties [3].

In 1340, cadaveric dissection was permitted at the University of Montpellier, but it was not officially sanctioned at the University of Paris until 1407. Thereafter it became a regular event at French universities. Initially dissections were authorized only for criminal cadavers, but later post mortem autopsy was also introduced in order to determine the cause of death which had received Papal sanction in the mid fourteenth century.

As anatomy became a more popular subject, Italian artists started to perform dissections to inform their works. Antonio Pollainolo (1432–1498), a Florentine artist performed produced a great body of work, as did Leonardo da Vinci (1452–1519) and Michaelangelo (1475–1564). More than 750 of Leonardo da Vinci's works have been preserved. These represent the skeleton, muscles, nerves, and vessels. His illustrations were often completed with annotations of the physiological type. Leonardo da Vinci was one of many who had to resort to grave robbing under cover of night to ensure a sure supply of cadavers to dissect for his artistic work and sculptures.

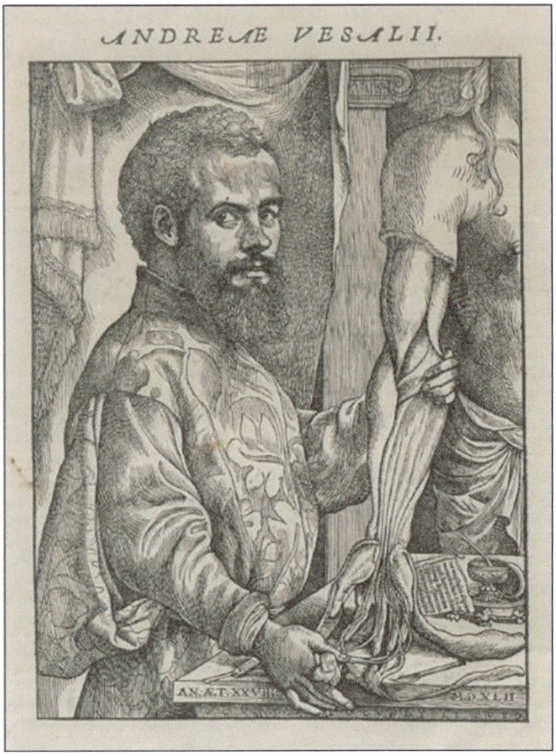

Fig. 4.3 Vesalius, Andreas, 1514–1564 Date: Anno salutis reparatae 1543. (This image is published with open access under the Creative Commons Attribution license. CC. https://en.wikipedia.org/wiki/Andreas_Vesalius#/media/File:Vesalius_Fabrica_portrait.jpg)

4.1.5 Anatomy in England

In 1565, King Henry VIII of England allowed the Royal College of Physicians of England (RCP) and Company of Barber-Surgeons (founded by Royal Charter in 1540) to dissect the cadavers of four executed criminals each year. This was later increased to ten each. John Caius (1510–1573) was President of the RCP from 1555 to 1560 and from 1562 to 1571 and popularized the study of anatomy by human dissection. In the seventeenth century there was even greater interest in anatomy (and thus a demand for cadavers) due to printed books from Italy and France. In 1752, the Murder Act, legalized the dissection of executed murderers by the University medical schools which were starting to grow in number.

In the seventeenth century, further discoveries were made in both anatomy and physiology.

4.1.5.1 William Harvey (1578–1657)

The next major step forward in medicine was to add to this growing anatomical knowledge, an understanding of physiology. William Harvey (1578–1657), an English physician with a doctorate from the then leading University of Padua, is credited with describing the body's full circulation for the first time. His *Exercitatio*

Anatomica de Motu Cordis et Sanguinis in Animalibus was first published in Latin in 1628, and then in 1653 in English (*Anatomical Exercise on the Motion of the Heart and Blood in Animals*). An understanding of the heart and circulatory system saw the emergence of physiology from an anatomical foundation, connecting structure and function. As has been said earlier, the Arab Physicians of the thirteenth century had already described the circulatory system but, by the seventeenth century, their works had been forgotten or overlooked.

Jan Swammerdam (1637–1680) was a Dutch anatomist and microscopist based in Amsterdam who first described the red blood cell.

Francis Glisson (1597–1677) described in detail the liver, stomach, and intestine. Although his views on biology were basically Aristotelian, he also conceptualized that nerve impulses were responsible for emptying the gallbladder.

4.1.5.2 John Hunter (1728–1793)

John Hunter was born in Scotland in 1728 and moved to London to pursue a career in medicine in 1748. He never studied at any University which was common for surgeons of his day. He was trained at the Chelsea hospital by the famous London surgeon, William Cheselden (1688–1752). Hunter initially worked in his brother's school of anatomy until appointed master of anatomy at Surgeon's hall in 1753. He practiced as a surgeon at St George's hospital and eventually became surgeon to King George III in 1776, the year the then 13 American States declared their independence from Great Britain. Hunter was known for his rigorous approach to scientific investigation and experimentation, which he applied to the study of anatomy, physiology, and surgery.

Hunter undoubtedly obtained many of his specimens by paying bodysnatchers which enabled him to amass a remarkable collection to inform his teaching and research. He also studied comparative anatomy and conducted experiments on animals to inform the development of surgical procedures. After his death his collection of anatomical specimens was purchased by the British government for the Royal College of Surgeons whose museum is now called the Hunterian museum. The reputation of surgery was very much better at the end of Hunter's life than it had been earlier in the eighteenth century.

During the eighteenth and nineteenth centuries, the study of anatomy continued to advance with the development of new techniques and technologies, such as the use of wax models, illustrations, and photography.

4.1.5.3 Histology

The work of Lyon anatomist, Jean-Marie-Francois X. Bichat, (1771–1802) laid the foundations for histology, describing 21 body tissue elements [4]. However, Bichat worked without a microscope.

In 1831, only 11 bodies were legally and "officially" available for dissection in London, while there were more than 900 students of anatomy. Desperation led some teaching centers to "ask no questions" about the bodies they were offered and grave-robbing became a growing trade. As surgeons sought to establish their credentials as professionals, their need for cadavers led them into nefarious relationships with so-called body snatchers. Sometimes poor people were even kidnapped and murdered so their bodies could be traded to the anatomy schools.

4.1.6 Anatomy in the Twentieth Century

By the end of the nineteenth century, the number of anatomical terms for body structures had accumulated to an unmanageable and confusing amount. Anatomical terms for the same structure often had multiple and sometimes different eponymous names, depending on the country of use, its original description, or subsequent interpretation of function. This led anatomists, animal morphologists, embryologists, and histologists to agree there was a need for an official standard of anatomical vocabulary for all health sciences. The German *Anatomische Gesellschaft* outlined a plan at their meeting in Leipzig, Germany in 1887, with further work continuing until their ninth meeting in Basle in 1894. In 1893, the Anatomical Society of Great Britain appointed a commission to adapt the suggestions of the German anatomists to an English nomenclature. An agreed list based on Latin anatomical nomenclature was published as the *Basle Nomina Anatomica* (BNA) in 1895. This reduced the number of terms from over 30,000 to 5528; an objective name was ascribed, sometimes with the eponym in brackets. The use of Latin was intended to eliminate international differences and create consistency but the BNA was not widely used, except by German, Italian, US, and Latin American anatomists [5, 6]. In 1903, an International Federation of Associations of Anatomists was founded which agreed to use a list of Latin terms to be translated into the vernacular of each nation. In Geneva, in 1905, during the first Federative International Congress of Anatomy, it was decided to review the BNA but little progress was made until a Birmingham revision was presented in 1933. The *Jena Nomina Anatomica* in 1936 incorporated proposals of the German, British and American Societies. Further revisions were then made through six editions of *Nomina Anatomica* between 1955 and 1989 [7]. A Federative Committee on Anatomical Terminology (FCAT) in conjunction with the International Federation of Associations of Anatomists (IFAA) published *Terminolgia Anatomica* in 1998 (second edition 2019), *Terminologia Histologica* in 2008, *Terminologia Embryologica* in 2008 (second Ed in 2017), and *Terminologia Neuroanatomica* in 2017 [8].

A Japanese version of anatomical terminology was published in 1895 by Suzuki which conformed to the BNA. Various versions of *Nomina Anatomica Japonica* were published between 1944 and 1982 (12th edition). A Japanese, English, and Latin version known as *Terminolgia Anatomica Japonica* was published in 2007. Similarly Chinese and Korean versions are available and revised at intervals.

Throughout the twentieth century, the study of anatomy continued to advance with the development of new techniques such as imaging technologies (CT, MRI, ultrasound) and computerized tomography, which allowed for non-invasive visualisation of the human body's internal structures including three dimensional (3D) imaging. 3D printing allows individual variance to be visualized and printed, to assist with operative planning and rehearsal.

4.1.7 Anatomy in the Twenty-First Century

In the twenty-first century anatomy education changed. Medical students no longer spent days and weeks dissecting cadavers. They either learned from prosections (previously dissected bodies or parts of bodies) but there was also increasing learning from imaging. 3-D reconstruction and the ability to view from inside a structure (e.g., a laparoscopic view of the abdomen) meant that even anatomy books needed to change. The former figures, drawn to depict anatomical parts, are less applicable when there can be a real-time still or videoscopic view. Computerized anatomical programs such as *Anatomedia* were designed to complement anatomy texts but their visual imagery enabled multiple views from different perspectives at the click of a mouse or finger on a touch-pad.

Anatomy is certainly the foundation of surgery and it is not possible to operate without a sound knowledge of anatomy and its variants. However, how students and trainees acquire this knowledge is changing. Reading a book and dissecting a cadaver for a year has served medicine well for five hundred years or more. However, now the anatomy and pathology are visible on CT, MRI, and other imaging modalities including ultrasound. Anatomy is not changing but how we learn it certainly is.

4.2 The Surgeon's Tools

The history of surgical tools dates back to prehistoric times (Fig. 4.4), when sharpened stone tools were used for surgical procedures. Over time, surgical instruments evolved to become more sophisticated, with the development of bronze and iron tools in ancient civilisations such as Egypt and Greece. In the medieval period, surgical instruments were made from steel and were often quite simple, such as scalpels and forceps. In the nineteenth and twentieth centuries, advances in technology led to the development of specialized instruments for specific surgical procedures, as well as the introduction of sterilisation techniques to reduce the risk of infection. Today, modern surgical instruments are often made from high-grade stainless steel or titanium and can be highly specialized, with a range of features designed to improve precision and minimise tissue damage during surgery [9].

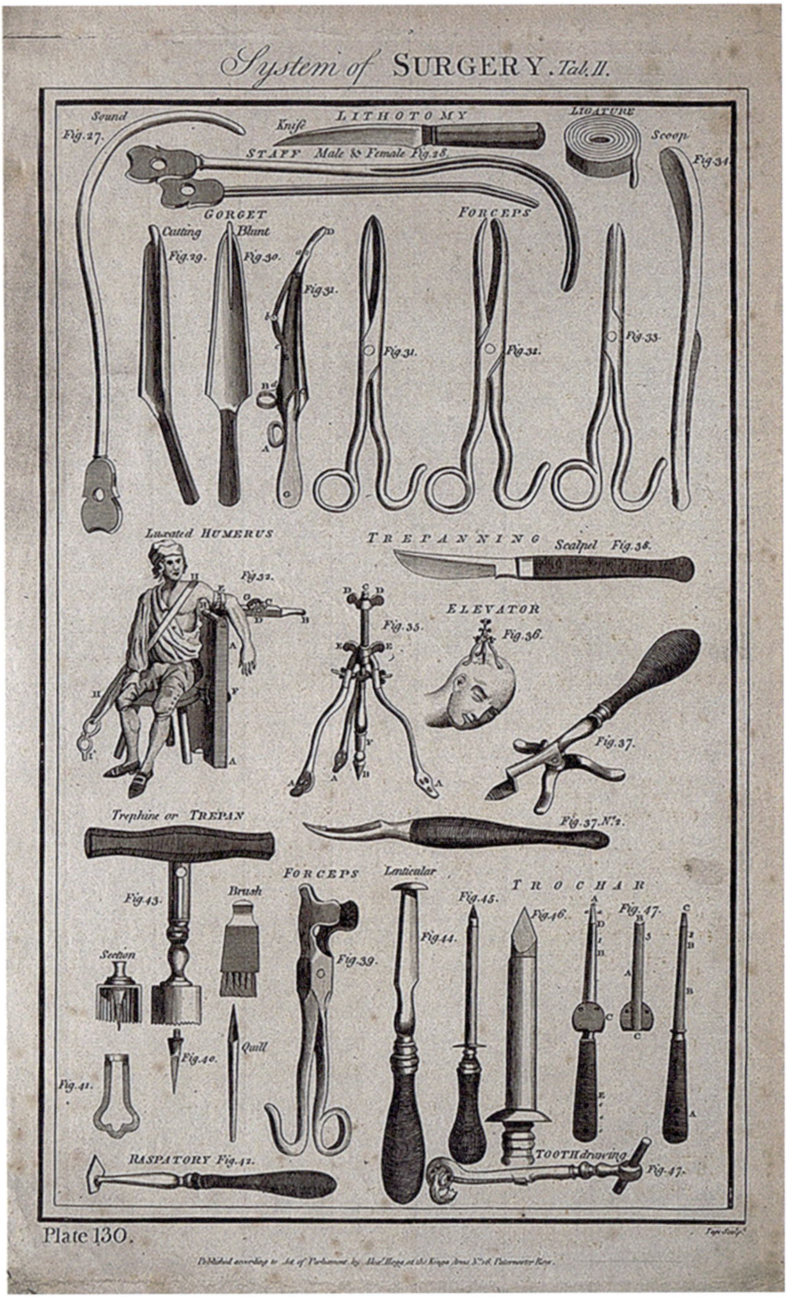

Fig. 4.4 Ancient surgical tools. (This image is published with open access under the Creative Commons Attribution license. CC. https://upload.wikimedia.org/wikipedia/commons/8/81/Surgical_instruments%2C_including_a_lithotomy_knife%2C_a_trepann_Wellcome_V0016416EL.jpg)

This chapter discusses key moments in the history of the scalpel, sutures and cautery, each critical to the skill of cutting, ligating, the arrest of bleeding and wound management (Figs. 4.5 and 4.6).

The Surgeons Knife

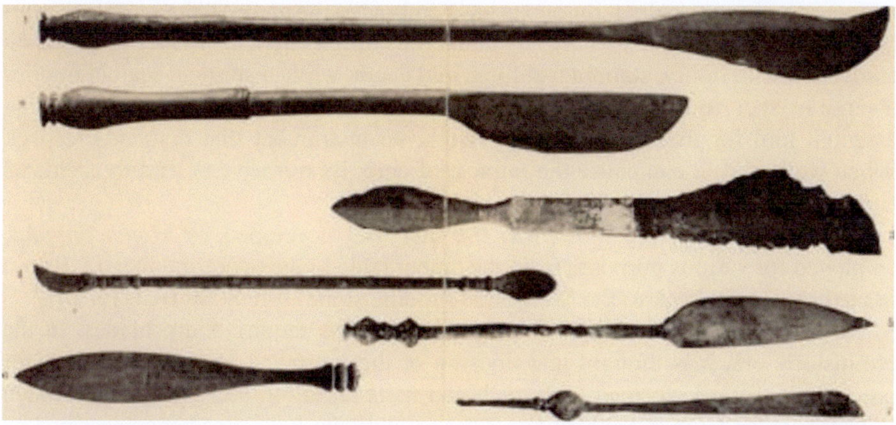

Fig. 4.5 Surgical blades. (This image is published with open access under the Creative Commons Attribution license. CC. https://commons.wikimedia.org/w/index.php?search=Surgical+blades+or+knife+&title=Special:MediaSearch&go=Go&type=image)

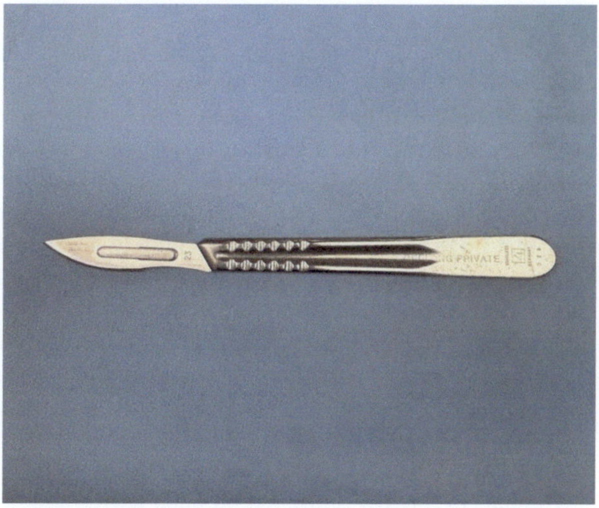

Fig. 4.6 Modern surgical blade. (Photo by the author SA)

4.2.1 The Surgical Blade: From Finger Nail to Carbon Fibers

I love thee, bloodstain'd, faithful friend!
As warrior loves his sword or shield; For how on thee did I depend When foes of Life were in the field!
To My Spring-Lancet. Snodgrass, 1841

The knife handle looks idle, a characterless object, but once its blade is attached, it comes to life as a scalpel. Surgeons have embraced the name scalpel, for the surgical knife. "Knife" signals something dangerous might happen. A knife is a weapon associated with injury, stabbing, cutting, and death, while a surgical scalpel implies a sense of security associated with a licence to cut for healing. The scalpel is an essential tool for the surgeon's daily work, an instrument that demands respect. When well used, it can cause the miracle of cure. Its misuse can lead to accidents and disasters, even for those wielding it.

It is thought that the knife was the first tool developed by *Homo Sapiens*, employed for various purposes from the dinner table to the operating theatre. Its use in medicine dates back to the Mesolithic (middle stone) Age 8000 BCE [9, 10].

Surgery requires planned incisions, and incisions require sharp blades. In the pre-historic era, it is thought that division of the umbilical cord and other minor procedures were performed with teeth and nails and flint, and later with wooden instruments, and mineral substitutes. These techniques have also been described by anthropological studies of primitive societies still surviving on the fringes of the world in remote villages of Melanesia, the Sub-Saharan desert or jungles in the Amazon [9, 10].

After the agricultural revolution and discovery of metals, sharper and more precise blades were produced to drain abscesses, perform circumcisions and other minor procedures. It is likely that some household utensils or tools were borrowed to perform surgical incisions. Traumatic wounds provided an opportunity for surgeons to dive deeper in human tissue mostly looking for retained foreign bodies that caused the injury. A lack of anatomical knowledge limited such explorations to the most superficial parts of the body, as our ancestors gradually enlarged the wound and devised new methods to cut [10].

Anthropological studies of primitive societies during the last two centuries make clear that fingernails were likely to be the first surgical knife ever used by Homo-Sapiens. The American aboriginal tribe of Klatsoops pinched through the umbilical cord with their fingernails until it was divided [10].

Jewish rabbi used sharp fingernails for performing circumcision on infants, whilst midwives grew long fingernails to cut the infant tongue tie. Traditional societies in Ethiopia also used fingernails to scarify or remove infected tonsils.

Some surgeons in the nineteenth century even suggested the use of metallic nail extensions to perform posterior nasal operations.

Humans eventually stumbled on plant leaves and branches that can be rendered razor sharp such as reed, bamboo, and palm. It has been documented that in the Kingdom of Loanga (today part of Democratic Republic of Congo), the umbilical cord was severed with the sharp palm leaves. Other tribes used bamboo. We now know that such leaves have a high concentration of silicate that makes them so sharp. Similar practices were seen in Polynesia and Melanesia using bamboo slivers and thorns. The Cherokee tribes in North America used blackberry thorns [9–11].

Later animal parts were exploited for similar reasons. Tohono O'odham, meaning "desert people" in Contemporary Arizona, were observed to cut the umbilical cord with shells. In Fiji there are reports of a contraceptive method that made a cut in the urethra with broken mussel shells. Shark teeth and river fish teeth were employed by the Karaya tribe in Brazil for scarification and by Ellice Islanders for venesection, drainage of abscess, and drainage of hydrocele. More efficient, hardier scalpels were developed made of flint, obsidian (volcanic glass), and other siliceous rocks that had been broken by natural forces and then sharpened by human effort [11].

Primitive venesection observed by explorers over the last century was performed with flint by American Cherokee and Alaskan Americans, or with lancets of jade cleft into wooden handles by Eskimos, and venesection was undertaken with flint lancets or arrow heads by American Chippewa and Mapuche. Perhaps male circumcision is the oldest elective surgical operation and was certainly performed by native Americans, native Brazilian, and Australian aborigines with stone knives. Volcanic glass (obsidian) has been used for similar purposes as it is sharp, enabling accuracy and some precision, but was superseded by the development of metal blades [10, 12].

About 3500 BCE, copper was discovered and after that the bronze alloy was manufactured which revolutionized the production of domestic tools and weapons. Bronze blades would have been used for surgical procedures throughout the bronze age. Iron smelting was discovered circa 1400 BCE, though the earliest description of a metal scalpel is in Hippocrates' bronze machairon (300 BCE). During Roman times there was large-scale steel production to provide armoury and weapons for the Empire's armies which spread the technology to over 60 m people. A variety of scalpel sizes and shapes were also produced, often with a bronze or copper handle and interchangeable blades. Despite many changes, the surgical blade has remained composed of a handle and a cutting edge on one side that is sharp and straight [13, 14].

Indeed the word scalpel is derived from the latin word "*scallpellus*," a term that appeared during the height of the Roman civilisation and the associated developments in medicine by Celsus, Galen, and others. The Romans borrowed extensively from Greek knowledge but took surgery to a new height that remained unmatched for many centuries. Surgical blades and lances of bronze and iron were discovered in the ruins of Pompeii, a city buried in lava from Mt. Vesuvius in 76 AD [13].

Among Roman archeological surgical finds, the "steel" scalpels had mostly disintegrated as a result of corrosion during the "dark ages" leaving only their bronze handles. The remaining records are very scant, rendering assessment of the use of "steel" surgical blades somewhat uncertain for over 1000 years. In Europe, during this medieval period, the craft of surgery was overtaken by religious orders, magicians, and fanatics. The prior Roman knowledge of surgery was lost to those who lived in its former Empire and, in Europe at least, advances in medicine came to a halt, understanding of medicine and surgery went backwards while superstition and religious beliefs led to scientific stagnation. Further advances in European surgery awaited the opening of Universities in the eleventh to thirteenth centuries [14].

Following the fall of Rome (476 AD), it fell to the blossoming Islamic World to take over the beacon of scientific surgery and technology. By the year 1000, the City of Damascus had perfected the art of Damascus steel—the finest steel the world had ever seen. These produced much stronger and sharper blades. Al-Zahrawi (aka Albucasis of Cordoba, 936–1063) was a prolific innovator—providing the first post-Roman illustrations of surgical instruments, many for novel procedures, such as the use of a copper and steel scalpel for the treatment of an imperforate urethral meatus in new-borns [15].

Progress continued in Europe during the Renaissance (fifteenth to sixteenth centuries,) when the increasing sophistication of weapons of war spurred the further development of surgical tools.

Scientific advances in chemistry and manufacturing during the seventeenth to nineteenth centuries enabled the quality of metals and crafting materials to be improved. Higher quality blades were produced, while the ability to exchange information progressed rapidly with the introduction of the printed press from the fifteenth century. The new alloys and manufacturing techniques allowed smaller, more portable instruments with sharper and more precise blades [15, 16].

Blades came in various shapes, for example a double-edged blade, an idea borrowed from swords and daggers, can cut on both sides. Modern urethrotomes, used to treat urethral strictures, are based on that idea. A particular problem faced barber surgeons for "lithotomy" or removal urinary bladder stones which was a common problem in that era. To address the difficult access, they produced a guarded, curved blade or lithesome, which was also used to divide hernia strictures and fistulas and to open peritonsillar abscess. To ensure the safe introduction of the knife, the cutting end was protected with a rounded probe to guard it during introduction and then exposed to incise as needed [16].

It was the mid-eighteenth century before the crucible steel process produced sharper, stronger, and more corrosion resistant surgical blades. Today these are superseded by plated or stainless steels, and dismountable crucible or carbon steel scalpel blades are widely available, easily mass produced, and safely disposed of before any corrosion occurs.

For millennia, surgical knives remained as single-piece instruments that needed to be sharpened after each use. In 1910, Murphy started experimenting with a replaceable blade. In 1915, Morgan Parker, an engineer, patented a locking scalpel handle and blade system that enabled easier mounting and removing of the blades that would be used once. He contacted Charles Russell Bard, a medical equipment supplier, and in 1915 the Bard-Parker company was founded. In 1932 the patent expired, and Swann-Morton Ltd., a razor blade manufacturer in Sheffield, in Britain began manufacturing scalpel handles and blades. With time, the original mechanism was modified to the one we currently use. That was followed by decades of further minor refinements including stainless steel and the introduction of titanium.

However, the surgical handle and disposable blade designed in the early twentieth century remains mostly unchanged in the twenty-first century [15, 16].

Today, the scalpel is a standardized medical instrument. The handles (often called "B.P. handles" after the Bard-Parker Company) are reusable, but the blades are only used once and then replaced. There are a variety of different blades, with a standard shape and specific use. For example, a No. 11 Blade has a triangular shape while a No. 12 blade has a curved, crescent shape. There are now several different standard scalpels in use in contemporary surgery.

Before the convenience of dismountable, disposable blades, scalpels were sterilized and reused but required constant resharpening. This task at times may have needed to be undertaken even during a difficult or prolonged surgical operation if the supply of sharp scalpels was exhausted. The invention of disposable blades in the late 1920s, thus made surgery safer, and ultimately proved to be more economic because the provision of sharpeners in the operating room proved more costly than replacing disposable blades. Today, the superior sharpness of carbon steel blades over stainless steel, which is not diminished by rusting, allows them to be disposed of and incinerated soon after being used.

During the twentieth century there were also developments in alternative cutting instruments using different energy sources such as electrocautery (1926), Laser (1964), Plasma (1980s), ultrasound (CUSA 1980), and waterjet (1990s) [18].

Electrocautery is covered in a separate section below as it offers coagulation and the sealing of vessels as well as cutting and dissection.

The harmonic scalpel is a surgical instrument that uses ultrasonic energy to cut and coagulate tissue. It was first introduced in the 1990s and has since become a popular tool in various surgical procedures, including general, gynaecological, and urologic surgery. The harmonic scalpel uses ultrasonic vibration to generate heat, which results in tissue coagulation and cutting without the need for direct contact with the tissue. This makes it useful for minimising tissue damage and reducing the risk of thermal injury during surgery. The harmonic scalpel is designed to be used in combination with traditional surgical instruments, such as scissors or forceps, to provide a versatile surgical tool for a range of procedures [17].

The history of the CUSA (Cavitational Ultrasonic Surgical Aspirator) is relatively recent, having been developed in the 1980s. CUSA is a type of ultrasound-assisted surgical instrument that uses high-frequency vibration to emulsify and aspirate tissue. It was designed to provide a minimally invasive alternative to traditional surgical techniques, such as electrocautery and manual dissection. The technology works by creating cavitation within tissue, which allows for the fragmentation and removal of tissue with minimal thermal injury. The first commercial CUSA systems became available in the 1990s, and since then the technology has been widely adopted in various surgical specialties, including liver surgery and brain surgery [18].

Waterjet dissectors, which had been used in industry since the 1930s, were introduced to surgery in the 1990s particularly for hepatic surgery [18].

4.2.2 Electocautery: From Hot Metal to Diathermy

Electrocautery, also known as diathermy or electrocoagulation (Fig. 4.7), is a surgical technique that uses an electric current to generate heat for cutting or coagulating tissue. In 1890–1891, a French physician and biophysicist named Jacques Arsene d'Arsonval and a Serbian American engineer named Nikola Tesla independently explored the therapeutic effects of high-frequency electromagnetic currents [19].

In 1908, the pioneering German physician, Karl Franz Nagelschmidt, coined the groundbreaking term "diathermy" and embarked on a series of extensive experiments with patients, which revolutionized the field. He described his findings in 1909 in a conference in Budapest.

His seminal work culminated in the publication of the first comprehensive textbook on diathermy in 1913, a seminal contribution that profoundly transformed the landscape of medical science.

The history of electrocautery can be traced back to the late nineteenth century, when doctors first began experimenting with electricity as a surgical tool [19].

In 1895, Dr. William Halstead, an American surgeon, performed the first recorded electrocautery procedure, using a direct current to cauterise a small blood vessel [20].

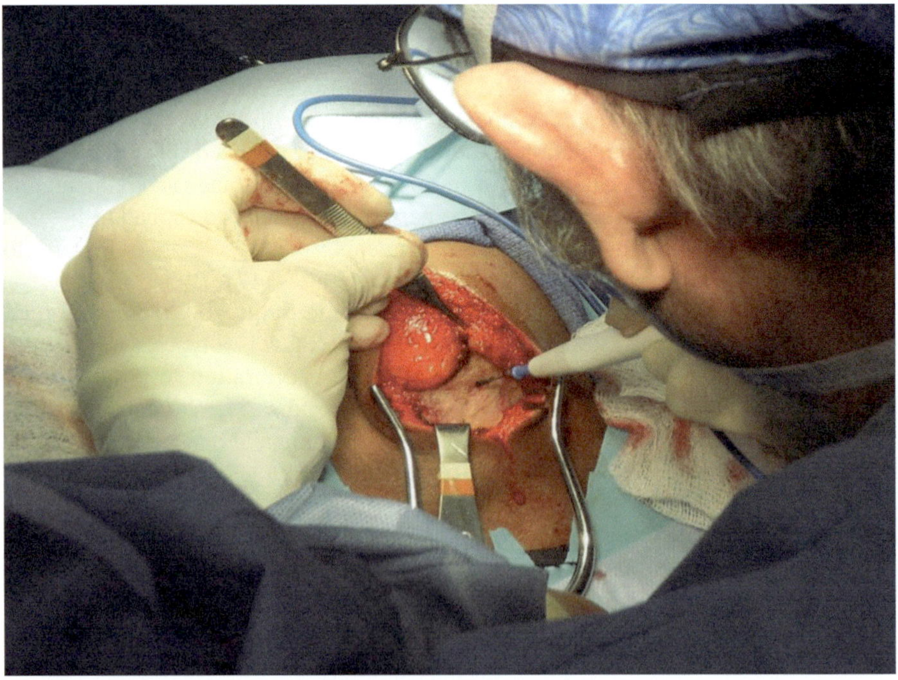

Fig. 4.7 Elecro-surgery. (This image is published with open access under the Creative Commons Attribution license. CC. https://upload.wikimedia.org/wikipedia/commons/1/14/Electrosurgery.jpg)

The use of electrocautery gained popularity in the early twentieth century, especially after the development of high-frequency alternating current electrocautery in the 1920s, which allowed for more precise and controlled cutting and coagulation. In the decades that followed, various types of electrocautery devices were developed, including bipolar and monopolar electrocautery, allowing for a wider range of surgical applications. Today, electrocautery is widely used in many surgical procedures, from simple biopsies to complex operations, and is an essential tool for many surgeons.

While diathermy is a fundamental tool of modern-day surgery, particularly for its role in hemostasis, cauterisation has been used since at least Egyptian times. It would be thousands of years from the inception of cautery in medicine until the birth of Dr. William Bovie and his device. However, his work in biophysics and collaboration with Dr. Harvey Cushing would revolutionize surgical practice in the early twentieth century [21].

An ancient aphorism describing the power of cautery proclaimed,

Those diseases which medicine does not cure, iron cures; those which iron cannot cure, fire cures; those which fire cannot cure, are to be reckoned incurable.

Its use has been described since 3000 B.C., Egyptians treated tumors and ulcers of the breast with the "fire-stick." 2600 years later, it was described by Hippocrates as a treatment for joint problems and hemorrhoids. By the seventh century CE., cautery would be identified not only as a therapy, but also as a hemostatic agent that used by Arabs to stop bleeding after life saving amputation and it would subsequently be used most commonly for that purpose [21, 22].

The first cited use of electricity in surgery was the year 1900, when a Parisian physician, Dr. Joseph Rivière, was using electrical currents to treat a patient for insomnia. During one of these sessions, a spark from an electrode generating his currents landed on his hand, and he realized its coagulating effects. He subsequently used this same current to successfully remove a carcinomatous ulcer off the hand of his patient. During the next decade, electricity was used and modified to treat minor lesions of the skin, oral cavity, bladder, and rectum. Approximately 1910, Dr. William L. Clark, of Clark Hospital in Philadelphia, made a major breakthrough in electrosurgery. He changed the design by increasing the amperage and decreasing the voltage of electrical current. This generated very high heat that was able to penetrating deeper into tissues and produce coagulation that reduced blood loss. This new design was found to shrink tissues from dehydration. Dr. Clark's improvements on the electrosurgical apparatus set the stage for the work of William T. Bovie. While Dr. Clark was experimenting with electrotherapy, William T. Bovie had just received his bachelor's degree from the University of Michigan in 1905. He then went on to attain a Masters in botany and a Doctorate in plant physiology from Harvard University. He stayed at Harvard and fortuitously partnered with Dr. Harvey W. Cushing, the "father of modern neurosurgery." From 1914 to 1927, William T. Bovie discovered that high-frequency alternating current ranging from 250,000 to 2,000,000 Hz could be used to cut through and seal bleeding tissue. At Harvard University, he developed the first commercially viable electrosurgical device.

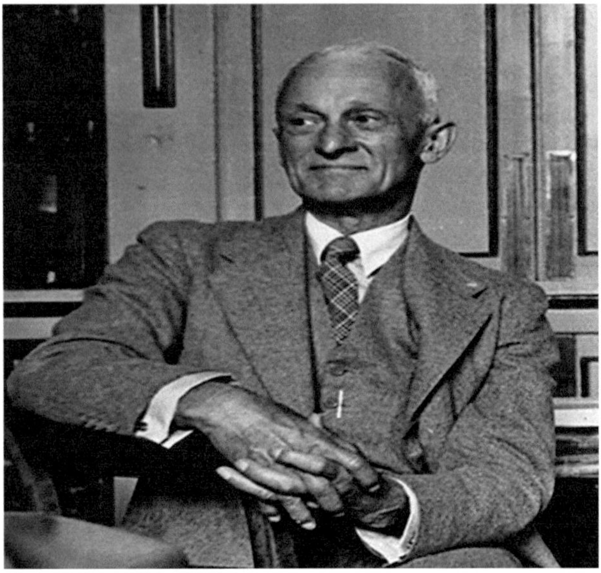

Fig. 4.8 Harvey Cushing. (This image is published with open access under the Creative Commons Attribution license. CC. https://upload.wikimedia.org/wikipedia/commons/7/79/Harvey_Williams_Cushing_1938b.jpg)

Harvey Cushing (1869–1939), (Fig. 4.8), a renowned neurosurgeon, played a pivotal role in popularizing the device within the field of neurosurgery. He first employed it in an operating room in 1926 and went on to use it in over 500 neurosurgical procedures. Following Cushing's lead, the device was subsequently adopted by other surgeons [23, 24].

His initial work revolved around the fundamentals behind electrotherapy rather than its clinical applications. By investigating the effects of different alternating currents, he eventually constructed what would become the prototype for all future electro-surgical devices.

This new apparatus produced a high frequency current delivered by a "cutting loop" that could either cut or coagulate depending on the type of current delivered.

The practice of electrosurgery slowly grew but was still limited to minor procedures because of an underlying skepticism within the surgical community. However, in 1926 when Dr. Harvey Cushing, expressed interest in Dr. Bovie and his work, the two established a well respected role for electrotherapeutics in surgery [23, 25].

Dr. Bovie's unit was put to the test on October 1, 1926, at the Peter Bent Brigham Hospital in Boston, Massachusetts. The patient was a 64-year-old who had possibly meningioma. Four days earlier, Cushing had tried but failed to remove it because of the tumor's high vascularity. Believing that the mass was a malignant meningioma, he sought the aid of Dr. Bovie and his electrical apparatus. He was able to resect the tumor without incident during the second attempt using Dr. Bovie's unit. Dr. Cushing was pleased with the results of Dr. Bovie's electrical device, and the pair continued to work on refining it. To make it widely available, Dr. Bovie sold his patent rights for just $1. Dr. Bovie's device allowed for minimal blood loss. Although not a surgeon himself, his work revolutionized surgical practice and the role of electrosurgery in medicine [24].

4.2.3 Sutures

Silk surgical suture is a non-absorbable type of suture material that has been used in surgery for many centuries. The use of silk as a suture material dates back to ancient times, when silk was first discovered in China. The first recorded use of silk sutures dates back to the Han dynasty (206 BCE to 220 CE), and silk sutures became widely used in Europe in the sixteenth century. The smooth texture and flexibility of silk make it a popular choice for suturing delicate tissues, and its tensile strength and biocompatibility make it well suited for use in surgery. However, silk sutures have largely been replaced by synthetic materials in modern surgical practice due to their superior durability, ease of handling, and reduced risk of infection.

Catgut sutures are an absorbable type of surgical suture that were commonly used for many years for closing wounds and incisions. They were named "catgut" because the material used to make them was derived from the intestines of domesticated animals such as sheep or horses, not cats. The use of catgut sutures dates back at least to the ancient Egyptians, who also used the material for musical instrument strings. The use of dried intestine as a suture goes as far back in history as the Papyrus of Ebers [circa 3750 BCE]. Egyptian surgeons at that time appear to have acquired considerable skills in wound repair. Gradually the use of catgut sutures became widespread, and they remained a staple of surgical practice even until the late twentieth century [26].

To return to catgut, it was in 1868, the year before he came to Edinburgh University as Professor of Clinical Surgery, that Joseph Lister experimentally tied catgut round the carotid artery of a calf. A month later the animal was sacrificed and Lister examined the suture which revealed the fact that the catgut was totally absorbed and had been replaced by a ring of living tissue.

In the mid-twentieth century, synthetic sutures began to replace catgut in many surgical applications, due to the greater consistency and durability of synthetic materials, as well as the increasing concern over the potential transmission of disease from animal-derived materials.

Though Lister was aware of the risk of infection and started the use of phenol as antiseptic to preserve the catgut sutures. Lister is mainly remembered for his introduction of antisepsis into surgery; his recognition of the absorbability of catgut has been of a fundamental importance in the successful modern use of this material.

References

1. Mummification in ancient Egypt. https://www.si.edu/spotlight/ancient-egypt/mummies.
2. Ghosh SK. Human cadaveric dissection: a historical account from ancient Greece to the modern era. Anat Cell Biol. 2015;48(3):153–69.
3. Ghosh SK. Henri de Mondeville (1260–1320) medieval French anatomist and surgeon. Eur J Anat. 2015;19(3):309–14.

4. Shoja MM, Tubbs RS, Loukas M, Shokouhi G, Ardalan MR. Marie-François Xavier Bichat (1771–1802) and his contributions to the foundations of pathological anatomy and modern medicine. Ann Anat. 2008;190(5):413.
5. Sakai T. Historical evolution of anatomical terminology from ancient to modern. Anat Sci Int. 2007;82:65–81.
6. Kachlik D, Baca V, Bzdechova I, Cech P, Musil V. Anatomical terminology and nomenclature: past, present and highlights. Surg Radiol Anat. 2008;30:459–66.
7. Warwick R. The future of Nomina Anatomica – a personal view. J Anat. 1978;126:221–3.
8. Di Dio LJA. History of international anatomical terminology. Federative International Program on Anatomical Terminologies. https://fipat.library.dal.ca/terminologies; Terminologia Embryologica. 2nd Ed., 2017. https://FIPAT.library.dal.ca; Terminologia Neuroanatomica. 2017. https://FIPAT.library.dal.ca
9. Ochsner J. The surgical knife. Bull Am Coll Surg. 1999;84(2):27–37.
10. Adams F. The genuine works of Hippocrates, vol. I. London: Sydenham Society; 1849. p. 808.
11. Englemann GJ. La Pratique des Accouchements Chez les Peuples Primitifs. Paris: Bailiere; 1886. p. 192–5.
12. Lillico J. Primitive bloodletting. Ann Med Hist 3rd Series. 1940;2:133–9.
13. Comey BG. Instruments from Fiji. In: Doran A, editor. Descriptive catalogue in the Museum of The Royal College of Surgeons of England, in manuscript, vol. XX; 1925. p. 20–3.
14. Oakley KP. Man the tool-maker. London: British Museum.
15. Kirkup J. Ann R Coll Surg Eng. 1995;77:380–8. 1961:5.
16. Forbes RJ. Metallurgy. In: Singer C, Holmyard EJ, Hall AR, Williams TI, eds. A history of technology, vol. I. Oxford:ClarendonPress,1956:41–80.
17. Ronald R Barbosa. Surgical scalpel handles and blades Br J Surg, 109, 10, 2022, 916–920, https://doi.org/10.1093/bjs/znac274.
18. Baer HU, Maddern GJ, Blumgart LH. Hepatic surgery facilitated by a new jet dissector. HPB Surg. 1991;4(2):137–44; discussion 144–6. https://doi.org/10.1155/1991/60679. Erratum in: HPB Surg 1994;8(1):following 76. PMID: 1931780; PMCID: PMC2443001.
19. Ho MW, Popp FA, Warnke U. Bioelectrodynamics and Biocommunication. World Scientific, 1994, ISBN 9810216653, 9789810216658 (436 pages) https://books.google.com.au/books/about/Bioelectrodynamics_and_Biocommunication.html?id=uxAfnxKMdPcC&redir_esc=y.
20. Carter PL. The life and legacy of William T. Bovie. Am J Surg. 2013;205(5):488–91. https://doi.org/10.1016/j.amjsurg.2012.12.005. PMID: 23592153.
21. Wangensteen OH, Wangensteen SD. The rise of surgery. St. Paul: University of Minnesota Press; 1978.
22. Goldwyn RM. Bovie: the man and the machine. Ann Plast Surg. 1979;2:135–53.
23. O'Connor JL, Bloom DA. William T. Bovie and electrosurgery. Surgery. 1995;119:390–6.
24. Massarweh NN, Cosgriff N, Slakey DP. Electrosurgery: history, principles, and current and future uses. Electrosurgery. 2006;202:520–9.
25. O'Connor JL, Bloom DA. William T. Bovie and electrosurgery. Surgery. 1996;119(4):390–6. https://doi.org/10.1016/s0039-6060(96)80137-1.
26. Dawson WR. Making a mummy. J Egypt Aust Archaeol. 1927;13:40–9.

Chapter 5
Blood, War and Trauma

5.1 A History of Blood, Blood Transfusion, and Anticoagulation

The modern practice of blood transfusion is little more than a century old, having been introduced during the First World War. However, the historical journey to do this safely begins in ancient times. The ancient Greeks from 300 BCE until the time of Galen believed that the arteries carried air from the lungs to the rest of the body, this theory was disproved by Galen. Galen thought that blood was generated by the liver and circulated in the vessels until consumed while being constantly replenished by the liver. The teaching of Galen prevailed for another fourteenth centuries until the Renaissance (fifteenth and sixteenth centuries) [1, 2]. The ancients believed, as many do today, that blood carried the vital forces of the body as well as the soul "the natural Balsam of life." It was thought that diseases and the ageing process were all due to exhaustion of this vital force. The use of blood as a therapeutic agent is as old as medicine itself. Some older people thought blood from young bodies would cure disease, so it wasn't surprising that there were early attempts to transfuse blood [1, 2].

Pliny the Elder [23–76 CE] reported that some suffering from epilepsy in Roman times believed they could get relief by drinking the blood of gladiators spilled in the arena. A number of ancient writers recommended this treatment, including Galen [2].

There are historical records of blood being transferred from one individual to another for medicinal purposes in various cultures, including the ancient Egyptians,

---

This should probably be discussed in three sections

5.1 Blood and Blood Transfusion

5.2 Surgery at War and Trauma Surgery

5.3 Amputation

These three sections cover the sixteenth to twentieth centuries for their relevant content. Blood and blood transfusion starts with some physiology and circulation and so probably deserves to go first as we planned.

S. Abbas, D. Watters, *The Road to Modern Surgery*,
https://doi.org/10.1007/978-981-96-4337-0_5

Greeks, as well as the Romans. However, these early transfusions were experimental and are likely to have been ineffectual at best, and sometimes would have led to serious complications or death. The idea of giving new blood to a sick person to help them recover is old, but until recently it was only in mythology. In fiction and in real life, people have long hoped to find a way to cure a person of sickness by transfusing blood from a healthy person [1, 2].

Blood was given orally in 1492 to Pope Innocent VIII, as he lay dying from old age. A Jewish physician tried to revive the Pontiff by oral transfusion with the blood from three little boys. The details are sketchy as no account of procedure was written down. Tragically, and probably criminally, the three boys died. The physician ran away as soon as possible after the failure of the experiment [1, 2].

It was an ancient tradition to treat a variety of ailments by letting out some "bad blood." Bloodletting started in ancient Egypt and lasted until the 1800s. It was used to treat everything from sore throats to the plague. In 1799, in his final illness, George Washington asked to be bled. The doctors, while prescribing other ineffective treatments, drained an estimated 80 ounces (40%) of his blood in less than a day, just before he died [3].

5.1.1 Early Experimental Transfusions

William Harvey's experiments leading to his description of the circulation in 1628 played a major role in providing a basis for experimentation with blood transfusion. In 1650, Blaise Pascal (1623–1662) [of Pascal's law] re-invented the syringe, though the introduction of a hollow needle to attach to a syringe would wait until the nineteenth century. Piston syringes had already been used in Roman times but later forgotten. However, suction syringes were used by Ammar ibn Ali al-Mawsili in the ninth century to suck out cataracts.

Pascal's rediscovery/reinvention enabled Richard Lower (1631–1691), an Oxford physician, to trial infusion in animals in the 1650s. In 1665, he transfused blood from one dog to another. He almost killed the first dog but was able to revive it. He injected blood and milk into the veins of dogs, and in the 1660s, Lower and Robert Boyle were almost the first to do an animal–human experiment but sought approval from the Royal Society. The Royal Society was faced with a difficult ethical decision, requiring someone who was clearly so ill that an experimental transfusion could be justified as a last resort, so the French beat the English to it [4].

5.1.1.1 Jean Baptiste Denys (1635–1704)

The first recorded human blood transfusion was thus performed by the French physician, Jean Baptiste Denys (1635–1704) collaborating with a barber surgeon, Paul Emmerez (d 1690). Denys transfused 12 oz. (about 350 mls as 1 fluid ounce = 29.5 mls) blood from a lamb into a 15-year-old boy who had suffered 2 months of fevers.

The boy survived and recovered from his fevers, perhaps because of the small amount transfused and lack of allergic reaction. Denys then performed a second transfusion on a middle-aged butcher who also survived [2–4].

5.1.1.2 Richard Lower (1631–1691)

With Royal Society approval, Lower performed the first human blood transfusion in Great Britain later in the same year, 1667. He transfused 9 oz. blood from a lamb into the bloodstream of a divinity student named Arthur Coga, who had agreed to the experiment for the price of a guinea (a coin worth 21 shillings = 1.05 pounds sterling). Lower described Coga as "the subject of a harmless form of insanity," "the perfect candidate for the experiment" as it was just such an unpredictable nature which Lower and his colleagues hoped to calm by the introduction of "the blood of a gentle lamb" (Fig. 5.1). This was on the surmise that madness is caused by blood that becomes overheated, either by illness or passion, with vapors rising to the brain to cause mental illness.

> *This was perform'd, November. 23. 1667. upon one Mr. Arthur Coga, at Arundel-house, in the presence of many considerable and intelligent persons, by the management of those two Learned Physicians and dextrous Anatomists Dr. Richard Lower, and Dr. Edmund King, the latter of whom communicated the Relation of it, as followeth* [to the Royal Society] [5].

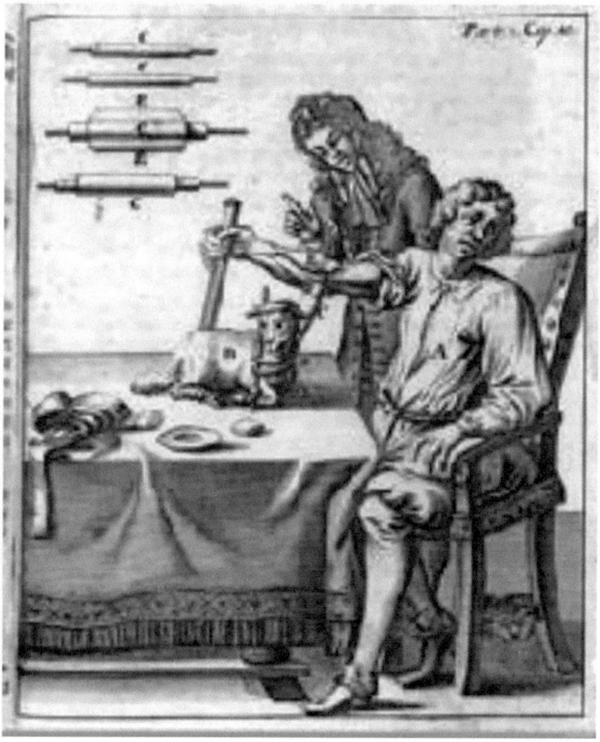

Fig. 5.1 First successful Human Blood Transfusion, June 15, 1667. Matthias Gottfried Purmann, Grosser und Gantz neugewundener Lorbeer-Krantz, oder Wund Artzney—Wellcome Library. (This image is published with open access under the Creative Commons Attribution license. CC. https://upload.wikimedia.org/wikipedia/commons/4/41/First_successful_Human_Blood_Transfusion.jpg)

"We opened the man's arm, easy as usual, and let 6 or 7 ounces of blood flow out. We planted silver Pipe into Incision, and inserted Quills between two Pipes. We were going to move arterial blood from sheep to man's vein". It was not clear how they kept the blood from clotting before transfusing. [5]

Both bloodletting and cold baths were prescribed to cool the body from excessive heat. Lamb's blood was thought to be cooler and purer than human blood. One doctor of the era said,

may, if it takes, be of mighty use to man's health, for the amending of bad blood by borrowing from a better body. [5, 6]

It is interesting that the first cases for transfusions were not for acute blood loss or anemia. Instead, they were for advanced lung or bowel disease, an attempt to restore youth, or bringing the insane to reason.

Denys' second patient, Antoine Mauroy, the provider of his lambs, was also an alcoholic. The transfusion was only successful in calming him for a short period before he returned to his drinking. Mauroy's wife persuaded Denys to perform another lamb blood transfusion which was shortly followed by Mauroy's death. Denys was accused of murder, but eventually, in a somewhat public trial, was exonerated by the court while Mauroy's widow was convicted of poisoning her husband with arsenic. The court records said, "Yes, the wife did it," but she had help from unnamed physicians [5, 6].

In addition the French judge ordered that

no transfusion should be made upon any human body but by the approbation of the physicians of the Parisian Faculty (of Medicine).

However, Denys had already ostracised the Parisian Faculty of Medicine by proceeding without their support. The practice of blood transfusion was then abandoned for several centuries. Denys' character and behavior were certainly questionable. He fell into the trap of becoming something of a showman, desperate for primacy. After establishing these animal-to-animal experiments in his home, all of his experiments were conducted in public in a carnival environment on the banks of the Seine. His descriptions of those experiments suggest they were done for excitement and entertainment [7].

5.1.1.3 Robert Boyle (1627–1691)

The Irish scientist, alchemist, and philosopher Robert Boyle (1627–1691) considered the effects of new blood on animals and humans. He is better known as the originator of Boyle's law which he had proposed in 1662 [the pressure exerted by a gas is inversely proportional to the volume occupied by it at a constant mass and temperature]. He formulated several questions to be examined in experiments on transfusion—some being whether it alters behavior, cures mental illness, transmits disease, or contains nutrients. In 1666, Boyle had injected broth into the vein of a dog and killed it, so wisely handed over the responsibility of further transfusion research to Lower through the Royal Society [8].

Specifically he asked: does transfusion change a dog's breed? Can a "fierce" dog be made into a "cowardly" one? Could repeated transfusions from untrained dogs change the learned behaviors? Boyle saw the potential for alchemical transformations in living organisms: when blood was transfused, he asked, what powers come with it? What makes a living creature unique? Are the physical and mental components of identity in the blood? However, these seventeenth century research questions posed by Boyle would not be answered till the nineteenth century [4–6].

5.1.1.4 Thomas Bartholin (1616–1680)

In 1673, Thomas Bartholin (1616–1680), a Danish physician, transfused cat's blood to an epileptic girl from Breslau, Poland, and reported her becoming "endowed with characteristics of a cat. Not content with climbing on the roofs of houses and imitating the manners of cat in voice, jumping, scratching and yowling, she would sit for hours gazing into a hole in the floor." Obviously any such behavior would have been random, or enacted, as neither the patient nor physician were blinded to the treatment being given. In response to the complications and death of blood recipients, the French Parliament, the Royal Society, and the Catholic Church banned further transfusions [9].

With so many bad cases for transfusion, few cures, severe reactions, and little understanding of what constitutes "bad blood", it was clear that something was wrong. But with no knowledge of how to prevent infection, how to ensure blood transfusion is safe, nor how to make sure blood doesn't clot during donation, further progress could not be made at that time. Attempts to transfuse blood to humans were ceased because of a lack of scientific support, a lack of legality, and church pressure. Although medical science was making progress there would be two centuries of further delay before the next major advance in blood transfusion [9, 10].

5.1.1.5 James Blundell (1790–1878)

The first blood transfusion of blood from one human to another was performed by James Blundell (1790–1878), an obstetrician at Guy's and St. Thomas' Hospitals in London. He found that dogs could be saved from hemorrhage by transfusion and that venous blood worked as well as arterial blood for resuscitation. He next reported a blood transfusion from a man to his wife, who suffered from postpartum bleeding. The case was published in a paper to the Medico-Chirurgical Society of London in 1818. This was the start of modern transfusion medicine [11].

5.1.1.6 Karl Landsteiner (1868–1943)

The next major breakthrough was achieved by an Austrian physician, Karl Landsteiner (Fig. 5.2), who observed that the addition of serum from some individuals would cause clumping of the red cells of others and he realized that this was an

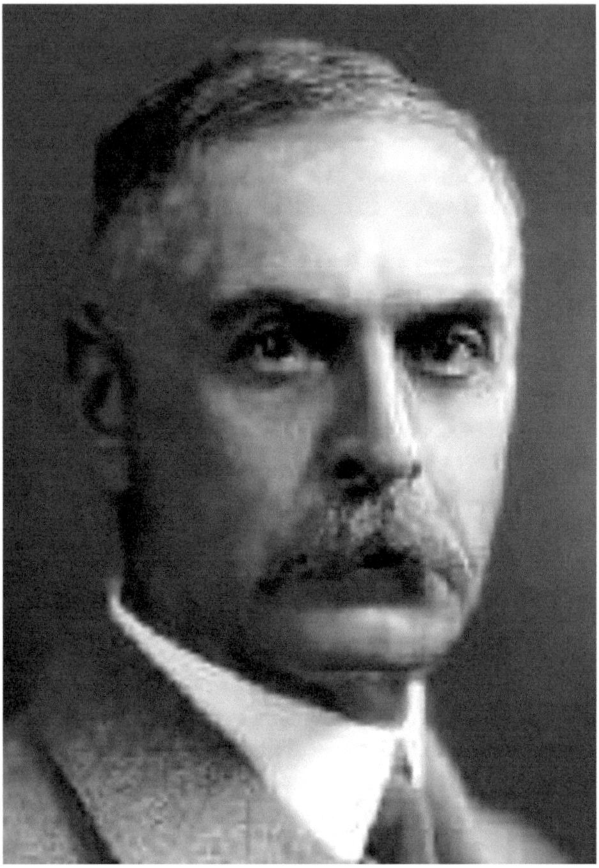

Fig. 5.2 Karl Landsteiner (1868–1943). Karl Landsteiner (June 14, 1868—June 26, 1943). (This image is published with open access under the Creative Commons Attribution license. CC. https://upload.wikimedia.org/wikipedia/commons/e/e0/Karl_Landsteiner_nobel.jpg)

immunological phenomenon. His work was conducted at the University of Vienna. Landsteiner is best known for his discovery of the ABO blood groups in 1900, though he initially called them A, B, and C. He later renamed type C to O. He recognized that transfusing the wrong blood group could result in intravascular hemolysis, a dangerous immune or transfusion reaction that can be fatal [12].

His work also paved the way for the development of blood typing and matching techniques, which are still used today to ensure the safe and effective use of blood transfusions. For his contributions to medicine, Landsteiner was awarded the Nobel Prize in Physiology or Medicine in 1930. However, he didn't talk at the presentation ceremony himself, but asked Sinclair Lewis to do it for him.

"You may call me the master of words, but what is he?" said Lewis, "he has been in a thousand cases the master of death."

He was described as a man of "military bearing but pervading simplicity and modesty." The discovery of the ABO blood group system was not limited to Landsteiner's work alone. Jansky in Poland, and Moss in Baltimore, also independently discovered the four blood groups around the same time. However, Moss's naming convention was different, while the current ABO terminology was adopted at the 1937 Congress of the International Society of Blood Transfusion in Paris to avoid confusion [12].

One of Landsteiner's first pupils at the Rockefeller Institute (1922–1943) was Philip Levine. In 1939, Levine published a case history of post-transfusion hemolysis in a woman with blood group O who had received blood from her husband and who also had blood group O. There was a history of stillbirth owing to erythroblastosis fetalis. Incubation of the woman's serum with red cells from her husband resulted in agglutination and, when her serum was incubated with 104 other ABO compatible samples, agglutination was seen in 80 cases. This was the first report of Rhesus antibodies and informed the initial description of foetal-maternal RH incompatibility that can lead to stillbirth [11, 12].

5.1.1.7 National Socialism and Implications for Blood Transfusion

During the period of national socialism in Germany, there was a deliberate manipulation of scientific data to fit into the ideological and political agenda of the regime. Blood group B was falsely identified as a marker for Slavic and Jewish races, and this became part of the Nazi's propaganda campaign. In contrast, group A was associated with positive traits such as intelligence and industry, which was also unsupported by scientific evidence. The Nazi regime used the ABO blood group system as a tool for eugenics and racial profiling, which resulted in the persecution and extermination of millions of people. The German army only accepted blood from "Aryan" donors [9].

The American Red Cross, like many organizations in the United States at the time, followed a policy of racial segregation. Blood donations from black donors were not accepted, and blood was segregated by race. This policy remained in place until the late 1960s, when it was finally abolished as part of the US Civil Rights Movement [9].

Ludvig Hektoen (1863–1951), a Norwegian-American pathologist and professor/chief of pathology at the University of Chicago and the Cook County Hospital, discovered that isoagglutinins were common in human serum. He thought that this could mean that transfusions might be dangerous, because erythrocytes might adhere and block vessels. This observation led to the understanding that matching donor and recipient blood would make it safer. This formed the basis for the blood cross match that we know today. In 1912, Doctor Roger Lee (1881–1964) showed that O blood can be given to anyone, while AB blood can receive blood from anyone, the respective universal donors and recipients [13–15].

5.1.2 Anticoagulation

The coagulation of blood, or the process by which blood forms clots, has been studied and understood for centuries. Ancient civilizations such as the Egyptians, Greeks, and Romans observed and described the process of blood coagulation. The

Greek physician Galen, who lived in the second century CE, wrote extensively about blood coagulation and described it as being related to the balance of the body's "humours." Galen based his observations on Hippocrates' theory of the four humours—black bile, yellow bile, phlegm and blood—each of which affected personality and health [1, 2].

During the Middle Ages, the understanding of blood coagulation advanced through the works of Arabic physicians such as Avicenna (980–1037), who wrote about the role of blood vessels in the coagulation process. In the seventeenth and eighteenth centuries, scientists and physicians began to understand the importance of platelets in blood coagulation, and the role of protease enzymes, such as thrombin, in the formation of clots [1, 2].

In the nineteenth century, the understanding of blood coagulation was further advanced by scientists such as the German physician and physiologist Carl Ludwig (1816–1895) who described the process of coagulation as a cascade of reactions involving several blood clotting factors. The French physiologist, Nicolas Arthus (1862–1945) identified the key role of calcium in coagulation [15].

The normal rapid coagulation of blood imposed a limit to the quantity of blood that could be transfused in the early days. In 1908, Alexis Carrel (1873–1944) developed a technique for suturing blood vessels together, which he called "the triangulation method." This allowed for direct blood transfusion of a large volume from one person to another by suturing the artery of the donor to the vein of the recipient. However, there were problems with this surgical approach. For example, you need a donor present at the time of transfusion and it's hard to tell how much blood is passing from donor to recipient. Another method was using defibrinated blood, blood that has been collected in an open vessel to promote clotting, then the clot was removed allowing the remaining fluid to be used for transfusion [14, 15].

Richard Lewinsohn (1875–1961), of the Mount Sinai Hospital in New York, introduced sodium citrate as an anticoagulant. One percent sodium citrate was used in laboratories as an anticoagulant but at this concentration was toxic to humans. In 1915, he published results showing that a 0.2% solution of sodium citrate was sufficient to be anticoagulant but not toxic. A year later it was reported that dextrose added to blood can be stored for 2 weeks in animal experiments and so could correct anemia after transfusion. This step allowed blood to be stored and given when needed. Dextrose was used to nourish red blood cells. Citrate- phosphate—dextrose (CPD) solution was then adopted as the anticoagulant of choice for storage, later for up to 28 days. These discoveries were made during World War I which incentivized their rapid uptake to treat the casualties of what was a brutal war then being fought on Europe's Western Front [16].

In 1916, Jay Mclean (1890–1957), then a John Hopkins' medical student working in the lab of William Henry Howell on pro-coagulants, discovered the anticoagulant properties of heparin, a powerful blood thinner that prevented blood clot formation. In 1918, Howell named heparin after the Greek word, *hepar*, meaning liver. It took another 20 years before its clinical value in preventing venous thromboembolism was recognized. Heparin was one of the necessary discoveries to enable cardiovascular surgery and hemodialysis to proceed, never mind the prevention of venous thromboembolism [17, 18].

By the mid-twentieth century, researchers had discovered the important roles of vitamin K and prothrombin in blood coagulation, and their discovery laid the foundation for the development of blood-thinning drugs such as warfarin. Warfarin was first marketed in 1948 as a rat poison and approved for medical use in 1954. Warfarin blocks vitamin K related enzymes responsible for blood clotting factors II, VII and IX and X and so is widely used to prevent blood clotting disorders. It requires medical monitoring to ensure safe usage as its main side effect is bleeding [18].

Today, scientists continue to study blood coagulation and the complex network of proteins and enzymes involved in the process, including fibrinogen, thrombin and factor XIII. These studies have led to the development of new blood-thinning drugs and oral treatments to prevent and treat blood clots [18], termed New Oral Anticoagulants (NOACs).

5.1.3 Blood Transfusion Advances During the World Wars

As discussed above, in the late nineteenth and early twentieth centuries, scientists and physicians began to understand the importance of matching blood types between donors and recipients in order to reduce the risk of complications and death. These were major breakthroughs that made blood transfusions safer and more effective [19].

Prior to World War I, blood transfusions were relatively rare, and often dangerous due to the risk of transfusion reactions and infections. However, the increased demand for blood on the battlefield led to a surge in research and innovation, resulting in significant improvements in the safety and effectiveness of transfusion practices [19, 20].

5.1.3.1 The Robertsons on the Western Front

Lawrence Bruce Robertson (1879–1935) was a Canadian surgeon serving on the Western Front during World War I. In 1915 he performed a life-saving direct transfusion of whole blood using a syringe from a donor to recipient. He had brought this technique from Canada where he had successfully used it on children. His first 36 published cases were accompanied by 3 fatalities due to hemolysis from blood transfusion reaction. However he succeeded in showing the effectiveness of blood for resuscitation rather than relying on saline infusion alone [13].

One of the leading surgeons of the era, George Crile, had previously argued against the use of whole blood transfusion, advocating instead for the continued use of saline solutions or other alternatives. Crile believed that whole blood transfusions were too risky and that the potential for transfusion reactions and other complications outweighed any potential benefits. He wrote in the British medical journal:

> *Excellent results were certainly obtained in some cases of shock, but in the treatment of this condition, and indeed, of all others in which intravascular infusion of some kind is clearly indicated, surgeons, we imagine, will find no good reasons given here for abandoning the safe and simple method of saline injection.* [16, 21]

In 1917, Osward Howard Robertson (1886–1966), an American who had worked with Pathologist, Peyton Rous (1879–1960), brought the techniques of cross matching to the Allied forces in Europe. He even set up a small scale blood bank and gave 22 transfusions in a casualty clearing station near the front line. The blood Robertson was given was also tested for syphilis. Robertson is best known for his development of the glass transfusion bottle, which he created using a solution of citrate and glucose developed by Rous and Turner. This solution proved to be an effective preservative, allowing for the safe and effective storage of blood for extended periods of time [13, 16].

The improved safety of blood transfusion rapidly overcame peer skepticism such that in October 2018, just before the war ended, Harvey Cushing wrote "*good hospitals are performing 50 transfusions a day.*"

5.1.3.2 Between the Wars

As the use of blood transfusions became more widespread in medical practice, the need for a reliable and efficient means of storing and distributing blood became increasingly apparent. This led to the development of the concept of blood banks, which were centralized facilities for collecting, processing, and storing blood products for use in transfusions. Bernard Fantus (1874–1940) and his family, originally from Hungary, emigrated to the USA when he was 15. He became a physician at Cook County Hospital in Chicago where he established the first blood bank in the United States in the 1930s. He developed a system for collecting and processing blood donations, and his efforts helped to establish the basic framework for modern blood banking practices [21, 22].

Around the same time, Carl Walter (1905–1992), a physician at the Peter Bent Brigham Hospital in Boston, also began working on developing a blood bank. However, his efforts were met with skepticism and resistance from some members of the medical community, who viewed the storage and use of blood as immoral and unethical. Despite these challenges, Walter persevered, and his work furthered the development of modern blood banking practices. Walter is also credited with inventing the plastic blood bag, though this was after WWII in the 1950s. This innovation provided a more efficient and reliable means of storing and distributing blood products and today plastic blood bags are the standard for blood collection and storage around the world [21, 22].

In Europe, Federico Duran-Jordan, a Barcelona physician, organized a blood bank with group O donors during the Spanish Civil War (1936–1939). After the Nationalists won the war, he went to London and helped Dr. Janet Vaughan establish a blood bank at Hammersmith Hospital in 1938. By then it was obvious that a war with Germany was inevitable. Behind the scenes, the Medical Research Council set up four London blood depots. The War Office created the Army Blood Supply

Depot (ABSD) in Bristol in 1938 to prepare for the demands for blood that World War II would bring [15, 16].

5.1.3.3 World War II

During World War II (1939–45), advances in blood banking and transfusion practices continued to evolve, driven by the urgent need to develop more effective treatments for combat injuries. In 1940, the US military began using frozen plasma as a treatment for combat injuries. However, this presented logistical challenges, as frozen plasma had to be stored at very low temperatures and was difficult to transport to the front lines [20, 21].

To address these challenges, the military began developing dried plasma, which could be easily stored, transported, and reconstituted when needed. Dried plasma became available for use in the field in 1944, and proved to be a highly effective treatment for combat injuries. In addition to the development of dried plasma, component transfusion therapy became more widely used during World War II. This approach involved separating whole blood into its individual components (red blood cells, plasma, and platelets), and transfusing only the component(s) needed to treat a particular condition. This approach allowed for more efficient and targeted treatment of combat injuries, and helped to save more lives [21, 22].

By the end of the war, the American Red Cross had collected over 13 million pints of blood for use by the military (1pint = 473mls). The success of the wartime blood program helped to establish the importance of blood banking and transfusion practices in the treatment of battle casualties.

5.1.3.4 Platelets and Plasmapheresis

In the 1960s, platelet concentrates were recognized as an effective treatment for reducing mortality from hemorrhage in cancer patients. This development was particularly important because cancer patients often experienced bleeding due to the side effects of chemotherapy.

In 1964, plasmapheresis was introduced as a means of collecting plasma for fractionation. This technique involves separating plasma from whole blood, and then processing it to create various blood products such as albumin, immunoglobulins, and clotting factors. Plasmapheresis allowed for more efficient production of these products, which were used to treat a variety of conditions including immune disorders and bleeding disorders [21, 22].

5.1.3.5 Minimizing the Risk of Transmitting Infection

During World War I blood began to be tested for syphilis as this was prevalent without effective treatments. In 1971, Hepatitis B surface antigen (HbsAg) testing of donated blood began, which helped to reduce the transmission of Hepatitis B through blood transfusions. Hepatitis B was not only a major risk associated with blood transfusions but also prevalent in many parts of the world particularly in sub-Saharan Africa and SE Asia [23].

During the 1980s a new acquired immune deficiency disease (AIDS), caused by a retrovirus HTLVIII, later to be termed HIV, was identified. By the time the first known 2000 persons (800 deaths) were infected between1981 and 1983, 74% of hemophiliacs who receive multiple blood transfusions had been infected. HIV screening for blood in addition to donor risk behavior deferral was introduced in the mid 1980s [3, 23].

Today, donor blood is tested for a wide range of incompatibilities and transmissible infections, making blood donation an extremely safe practice with a very small risk of transfusion reaction or infection.

5.2 Surgery at War and the History of Trauma Surgery

Towards the end of the twentieth century, trauma surgery grew to become a surgical specialty, particularly in the United States and other Western countries. Prior to that, trauma surgery was the domain of surgeons at war, as well as general and specialist surgeons in peace-time. Usually general surgeons coordinate the management of injured persons requiring admission to hospital, while orthopedic surgeons treat the musculoskeletal injuries, plastic surgeons manage wounds and tissue defects (including reimplantations), and neurosurgeons manage head injuries. Other specialists such as urologists, oro-facio-maxillary, or cardiothoracic surgeons manage respective injuries to the urogenital system, face, and thorax. In LMICs, or at remote and regional hospitals, a medical officer or general surgeon may treat injuries affecting all body systems [24, 25].

The Advanced Life Trauma Support (ATLS) course was launched in 1978. It followed a 1976 plane crash involving a pilot orthopedic surgeon, James Styner FACS (1934–2024), and his family. Styner's wife, Charlene, was killed instantly and his four children were injured, three of them critically. Styner was critical of the early management at the Lincoln, Nebraska hospital. Dr. Craig MD, a general practitioner later agreed to establish an early trauma management course, and the first drafts were compiled around the kitchen table by Styner and Craig (they went to the same church), as well as a Lincoln general surgeon, Dr. Collicot, who was also a Vietnam war veteran. They, and others, ran the first course in 1978, and soon, through Dr. Collicot, the American College of Surgeons Committee on Trauma, agreed to endorse and manage the course.

Today, ATLS has been taught in many countries of the world, with regional infrastructure across the various WHO regions. In many surgical education and training programs across the world, completion of the course, which has undergone a series of revisions over almost five decades, is a requirement for entry to, or completion of, training.

5.2.1 The Management of Injuries in Ancient Times

From the earliest human times, the consequences of battle required wound care, setting of fractures and at least some form of trauma management which might have been limited to debridements, amputations, removal of arrows, or palliation.

Trepanation, or drilling holes in the skull, dates back thousands of years. Archaeological evidence shows it was practiced in the Tigris-Euphrates Valley, the Mediterranean, and Mesoamerica. An example dating back to around 5000 BCE was found in France. Trepanation was also used in ancient Egypt to treat (misguidedly) epilepsy and headaches, as well as the elevation of skull fractures or drainage of hematomas to relieve pressure on the brain. Trepanation was common among the Maya and other ancient Mesoamerican cultures. Trepanation was also, more appropriately, used to treat head injuries in warfare. In addition to physical ailments, trepanation was believed to have spiritual benefits. It was thought that drilling a hole in the skull could release evil spirits, heal mental disorders, and bring good fortune, hence its spurious use also for conditions such as epilepsy and headache.

The Sumerians, who lived in what is now Iraq and credited with inventing writing, were one of the earliest cultures to document their treatment of the wounded. Similar records exist on the trauma care provided in ancient Egypt, ancient China, India, and throughout the Greek and Roman Empires. For example, in Homer's *Iliad* (Ancient Greece), there are accounts of wounds sustained by soldiers in battle and a well-organized system for their treatment, while Hippocrates described treatments for hemorrhage.

The Edwin Smith Papyrus (dated c 1600 BCE) contains case scenarios describing the clinical assessment, diagnosis, and treatment of 48 cases of trauma. Those relevant to head and spine injuries are discussed in the chapter on the history of neurosurgery. The Egyptians also were capable of wiring a jaw and even used leather as an external splint for broken mandibles.

The Greeks used a towel dipped in cold water to control hemorrhage, followed by a white bandage soaked in red wine to wrap the wound. They also used the juice of the fig tree (from the fruit, leaf, or root) medicinally, including to stop bleeding. Homer's Iliad described the somewhat unsuccessful management in the Trojan war (fifth century BCE), in which, reputedly, the 147 injured suffered a 77% mortality rate 31 head (21%), 16 neck (11%), 79 trunk (54%), 10 upper extremity (7%), and 11 lower extremity wounds (7%). Only 21 wounds were treated by the surgeon (Machaon), physician (Podalirius), paramedics (Mecisteus and Alastor), and other warriors (Sthenalus, Diomed and Nestor). The mortality was 5% for those treated with arrow, spear and stone wounds, though the triage process as to who was treated meant that wounds of the head (31 cases—87% mortality) and thorax (54 cases—78% mortality) tended to be left alone, while one of two spear wounds to the abdomen survived. Most survivors had wounds of the extremities. Homer's descriptions of injuries suggest he was well acquainted with anatomy and, perhaps, medical/surgical treatment of his period [26–29].

5.3 War and Trauma Surgery in the Sixteenth to Nineteenth Centuries

5.3.1 *Ambrose Paré (1510–1590)*

Ambroise Paré was a French barber-surgeon who made several important contributions to the field of trauma surgery during the Renaissance period. One of his most significant innovations was the use of ligatures to control bleeding during surgical procedures. At the time, the prevailing method for controlling bleeding was to use a hot iron or cauterise the wound, which was agonising and often ineffective. However, in 1536, while treating soldiers wounded in battle, Paré ran out of the hot oil used for cauterization and instead used silk threads to tie off the blood vessels and stop the bleeding. This technique, known as ligation, proved to be much more effective and far less painful than cauterization. Paré also introduced other important surgical techniques, such as improving the design of artificial limbs and developing better, less painful methods for treating gunshot wounds.

5.3.2 *John Hunter (1728–1793)*

John Hunter was a Scottish surgeon, based in London, who made many contributions to surgery in the eighteenth century. Although Hunter is famous for his contributions to anatomy and comparative anatomy, he also made contributions to military surgery. He joined the British army in 1760, aged 32, during a war with France in support of Frederick the Great of Russia. In 1761, being posted to Belle Isle, on the coast of Brittany, he gained considerable experience of gunshot wounds due to some 700 British soldiers being wounded or killed during the campaign. At the age of 40, he was appointed to the staff of St George's Hospital where he remained for the rest of his life. In 1792, he was appointed Inspector General of Hospitals and Surgeon General to the Army. Harold Ellis describes Hunter's dissatisfaction with the Army surgeon's management of gunshot wounds which involved bloodletting, dilating the wound, over probing/exploring for bullets and shrapnel, and an over-tendency to amputate.

His early experience at Belle Isle taught him to be conservative and he was unimpressed with his surgical colleagues. He recognized that gunshot wounds were contused in relation to their velocity and that wounds needed to be allowed to suppurate (and drain). Most of his experience during the early 1760s was in wounds caused by low velocity musket and pistol shots. He advocated surgery to remove superficial bullets, to arrest (ligate) bleeding, for protruding omentum from an abdominal wound, trephination of a depressed skull fracture, or to relieve pressure. With only the medical knowledge of the eighteenth century, Hunter's contemporaries were in practice introducing further contamination to the wounds from their fingers and contaminated instruments. A treatise on *Blood, Inflammation and Gunshot wounds* was published posthumously by Hunter's brother in 1794 [27].

5.3.3 Dominque Larrey (1766–1842)

Where Hunter was conservative in his approach to amputation. Dominque Larrey was aggressive. He once performed 200 amputations in a day in the Battle of Borodino (1812) during Napoleon's unsuccessful invasion of Russia. However, Larrey is also credited with introducing the concept of the "flying ambulance" (*ambulance volante*) which was essentially a mobile medical unit designed to provide rapid evacuation of wounded soldiers from the battlefield to field hospitals where they could receive more extensive medical care. Prior to that wounded soldiers were left on the battlefield until the fighting ended for the day. This concept helped to revolutionise battlefield medicine and reduce mortality rates among wounded soldiers. Before the Russian campaign, he established a system of triage that classified wounded soldiers according to the severity of their injuries, which helped prioritise their treatment and transport [28].

5.3.4 The American Civil War (1861–1865)

During the American Civil War and the Franco-Prussian War (1870–1871), field hospitals were established to treat the large number of wounded soldiers. Surgeons working in these hospitals developed better techniques for treating injuries including the importance of rapid transport and treatment of injured individuals. The mortality rate for penetrating wounds of the abdomen was very high during both the Crimean War (1853–56) and the American Civil War which was around 90%. During the Crimean War, Florence Nightingale emphasized sanitation and humane nursing care for combat casualties. The American Civil War had a high death rate among soldiers. The Union enlistments totalled 2,893,304 soldiers. The Confederacy enlistments were between 1,277,890 and 1,406,180 soldiers. Out of 246,712 wounds from weapons of war, 245,790 were gunshot wounds, while only 922 were saber and bayonet wounds. The average Union mortality rate from gunshot wounds to the chest was 62%. However, as in most wars, more soldiers died from medical diseases than from direct injury. Gangrene was a major cause of death, both the Confederate Army's surgeons and the Union Army's surgeons had very little experience in military surgery. The grim reality was that the only real way to reduce the number of cases of gangrene and erysipelas was to fumigate the wards and even entire hospitals, but this did little to improve the situation. Surgeon General William A. Hammond is credited with organizing the medical efforts for the Union side, At Gettysburg, every division had its own hospital. The results were superior to those reported for soldiers in the Franco-Prussian War, which was fought several years later, it is noteworthy that antiseptics were routinely used in the American civil war, prior to Lister's 1868 Lancet paper. One study, conducted by Goldsmith in 1863, showed that bromine reduced wound sepsis mortality to 2.6%. A group of 30 patients who weren't treated with the antiseptic had a 43.3% mortality rate [38–40, 41].

5.3.5 The Franco-Prussian War (1870–1871)

The Franco-Prussian War (1870–1871) saw terrible mortality, in part due to the reluctance of some surgeons to use the then known antiseptics for thigh fractures. The mortality rate for femoral fractures ranged from 54.2% to 91.7%. Lister and others' recommendations on antiseptic surgery were initially met with skepticism and resistance. During the war, pathologist Edwin Klebs (1834–1913) described bacteria in purulent gunshot wounds as a constant, associating their presence as the cause of specific wound infection, gangrene and necrosis. This convinced some surgeons to adopt Lister's methods and to experience a significant reduction in mortality rates.

Other than the major introduction of the principles of antisepsis, there were few other advances in the development of trauma care during the periods of the American Civil War, the Franco-Prussian War, the Sino-Japanese Russian War (1894–5), Spanish-American War (1898), and the Boer War (1898–1901 until World War I. For example, with regards abdominal injuries, the medical teams attending the Sino-Japanese (1894–95), and Spanish-American wars (1898), and the British in their campaigns including the Boer Wars adopted a conservative approach. However, there were advocates emerging that promoted more intervention [35, 37, 38].

5.3.6 Laparotomy for Penetrating Abdominal Injuries

During the Franco-Prussian war, J Marion Sims (1813–1883), an American surgeon, also advocated for laparotomy in an attempt to stop bleeding, repair damage and drain the wound. Although many cases died, he did, nonetheless save some patients whose survival would not have been expected. However, the French were strong proponents of expectant management, based on evidence from Parisian surgeon, Paul Reclus (1847–1914), who had performed dog experiments to justify his conservative approach, which was then reinforced by a series of 88 abdominal wounds treated expectantly with 66% patient recovery.

In the late nineteenth century, laparotomy for war wounds was considered disastrous and was forbidden by the respective army medical departments. The Anglo-Boer and Russo-Japanese wars saw a continuation of these policies, reported as achieving "excellent results" [34, 39].

5.3.6.1 Sir William MacCormac (1836–1901)

William MacCormac (Fig. 5.3) was a graduate of Queen's College, Belfast. He studied medicine in Dublin and Paris and did postgraduate studies in Berlin. His travels enabled him to establish a network that included Langenbeck, Billroth and von Esmarc. He was consultant surgeon in Belfast from 1864 to 1870. When the FrancoPrussian war broke out, he volunteered to undertake hospital duties in Metz.

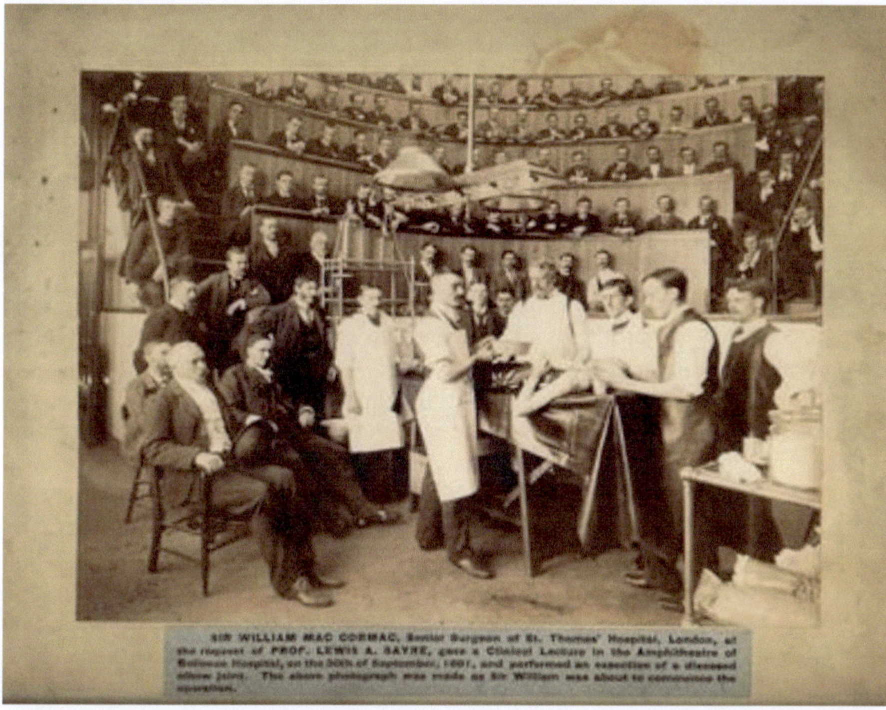

Fig. 5.3 Sir William MacCormac (other side of table) of St Thomas' hospital, London, about to undertake a surgical procedure at Bellevue hospital, New York, Wellcome Collection. (This image is published with open access under the Creative Commons Attribution license. CC. https://upload.wikimedia.org/wikipedia/commons/0/04/Sir_William_MacCormac_about_to_perform_a_surgical_operation_Wellcome_V0029748.jpg)

However, he was treated as a spy and returned to Paris. After the war he took up practice in London, including being a surgeon at St Thomas' from 1873, two years after being awarded his FRCS ad eundem (literally = "to the same" or without examination). He was made a baronet in 1897, and knighted in 1898, being surgeon to the Prince of Wales, who was later to become King Edward VII, after the death of Queen Victoria, who died the same year as MacCormac in 1901 [28].

MacCormac was a sometimes protagonist of intervention, based on his experience obtained in the Franco-Prussian war, but summarized the "to do or not to do" laparotomy dilemma that influenced British thinking. The statement below became known as the 'MacCormac aphorism' and became so instilled in British Army thinking that it remained standard practice until well into World War I.

> *In this war [the South African] a man wounded in the abdomen dies if he is operated upon and remains alive if he is left in peace.*

Although the statistics of the British South African War are severely defective, the official history collected 207 cases of abdominal wounds, 26 received laparotomy, with 18 deaths; a mortality of 69%. The total death rate of all abdominal cases was 30.4%. Clearly the laparotomy cases and the non-laparotomy cases were not risk adjusted, so like was not compared with like and it is difficult to draw any conclusions because of the selection bias.

5.3.7 Chest Injuries

Prior to WWI the approach to chest injuries took a similar approach to abdominal injuries. However, it was soon appreciated that a hemothorax should be drained and that the accompanying problems of pneumothorax, open chest wounds, and clotted hemothorax needed to be addressed.

At the start of WW1, prevailing wisdom suggested that penetrating wounds of the chest should be managed conservatively, with hemothorax drained by aspiration as necessary. Penetrating chest wounds incurred a 27% mortality in the Boer War which was then thought to be quite good, despite being three times more than the average 9% for all wounded.

During WW1, Hutchison reported his experience of aspiration in 368 cases out of 450 chest wounds with only 27 deaths, most of which were due to septicemia or underlying pneumonia. Aspiration was undertaken only on clinical grounds, and only if there were more than two fingerbreadths of dullness by percussion.

> *At the beginning of the war we were interested merely in the question of the diagnosis of haemothorax and whether or not aspiration of the blood was worthwhile. Fortunately it did not take very long to settle this latter point, and aspiration very quickly became a routine procedure.*

> *Simple aspiration very soon was followed by replacing the aspirated blood with oxygen in order to do away with the disagreeable symptoms sometimes produced by the rapid removal of a large quantity of blood from the pleural cavity... the problems with which we were [then] confronted were three in number: how to deal with an open pneumothorax...an infected haemothorax...a foreign body in the lung.*

However, it was soon appreciated that there were indications for surgical intervention including the presence of a foreign body in the chest that was accessible to being removed safely, a significant hemothorax, any rent in the diaphragm, or internally facing rib fragments. Smaller collections could be aspirated while open drainage was employed for empyema. At the time there were no underwater seal drains. Significant volumes of retained hemothorax was recognized to be responsible for collapse of the lung, which later became infected resulting in empyema. Empyema, depending on its consistency and the condition of the patient, could sometimes be managed by aspiration, but more commonly, by open drainage.

Chapter 4 of *ANZAC Surgeons of Gallipoli*, covers some of the main surgical advances of WWI with regards chest injuries [29–34]:

> *It was not until 1916–1917 that a more aggressive and successful approach to penetrating chest injuries was adopted. It was appreciated that operation needed to be performed at the Casualty Clearing Station, so cases needed to be sent on promptly by the Field Ambulances if surgery was to be conducted within a few hours and have a chance of success.*

In 1916, the first chest procedures were being performed in France. Major Don observed that patients with penetrating wounds of the chest often died of severe haemorrhage within a few hours, and that, in early 1916, little success had been achieved in checking this mortality. His view was that the bleeding lung needed to be collapsed to help arrest the bleeding, and that a persistent haemothorax was likely to become infected, particularly because the thoracic cavity was infected. Therefore debridement of the chest wound together with sufficient thoractomy to collapse the lung, and to evacuate the haemothorax and any other foreign matter would be beneficial. He described a thoracotomy, evacuation of haemothorax and postoperative drainage by tracheotomy tube for 24–48 hours....

Roberts and Craig wrote in 1917: ...there is no defensible reason why chest injuries should not be treated at the earliest moment on exactly the same principles as wounds of other parts. They advocated operating [early], ... excision of all infected tissues, removal of foreign bodies, cleansing of the pleural cavity (sometimes using Daikin's or flavine solution) and suturing the ...[pleural] membrane over it, whenever possible without drainage. A series of 199 cases was presented, sub-classified into open or sucking wounds (39), closed wounds with large septic laceration of the parieties (32), closed wounds with early signs of infection (20) and closed wounds with no signs of infection (108). This last group of 108 cases was sent from the CCS to base without surgery. Twenty four patients died without surgery and 67 were operated on, with 34 surviving to be evacuated. Half of the 33 deaths were also suffering from other significant injuries. Herringham reported a 7–25% mortality for penetrating chest wounds in the same edition of the BMJ (November 1917), and concluded that more surgery would result in better outcomes. Concerns about the dangers of anaesthesia, lack of experience in chest surgery, and the complexity of chest surgery in civilian practice were regarded as 'phantom'. Instead, many of the procedures could be done under intercostal block, excising the wound, removing loose and sharp rib fragments, evacuating haemothorax and once the lung was collapsed removing foreign matter. If fragments needed to be removed from the lung, this could then be sutured.

5.3.8 Neurotrauma in World War I

[This account is adapted from Chapter 4 ANZAC surgeons of Gallipoli and as section written by Major General JVR Rosenfeld AC OBE.]

WWI's trench warfare gave rise to a high proportion of bullet wounds to the head. Generally it was soldiers with more superficial shrapnel wounds, compound fractures of the skull, and concussion who reached the care of the military surgeons at this time. More severe grades of neurotrauma due to penetrating cranio-cerebral bullet wounds would have likely died on the battlefield. Even today a high mortality for gunshot wounds to the head prevails.

In 1915, neurosurgery was not a distinct surgical subspecialty. General surgeons managed penetrating head and spine wounds. Interestingly, Sir Victor Horsley (1857–1916), of University College Hospital, London, a pioneer of neurosurgery and a consulting surgeon in Egypt, had given an address to the Medical Society of London in February 1915. In it he described the ballistics of high velocity bullets passing through scalp, skull meninges, and brain, as well as the complications ensuing such as bleeding, raised intracranial pressure, and sepsis. He advocated early intervention for bullet wounds to the head, rather than the conservative approach which had largely failed during the Boer war. To avoid sepsis arising from bullet wounds to the head, Horsley advocated excision of necrotic brain and the use of absolute alcohol, but where pus was already present on debridement, he practiced irrigation with hydrogen peroxide and weak carbolic lotion [38–40].

Surgeon, George Syme, who would later become the first President of the Royal Australasian College of Surgeons had read Horsley's BMJ address, so decided [36]:

> *...every gunshot wound on the Gascon [a ship evacuating the wounded ANZAC soldiers from Gallipolit to Egypt] was operated on. The hair and wound were painted with benzene and iodine, the wound protected with gauze, the scalp shaved, and again painted, and the scalp wound freely cut out. A big flap was then turned down and the bone thoroughly exposed. It frequently transpired that in what appeared a mere glancing scalp wound the bone was fractured—a small gutter or merely a crack. This was then trephined and invariably the inner table was found extensively splintered and fragments driven through the dura matter and into the brain. These were picked out with forceps, the whole area well flushed with hot sterile saline solution, the original wound drained and the flap sutured... when a bullet had penetrated, if it was easily accessible, it was removed also. When it was deep and not localizable it was left... We found it difficult to get satisfactory X-ray photographs of the skull owing to the vibration and movement of the ship.*

Once the Americans entered the war in 1917, Dr. Harvey Cushing (1869–1939) was posted to the Western Front and had a profound influence on the management of penetrating cranio-cerebral head injury. He played a major role in the development of neurosurgery as a specialty and was also a pioneer of mission rehearsal by setting up a military hospital in Boston before deployment. Cushing advised shaving the scalp, the use of wet antiseptic dressings and evacuation to base hospitals. There he recommended local anesthesia for most cases, with or without morphine supplement. A number of surgical techniques including craniectomy, cerebral debridement, and techniques of haemostasis were developed by him, together with the practice of not opening the dura unnecessarily but, only when indicated, to "evacuate clot or disorganized brain tissue," and then to be followed, if possible, by dural closure.

Cushing brought neurosurgery close to the frontline and developed the "all or nothing rule." He believed a delay of 2–3 days to get to specialist was better than recovering from an incomplete procedure before transportation. The Base or General Hospitals had X-ray machines, and better anaesthesia and instruments than the casualty clearing stations. .... During the later years of the war, Cushing, employing his meticulous methods, reporting that the mortality of penetrating brain injury fell from 78% to 28.8%, a remarkable achievement in the pre-antibiotic era and before the introduction of bipolar diathermy. Cushing was a careful and precise operator, marvellous to observe, but one who did not necessarily consider the amount of work building up nor the congestion his slow operating was causing.

WW Keen (1837–1932) had performed surgery during the American Civil War and published "*The treatment of war wounds*" in 1917. He endorsed Cushing's teachings which included the use of muscle for haemostasis (Horsley's technique), dural closure, cranial decompression, siting surgical entry wounds away from the bullet or shrapnel entry wounds and the extraction of foreign bodies lodged in the brain, albeit within limits. Many of Cushing and Keen's principles are still followed today. Keen cited Cushing's recommendations as follows: There is fairly universal agreement that almost all cranial wounds produced by projectiles, even though they appear trivial, require surgical investigation, with the possible exception

1. Of certain of the tangential longitudinal sinus injuries, which according to Sargent and Holmes, have a high degree of spontaneous recoverability, and which when investigated [interfered with], present unusual surgical risks;
2. Of certain of the fractures of the base due to perforating wounds, owing to their inaccessibility…

With the exception of the more serious injuries with extensive haemorrhage, in which surgical measures are practically unavailing, craniocerebral wounds, as a rule, present no immediate urgency, for as a tissue the brain is notably tolerant of contusions and infections. Hence a delay of 2 or 3 days in forwarding this class of wounded with expedition to a suitable base is preferable to…an incomplete procedure.

A 6 week neurosurgical course for 230 American military surgeons was developed during WWI. The civilian neurosurgical training system in the USA evolved from this course [43, 44].

5.3.9 World War I and Advances in Wound Management, Injuries, and Resuscitation

Airplanes, tanks, machine guns, and phosgene gas resulted in high rates of complex and lethal injuries during World War I. Sequential Allied health conferences throughout the war led to consensus on resuscitation, management of wounds, splintage of fractures, body cavity and head injuries, transportation, and field hospitals closer to the front.

5.3.9.1 Wound Management

Early in the war, the principles for managing wounds sustained in battle in 1915 were influenced by those of earlier conflicts, most recently the Boer (1899–1902) and Russo-Japanese (1904–1905) wars. However, it was soon recognized that delay in surgical management of the wound, in the form of debridement and excision, particularly for contaminated and high velocity wounds, meant a higher risk of gangrene, necessitating amputation, and a higher likelihood of death.

British Surgeon John Morley, working at Cape Helles in the Gallipoli campaign 1915, wrote:

> *In a contused and lacerated wound …nothing short of complete excision of the soiled and devitalized tissues can be relied on to secure the healing by first intention that should*

always be regarded as ideal. This local excision of soiled tissues is of no avail when once enough time has elapsed to permit the multiplication of organisms in the wound, and then invasion of the lymphatics; to put it another way, the prospect of securing primary healing of these wounds varies inversely with the time that elapses between the infliction of wound and operation…if the presence of some important vessel, nerve, or other organ in the wound prevents complete excision, results become less satisfactory at once.

However, when wounds could be promptly surgically debrided and/or excised so that contamination was removed, they were often rendered clean, suitable for either primary or, at 2–5 days, delayed primary closure and earlier return to the battlefield.

During 1915, the majority of war wounds were managed without immediate primary suture as they were rightly considered as contaminated or infected. The longer the time since wounding the more infected the wounds were likely to be. Thus treatment of a wound was directed at the prevention or management of infection. Suture and closure was advised only when a wound was clean. As wounds were much more contaminated than they might appear to the naked eye, adequate debridement and excision; widening the wound if necessary to remove foreign matter and devitalized tissue, was the standard practice. The campaigns in France and the Dardanelles taught surgeons how important it was to avoid delay in performing debridement and/or excision. Through the early years of the war, surgery began to be performed earlier, closer to the frontline, to lessen the risk of gangrene…. By the end of 1917 there was consensus that primary or delayed primary suture was safe for selected wounds that had been well managed surgically. The emphasis was placed on thorough debridement and excision –cleaning, irrigating and removing foreign matter such as clothing, shrapnel and the contents of a soldier's pocket. The various chemical treatments aimed at 'sterilization' were regarded as supportive. If wounds were to be immediately sutured, this was only advised where a patient could be monitored for some 15 days. The evidence mounted that soldiers with sutured wounds healing without infection, were returned to active combat much quicker than those whose wounds were left open to heal by secondary intention.

This shift in the management of clean or clean, surgically debrided wounds was accepted over the course of five Inter-Allied Surgical Conferences between 2016 and 2018. There was also additional information provided from wound swabs and bacteriology results that had not been available in earlier conflicts.

It should be noted that there were no antibiotics until the introduction of sulphonamides in the late 1930s and penicillin in the early 1942s during World War II. Instead, additional disinfection was provided chemically. Henry Dakin (1880–1952) also worked with Alexis Carrel (1873–1944), a French Nobel laureate of 1912, using a mixture of hypochlorite and boric acid to chemically disinfect wounds utilizing wound catheters and continuous irrigation. This reduced the presence of *Cl Welchii* (the organism responsible for gas gangrene) in WWI wounds from 80% to 20%. The hypochlorite also did not impair healing, unlike carbolic acid. Other chemical agents used were liquid paraffin and, in 1915, a Parisian Professor, Pierre Delbet, recommended magnesium chloride, the active ingredient of the Epsom salts. However, once France was occupied there was no opportunity for Delbet's solution to be studied by the Allies so there was little recognition of its effectiveness.

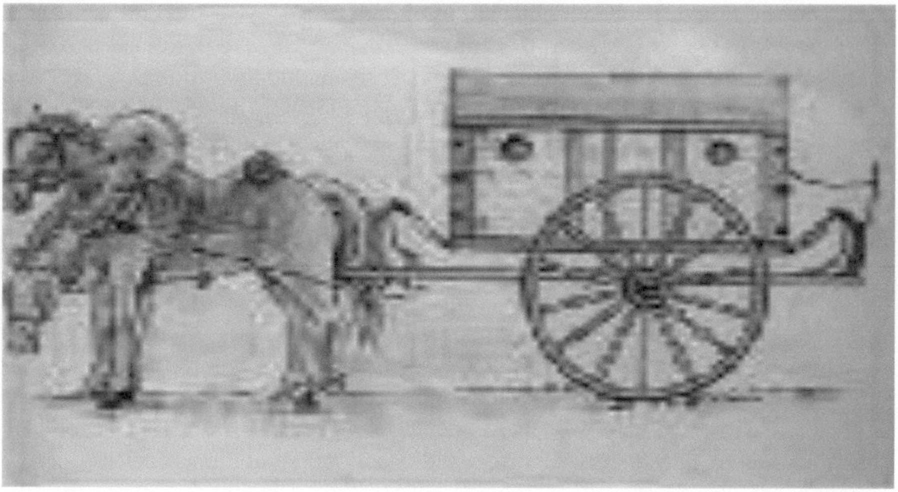

Fig. 5.4 The first ambulance. (This image is published with open access under the Creative Commons Attribution license. CC. https://upload.wikimedia.org/wikipedia/commons/c/cd/The_first_ambulance_carriage_in_Vilnius%2C_1903.jpg)

5.3.9.2 Field Ambulances

Although the advent of ambulances was considered a major step forward during WWI, care was often delayed by as many as 12–24 h after injury due to a lack of standardized protocols (Fig. 5.4).

5.3.9.3 Fracture Management

Femoral fractures are associated with a high blood loss, in the range of 1–2 liters, but even greater volumes if subjected to constant rocking and rolling being carried by stretcher without splinting. The mortality of open femoral fractures, also subject to contamination complicated by infection, approached 50–80% mortality at the start of the war, and surgeons were often prone to amputate, as in previous wars.

5.3.9.4 Robert Jones (1857–1933)

Robert Jones was a Liverpool based orthopaedic surgeon, who founded the British Orthopaedic Society in 1894. He was Welsh, the nephew of Liverpool orthopaedic surgeon, Hugh Owen Thomas (1834–1891), the inventor of the Thomas splint. Thomas also introduced the Thomas test for contracture of the hip (patient lies flat, opposite hip is flexed to chest and if a contracture then the hip being tested cannot remain straight). Jones had gained considerable experience in orthopaedics and trauma as surgeon to the Manchester Ship Canal after appointment in 1887. In 1896,

Jones was the first to publish a clinical radiograph of a 12-year-old boy who had a bullet lodged in his wrist around the third metacarpal. He also described the Jones fracture of the fifth metastarsal describing six cases including himself.

In 1914, Jones was asked by Sir Alfred Keogh, Director of Medical Services for the British Army, to carry out an inspection of the management of wounds in France. He reported to the British War Office that a Thomas' splint would greatly improve femoral fracture transport and management. Three Australian surgeons read the report and purchased Thomas' splints privately before heading to war. One was an unnamed RMO, possibly Butler who compiled the Australian Medical History of World War I, another was Fred Bird from Melbourne and the third was Alexander McCormick from Sydney. These splints reduced the mortality of an open femoral fracture from 80% to 20%. Unfortunately it took 3 years before the British War Office acted officially on Jones' advice. Jones was responsible for 30,000 beds as Inspector of Hospitals. He was also allocated 400 beds at Alder Hey hospital in Liverpool where he supervised orthopaedic and rehabilitation services for the wounded. He also worked in Shepherds Bush hospital in London. After the war Jones was knighted and made a Baronet [43, 44, 45, 46].

5.3.9.5 Resuscitation

At the start of WWI shock was not well understood. The importance of restoring adequate blood volume and therefore maintaining or supporting blood pressure in contrast to restoring blood was appreciated in early resuscitation. The impact of the cold and peripheral vasoconstriction was appreciated with the need to warm hypothermic patients. There was debate as to whether, in a shocked patient, resuscitate or operate first, with the evidence mounting that generally where there was not active blood loss it was better to resuscitate first and then operate. By the end of the war specific resuscitation teams had been established to provide resuscitation as close as possible to the front lines.

A commission was appointed to study shock and resuscitation in order to find a solution to the problem of how to save lives in an emergency situation. The commission examined research from around the world, including existing methods and techniques, and developed a set of recommendations for first responders. These recommendations included the use of warm blankets, IV fluids, and drugs such as adrenaline (epinephrine) and atropine to help restore the patient's circulation.

The administration of blood transfusions, initially given by the direct method in 1915 [cross-ref], was facilitated by advances made in preventing stored blood clotting and in improved methods of storage [cross-ref]. Initially there was opposition to blood transfusion, given the risk of reactions. Leading surgeons preferred intravenous saline for resuscitation, an infusate with which they were familiar.

The seminal work on shock came in 1918 when Walter B. Cannon (1871–1945), a Harvard medical physiologist, studied the signs of shock in casualties at Clearing Station 33 during World War I. His definition of shock is applicable even today:

Wound shock occurs as a consequence of physical injury. It is characterised by a low venous pressure, a low or falling arterial pressure, a rapid, thready pulse, a diminished blood volume, a normal or increased erythrocyte count and haemoglobin percentage and peripheral blood (thereby differing from simple haemorrhage), a leukocytosis, an increased blood nitrogen, a reduced blood alkali, a lowered metabolism, a subnormal temperature, a cold skin moist with sweat, a pallid or greyish or slightly cyanotic appearance, also by this, by shallow and rapid respiration, often by vomiting and restlessness, by anxiety, changing usually to mental dullness, and by lessened sensitivity.

Cannon classified shock into three groups: compensated, partially compensated, and uncompensated, observing that all organs respond to a shock by regulating blood pressure. He thought that if the blood pressure could be kept above 80 mm Hg, the patient could be taken to the operating room and the bleeding could be controlled. He also recognized that delay in proceeding with surgery as a result of cold weather increased mortality rates [46–48].

5.3.10 Between the Wars

Cannon postulated that shock involved a depletion of the extracellular space, yet it was only in 1964 that his hypothesis was proven correct. Through studies of body fluid volume of distribution, he was able to conclusively show the extent of the fluid loss in patients suffering from severe shock. His work built upon that of British physician Sidney Ringer (1835–1910), who in 1880–82, reported that potassium was a normal constituent of physiologic fluids and was later to introduce Ringer's Lactate. Nine years later, Rudolf Matas (1860–1957), Professor of Surgery at the University of Louisiana, reported success with intravenous fluid administration again for resuscitation following the ECF loss due to diarrhoea from cholera [49–51].

5.3.10.1 Intravenous Fluids

In 1915, the chemical composition of diarrhoea fluid in infants was described. Thirteen years later, an American paediatrician, Alexis Frank Hartmann (1898–1964), [not the French Henri Albert Hartmann (1860–1952) who gave his name to sigmoid resection and the gall bladder pouch], described the chemical changes in the body as the result of certain diarrhoeal diseases and developed fluid therapy based on the 1915 works. He could not dissolve bicarbonate; therefore he replaced it with lactate. He gave this solution to seven medical students, and they had no undesirable side effects. Six years later, it was used in children suffering from cholera and dysentery, with a remarkable reduction in mortality from 60% to 10% [42–44].

The next major hurdle was to use blood. Work by Nuttal, identified the blood groups. Arthus and Pages showed that calcium was necessary for clotting, and

Hustin described citrate anticoagulation. It was Robinson who used citrated blood for combat casualties in World War I. By the end of WWI, blood transfusions were commonplace and blood banks had started to form. These blood banks formed the basis of a safe, viable and efficient system for the collection, storage and distribution of blood, which is still in use today. However, it was not until the discovery of antibiotics and the development of methods to test for and eliminate infectious agents from donated blood.

In Austria, Böhler started the first trauma care system for civilians in 1925. The original aim was work-related injury, but it has since grown to include all accidents. Routine blood banking and Fleming's penicillin discovery both happened in the 1930s. But excellent trauma care still wasn't consistent. The discovery of antibiotics was to make a huge contribution to reduce death from trauma by preventing and treating sepsis. The effectiveness of penicillin was first trialed during World War II and available to the Allied troops from 1943 [52, 53].

5.3.11 After World War II

5.3.11.1 Systems to Manage Civilian Trauma

In the 1960s, more Americans were killed on highway accidents than during the Vietnam conflict. It wasn't until the 1970s that civilian trauma care saw some major systematic changes. The American College of Surgeons created the Committee on Trauma, which later became the American Association for the Surgery of Trauma, and published the first Advanced Trauma Life Support manual in 1983. This manual is still used by trauma care providers today. In addition, the federal government passed the Emergency Medical Treatment and Labor Act in 1986, which ensured that all patients needing emergency medical care would be seen and treated regardless of their ability to pay.

In the post-war period, the field of trauma surgery continued to develop with the establishment of trauma centers, facilities designed to provide rapid and comprehensive care for injured individuals. The lessons learned and the changes in trauma care that have occurred in military conflicts over the last century have been applied to civilian trauma care. The concept of "damage control surgery" was also developed, which focused on the primary care of injuries, the control of bleeding before performing definitive procedures and avoidance of hypothermia.

In recent years, advances in imaging technology, such as computed tomography (CT) and magnetic resonance imaging (MRI), have greatly improved the diagnosis and management of traumatic injuries. Additionally, advances in surgical techniques, such as minimally invasive surgery, have improved outcomes for patients with traumatic injuries.

Trauma surgery as a field continues to evolve and improve with the integration of new technologies and research, whilst protocols for the management of traumatic injuries are constantly being developed and improved. Today, the field of trauma surgery is an important and rapidly developing field that continues to save lives and improve the quality of life for individuals who have suffered traumatic injuries from motor vehical crashes, falls, assaults, missiles, land mines and falling objects [46–48].

5.4 Amputation

In certain cases, the extremities may develop gangrene. In such situations, it is necessary to amputate the affected limb to the extent of the disease's reach, in order to prevent the patient from succumbing to death or suffering even more severe consequences than the loss of the limb. Albucasis, c1000 CE

Removing a body part that doesn't have enough blood flow (an ischaemic limb) is one of the earliest and riskiest surgeries.

Even though it may seem brutal, it's sometimes needed to save a person's life, often in times of war. There are cultural views about amputation that were considered taboo and against certain religious convictions. In ancient Egypt, and in many cultures, people were/are terrified of losing a limb. It can be perceived as a fate worse than death, particularly to continue to be dismembered in the afterlife. It has been reported that in the United States, around 150,000 people undergo lower limb amputations annually. This is primarily because of diabetes vasculopathy and other causes of peripheral vascular disease (usually smoking-related), impairing peripheral blood flow, eventually causing ischaemia, ulceration, and gangrene. Other pathologies that lead to amputation are cancer, and trauma [52, 53].

5.4.1 Amputation in the Ancient World

The first recorded therapeutic amputation in history dates back to 31,000, discovered in Borneo on an individual who lived for another 6–9 years. Before that, the oldest human remains that showed signs of amputation were found in the Neolithic site of Buthiers-Boulancourt, near Paris, France. These remains date back to around 4900 BCE. They belonged to an adult male who seemed to have had his forearm amputated [54–56].

In the Babylonian era, surgeons were very hesitant to perform an amputation. The operation may have been partly attributed to medico-legal regulations of the time. King Hammurabi of Babylon (c1900 BCE) codified the laws of the land onto the pillar of the main temple. This equates to a doctor's failure leading to losing a patient to be as significant as a doctor sacrificing their own hand.

If a physician shall make a severe wound with an operating knife and kill a patient or destroy an eye, his hand shall be cut off ~Code of Hamurabi. [54–56]

Hippocrates (460–380), who described amputation for vascular gangrene first described the procedure in ancient Greece. They removed the black tissue at the joint above the line of demarcation. They wrote

> *Even when a part of the thigh comes away, or of the arm, both bones and flesh, but less as in this case, and when the forearm and leg drop off, the patients readily recover.*

At that time, surgery in Greece was relatively advanced. Surgeons described tourniquets, drains, cautery, and wound cleanliness. They used honey, wine, and vinegar as antiseptics [44].

In Roman times, Celsus in the first century CE described amputating the leg by cutting in the healthy tissue just above the line of demarcation. He described ligation of the blood vessels, dividing the bone at a proximal level. Also smoothing of the bone, skin flap to cover the bone, and packing with lint and vinegar. He wrote,

> *Amputation involves a very great risk for patients who often die under the operation, but it does not matter if the remedy is safe, since it is the only option, Therefore, between the sound and diseased part, the flesh is to be cut through with a scalpel down to the bone…it is better that some of the sound part be cut away than any of the diseased part should be left behind.*

Roman texts also mention the criminal penalty of amputation, which involves the removal of one's hands. Roman surgeons of the time had developed a wide range of forceps, blades, and saws to operate with. Examples of such instruments, dated to 79 CE were later found at the surgeon's house in the volcanic ruins of Pompeii, Italy [54, 56].

Albucasis (926–1013) employed amputation in the treatment of congenital malformations such as polydactyly and gangrene secondary to poisonous reptile and spider bites. He applied tourniquets proximal and distal to the site of transection to tense the soft tissue, which linen dressings then protected to avoid saw injury. He also was the first to advocate for double suture, which is still used today for high-tension closures.

Just as amputation began the transition from an art to a medical science, its progress was stifled by the Catholic Church. Between 1130 and 1247, "Ecclesia abhorret a sanguine," a decree by the church prohibiting bleeding served to discredit surgery and surgeons. Due to the feudal system of the Dark Ages, Europe was divided into kingdoms that became isolated from parts of the world that had a better knowledge of science and medicine such as the Arab world in the Middle East, North Africa, and Spain. This further slowed innovation and dissemination of surgical knowledge. Technical advances from Hippocratic, Roman, and Greek times were either forgotten or abandoned in Europe to the detriment of the medical management of its citizens. With the advent of gunpowder from China, and the introduction of firearms in France in 1346, these quickly spread throughout Europe. However, it was to be more than a century until amputation was reemployed to treat battlefield wounds caused by the new, higher velocity and tissue compromising firearm injuries. Still, the complication rate of amputation was very high, something that haunted the consciences of surgeons for a long time [57, 58].

5.4.2 Amputation in Europe in the Thirteenth to Eighteenth Centuries

5.4.2.1 Ambrose Paré (1510–1590)

Ambrose Paré spent many years as a barber surgeon apprentice before becoming a French army surgeon. He also served under several French kings. Paré described many amputations on the battlefield. They reintroduced ligation of the blood vessels instead of hot oil or hot iron to stop the bleeding. From then on, amputation was regarded as the limb excision that would save a life. Despite that, the death rate by hemorrhage or sepsis was extremely high. The high mortality of amputation wouldn't decrease until the advent of aseptic technique and general anesthesia in the mid-nineteenth century.

Paré was eventually to advocate against hot iron application for a wound or an amputee, because it led to eschars that eventually became infected, or sloshed and caused secondary hemorrhage or non-healing chronic ulcer. Instead, he reintroduced the ligation of the arteries and the application of a tourniquet. He introduced the artery forceps that's used to day to ligate blood vessels also known as the hemostat. He also introduced the idea of prosthetic replacement to help regain some function and designed a few forms of prostheses. One of Pare's most famous "Le Petit Lorrain," was a mechanical hand that a French army captain wore into battle. They revolutionized the field of amputation and made the bases for modern practise and also set the stage for vascular surgery.

In 1616, William Harvey's discovery of the circulatory system led to the further development of the tourniquet. This led to identifying the bleeding vessels and ligating them that meant a dramatic reduction in blood loss after amputation. These improvements made it easier for surgeons to identify blood vessels and nerves, but building a stump was still a difficult problem for them and the healing process often had high rates of infection after surgery. Jean Louis Petit, whose tourniquet in 1718 stood the test of time, reintroduced the skin flap by cutting the bone proximal to the skin [54, 56, 57].

In the year 1810, Bernhardt von Langenbeck masterfully revolutionized the prevailing surgical technique through the groundbreaking employment of a meticulous and intricately crafted soft-tissue flap. This innovative flap delicately embraced the vulnerable bone, making sure a remarkably gentle and tension-free coverage.

In the Napoleonic Wars, a skilled and caring doctor named Dominique Jean Larrey rose to the rank of Surgeon Major in the powerful Army of the Rhine. This was a time of constant fighting and new medical discoveries. Larrey witnessed with horror the low value of soldiers and how they were treated by high-ranking officers of the army. They were treated as dispensable commodities. The wounded lost their humanity and were often abandoned on the battlefield to avoid slowing military progression. Injured soldiers during combat were left on the battlefield until the end of the engagement. Battles often raged on for hours. The lucky ones would then be collected and treated. During his 18-year service to Napoleon, Larrey witnessed 25 campaigns, 60 battles, and more than 400 engagements. They honed their skills in wound management and amputation. Amidst the tumultuous retreat from the formidable Russian forces in the aftermath of the cataclysmic battle of Borodino. Larrey is renowned for accomplishing the astounding feat of performing no fewer than 200 intricate amputations within a remarkably compressed span of 24 h. To avoid death from haemorrhagic shock, he advocated early amputation in the field [58–60].

5.4.3 Amputation in the Nineteenth Century

5.4.3.1 Joseph Lister and Asepsis (1860s)

Lister hypothesized that the septicemia and putrefaction process closely resembled the fermentation process described by Louis Pasteur in the 1860s. Convinced that living organisms were responsible for wound sepsis, he began surgically debriding his amputees' limbs and applied carbolic acid (phenol). He was eventually able, after initial setbacks, to drop the death rate from 45% to 15%. Despite his evidence-based approach, the surgical world was slow to adopt his aseptic technique.

5.4.3.2 The American Civil War (1861–5)

The American civil war led to an unbelievably higher incidence of amputation than any war before, created by the firearms used by the two sides. Rifled muskets fired lead bullets that travelled relatively slow but with accuracy up to a half mile away. Once it hits the body, it drives with it, clothes and dirt that lead to rapid-onset infections. To reduce deaths from septic shock, amputation was employed as the most common operation in the civil war. That was all before Lister's aseptic procedures were employed as a standard surgical technique [60, 61].

According to William Keen, a Union Army surgeon, "it was seven times safer to fight through all three days of Gettysburg rather than undergo an amputation." The surgeons didn't recognize the need for cleanliness and sanitation. Little was known about bacteria and germs. For instance, bandages were repeatedly employed on various individuals without undergoing any form of sanitization, contributing to the development and spread of infections.

There were so many wounded soldiers that surgeons didn't have time to be careful when fixing their injuries. Many wounds that could be treated easily today with simple methods got infected. So the army surgeons amputated a vast number of arms and legs. About three out of four surgeries during the civil war were to take off limbs.

5.4.3.3 Theodor Billroth at the Franco-Prussian War (1870–71)

A decade later, the Viennese Professor, Theodore Billroth, was one of the early adopters of Lister's recommendations, when he served a few months in 1870, as a military surgeon during the Franco-Prussian War. They utilized aseptic technique and worked meticulously to achieve haemostasis and soft tissue approximation. Instead of suturing amputation stumps closed, he used the technique of open drainage and healing by secondary intention. Using this approach, it's reported that Billroth audited the results of almost 100 patients, reporting that none of them developed gangrene [62–64].

5.4.4 Amputation in the Twentieth Century

World War One was a static warfare that meant soldiers spent days on end in cold flooded trenches that led to the syndrome known as trench foot, which was caused by skin damage by ischaemia from vascular spasm and superseded infection.

The highly explosive shell took the destruction of limbs to a new level that led to mass casualties. General Norman Kirk carefully reviewed the surgical approaches of amputation. Many old techniques were discarded. Innovations were developed, and the surgical approach to amputation was simplified to preserve limb functionality.

5.4.4.1 Antibiotics

In 1928, Alexander Fleming discovered Penicillin, which in the 1940s was manufactured in massive quantities. In 1938, sulfonamides, became available as a new antibacterial drug. At this stage, hemorrhage, pain, and infection became under control. New weapons designed to inflict increasingly destructive wounds were to further challenge the management of injuries and the practice of amputation.

5.4.4.2 The Myoplastic Approach

Felix Mondry in 1952 refined amputation by employing a myo-plastic approach. During the amputation, muscles were transected according to their natural tension and stitched together carefully to cover the bone and reduce tension to provide an adequate blood supply. As a result, amputation changed from the most gruesome form of traumatic surgery to a life-saving operation focused on regaining patient independence [64, 65].

5.4.5 *Limb Prostheses*

One of the earliest examples of limb prosthesis comes from the 18th dynasty of ancient Egypt in the reign of Amenhotep II in the fifteenth century BCE. The Cairo Museum houses a mummy with a prosthetic toe made of leather and wood, replacing the amputated great toe on the right foot.

In ancient Rome, a Persian soldier escaped imprisonment by cutting off his own leg. He then replaced it with a wooden one and travelled 30 miles to Tregea, where he was caught by Zaccynthius and killed. In 1858, a copper and wood leg was found in Capri, Italy that dated back to 300 BCE and matched the prosthetics used during that time.

The first real tools that could be called prostheses were made in ancient Greece and Rome. These early prosthetics weren't very good. They were made of whatever materials were available, like wood, metal, or leather. They were often uncomfortable and didn't work well.

During the mediaeval period, knights used iron prosthetics to conceal amputated limbs. Some pirates did wear poorly designed hooks and peg legs.

Fast forward to more recent history, one of the earliest written reports of prosthetic limbs is found in a book published by a French surgeon Ambroise Paré (1510–1590), part of which described the artificial limbs he fitted on his amputees.

After the American Civil War, on January 23, 1866, North Carolina became the first of the former Confederate states to offer artificial limbs to amputees. It contracted with Jewett's Patent Leg Company, with a temporary factory set up in Raleigh. A system was developed whereby amputees could get an artificial limb at no cost for 5 years. Many took up the offer [64–66].

References

1. Fastag E, Varon J, Sternbach G. Richard lower: the origins of blood transfusion. J Emerg Med. 2013;44(6):1146–50. https://doi.org/10.1016/j.jemermed.2012.12.015. Epub 2013 Mar 15. PMID: 23499352.T.
2. The history of blood transfusion. Bull Med Libr Assoc. 1942; 30: 105–112. The Method Observed in Transfusing the Blood out of one Animal into Another. By: Richard Lower. Philosophical Transactions, Vol. 1 (1665–1666), pp. 353–358. Royal Society. New England Journal of Medicine in 1999. (1999; 341: 1845–1849).
3. Morens DM. Death of a president. N Engl J Med. 1999;341(24):1845–9. https://doi.org/10.1056/NEJM199912093412413. PMID: 10588974.
4. An Account of the Experiment of Transfusion, Practiced upon a Man in London. By: Edmund King. Philosophical Transactions, Vol. 2 (1666–1667), pp. 557–559. Royal Society.
5. Lower R. An account of the experiment of transfusion, practiced upon a man in London. 1667. Yale J Biol Med. 2002;75(5–6):293–7; discussion 292. PMID: 14580110; PMCID: PMC2588804.

6. Blakemore C, Jennett S, editors. The Oxford companion to the body. New York: Oxford University Press; 2001.
7. Tucker H. Blood work: a tale of medicine and murder in the scientific revolution. W. W. Norton & Company; 2012. ISBN 978-0393342239.
8. https://royalsocietypublishing.org/doi/10.1098/rstl.1665.0147
9. Learoyd P. A short history of blood transfusion. National Blood Service; 2006.
10. Blundell. Observations on transfusion of blood. The Lancet. 1829;2(302):321–4. https://doi.org/10.1016/S0140-6736(02)92543-2. ISSN 0140-6736.
11. History of Blood Transfusion. American Red Cross.
12. Schwarz HP, Dorner F. Karl Landsteiner and his major contributions to hematology. Br J Haematol. 2003;121(4):1365.
13. Stansbury LG, Hess JR. Blood transfusion in World War I: the roles of Lawrence Bruce Robertson and Owen Hope Robertson in the "most important medical advance of the war". Trans Med Rev. 2009;23(3):232–6.
14. Stansbury LG, Hess JR. Putting the pieces together: Roger I. Lee and modern transfusion medicine. Transfus Med Rev. 2005;19(1):81–4. https://doi.org/10.1016/j.tmrv.2004.09.003. PMID: 15830330.
15. Levine P, Stetson RE. An unusual case of intragroup agglutination. J Am Med Assoc. 1939;113:126–7.
16. Maxwell A. Dr. Lawrence Bruce Robertson and blood transfusion in the trenches of World War I. Canadian Blood Services. https://blood.ca/en/research/ourresearch-stories/research-education-discovery/dr.lawrence.b.robertson.
17. Dinis da Gama AA. histróia ignorada da descoberta da heparina [The unknown history of heparin's discovery]. Rev Port Cir Cardiotorac Vasc. 2008;15(1):25–30. Portuguese. PMID.
18. Mclean J. The discovery of heparin. Circulation. 1959;19:75–8. Originally published 1 Jan 1959. https://doi.org/10.1161/01.CIR.19.1.75.
19. Crile GW. The transfusion of blood. Br J Med. 1907;2:1007.
20. Cushing H. From a Surgeon's Journal. Boston Little Brown and Co; 1936.
21. Obituary- Dr. Carl W. Walter; Inventor of Blood Bag. Los Angeles Times, May 10, 1992.
22. Lewinsohn R. Blood transfusion by the citrate method. Surg Gynecol Obstet. 1915;21:37–47.
23. Rous P, Turner JR. Preservation of living red blood corpuscles in vitro. II. The transfusion of kept cells. J Exp Med. 1916;23:219; New England Journal of Medicine in 1999. (1999; 341: 1845–1849).
24. Koutserimpas C, Alpantaki K, Samonis G. Trauma management in Homer's Iliad. Int Wound J. 2017;14(4):682–4. https://doi.org/10.1111/iwj.12672. Epub 2016 Sep 9. PMID: 27611659; PMCID: PMC7949588.
25. Kayhanian S, Machado RJ. Head Injuries in Homer's Iliad. World Neurosurg. 2020;143:33–7. https://doi.org/10.1016/j.wneu.2020.07.037. Epub 2020 Jul 13. PMID: 32673804.
26. Basma J, Kayssi AR, Zein R, Krisht AF. Meges of Sidon: the most learned of surgery's founding fathers. World Neurosurg. 2023; https://doi.org/10.1016/J.WNEU.2023.07.044.
27. Ellis H. John Hunter on gunshot wounds. J Roy Soc Med. 2001;94:43–5.
28. Royal College of Surgeons of England. William MacCormac (1836–1901). Plarrs Lives of Fellows. https://livesonline.rcseng.ac.uk/. Last accessed 15/5/2024.
29. Stewart G. ANZAC Surgeons of Gallipoli. Chapter 4: abdominal injuries. Royal Australasian College of Surgeons; 2015.
30. Hutchinson W. Treatment of wounds of the chest. BMJ. 1918;1:196–8.
31. Don A. Perforating and penetrating wounds of the chest with severe haemorrhage. BMJ. 1916;1:1816–7.
32. Roberts JE, Craig JG. The surgical treatment of severe wounds of the chest. BMJ. 1917;2:576–9.

33. Herringham W. Penetrating wounds of the chest at the casualty clearing stations. BMJ. 1917;1:721–2.
34. Zisis C, Tsirgogianni K, Lazaridis G, Lampaki S, Baka S, Mpoukovinas I, Karavasilis V, Kioumis I, Pitsiou G, Katsikogiannis N, Tsakiridis K, Rapti A, Trakada G, Karapantzos I, Karapantzou C, Zissimopoulos A, Zarogoulidis K, Zarogoulidis P. Chest drainage systems in use. Ann Transl Med. 2015;3(3):43. https://doi.org/10.3978/j.issn.2305-5839.2015.02.09. PMID: 25815304; PMCID: PMC4356865.
35. Aarabi B, Tofighi B, Kufera JA, et al. Predictors of outcome in civilian gunshot wounds the head. J Neurosurg. 2014;120(5):1138–46.
36. Horsley V. Gunshot wounds of the head. BMJ. 1915;1:321–3.
37. Syme GA. MJA. 1915;1:277–9.
38. Hanigan WC. Neurological surgery during the Great War: the influence of Colonel Cushing. Neurosurgery. 1988;23:283–94.
39. Keen WW. The treatment of war wounds. Philadelphia/London: W.B. Saunders Co; 1917. p. 100–1.
40. Dowdy J, Pait TG. The influence of war on the development of neurosurgery, Historical vignette. J Neurosurg. 2014;120(1):237–43.
41. Keen WW. Treatment of war wounds. Philadelphia and London: W. B. Saunders Co; 1918. [Google Scholar].
42. Jones R, Lodge O. The discovery of a bullet lost in the wrist by means of the Roentgen rays. Lancet. 1896;147(3782):476–7. https://doi.org/10.1016/S0140-6736(01)93204-0.
43. Lee JA. Sidney Ringer (1835–1910) and Alexis Hartmann (1898–1960). Anaesthesia. 1981;36:1115–21.
44. Homer. The Iliad. Translated by Robert Fagles. New York: Penguin Books Ltd.; 1990.
45. Calne Sir Roy. The Illustrated Hsitory of Surgery. Calne Sir Roy. 2nd ed. Barbican, London: Harolde Starke Publishers Ltd.; 2000.
46. Woodward JJ. The medical and surgical history of the war of the rebellion. Washington, DC: Government Printing Office; 1875.
47. Mullins RJ. A historical perspective of trauma system development in the United States. J Trauma. 1999;47:S8–S14.
48. Shackford SR. The evolution of modern trauma care. Surg Clin N Am. 1995;75:147–56.
49. Optimal hospital ressources for care of the seriously injured. Bull Am Coll Surg. 1976;61:15–22.
50. Detmer DE, Moylan JA, Rose J, Schulz R, Wallace R, Daly R. Regional categorization and quality of care in major trauma. J Trauma. 1997;17:592–9.
51. West JG, Trunkey DD, Lim RC. Systems of trauma care. Arch Surg. 1979;114:455–60.
52. American College of Surgeons. Advanced trauma life support for doctors (ATLS). 6th ed. Chicago: American College of Surgeons; 1997.
53. MacKenzie EJ, Rivara FP, Jurkovich GJ, Nathens AB, Frey KP, Egleston BL, Salkever DS, Scharfstein DO. A national evaluation of the effect of trauma-center care on mortality. N Engl J Med. 2006;354(4):366–78. https://doi.org/10.1056/NEJMsa052049. PMID: 16436768.
54. Maloney TR, Dilkes-Hall IE, Vlok M, et al. Surgical amputation of a limb 31,000 years ago in Borneo. Nature. 2022;609:547–51. https://doi.org/10.1038/s41586-022-05160-8.
55. Isherwood PA. The controlled pressure distribution system for prosthetic casting. PhD thesis, University of London; 1980.
56. Butler CM. The vascular amputee. MS thesis, University of London; 1986.
57. Bennett-Wilson A. Limb prosthetics-1970. Artif Limbs. 1970;14:1–52.
58. Spink MS, Lewis GL. Albucasis on surgery and instruments. London: Wellcome; 1973.
59. Kirkup J. A history of limb amputation. London: Springer-Verlag; 2007.
60. Thurston AJ. Paré and Prosthetics: the early history of artificial limbs. ANZ J Surg. 2007;77:1114–9.

61. Magee R. Amputation through the ages: the oldest major surgical operation. Austr NZ J Surg. 1998;68:675–8.
62. Larrey DJ. Memoirs of military surgery, and campaigns of the French armies, on the Rhine, in Corsica, Catalonia, Egypt, and Syria; at Boulogne, Ulm, and Austerlitz, in Saxony, Prussia, Poland, Spain, and Austria. Joseph Cushing: Baltimore; 1814.
63. Lister J. On the effects of the antiseptic system of treatment upon the salubrity of a surgical hospital. Lancet. 1870;1:84–101.
64. Keen WW. The contrast between the surgery of the civil war and that of the present war. NY Med J. 1915;101:817–24.
65. Bilguer JU. A dissertation on the inutility of the amputation of limbs. (English translation). London: R. Baldwin; 1764.
66. Ham R, Cotton L. Limb amputation: from aetiology to rehabilitation. London: Chapman and Hall; 1991.

Chapter 6
The Nineteenth Century: Anti-sepsis, Asepsis, Antibiotics and Anaesthesia

The value of cleanliness in the conduct of examination and surgical procedures had been recognized since ancient times and was also strongly promoted by the writings of Guy de Chauliac and others. However, the re-introduction of cadaveric dissection and the role of the autopsy (often carried out in the operating theatre) to identify the cause of death introduced a carelessness (or unwillingness to recognize the risks) as to how a lack of cleanliness might promote infection. Even in the 1870s surgeons were want to wear a jacket stained with blood from previous operations and the same jacket would be worn with pride, the more stains the greater the prowess of the surgeon!

There were three principle developments that spanned the nineteenth century in relation to infection. The first was the use of anti-septics for the surgical environment, the instruments and on the wound; the second was a recognition that infection could be transmitted by doctors, nurses, and midwives and not through bad odor in the air (miasma theory); the third was a recognition that microbes which had been first discovered in the seventeenth century were the cause of infectious disease including surgical infections (contagium vivum).

6.1 Microscopes and Micro-organisms

Girolamo Fracastoro (1484–1553), Fig. 6.1, was a physician, poet, and geographer. He is credited with giving syphilis its name through a poem he wrote focused on a Greek shepherd named Syphilus. He provided the first accurate clinical description of the disease typhus and came close to suggesting that contagious diseases were

This chapter covers asepsis, handwashing, rubber gloves, antibiotics, and the introduction of general, local, and intravenous anesthesia in modern surgical practice. It covers ICU, airway management, ventilation, and tracheostomy.

S. Abbas, D. Watters, *The Road to Modern Surgery*,
https://doi.org/10.1007/978-981-96-4337-0_6

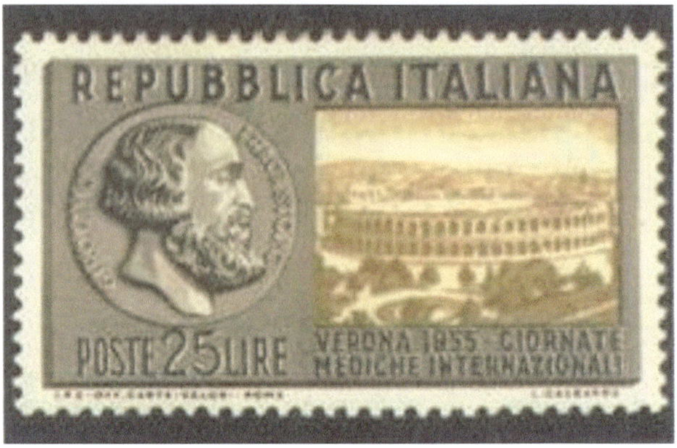

Fig. 6.1 Italian postage stamp commemorating Girolamo Fracastoro issued in 1955, public domain. https://upload.wikimedia.org/wikipedia/commons/5/5d/Redenti_-_Girolamo_Fracastoro.jpg

spread by some "seed" or infective agent by direct contact, contamination of the environment or through the air. This was contrary to the miasma theory of disease that had persisted for centuries and would remain prevalent until the late 1900s. Dutch spectacle maker Zacharias Janssen (1585-c1632) is credited with making one of the first compound microscopes (ones that used two lenses) in the early 1600s, allowing a magnification of 20-30 times normal size.

Athanasius Kircher (1602–1680) was a Jesuit and polymath. Among his many interests, he was one of the first to observe micro-organisms under the microscope in 1658, and so proposed that the plague might be spread by a micro-organism. Robert Hooke (1635–1702) described a microscopic fungus in 1665. Another Dutchman, Antoni van Leeuwenhoek (1632–1723), ground his own lenses to achieve a magnification of up to 200 fold. Initially he studied plants, animal tissue, minerals, fossils, sperm and blood but later described protozoans and bacteria which he called "animacules" or "little eels" in 1676. Hooke subsequently verified van Leeuwenhoek's findings and presented them to the Royal Society. In 1680, van Leeuwenhoek also performed an experiment in which he cultured anaerobic bacteria almost two centuries before their later re-discovery by Pasteur in 1862. However, others in the intervening years also deserve credit for the recognition that infectious diseases are indeed transmitted by micro-organisms [1–3].

6.1.1 Agostino Bassi (1773–1856)

Agostino Bassi, Fig. 6.2, was an Italian scientist who in 1826 reported that fungi caused silk worm disease and its contagiousness. In 1844 he went on to postulate that other human diseases such as measles and cholera were also transmissible, a somewhat radical view at the time and one that was only accepted slowly over the subsequent decades of the nineteenth century.

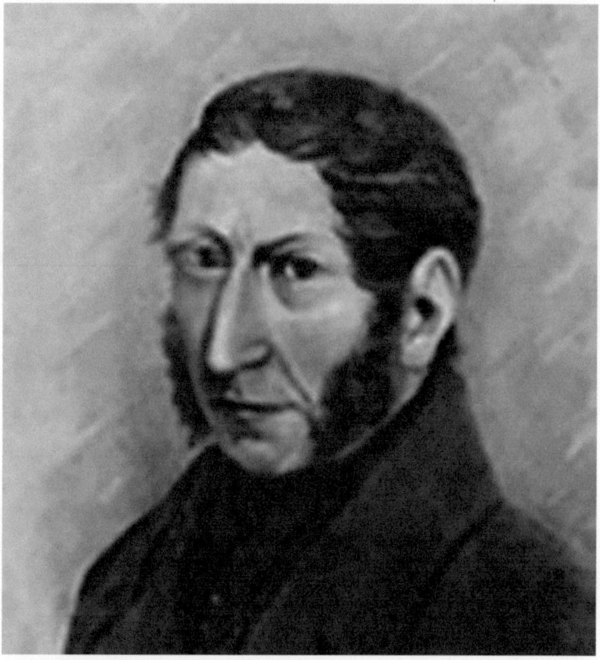

Fig. 6.2 Agostino Bassi by G.C Ainsworth Wikicommons, no restrictions. https://en.wikipedia.org/wiki/Agostino_Bassi#/media/File:Agostino_Bassi_by_G.C._Ainsworth.jpg

6.1.2 Miasma Versus Contagium Vivum Theory

In the mid-1800s, the germ theory of disease had not yet been established, and the miasma theory was still strongly supported by the scientific community. The miasmatic theory was a hypothesis that was popular during the nineteenth century, which suggested that diseases such as cholera, yellow fever, and the bubonic plague were caused by a "bad air" or miasma, emanating from decaying organic matter.

However, Giovanni Rasori (1766-1837), Professor of Pathology in Pavia, was a supporter of the less accepted contagium vivum theory (i.e., the theory that epidemic diseases was generated by microscopic agents transmitted by a patient to a healthy individual), at that time not so considered [3, 4].

6.1.3 Louis Pasteur (1822–1895)

Louis Pasteur was responsible for popularising "germ theory." His early studies were based on fermentation. His paper on spontaneous generation described *"les corpuscles organises dans l'atmosphere"* was focused on wine, but would have far wider implications ever after. Pasteur's later work progressed to study fowl cholera before he successfully introduced vaccination for rabies post exposure, possible because of its long latent period.

6.2 Surgical Infection

> *A man laid on the operating table of one of our hospitals is exposed to more chance of death than the English soldier on the field at Waterloo.* (Sir James Simpson, 1869)

In the early nineteenth century, doctors did not know about the role of microorganisms in causing infections and, as a result, they did not take the necessary measures to prevent the spread of disease. This is in spite of De Chauliac's and others' advocacy for cleanliness. There were high rates of infection and death, never mind that their bare hands transmitted infection between cases, and nowhere more so than the maternity ward [5].

In 1841, in Paris, Joseph-Francois Malgaigne (1806–1863) reported a mean mortality of 60% for amputations. These poor outcomes were attributed mainly to hospital-acquired diseases which included five infective nosocomial entities, which at that time were diagnosed more frequently: erysipelas, tetanus, pyaemia, septicemia, and gangrene. At the time surgeons believed that surgical site infection was inevitable and necessary to promote successful wound healing. James Syme (1799–1870) calculated a mortality rate of 43% among amputated patients in Edinburgh, and there were reports of 26% in Boston and 23% in London. In Munich, the mortality for nosocomial gangrene reached 80% in some periods, and 46% in Zurich [5].

Although micro-organisms had been discovered by the 1860s, any general acceptance of their connection to disease was to follow Louis Pasteur's and Robert Koch's work. However, there were still those in the eighteenth and early nineteenth centuries appropriately advocating for cleanliness, even without a knowledge of microbes. Their work, based on observation and protocol, was rewarded by lowering maternal mortality without being able to provide the scientific evidence as to what was causing puerperal sepsis, nor how doctors, whose overcoats were often smeared with blood, pus, and other bodily matters, were responsible for transmitting it. Similarly without understanding what it was that caused infection in an amputation, Joseph Lister and others were still able to show how carbolic acid significantly reduced the incidence of postoperative infection.

6.2.1 Chlorine and Putrefaction

Chlorine had been discovered in 1775 by Swedish chemist, Carl Wilhelm Scheele (1742-1786). In 1789, Claude Berthollet (1748–1822) introduced the antiputrifying agent, sodium hypochlorite, "*eau de Javel*." Then in the 1820s, Antoinne Labarraque (1777–1850), a Parisian chemist and pharmacist, developed chloride of lime (calcium hypochlorite) solution as a novel and better method of preventing putrefaction in the animal gut required for the making of musical instrument strings. He then reported its use in removing the putrid smell from morgues, sewers, and hospital wards. Parisian surgeons then found chloride of lime (calcium hypochlorite) an efficacious method for cleaning carbuncles, ulcers, and necrotic or gangrenous wounds.

During General Custer's campaigns in North Dakota (1873–74), the chief surgeon, Dr. Henry H Ruber, would later use chloride of lime, or *"eau de Labarraque,"* as it was then called, to prevent further deterioration in cases of frostbite [5, 6].

6.2.2 Preventing Puerperal Sepsis

Puerperal sepsis was an all too common complication of childbirth throughout the ages. Epidemics came in waves and are now recognized to have been the result of health care worker transmitted infection, crowded lying-in hospitals and unsanitary conditions.

6.2.2.1 Alexander Gordon (1752–1799)

Alexander Gordon was a Scottish obstetrician who demonstrated by meticulous record keeping of puerperal sepsis cases, that puerperal fever was contagious, albeit that the underlying means of contagion was unknown. He showed that the disease was being spread from woman to woman by the midwife or doctor, and so recommended fumigation of clothing, burning of the bed linen and cleanliness of the woman's attendants could control the disease [7].

His 1795 epic *Treatise on the Epidemic of Puerperal Fever of Aberdeen* which had begun in 1789, included 7 chapters. It was reprinted 3 times over the next 55 years in Edinburgh, London, and Philadelphia. Gordon stated:

> *It is a disagreeable declaration for me to mention that I myself was the means of carrying the infection to a great number of women.* [8]

He also recognized a connection between the skin infection, erysipelas, and puerperal fever, although the causative micro-organism *Streptococcus pyogenes* was yet undiscovered. Somewhat radically, Gordon proposed the disease was caused by "contagious particles" rather than the more widely accepted "noxious atmosphere." Gordon's hypothesis was not accepted widely in his day, so he suffered much criticism, and it was to take a further century before the causative organism was identified. It is likely that both Oliver Wendell Holmes and Ignac Semmelweis were aware of his work. Gordon's advocacy for cleanliness resulted in only 28 of 77 women with puerperal sepsis dying. In addition to prevention, his recommended treatment for established puerperal sepsis were bleeding and purging which are highly likely to have been unhelpful and, for some of the unlucky, may have hastened death [6–8].

6.2.2.2 Oliver Wendell Holmes (1809–94)

The high incidence of nosocomial puerperal sepsis during the mid-nineteenth century prompted Harvard's Oliver Wendell Holmes in 1843, to pen a classic essay on *The Contagiousness of Puerperal Fever* with rules for the obstetrician to mitigate this risk including hand washing, changes of clothing, and avoidance of autopsies when managing obstetric cases.

His views were bitterly opposed by the then famous Charles Meigs (1792–1869) who declared:

Doctors are gentlemen and gentlemen's hands are clean

Meigs also opposed the use of chloroform for women in labor.

6.2.2.3 Ignaz Philipp Semmelweis (1818–65)

On the other side of the Atlantic, Hungarian Ignác Semmelweis—never one for conducting laboratory research or showing respect to colleagues with whom he disagreed—reduced the Maternal Mortality in Vienna's Allgemeine Krankenhaus in 1847 from 16% to 2% by enforcing hand washing with *chlorina liquida* in the obstetrics ward [5, 9, 10] (Fig. 6.3).

Other pioneers in the first half of the nineteenth century who advocated for hand hygiene included Semmelweis's own disciples, Routh (1848), Weiger (1848) and Skoda (1849). Another brave advocate was Thomas Watson in London (1842). These pioneers and champions suffered ridicule, professional isolation and, in

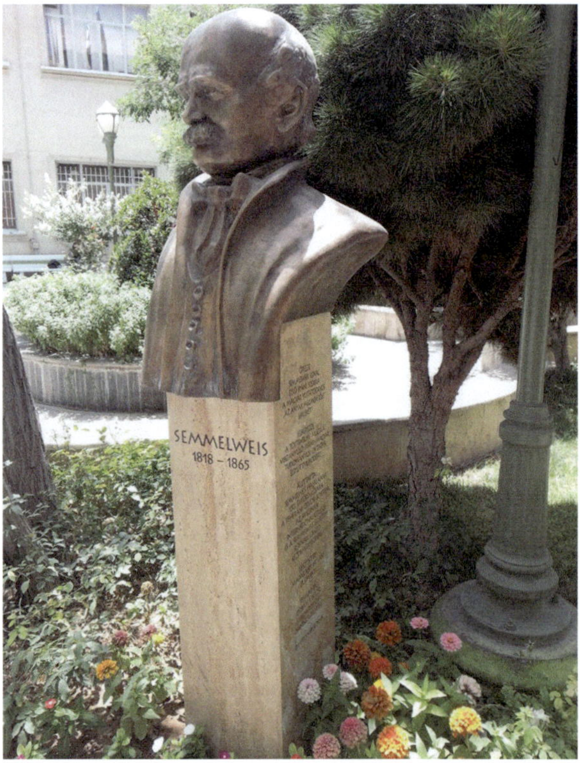

Fig. 6.3 Semmeleweis. A bust honouring Ignác Semmelweis located in the the grounds of the original Allgemeine Krankenhaus (General Hospital) in Vienna. Wikicommons, no restrictions. https://upload.wikimedia.org/wikipedia/commons/f/f8/Ignaz_Semmelweis_1860.jpg

Semmelweis' case, non-renewal of contract [4]. Semmelweis was forced to return to his native Hungary and so that the women of Budapest became the beneficiaries of his hand hygiene practice where, as in Vienna, his strict protocols greatly reduced the death rate from puerperal sepsis [11–13].

6.3 Surgical Asepsis

Asepsis is the practice of using chemical agents to reduce or eliminate harmful microorganisms on living tissues, such as skin or mucous membranes and deep tissues. The goal of asepsis is to minimize the risk of infection particularly in surgical procedures.

The introduction of asepsis to surgery represents a crucial milestone in the history of medicine. Though widely attributed to the work of Joseph Lister in the 1860s, it should be recognized for historical accuracy that Lister was not the first to use carbolic as he was prompted to acknowledge late in 1867, responding to James Simpson's correspondence on the topic in Lancet. Simpson's letter provides a detailed account of the discovery of carbolic, its use in sanitation and application in medicine, as does Ehrhardt et al.'s review of the topic in the American Journal of Surgery in 2020. The following section briefly covers the contributions of those preceding Lister before addressing Lister's systematic approach that provided the evidence for both asepsis and disinfection of surgical instruments and the surgical environment [14, 15].

6.3.1 Coal Tar, Carbolic Acid, and Phenol

In 1834, Friedlieb Ferdinand Runge (1795–1872) distilled coal tar to obtain carbolic acid. The oil produced was used to preserve wood from rotting on railway tracks. Then Frederick Calvert (1819–1873), an English chemist, who studied in Paris in 1835 brought the discovery back to England. When appointed as an industrial chemist in Manchester in 1846 (and later honorary chemist to Manchester Royal Infirmary), he also introduced carbolic acid to the anatomy department, for the preservation of cadavers. Injecting cadavers with dilute carbolic resulted in their being preserved for up to a month [16, 17].

Calvert linked up with Robert Angus Smith (1817–1874), later to discover acid rain, and Alexander McDougall who took an interest in linking chemistry to public health by using carbolic to reduce the stench of sewage and farm manure in English towns and their rivers. McDougall pursued a career in chemical sanitation and marketed a compound containing carbolic acid and lime as "McDougall's powder." Then Thomas Anderson (1819–1874), an Edinburgh medical graduate (1841) who pursued postgraduate studies in Chemistry in Europe, was appointed Professor of Chemistry in Glasgow. In response to problems with Glasgow's sanitation, Anderson recommended the use of McDougall's powder in 1858 although it proved toxic to the River Clyde's trout. It was to be Thomas Anderson that guided Joseph Lister to trial carbolic acid as an antiseptic in Glasgow when he took up his post there in 1860 [18–20].

6.3.1.1 Jules Lemaire (1863)

The clinical use of carbolic preceded Lister by almost a decade, at least in France, Italy, and Germany. Jules Lemaire (1814–1873) was a French chemist and pharmacist, who published a 795 page treatise *De l'acide phénique* that reported the antiseptic properties of carbolic acid in 1863. He observed that phenol was good for wounds and postulated that this may be because it would be toxic to any germs that may be present. His work and that of Pasteur also provided the basis for Joseph Lister to trial carbolic with surgical wounds, though Lister was not aware of the Lemaire's treatise when he started.

6.3.1.2 French Pioneers Corne, Demeaux and Velpeau (1858–60)

French physician, Edmond Corne, developed a coal tar and plaster compound for use in the sanitation of the stinking River Seine. In 1858, Jean Baptiste Demeaux used Corne's carbolic powder in his private clinical practice where it proved efficacious, though being a private practitioner his case numbers were limited. He then shared his experience with Alfred-Armand-Louis-Marie Velpeau (1778–1867), chief surgeon of Hôpital de la Charité where there was a large case volume of suitable wounds for clinical study. Velpeau, with detailed knowledge of anatomy and embryology, would amass some 340 publications during his career and at the time a femoral hernia was termed the "Velpeau hernia." He also gave his name to the Velpeau arm sling which is used today to immobilize shoulders. Velpeau and Demeaux observed marked reductions in suppuration when it was already present, but also reported that the compound was effective at preventing suppuration in the first place. Corne's coal tar powder was soon used by Napoleon III's military surgeons during the second Italian war of independence in 1859. Ferdinand Le Beuf, a pharmacist, isolated carbolic acid from coal tar and saponified the solution to form a carbolic acid lotion. This was used by Jules Lemaire to successfully treat a necrotic wound of the gluteal cleft. His results with Le Beuf's solution were published in 1860 in a book, *Du coaltar saponiné, désinfectant énergique* [21–23].

Velpeau presented their clinical experience of coal tar at the 1860 Parisien Academie de Sciences. Despite its efficacy he still was concerned as to adverse effects [22–24].

> *The powder is dirty, ill-coloured, and stains the patient's linen. It hardens, causes pressure on and around the wounds dressed with it. It stains the compresses also, and requires to be frequently renewed; moreover, although it does destroy the putrid odor of suppuration, yet it leaves behind a bituminous flavor which may not be pleasing to everybody.*

6.3.1.3 Enrico Bottini (1862–66)

Lemaire published an account of 26 cases treated with saponified coal tar in 1861, six years before Lister's paper in the Lancet. At the Great Exhibition in London (1862) an Italian physician, Carlo Pavesi, inspired by Lemaire's lectures, returned to Piedmont and encouraged Enrico Bottini to trial Lemaire's techniques. By 1866 Bottini had used carbolic in 600 cases, reporting impressive results. James Simpson also noted that by 1860, carbolic was also being used in Germany by a Dr. Küchenmeister of Dresden who had applied the carbolic acid to wounds and ulcers [23]

> *with the most satisfactory results both in medical and surgical practice, and as a means of arresting putrefaction and preventing the development of fungi.*

In his letter to the Lancet, Simpson goes on to note the medical publications in English that prior to Lister's papers already presented clinical outcomes of coal tar or carbolic [14]. He referenced the use of creasote, an impure form of carbolic acid and hydrate of cresyle in wounds and burns in the Edinburgh Royal Infirmary in 1842 by a Dr. Handyside. This followed an earlier Treatise on Creasote by Dr. Cormack (Edinburgh 1936). It was also used as an anti-septic in Leeds Hospital in 1964 [Sixth Report of the Officer of Health] [24].

6.3.2 Joseph Lister (1827–1912)

Lister was born on October 12, 1827 (Fig. 6.4), in West Ham, Essex, to Joseph Jackson and Anne Lister. He was the son of an amateur scientist who was very influential in the development of achromatic lenses for microscopes. He was a gifted student with a voracious appetite for learning with a passion for literature and the arts, but somewhat of a social outcast at school. His parents encouraged him with his schoolwork, especially with microscopy [25, 26].

Lister went to University College London from where he first obtained BA honours in classics and botany in 1847. He studied medicine from 1848 to 1852, graduating with honours, before becoming house surgeon at University College Hospital. He passed his MRCS and FRCS to become a Fellow of the Royal College of Surgeons in 1852 [25, 27].

His physiology tutor, Professor Sharpely, recommended he study with the great surgeon, James Syme, in Edinburgh. Syme was famous for being regarded as the best surgical tutor in the country. Syme had a great influence on Lister's surgical outlook and Lister married Syme's eldest daughter, Agnes. Some months later, in October, he was appointed surgeon to the Edinburgh Royal Infirmary where he worked under Syme (1853–1860). Then at just 33 years of age, he was appointed Regius Professor of Surgery at the University of Glasgow and Glasgow Royal Infirmary. There he noted that 16 of 35 amputations performed died between 1864 and 1866. He believed that infections were caused by some *influence in the atmosphere* and that by disinfecting/sterilising surgical instruments, wounds, and even

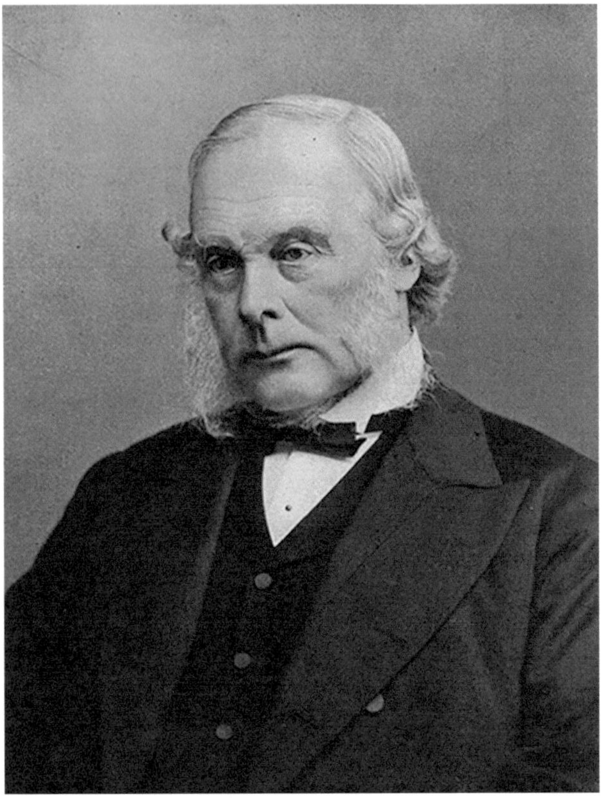

Fig. 6.4 Baron Lister of Lyme Regis (1897), Order of Merit (1902) and Privy Councillor (1902). (Image from Wikicommons (License type: no restrictions.https://upload.wikimedia.org/wikipedia/commons/a/a1/Joseph_Lister_1902.jpg)

the air in the operating room, he could prevent infections and improve patient outcomes [28].

On the advice of Thomas Anderson, then Professor of Chemistry, Lister began using carbolic acid (phenol), as an antiseptic during surgical procedures. He soaked his surgical instruments in a carbolic acid solution and sprayed the air in the operating room with a nebulized solution. He also used the carbolic to clean wounds before and then dress them after surgery. His first case series involved 12 compound fractures (8 of whom survived) before extending his techniques to amputations, 34 of 40 surviving between the years of 1867–1869 [29].

In a report in the Lancet in 1867, Lister described his findings [28].

> *Previous to its introduction, the two large wards in which most of my cases of accident and of operation are treated were amongst the unhealthiest in the whole of surgical division at the Glasgow Royal Infirmary, but since the antiseptic treatment has been brought into full operation, my wards have completely changed their character; so that during the last 9 months not a single instance of pyaemia, hospital gangrene or erysipelas has occurred in them.*

In 1869, Lister went back to Edinburgh to succeed his mentor and father-in-law, James Syme. Slowly, a few surgeons started incorporating carbolic acid and antiseptic techniques into their practice. At University College Hospital London, Marcus Beck adopted Lister's ideas, publishing a textbook on aseptic practice. However, it was only in 1879, when Lister took up the Chair at King's College hospital that the Kings' surgical department adopt his aseptic techniques.

Lister retired from practice in 1893 after his wife Agnes died. He came out of retirement briefly in 1902, when King Edward VII developed appendicitis. Appendicectomy was then still a risky procedure. The surgical team consulting him about the King were anxious. Lister advised them on the use of aseptic techniques. The surgery went well and the King survived. Edward VII later told Lister,

> *I know that if it had not been for you and your work, I wouldn't be sitting here today.*

Lister's use of aseptic techniques in surgery was initially met with resistance and skepticism from his peers, but his success rate in preventing infections and improving patient outcomes soon became renowned. His methods were to become widely adopted in the medical community throughout Europe and the USA, and by the early 1900s, aseptic techniques had become standard practice in surgery. Lister was not the first to use carbolic on wounds but the completeness of his aseptic approach using carbolic of lime as a disinfectant for instruments, disinfecting the theatre environment in addition to wound dressings may have been the advance that led him to be accredited as a major pioneer in its use. His influence on surgical trainees and surgical practice resulted in asepsis being widely practiced by those who trained under him but also on those who visited or read his papers [28–31].)

6.3.2.1 Edwin Klebs and Richard von Volkmann (1870–71)

In the Franco-Prussian war of 1870–71, pathologist Edwin Klebs (1834–1913) had described the presence of bacteria in purulent gunshot wounds as a somewhat constant finding. The following year in Germany, where an increase in work related injuries as a result of industrialization was occurring, 37–41% of patients with fractures died with pyaemia. Rather than closing his Halle institution, surgeon Richard von Volkmann (1830–1889) chose to adopt Lister's methods and was pleased to observe his patients' wounds heal without problems in response to being dressed with carbolic acid. The healing process under a Lister dressing was different from what surgeons had seen before. Wound secretion was minimal, healing by first intention was common, and wound infection was rare. Volkmann reported that more patients survived thigh amputations in one year than had done in his career up to that point. For him, antisepsis was the greatest progress in surgery since he had become a surgeon. Speaking at an International Medical Congress in London in 1881 he stated:

> *Until very recently the surgeon, at the moment of having skillfully finished his operation, was in the same position as the farmer after cultivating his land, only able to await the harvest and accept whichever way it turns out—sunshine, storm or hail—whereas today the surgeon is more like the manufacturer from whom, come what may, the public expects high quality products.* [32, 33]

6.3.2.2 Karl Thiersch in Leipzig (1867)

In Leipzig, Karl Thiersch (1822–1895) adopted the technique immediately after the publication of Lister's first article in 1867. Being the head of an academic department and thus a typical exponent of the German system, he had the authority to ensure that his students' learning and academic success would not be compromised during the transition. He also had one of his students write his doctoral thesis on a case series of complicated bone fractures and abscesses successfully treated with Lister's antiseptic techniques.

6.3.2.3 Von Nussbaum in Munich (1875)

Johann Nepomuk Ritter von Nussbaum (1829–1890) in Munich started using Lister's method in surgery in 1875, publishing a textbook in 1882, in which he said that not a single case of hospital gangrene, pyaemia or erysipelas had occurred, and general mortality had been cut in half. For von Nussbaum, Lister's antisepsis was also the greatest invention ever made in surgery. It had eliminated all the problems of wound disease *"as if by magic"* and *"saved the lives of thousands*." Though true, he may have been somewhat under-rating the impact of anaesthesia on surgical practice.

6.3.2.4 Giuseppe Ruggi in Bologna

Despite the earlier Piedmont use of carbolic acid by Bottini, it was Giuseppe Ruggi's (1844–1925) adoption of Lister's aseptic methods in the Surgical Department of the Maggiore hospital in the Italian city of Bologna that led to improved disinfection of instruments and wound management. In 1825, he observed:

> *Of all countries, Italy is the most indifferent and uninterested in experimenting this method, which has been so favorably judged from the greatest surgical societies in Germany.*

6.3.2.5 Modern Antiseptic Solutions

In the following years, other antiseptic agents such as hydrogen peroxide and mercuric chloride were also introduced to surgery, but carbolic acid remained the most widely used antiseptic in surgery for many years.

As understanding about the cause of infection and surgical sepsis grew, carbolic acid was replaced by more effective and less toxic antiseptic and disinfectant solutions, such as iodine and alcohol. Edinburgh University solution (Eusol), based on chloride of lime and boric acid was introduced in 1916 during WW1 as a wound disinfectant. Today, the most widely used topical antiseptics are povidone iodine, chlorhexidine (in alcohol or acqueous) while glutaraldehyde and hypochlorite are used for instruments that cannot be autoclaved. However, clinical trials have shown that some of the ancient recipes involving honey or yoghurt have similar efficacy on wounds and ulcers even though they may be more messy to use.

6.3.3 From Antisepsis to Asepsis

Between the 1840s and 1870s, research on infectious disease became a science that was based in the laboratory. This was due to the increasing use of microscopy, culture, and, above all, animal experiments. Scientists carried out the research to demonstrate causality relationships between specific microorganisms and disease.

The arrival of new culture and staining methods in the 1870s allowed them to distinguish bacterial species and link them to specific diseases, following the approach of German botanist Ferdinand Cohn (1828–98).

In 1872, Casimir Davaine (1812–82) in France transmitted septicemia in rabbits with very small amounts of bacteria. Koch had proved infectious diseases were caused by specific micro-organisms in his previous work on anthrax. His next research area was wound infections. He injected putrid fluids into mice and got six different wound infections, linked to specific identifiable bacteria.

Koch used another animal to separate bacterial species that cause specific infectious diseases. He would inoculate an animal with infectious material, then allow the bacteria to multiply in the new organism before transferring it back. This method allowed Koch to separate specific bacteria from others.

These new research methods allowed Koch to forge the causal link between identifiable microorganisms causing wound infection.

In 1881, Koch investigated the efficacy of antiseptics using his bacteriological toolset [1, 16]. Most importantly, Koch found in his studies on wound infection that carbolic acid, used in antisepsis, was almost useless in the laboratory. All of this was not lost on surgeons, who were already wary of Koch's conversion of germ theory into a series of demonstrable bacterial aetiologies. However, Koch's evidence based on sound bacteriological evidence made the adoption of antibacterial measures difficult to resist, given the many complications that could arise from a bacterial infection. The antibacterial measures became a declared strategy of "asepsis" rather than "antisepsis" were initially quite crude and unsophisticated, but as time went on, they became more and more refined and efficient. It put surgery in alignment with the scientific evidence.

The most influential proponent of the realignment strategy was Ernest von Bergmann, Professor of Surgery in Berlin (see below under Sect. 6.4.2) who was committed to making laboratory science the basis of surgery. Before antisepsis, he said, surgeons controlled only the "*bloody act*" of the operation, such as the size of the cut, hemostasis, and so on. After the operation, the surgeon didn't know if his patient would die or survive for previously surgeons could only tell patients "*the operation is complete*." He recognised surgeons were not as affected by chance, and that the new power that surgeons acquired came from the lab. "*Only laboratory science can help with clinical world's messiness and give clinicians certainty to do their tasks with confidence."*

Karl Garre a Swiss surgeon, used himself as an experimental subject. He inoculated bacteria from the Staphylococcus culture obtained from osteomyelitis cases into the skin of his own arm. The infection that occurred was difficult to control. Experiments like that confirmed the germ theory of wound infection beyond doubt. That led to the idea of sterilization of wound dressings, instruments, and surgeon gloves, the process was achieved by heat and steam using, initially, steam cookers. Scientists and surgeons devised various protocols for stringent care taken in the operating theatre to keep wound sterility as perfect as possible for the fear of infections. Surgeons began to sterilize tools and wear masks, gloves, and gowns to protect themselves, as well as their patients, from any potential germs and infections that could be transmitted from one to the other. Instead of everyday clothes, operating teams began to wear a special outfit that was a linen gown and long boots. Many of the cutting-edge, lab-driven elements of today's surgical paraphernalia were added in the search for weak points in the aseptic all-or-nothing system of preventing wound infection. Two years after publishing his wound infections study, Koch moved to Berlin to work at the Imperial Health Office. The Office had a laboratory set up for him and a research group of young doctors working on infectious disease. Koch's bacteriology was based on practices that had always had a pragmatic medical use. With his staining and culture techniques, Koch made the world of the "invisible" visible, observable, and thus potentially controllable for surgeons.

By the end of the nineteenth century, Robert Koch had developed his four postulates that must be fulfilled before proving that a disease is caused by a specific micro-organism.

(1) The microorganism must be found in diseased but not healthy individuals;
(2) The microorganism must be cultured from the diseased individual;
(3) Inoculation of a healthy individual with the cultured microorganism must reproduce the disease; and finally,
(4) The microorganism must be re-isolated from the inoculated, diseased individual and matched to the original microorganism.

Despite some modifications during the twentieth century—such as healthy carriers versus those with disease (e.g., *Vibrio cholerae*)—his postulates still hold true today.

Antiseptics began to be used to clean the wound area before surgery. This method significantly reduced the risk of infection after surgery and allowed surgeons to confidently perform increasingly complex operations. In the late 1890s, people said surgeons were becoming nervous. With so many wound treatments to perfect, they were worried about their practice. Despite all these measures there was still the risk of infection because it is not possible to guarantee wounds were germ-free. This leads some to doubt the benefit of antisepsis. One of the primary reasons for surgeons' uncertainty in determining whether or not a patient has been adequately disinfected stems from the fact that asepsis was often difficult to monitor. It depended on an absence, not a presence.In antisepsis, surgeons knew when they had disinfected an object. This was easier to control. In asepsis, which was more elusive, it was more difficult to know when you had done enough. There was a period of improvement and simplification, until bacteriological science showed the errors of Lister's theories. Thus convinced surgeons to replace antisepsis with asepsis. Antisepsis and asepsis were pitched against each other to control wound infection. The British champion of asepsis, Charles B. Lockwood, put it well: "The people who do it are the ones who win." It's a matter of character and determination "resistance of healthy living tissues to bacterial invasion cannot be relied upon. It is beyond the control of the surgeon, while asepsis is not. No one would exchange a certainty for an uncertainty." In the meantime, bacteriology had become more complex. While Koch's success reached its apogee in the 1890s, other scientists had started adding another layer of complexity to the master's original concept of a simple bacterial invasion: They realized that not all bacteria were the same, and that different types of bacteria could infect different host species. So, on the one hand, Koch showed the success of his simplistic strategy of pursuing the infectious agent "into its remotest nook" during the 1892 Hamburg cholera epidemic.In his manual *Antisepsis and Antiseptics* of 1895, Charles Buchanan called modern bacteriology "the legitimate offspring of antiseptic surgery" [34, 35].

6.4 Sterilization

With the recognition of the existence and role of germs or microbes, there was a greater recognition that sterilization of instruments would help to prevent infections. In the late nineteenth century new methods of sterilization were introduced, such as the use of heat, steam and pressure as well as chemical disinfectants. As bacteriology labs did the experiments to show how to kill the micro-organisms, surgeons applied the evidence to develop rigorous protocols to clean and sterilize their surgical instruments and equipment [36].

6.4.1 Pasteurization

Louis Pasteur demonstrated that bacteria could be killed by heat, and "pasteurization" is a process for milk that still bears his name today. The milk is heated to a temperature of at least 72C for at least 15 seconds. Pasteur also showed that moist heat was more lethal than dry heat in killing bacteria [37].

6.4.2 Dry Heat and Steam Sterilization

Robert Koch (1843–1910), who was the first to identify *Mycobacterium tuberculosis as the cause of TB*, demonstrated that dry heat and steam sterilization could kill bacteria. Ernst von Bergmann, (1836–1907), was a German Surgeon who had studied in Dorpat (1860), was Professor there from 1870-78, and became Professor in Wurzburg (1878-82) before suceeding Bernhard von Langenbeck in Berlin (1882 onwards). He was the first surgeon to use heat sterilized surgical instruments, and demonstrated the efficacy of steam sterilized dressing materials versus chemical antisepsis. He was also an early adopter of the white coat.

6.4.3 Steam Under Pressure: The Autoclave

The pressure cooker had been introduced to cooking in the late seventeenth century by Denis Papin and was called a "Digester." The first autoclave (latin for auto = self and clavis = key) was built by Pasteur's pupil and collaborator, Charles Chamberland, in 1876.

> *Koch, Gaffsky and Loeffler in 1881 published a description of a steam-heated sterilizer. von Bergmann of Berlin was one of the first to use steam to sterilize surgical materials in 1886. Schimmelbusch, von Bergmann's chief assistant, had a modified Koch steam sterilizer built by Rietschel and Henneberg of Berlin.* [37]

In 1886 Bedard, a French surgeon, designed an autoclave and had Weisnegg build it for use in the operating room. Bedard evidently was the first to use steam under pressure to sterilize operating-room supplies.

Ferdinand Cohn (1828–1898), Professor of Botany in Breslau in the Prussian State of Silesia, was the first to classify bacteria according to their shape but also described how a bacillus in a vegetative state can transform itself to an endospore in response to a deleterious environment. This is of particular significance for sterilization, and the need for steam under pressure as provided in an autoclave [16, 37].

Other methods were developed during the twentieth century to sterilize surgical devices by ethylene oxide, gamma irradiation, X-ray, E-beam, or low temperature hydrogen peroxide. Instruments such as endoscopes dialysis and cardiac by-pass machines require chemical sterilization. However, the autoclave remains the most common method used for metallic surgical instruments.

Florence Nightingale (1820–1910), Fig. 6.5, was an English social reformer and statistician, best known for her pioneering work as a nurse during the Crimean War (1853–1856). She collected data on the cause of death in war injuries and concluded that most deaths were caused by infections and potentially avoidable. She implemented nursing and sanitary changes that saved the lives of many people, earning her the nickname, "the Lady with the Lamp." Nightingale is considered the founder of modern nursing and was instrumental in transforming nursing into a profession for educated women. She made significant contributions to public health, using statistics to demonstrate the need for sanitary reforms and better living conditions. She wrote several books on nursing, healthcare, and social [38].

The science of Bacteriology made a big change to surgical practice. Now we can do more complicated operations, which lets us try new and more invasive surgical

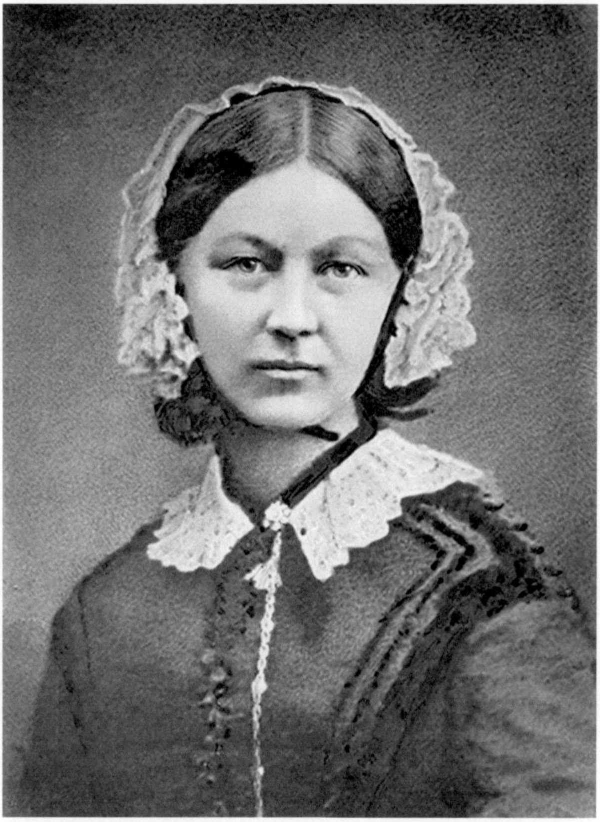

Fig. 6.5 Florence Nightingale. Wikipedia, public domain.CC. https://upload.wikimedia.org/wikipedia/commons/a/ab/Florence_Nightingale_%28H_Hering_NPG_x82368%29.jpg

procedures. In the twentieth century, surgeons improved surgical techniques using asepsis and laboratory science [30, 39, 40]. In his manual Antisepsis and Antiseptics of 1895, Charles Buchanan called modern bacteriology "the legitimate offspring of antiseptic surgery" [34, 35].

6.5 History of Rubber Gloves

Today any operative procedure at risk of contamination with micro-organisms is conducted with the surgeon and their assistants gloved. This acts to protect both the patient from the transmission of infection but also to protect the surgical/ perioperative team from inadvertent injury. This is particularly important since the recognition that viruses are transmitted through body fluid contact and needle-stick or scalpel injuries, with hepatitis B, C, and HIV viruses being the most common. Viral transmission and occupational health exposure are dealt with in a separate section that belongs to the twentieth century. This section considers the introduction of gloves to surgery, an innovation which, in the late nineteenth century, was met with skepticism, but first let us cover the discovery of rubber gloves [41, 42].

6.5.1 Discovery and Early Industrial Use of Rubber

Surgical gloves are no longer made of latex rubber, given the emergence of latex allergies and the need to ensure that hospitals are latex-free for the protection of their patients and staff. However, the story of surgical gloves begins with the European discovery of rubber. In central and southern America, the Mayans played a game with a rubber ball and Columbus' second voyage in 1496 gave an account of their game with a ball that bounced. In 1528, Hernán Cortés brought some of the Aztec players and balls back to Spain to perform at the Court. The Mayans obtained their rubber from the plant *Castilla elastica* which was described as the rubber producing tree in *Rerum Medicarum Novae Hispaniae Thesaures* published by Court physician, Francisco Hernández, in 1649. In 1736, Charles Marie de la Condamaine (1701-1774) discovered the inhabitants of the Amazon using waterproof dishes and wearing footwear made of rubber sap obtained from rubber trees (*Hevea brasiliensis*).

Western Europe was undergoing industrialization in the 18th and 19th centuries when Thomas Hancock (1786–1865) developed machines to soften, mix, and shape rubber. A Scottish Industrial Chemist, Charles Macintosh (1766–1843), found rubber was soluble in hexane and invented the "Mackintosh" in 1823. In 1839, Charles Goodyear (1800-1860) in Boston incorporated sulphur atoms to create cross linkages to improve rubber's strength and elasticity, a process called vulcanization. The commercial value of rubber was by then well appreciated and in 1877, Sir Henry Wickham (1846-1928) planted rubber plantations in the East Indies to secure sufficient supply [41–43].

6.5.2 The Use of Gloves in Surgery

The first gloves in surgery were not made from rubber. In 1758, Johann Walbaum fashioned a glove from a sheep's caecum to enable the turning and drawing out of a retained child. The intestinal glove was softened with lukewarm water, only covered 3 fingers while the hand was smeared with oil. Joseph Jakob Plenck (1738–1807), an Austrian Dermatologist was an early advocate for gloves to protect the hand of the examining doctor from contracting syphilis which is transmissible through the skin. Early in the nineteenth century the options for glove manufacture were either the sheep's caecum or gloves made of material such as linen, silk, cotton, or leather. It was only in 1834, that a young doctor, Richard Cooke conceptualized that "*a pair of rubber gloves would be perfectly impermeable to the most malignant virus.*" In

England, Sir Thomas Watson (1792–1882), who lost his wife to puerperal sepsis in 1843, reflected

an accoucheur might with advantage wear a glove, impervious to fluids for the safety of the mother in labour.

Maurice Gariel introduced a rubber glove for anatomical dissections and autopsy to "guarantee the hands against all bad odours and against infection."

In 1867, rubber gloves were advised for those who have to dip their hands into corrosive solutions and in 1887, a French surgeon, Jalaguier started using gloves because of dermatitis.

Slowly a small number of surgeons began to use gloves. The first reported use in America was the assistant of a Dr. Thomas in New York in 1878. Papin, a St Louis graduate, was reported wearing rubber gloves in 1880.

6.5.2.1 William Halsted and Caroline Hampton (1889)

However, rubber gloves were not manufactured until William Halsted negotiated with the Goodyear rubber company to make surgical gloves in 1889, because his scrub nurse and lover, Caroline Hampton, was suffering dermatitis from the mercuric chloride used to sterilize the instruments. Halsted's house surgeon, J C Bloodgood then reported a reduced infection rate due to the use of gloves, with only 1 infection in 100 hernia repairs. [J Hopkins Hosp Rep 1899;223–63.]

Glove advocates such as Werner Zoege von Manteuffel (1857–1926), surgeon to the Tsar, stated in 1897 of their ability to protect the patient from infection. Jan Mikulicz -Radecki (1850-1905), was an asepsis champion who had trained under Bilroth, and worked in Königsberg before taking up his final position in Breslau. He was the first surgeon to abandon the operating theatre and to perform surgery in a purpose built operating room to facilitate aseptic surgery rather than performing under the gaze of an audience. He also promoted the wearing of gloves, trialing cotton, silk, and eventually rubber gloves. His name is associated with the Heinecke-Mikulicz, Mikulicz disease and he was the first to perform a gastroscopy [45, 46].

to have boiled rubber gloves is to have boiled hands.

Henri Chaput (1857–1919), Fig. 6.6, was a French surgeon advocate for surgical asepsis and aseptic techniques, one who also recommended the use of rubber gloves. This was despite his mentor, Octave Terrillon (see below), objecting to their ability to impair his sense of touch.

A senior French surgeon at the Salpêtrière Hospital, Octave

Terrillon (1844–1895), despite being an advocate for asepsis, Lister's techniques and the autoclave, decried the impact of gloves on the practice of surgery:

On the other hand patients could not gain by it because I would diminish the sense of touch of which I have the greatest need when, in an abdominal cavity, away from view, I examine all the organs attentively with my fingers. [44, 45]

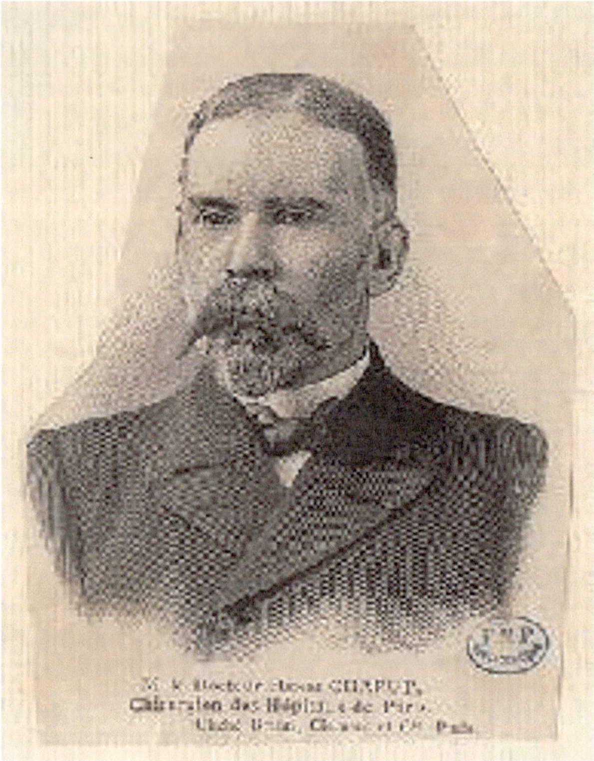

Fig. 6.6 Henri Chaput, Wimedia, public Domain. No restrictions. https://en.wikipedia.org/wiki/Henri_Chaput#/media/File:Chaput,_Henri_Victor_A._(1857-1919)_CIPA0130.jpg

RI Morris complained (in 1907),

> *The use of gloves made it necessary to use such long incisions that we could work by sight.... Long incisions are used for killing bears... the coming generation will not do the wizardlike work that was done by other operators.*

In 2023 Hernigou et al. reviewed operation photographs for the frequency of glove use and found that it took until 1950 for gloves to become ubiquitous and widely accepted in surgery [46, 47].

Today surgical gloves are made by a variety of manufacturers but the Australian company, Ansell, established in 1905 began producing rubber gloves in 1920 and in 1965 introduced gamma irradiation to enable the gloves supplied to be sterile. Alternatives to latex have been developed because of latex allergies and in the twenty-first century many surgical gloves are made of vinyl or nitrile products. And to mitigate the potential risk of transmission of viruses, most surgeons and their surgical teams wear two pairs of gloves. Not to wear gloves at all would, most probably, today generate an incident report.

6.6 The Discovery of Antibiotics

For most of the history of humanity we remained ignorant about the 99.99% of organisms on the planet, those unicellular organisms that inhabit and form our microbiome. They help us digest food and produce certain nutrients. Our microbiome protects us from other microbes and is directly associated with our health including our mental health. Some microbes have proved to be our best friends while others are a dangerous enemy.

6.6.1 Antibiotics in Ancient Times

The use of antibiotics dates back to millennia. The ancient Egyptians, for example, used moldy bread to treat infected wounds. The mould on the bread was actually a strain of Penicillium, which produces penicillin, one of the first antibiotics discovered in the modern era. However, the discovery and development of antibiotics as we know them today didn't occur until the early twentieth century, with the discovery of penicillin by Alexander Fleming in 1928 (Fig. 6.7) [48, 49]

In 2010, a study published in the journal *Nature* reported that traces of tetracycline, an antibiotic, were found in bones from ancient Sudanese Nubia, believed to date back to the period of 350–550 CE. The discovery suggested that the Nubians had been using tetracycline-containing plants to treat infections long before the modern discovery of antibiotics.

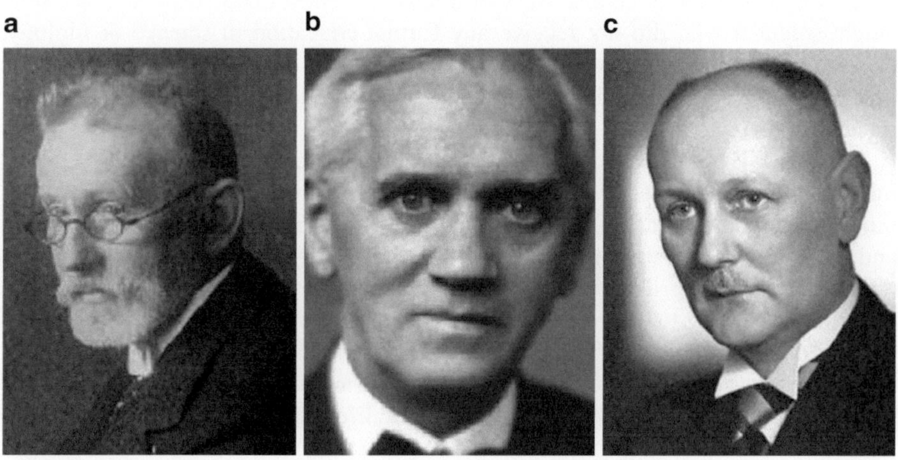

Fig. 6.7 (**a**) Paul Ehrlich, https://en.wikipedia.org/wiki/Paul_Ehrlich#/media/File:Paul_Ehrlich_1915.jpg and (**b**) Alexander Flemming, https://simple.wikipedia.org/wiki/Alexander_Fleming#/media/File:Alexander_Fleming_1945.jpg and (**c**) Gerhard Domagk, https://en.wikipedia.org/wiki/Gerhard_Domagk#/media/File:Gerhard_Domagk_nobel.jpg

Another study published in the journal *Lancet* in 2010, reported evidence of tetracycline use in ancient Egypt, identified by examining bone samples from several human remains. These dated to the late Roman period, around 350 to 550 CE. The study also found that the bones showed signs of tetracycline exposure. The tetracycline may have been obtained from the soil or the food supply, possibly through the consumption of moldy bread [49, 50].

Researchers have found that the red soils of Wadi Araba in Jordan have been used for centuries by Bedouin tribes as a remedy for skin infections. In recent years, scientists have discovered that these soils contain a number of bacteria that produce antibiotics, including some that are effective against antibiotic-resistant bacteria. This has led to increased interest in exploring natural sources for new antibiotics [48, 51].

Herbs used in traditional Chinese medicine have also been found to have antimicrobial properties. For example, extracts from plants like honeysuckle, *Scutellaria baicalensis*, and *Andrographis paniculata* have been shown to have antibacterial activity against a range of pathogens. Additionally, traditional Chinese medicinal formulas often include multiple herbs, some with antimicrobial properties to treat infections [52].

6.6.2 Anton van Leeuwenhoek

Surgery in the past was risky because it breaks tissue barriers so allows bacteria to gain access to sterile tissues which may succumb to infection and sepsis. Bacteria were first seen by Anton van Leeuwenhoek (1632–1723), a Dutch scientist famous for his contributions to the discovery of microorganisms. Leeuwenhoek was a self-taught scientist who did not receive any formal education in science or biology. Despite this, he made numerous advances in the field of microscopy and was the first person to observe and describe in detail, single-celled organisms such as bacteria and protozoa.

This discovery of small living creatures, which he called *animalcules*, using microscopes he designed himself was a major breakthrough in the study of microbiology. He communicated his findings to the Royal Society of London in 1676, and his work was subsequently published in the society's journal. Leeuwenhoek's observations of bacteria and other microorganisms laid the foundation for the study of bacteria, helping to establish the field of microbiology. Leeuwenhoek's discovery was also significant because it challenged the prevailing belief at the time that all living things could be seen with the naked eye, and it opened up new avenues of scientific inquiry into the world of microscopic life [53, 54]. It would be two centuries before it was understood that these bacteria that Leeuwenhoek had identified were the cause of surgical sepsis and many other infectious diseases.

It was in the late nineteenth century that the antibacterial properties of some chemicals were appreciated. Paul Ehrlich, a German physician and microbiologist (Fig 6.7a), noticed in that certain chemical dyes (synthetic aniline) coloured some bacterial cells but not others. He came to the conclusion that, according to this principle, it must be possible to create chemicals that can kill certain bacteria without harming other cells [54, 55].

Pyocyanase is an enzyme produced by the bacterium *Pseudomonas Aeruginosa*. It was first discovered by French biologist Ernest Duchesne (1874-1912) in 1894. This enzyme is involved in the breakdown of red blood cells and has been used in the past as a treatment for bacterial infections. It was first used as a topical application as it is toxic while its benefit was not proven.

6.6.3 William Osler (1892)

William Osler (1849–1919), a Canadian physician and one of the founding four Professors of Johns Hopkins Hospital, described the use of antistreptococcal serum for bacterial endocarditis. The serum was obtained from rabbits that had been immunized against streptococcal bacteria [55, 56].

In the late 1800s, bacterial endocarditis was a common and often fatal disease that affected the heart valves. Osler recognized that the disease was caused by bacteria and that the use of antiserum could potentially help to treat it. In collaboration with bacteriologist J.W. McFarland, they developed an antiserum against streptococci, obtained by immunizing rabbits. In 1892, Osler reported the first successful use of antistreptococcal serum to treat bacterial endocarditis in a patient at Johns Hopkins Hospital. The patient, a young woman with a history of rheumatic fever, had developed the disease and was not responding to any other treatments. After receiving the antiserum, her condition improved dramatically, and she eventually made a full recovery [54].

6.6.4 Ernest Duchesne (1897) MD Thesis on Penicillium glaucum

In 1897, Ernest Duchesne (1874–1912), a French medical student in Lyon, France, observed Arab stable boys treating saddle sores with mould that was propagated on their saddles. He took the mould *(Penicillium glaucum)* and used it to successfully treat induced typhoid in guinea pigs. His MD thesis was titled,

> *Contribution à l'étude de la concurrence vitale chez les micro-organismes: antagonisme entre les moisissures et les microbes*. (Contribution to the study of vital competition in micro-organisms: antagonism between molds and microbes).

However his work was largely ignored at the time and only rediscovered after Fleming's discovery of penicillin in 1928 [52, 53].

6.6.5 Paul Ehrlich and Salvarsan (1910)

Paul Ehrlich (1854-1915) (Fig. 6.7), Alfred Bertheim (1879-1915), and bacteriologist Sahachiro Hata (1873-1938) synthesized a large number of organo-arsenic derivatives from a toxic drug called Atoxyl in the early 1900s. They tested these derivatives on syphilis-infected rabbits. Syphilis is caused by the spirochete *Treponema pallidium*. The treatment at the time was inorganic mercury salts, but had unpleasant side effects and wasn't very effective. They eventually discovered a compound called arsphenamine, also known as Salvarsan, which was effective in treating syphilis. This became the first modern antibiotic. Salvarsan was marketed by the German pharmaceutical company Hoechst under the name Neosalvarsan (less toxic) and became a widely used treatment for syphilis until the availability of penicillin in the early 1940s. The mode of action of Salvarsan is still not fully understood despite its being over 100 years old.

Paul Ehrlich's discovery of arsphenamine in 1909 was the first modern antibiotic, although he referred to its use as "chemotherapy" rather than "antibiotic therapy." Because arsphenamine was effective against a bacteria it paved the way for the search for other antibiotics in the years to come.

Paul Ehrlich's systematic screening approach was a major milestone in drug discovery and development, with profound implications for the pharmaceutical industry. It laid the foundation for modern drug screening methods that led to the identification of many drugs, including antimicrobials.

6.6.6 Gerhard Domagk and Sulfonamides (1935–1939)

Gerhard Domagk (1895–1964) (Fig. 6.7) was the discoverer of the antibacterial activity against Streptococcus pyogenes of a sulfa drug, sulfonamidochrysoidine in 1935. That year, his daughter developed a Strepococcal infection in her arm which was about to lead to amputation. In desperation, Domagk gave her the sulfonamide he was working on and she recovered. It was first marketed as Prontosil in 1939, the first antibiotic to be released. Domagk received the 1939 Nobel prize in Physiology or Medicine. Sulphonamides allegedly saved the life of Winston Churchill [53, 56].

Sulfanilamide was relatively cheap to produce and off-patent, with a molecular structure that can be modified to create new derivatives offering the potential for improved properties. As a result, many companies started mass production of sulfonamide derivatives, leading to the widespread use of these drugs in the mid-twentieth century. The combination of a sulfonamide, sulfamethoxazole, with trimethoprim is still in use today.

While Alexander Fleming (1861–1955) is credited for discovering penicillin, Sir John Scott Burdon-Sanderson (1828–1905), a British physiologist, first described in 1870, how culture fluid covered in mould inhibits the growth of bacteria, although he did not investigate the mould further.

In 1871, Joseph Lister, a British surgeon and pioneer of antiseptic surgery, found that *Penicillium glaucum* had an antibacterial effect in human tissues. However, he did not pursue the research further. In 1875, John Tyndall, a British physicist and microbiologist, presented his experiments with *Penicillium notatum* to the Royal Society. He showed that the mould could kill some types of bacteria, but he also did not investigate the mould's antibacterial properties further [54, 57].

6.6.7 Alexander Fleming, Howard Florey, and Ernest Chain: The Discovery and Manufacture of Penicillin (1928–1941)

Alexander Fleming (Fig. 6.7) was a Scottish biologist and pharmacologist who is credited with discovering the first antibiotic, penicillin, in 1928. Fleming was studying bacteria in his laboratory at St. Mary's Hospital in London when he noticed that a mould, *Penicillium notatum*, had contaminated one of his petri dishes and was killing the bacteria growing in it. He concluded that the mould must be producing a substance that had antibacterial properties. Fleming named this substance penicillin and conducted further research to isolate and purify it. The fungus had created bacteria-free zones wherever it grew on the plate. Fleming isolated and grew the mould in pure culture. He discovered that *P. notatum* was highly effective even at very low concentrations, preventing S. aureus growth even when diluted 800 times, and was less toxic than the antiseptic agents used at the time [52, 58, 60].

However, it was not until the 1940s, when Australian, Howard Florey (1898–1968), and German, Ernst Chain (1906–1979) (who had fled Nazi Germany in 1933), at the University of Oxford developed methods for mass-producing penicillin, that penicillin became widely available for medical use. Howard Florey, Ernst Chain, and their colleagues at Oxford University made penicillin into a drug that saves lives. Their work on penicillin started in 1939 when wartime conditions were getting worse. The team needed to process 500 liters a week of mould filtrate. They did this by using animals and clinical trials. They began growing it in a variety of culture vessels such as baths, bedpans, and food tins. A team of "penicillin girls" was employed to look after the fermentation. In effect, the Oxford laboratory was being turned into a penicillin factory.

A 43-year-old policeman named Albert Alexander became the first recipient of penicillin from the Oxford University Hospital on February 12, 1941. He had cut himself while trying to prune some roses, and now he had a scratch on the side of his mouth, had developed a life-threatening infection with huge abscesses affecting his eyes, face, and lungs. He had been left in complete darkness, unable to see, and barely able to breathe. Penicillin was injected and within days he made a remarkable recovery [58, 60].

Penicillin revolutionized the treatment of bacterial infections and saved countless Allied lives after being trialled in World War II. By 1944, penicillin was used to treat infections in both the field and hospitals in Europe. Penicillin was dubbed "the wonder drug" at the end of World War II. Alexander Fleming shared the 1945 Nobel Prize in Medicine with Howard Florey and Ernst Chain for creating the first mass-produced antibiotic [58, 59].

6.6.8 Selman Waksman and Streptomycin (1943–1946)

The term antibiotic was first suggested by Jewish, Ukranian-born, Selman Waksman (1888–1973) at Rutgers University, New Jersey. His team discovered or developed several antibiotics, including streptomycin (and other aminoglycosides), the first effective treatment for tuberculosis.

Waksman, who had been studying soil microbes as a potential source of antibiotics, isolated streptomycin from a soil-dwelling bacterium called *Streptomyces griseus*. Streptomycin was the first antibiotic that was effective against tuberculosis, a disease that had long plagued humanity and had been responsible for millions of deaths over the centuries.

Streptomycin was actually discovered by Waksman's PhD student, Albert Schatz (1920–2005) in 1943. In 1944, Waksman and his team published a landmark paper describing the discovery of streptomycin and its effectiveness against tuberculosis in laboratory animals. Clinical trials of streptomycin in humans began soon after, and the results were promising. In 1946, the antibiotic was approved by the U.S. Food and Drug Administration for the treatment of tuberculosis, and it was quickly adopted as the standard treatment for the disease.

Streptomycin marked a major breakthrough in the fight against infectious diseases and sparked a new era of antibiotic research and development. It also earned Waksman the Nobel Prize in Physiology or Medicine in 1952. However, Schatz was never duly acknowledged for his discovery and this led to a legal challenge and change in US legislation.

Today, streptomycin is still used as a treatment for certain types of bacterial infections, although its use is often limited due to concerns about antibiotic resistance and potential side effects.

In total, Waksman's team discovered over 20 antibiotics [55].

6.6.8.1 Vancomycin (1952)

In the early 1950s, the pharmaceutical company Eli Lilly launched a program called the "Antibiotic Screening Program" to discover new antibiotics. As part of this program, the company solicited soil samples from around the world, including samples from remote and exotic locations. Christian missionaries were among the people recruited to collect soil samples, as they travelled to many remote areas and were often willing to participate in the program. In 1952, a soil sample collected from the island of Borneo by a Christian missionary named Father Edward J. McHugh was found to contain *Streptomyces orientalis*, a bacterium that produced a potent antibiotic called vancomycin. Vancomycin became an important antibiotic for the treatment of serious infections, particularly those caused by antibiotic-resistant bacteria, and is still used today in clinical practice.

6.6.8.2 Macrolide Antibiotics and Erythromycin (1950s)

Macrolide antibiotics were discovered in the 1950s, following the work of Filipino scientist Abelardo B. Aguilar (1917-1993). Aguilar was working as a researcher at the Philippine General Hospital when he discovered erythromycin, the first macrolide antibiotic.

6.6.8.3 Methicillin (1959)

In the late 1940s and early 1950s, resistance to penicillin and other antibiotics became a significant problem, leading to a search for new antibiotics and modifications to existing ones. In 1959, Beecham scientists developed methicillin, a β-lactam antibiotic that was resistant to the penicillinase enzymes that many bacteria produce to inactivate penicillin. Methicillin was one of the first members of a new class of antibiotics called the methicillin-resistant staphylococcus aureus (MRSA) antibiotics. Unfortunately, MRSA strains quickly emerged that were resistant to methicillin and other β-lactam antibiotics, leading to the use and/or development of new classes of antibiotics, such as vancomycin and linezolid, to treat these infections. The widespread use of antibiotics in the following decades led to the emergence of resistance in many other bacterial species, including *Streptococcus pneumoniae*, *Escherichia coli*, and *Neisseria gonorrhoeae*. To combat this growing problem, in addition to methicillin and other penicillinase-resistant β-lactams mentioned above, the tetracyclines, macrolides, aminoglycosides, and their derivates were developed. However, the bacteria, in their struggle for survival, continued to evolve and develop new mechanisms of resistance, so the ongoing search for new antibiotics remained a constant challenge for scientists and clinicians.

6.6.8.4 Cephalexin and the Cephalosporins (1948–1967)

Cephalosporins are a class of antibiotics that were first discovered in 1948 by Italian microbiologist Giuseppe Brotzu (1895–1976). *Cephalosporium acremonium*, which was found in a sewage outfall off the coast of Sardinia. However, it was not until the 1960s that the cephalosporins were purified and further developed for clinical use. Cephalexin, a first-generation cephalosporin, was introduced in 1967 and became widely used for the treatment of a variety of bacterial infections. Other cephalosporins followed, including cefazolin, a first-generation cephalosporin that is commonly used as prophylaxis against infections in surgical procedures. Ceftazidime, a third-generation cephalosporin antibiotic with activity against *Pseudomonas aeruginosa*, was introduced in the late 1970s. It was one of the first antibiotics specifically designed to target this difficult-to-treat bacterium, which is a common cause of nosocomial infections in hospitals [52, 55].

Cephalosporins are structurally similar to penicillin, and like penicillin, they work by inhibiting bacterial cell wall synthesis. However, cephalosporins are more resistant to bacterial enzymes that break down penicillin, making them effective against a wider range of bacteria. Today, cephalosporins are an important class of antibiotics and are used to treat a variety of infections, from mild to severe.

In 1975, the Journal of Antimicrobial Chemotherapy published a paper describing the antimicrobial activity of cefamandole, another cephalosporin antibiotic. The discovery of cefamandole's activity against *Pseudomonas aeruginosa* was serendipitous, as the drug was originally developed for its activity against Gram-positive bacteria. Cefamandole's activity against *Pseudomonas aeruginosa* paved the way for the development of other cephalosporin antibiotics with similar activity, including ceftazidime. Today, third- and fourth generation cephalosporins remain an important class of antibiotics used to treat a wide range of bacterial infections, including those caused by *Pseudomonas aeruginosa* [52, 57, 59].

6.6.8.5 β-Lactamase Inhibitors (1976)

Bacterial β-lactamase inhibitors were first discovered as a byproduct of Streptomyces in 1976. These inhibitors, including clavulanic acid, can help to restore the activity of βlactam antibiotics, such as penicillins and cephalosporins, against bacteria that produce β-lactamase enzymes that would normally inactivate these antibiotics [55, 57, 58, 60].

6.6.8.6 Imipenem and the Carbapenems (1980s)

Thienamycin is a naturally occurring antibiotic produced by the bacteria *Streptomyces cattleya*. It was discovered in the 1970s and was found to be highly effective against a broad spectrum of bacteria. However, it was not suitable for use in humans due to its rapid degradation in the body. In the 1980s, researchers modified the structure of thienamycin to create imipenem, a semi-synthetic antibiotic that is more stable in the body and has a longer half-life. Imipenem is part of the class of antibiotics known as carbapenems, which are highly effective against many types of bacteria, including some that are resistant to other antibiotics. It is commonly used to treat serious bacterial infections, such as sepsis and pneumonia, and is considered a "last resort" antibiotic for the treatment of antibiotic-resistant infections [58].

6.6.8.7 Nalidixic Acid

Nalidixic acid (accidentally discovered in the 1960s by George Lesher) is an antibiotic that belongs to the class of drugs known as quinolones. It was the first synthetic quinolone antibacterial to be developed and was introduced for clinical use in the 1960s. Nalidixic acid is primarily used to treat urinary tract infections caused by susceptible strains of bacteria, including *Escherichia coli, Klebsiella pneumoniae, and Proteus mirabilis*. It works by interfering with the DNA synthesis of bacteria, thereby preventing their growth and replication [60, 61].

6.6.8.8 Oxazolidinone Antibiotics

Cycloserine, the first oxazolidinone antibiotic to be discovered, was approved for the treatment of tuberculosis in the 1950s. However, it is no longer a first-line treatment due to its toxicity and the development of drug-resistant strains of the bacteria that cause TB. Linezolid is a newer oxazolidinone antibiotic that was approved in 2000. It is active against a broad range of Gram-positive bacteria, including MRSA and VRE. Linezolid inhibits bacterial protein synthesis, which kills bacteria. It's used to treat pneumonia, skin and soft tissue infections, and certain bloodstream infections [60, 61].

In recent years, the emergence of multidrug-resistant bacteria has become a major challenge for clinicians, particularly in the intensive care setting, where patients are often more susceptible to infections and have weakened immune systems. Infections caused by pan-resistant bacteria, such as Acinetobacter, Enterobacteriaceae, and Pseudomonas, are particularly difficult to treat because they are resistant to multiple classes of antibiotics, leaving clinicians with few options for effective treatment. As a result, the development of new antibiotics and alternative treatments has become a critical area of research in the field of infectious diseases [61, 62].

6.7 The History of Anaesthesia

6.7.1 Introduction

Through the ages human have used many methods to get rid of the pain inflicted by a surgical procedure. The Sumerian 3000 BC resorted to compressing the carotid arteries to make the patient unconscious so they don't feel the pain. Ancient Egyptian used snow to cause analgesia by hypothermia; the Chinese developed acupuncture to treat pain. Other methods like knocking-down and physical restraint were cruel measures that had been tried.

In the medieval times, potions for pain control included alcohol plant extracts, such as mandrake root. Opium was widely used, particularly in China, and the first documented intravenous injection of opium was recorded in the 1660s. Pain relief in an arm or a leg was produced by squeezing the nerves in the upper part of the limb and also by applying snow. Hypnosis was often used for pain control in the eighteenth century.

There was no real anaesthesia until the middle of the nineteenth century, these developments happened owing to progress in science, particularly in chemistry and human physiology.

It had been argued that modern surgery began in 1846 in Boston when it then became possible to induce reversible unconsciousness by inhalation of a volatile chemical gas. Hence the 16th of October 1846, was the day that revolutionized surgery, at Massachusetts General Hospital. This was the day that dentist William Morton, (Fig. 6.8), in front of an audience, used ether to painlessly extract a tooth. This demonstration sparked off considerable controversy regarding who was the first to use an anaesthetic gas for medical purposes. As with many medical advances there were others less willing or less able to promote themselves in surgical history [63].

It is difficult to understand today how major this advance was. Before this, surgery was a terrifying last resort in a final attempt to save life and associated with intense suffering. The operations performed were limited to skin surgery, limb amputation, excision of ulcerating tumors, and removal of bladder stones. The inside of the abdomen, chest and skull were "no go" zones. Speed was an essential factor for success. Most patients were held or strapped down, many of them died on the table or shortly after. Major surgical procedures were for the desperate or dying.

The New York Herald reported a terrifying account of an amputation performed before the introduction of anaesthesia on 21 July 1841:

> *The case was an interesting one of a white swelling, for which the thigh was to be amputated. The patient was a youth of about fifteen, pale, thin but calm and firm. One Professor felt for the femoral artery, had the leg held up for a few moments to ensure the saving of blood, the compress part of the tourniquet was placed upon the artery and the leg held up by an assistant. The white swelling was fearful, frightful. A little wine was given to the lad; he was pale but resolute; his Father supported his head and left hand. A second Professor took the long, glittering knife, felt for the bone, thrust in the knife carefully but rapidly. The boy screamed terribly; the tears went down the Father's cheeks. The first cut from the inside was completed, and the bloody blade of the knife issued from the quivering wound, the blood flowed by the pint, the sight was sickening; the screams terrific; the operator calm.* [63, 64]

6.7.1.1 The Discovery of Anaesthetic Gases

The end of the eighteenth century saw increasing research in the field of chemistry including gases. Joseph Black discovered carbon dioxide, Henry Cavendish discovered hydrogen, Antoine-Laurent de Lavoisier nitrogen and oxygen.

Among his many achievements, Joseph Priestley (1733–1804) discovered nitrous oxide (NO) and its analgesic effects were recognized shortly after. Priestly also described its use for headaches and other pains as a cold application as early as 1794. That was accompanied by increasing knowledge of the physiology of the heart and lungs. The therapeutic possibilities for gases were explored, although many of its practitioners were charlatans happy to defraud a gullible public. However, Thomas Beddoes (1760–1808), once Black's student, a physician and public health advocate, established a Pneumatic Institute near Bristol in 1798, to study the medicinal effects of inhalation of different gases on tuberculosis.

In 1799 Humphrey Davy (1778–1829), who was studying nitrous oxide at the Bristol institute, coined the term "laughing gas" after inhaling it himself at the encouragement of Beddoes. In the nineteenth century, laughing parties became popular in Britain through inhalation of nitrous oxide gas.

In 1800, he also suggested inhalation of nitrous oxide might be used during surgical operations, but this was not followed up.

> *As nitrous oxide in its extensive operation appears capable of destroying physical pain, it may probably be used with advantage during surgical operations.*

Nitrous oxide was the first gas to be used for pain reduction and induction of sleep in animals.

In 1818, Michael Faraday (1791–1867) discovered that ether had similar, but better, analgesic properties to nitrous oxide.

Ether had been originally synthesised (by the action of sulphuric acid on ethanol) in the 13th century by a Catalan monk, Ramon Llull. He called this liquid "sweet vitriol," the effects of which were studied on chickens in the renaissance by a Swiss doctor, Paracelsus (1493-1541). Then in 1730, a German chemist, August London Sigmund Frobenius, gave the compound ether (Greek = heaven) its name. Ether was originally a term used to describe all volatile gases. Sulphuric (di-ethyl) ether (CH_3-CH_2-O-CH_2-CH_3) is what is known as ether today, and Chloric ether ($CHCl_3$) is now known as chloroform. Muriatic ether (CH_3-CH_2-Cl) was recognized for its cold, temporary, local anaesthetic properties and is still in use in emergency departments today as ethyl chloride.

6.7.1.2 Ether Anaesthesia

A review of the Boston Medical and Surgical Journal (the forerunner of the New England Medical Journal) from its first issue in 1824 to 1846 show there were a number of isolated case reports of medicinal ethers generally applied topically, sometimes ingested, particularly for a cold application for headaches.

The first deliberate use of surgical anaesthesia was in January 1842. William E. Clarke (1819–1898), while a medical student in Rochester (NY), provided dentist, Elijah Pope (1818–1856), with ether to extract a tooth. Clarke did not graduate in medicine until 1849. Clarke's professor believed the female patient, a Miss

Hobbie, had had a hysterical attack and so Clarke, who went on to become a surgeon in Michigan and Chicago, was never fully aware of his role in the discovery of anaesthesia. The Clarke/Pope procedure was, however, observed by one William Thomas Green Morton who was also at the time a medical student.

The next use of surgical anaesthesia using ether was by Crawford Williamson Long (1815–1878) practicing in Jefferson, Georgia, USA, on 30th March 1842. This was four years before William Morton's demonstration of ether anaesthesia in Boston. Clarke removed a tumour painlessly from the neck. He performed a second operation two months later and then amputated a burned toe on July 3rd of 1842. However, Long was discouraged from continuing his use of anaesthesia by a fear of being regarded as a quack and a concern that potential side effects might end his career and jeopardise his livelihood. He also felt he hadn't accumulated enough evidence despite doing a further 8 minor procedures. He did not publish his findings until 1849 by which time anaesthesia with both ether and chloroform were a worldwide innovation. It was only in 1990, that the 30th March became known as "Doctor's Day" in honour of Crawford Williamson Long, with the official sanction for the holiday signed into law by President George Herbert Walker Bush.

In 1844, in Boston, G.Q. Colton and the dentist, Horace Wells (1815–1848), successfully used nitrous oxide as an anesthetic for tooth extraction.

Elton Romeo Smilie (1819–1889) qualified from Vermont's Castleton Medical College in 1842 and started practice in Derry, New Hampshire. Tooth extraction was the commonest surgical procedure performed at that time. Smilie's technique was to mix opium in ether in a glass retort and heat the solution to cause slow evaporation which the patient then inhaled. Smilie wrongly assumed it was the opium that was providing the anaesthesia when it was in fact the ether which boils at 35 °C. He wrote to the Boston Medical and Surgical Journal on October 28th prior to the publication of Bigelow's (November 18th) and Warren's (December 9th) accounts of William T G Morton's ether anaesthetic given on 16th October.

William Thomas Green Morton (1819–1868), Fig. 6.8.

Morton was someone from a farming background who exuded confidence and could persuade people to trust him. This was somewhat surprising in that he was wanted by the law for fraud and embezzlement of funds. This did not stop him from beginning dental studies in Baltimore in 1840. He then moved to Connecticut to study under Horace Wells. He and Wells moved to Boston to market a dental prosthesis they had designed. He started as a medical student at Harvard in 1844 but would not graduate, only receiving an honorary MD from Baltimore in 1852. He received advice from Charles Thomas Jackson (1805–1880) a chemist and prominent physician. He had watched Wells administer nitrous oxide and also that Clarke had used ether. At the time of the demonstration, Morton tried to conceal that his anaesthetic agent was ether, hoping to gain financial rewards.

However, at the Massachusetts General Hospital in Boston, on October 16th 1846, Morton successfully used ether as an anaesthetic during a surgical operation. The operation, per- formed by the Boston surgeon John Collins Warren (1778–1856), was to remove a tumor from a man's lower jaw *making "….an incision some inches in length,"* marking the first recorded use of general anesthesia in surgery. The

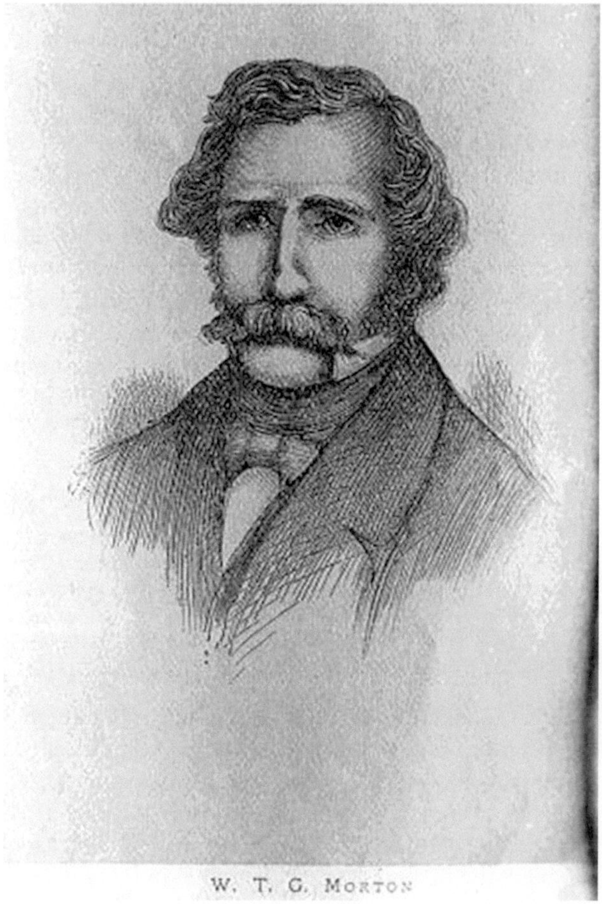

Fig. 6.8 William Thomas Green Morton (1819–1868) Merton. Wikicommons, licence: public domain. https://commons.wikimedia.org/w/index.php?search=Wtg+Morton&title=Special:MediaSearch&go=Go&type=image

following day *"a fatty tumour of considerable size was removed by Dr Hayward [1791-1863], from the arm of a woman near the deltoid muscle."* A third operation, an amputation, was performed by Hayward on November 7th. A few weeks later Oliver Wendell Holmes coined the word "anaesthesia." He used the word to describe "insensibility."

Jurgan Thorwald wrote in the "Century of the Surgeon."

> *A young man lay quietly under Warren's knife, uttering not a sound, unstirring, in a state of merciful insensibility, feeling none of the inconceivable pain that countless human beings had endured before him. Our whole world was transformed by an operation that lasted only a few minutes. A light burst forth from the darkness of those days, so bright that its first flash blinded us.*

Morton claimed to be the discoverer of anaesthesia, something which was later vigorously contested by Wells and Jackson. This led to series of legal cases. Bigelow supported Morton's on the basis that Morton had demonstrated ether as an agent possessed the three necessary qualities—completeness, inevitability, and safety.

Henry Jacob Bigelow (1818–90) graduated from Harvard Medical School in 1841 and, in 1844, set up practice in Boston and was appointed a visiting surgeon to MGH in 1846. Bigelow had already experience of publishing papers and he was the first to formally publish an account of *"Insensibility during surgical operations produced by inhalation"* in the Boston Medical and Surgical Journal.

From 1821 to 1846 the annual reports of MGH recorded on 333 surgeries, representing about one per month. With Morton's demonstration, anaesthesia had come alive, (Fig. 6.8), and Bigelow was to be the one giving the anaesthesia in subsequent years. The first successful hysterectomy was performed in 1855 (under chloroform), the first gall bladder lithotomy in 1868, the first thyroidectomy in 1880, and the first brain tumor resection in 1884. There was considerable bias, controversy, and sectarian division concerning the safety of ether as an anaesthetic agent, particularly when rendering the patient unconscious. For example, in Philadelphia anaesthesia was regarded as a "Boston phenomenon" and banned for some seven years. The agent was sometimes blamed for surgical deaths even days after the operation.

Following Bigelow's death Oliver Wendall Holmes (1809–94) said of the surgeon

> *No person took hold of Dr Morton's discovery with such far-seeing, almost prophetic appreciation, as the young surgeon who had been but a few years in practice, and threw all the energy of his early manhood into his advocacy of the new and starling innovation which was destined to change the whole impact of surgery. It was not merely his sagacious foresight that he recognized the importance of this epoch-making novelty, but throughout its subsequent history he was the foremost champion of artificial anaesthesia.*

Ether quickly became the most commonly used anaesthetic in the United States and Europe, and general anaesthesia rapidly spread throughout the world. In December that year Dr. Francis Boott has a tooth extracted before a group which included Robert Liston (London leading surgeon). Liston was so impressed he arranged to perform an amputation under ether vapour on at University College Hospital, the first public demonstration in Britain.

6.7.1.3 Chloroform Anaesthesia

Chloroform was first produced in 1831, by both Samuel Guthrie in the USA and Eugene Soubeiran in France. As discussed above, it was originally called chloric ether (CHCl3).

On 19th January, 1847, James Simpson (1811–1870), an Edinburgh Obstetrician used ether to manage an obstructed labor achieving a version and breech extraction. In November 1847, he was the first to use chloroform, another etheric volatile compound.

> *Three and half hours after [labor] commenced, and ere the first stage of labor was completed, I placed her under the influence of chloroform, by moistening, with half a teaspoonful of the liquid, a pocket handkerchief, rolled up into a funnel shape, and with the broad or open end of the funnel placed over her mouth and nostrils. In consequence of the evaporation of the fluid, it was once more renewed in about ten or twelve minutes. The child was expelled in about twenty-five minutes after the inhalation was begun. The mother sub-*

sequently remained longer soporose that commonly happens after ether. The squalling of the child did not, as usual, rouse her; and some minutes elapsed after the placenta was expelled, and after the child was removed by a nurse into another room, before the patient awoke. She then turned round and observed to me that she had 'enjoyed a very comfortable sleep....'

Chloroform relieved labour pain though some objected on religious grounds that God had intended women to suffer pain in child bearing (Genesis 3). However, chloroform became the anaesthetic of choice in many countries, particularly in the United Kingdom and Germany. Simpson also described the first anaesthetic death in 1848, the patient being a 15-year-old girl, Hannah Greer. She was the first of many who suffered sudden heart failure under chloroform, although for decades clinicians were unsure whether chloroform exerted its adverse effects through the respiratory system or on the heart. Despite a number of inconclusive commissions into the safety of chloroform in the UK between 1864 and 1910 it was only in 1911, that animal experiments demonstrate that chloroform can cause fibrillation. Between 1865 and 1920 chloroform was used for over 80% of all general anesthesia in both UK and Germany [65–67].

Velpeau, Professor of Surgery in Paris, stated:

On the subject of ether ... it is a wonderful and terrible agent.
I will say of chloroform that it is still more wonderful and more terrible!

Chloroform proved highly addictive for those who chose to use it for comfort, pleasure, or entertainment. Soon after the introduction of chloroform, the dentist of nitrous oxide fame, Howard Wells (1815–1848), died from the adverse effects of chloroform [68].

Robert M Glover (1815–1859) in UK suffered a similar fate a decade later. Glover trained in Edinburgh becoming a Licentiate of the Royal College of Surgeons in 1837, studying in Paris in 1838 and gaining an MD in 1840. His thesis was on the medical and physiological properties of bromine and its compounds. From 1839, he taught in the Newcastle school of medicine. His research was focused on bromine, iodine, and chlorine compounds including chloroform and dichlorethane. He won the Gold Medal of the Haverian society in 1842, describing the pharmacological action of chloroform, 5 years before J P Flouren's report of the anaesthetic action of ether and chloroform on dogs. Glover also injected chloroform into the jugular veins of two dogs who became transiently unconscious. He missed the significance of this effect and was more concerned about the engorgement of the pulmonary veins and capillaries he found at autopsy. James Simpson was not aware of Glover's paper on the topic, written in 1842, when he gave the first chloroform anaesthetic as described above but acknowledged Glover's research when made aware of it (by Glover). Glover later gave anaesthesia for surgeons at Newcastle Royal Infirmary and wrote articles on chloroform. He also assisted with the autopsy of Hannah Greener, the first victim of chloroform, in January 1848, noting the same pulmonary congestion in her autopsy that he had found in the dogs six years earlier. Glover left Newcastle in 1853, after an unhappy period involving the dissolution of the medical school with two rival schools established in their place, one led by Glover. He moved to London, taught chemistry at the Royal Free Hospital Medical School and may have given chloroform anaesthesia there for surgeons Frederick J Gant and Thomas H Wakely, the latter the founding editor of the Lancet. However, his clinical work was by then deteriorating, and the Medical Committee sent him a reprimand, censuring him for not taking his LRCP. Glover and Gant then joined the British forces in the Crimea during 1855–1856. He returned having suffered severe dysentery for which he had taken opium and chloroform, then commonly prescribed to treat bowel conditions. However, his return to London found him addicted to both. Despite this he passed the LRCP in July 1856, and continued to publish papers and books while his life and finances deteriorated. He died in 1859 from an overdose of chloroform. Surgeons Gant and Wakely performed his autopsy.

The first ether anaesthetic in England was administered by a London dentist, James Robinson on 19th December 1846. In 1843, John Snow (1813–1858), a London physician, was already experimenting with ether in his laboratory. Within 2 years of Robinson's demonstration, Snow was the most accomplished anaesthetist in the British Isles and published a practical guide *On the Inhalation of ether* in 1847. He developed an apparatus to more accurately administer ether that took account of the temperature. In 12 years of practice he recorded more than 5000 anaesthesia cases, that included dental extractions, lithotomy, lithotripsy, excision of breast tumors, treatments of haemorrhoids, repair of anal fistulae, repair of cleft lips, and anaesthesia for childbirth. He studied chloroform as well as ether. In 1853, he was asked to provide a chloroform anaesthetic in 1853 during the birth of Queen Victoria's eighth child, Prince Leopold, and again 3 years later with Princess Beatrice [69–72].

John Snow (1813–1858) inhaled chloroform and also performed assays on the gas in his exhaled breath. At a similar time, Claude Bernard (1813–1878) in France developed a silver nitrate assay to study chloroform levels in blood and urine. John Snow was not only an anaesthetist, but a physician and one of the fathers of epidemiology. He is famous for his investigation into the 1848 cholera outbreak in London when his pioneering work recording cholera's incidence in London's 32 subdistricts and led to his proposing that cholera was a water-borne infection in a paper *On the Mode of Communication of Cholera*. During the 1853–54 outbreak he correctly identified the source of cholera to be the Golden Square water pump on Broad Street which had even developed an offensive smell. His view on the spread of cholera was contested until after his death, when during the 1866 outbreak of cholera, his theory was finally accepted [68, 73, 74].

Late in the century, clinicians learned the hard way that although chloroform decomposes at flame temperatures, in the vicinity of flames and lit candles it liberates the toxic phosgene gas. In 1899 two physicians and a nurse were attending a forceps obstetrical delivery under chloroform while the room was lit by three gas flames. All of the attendants other than the patient suffered choking, stinging respiratory symptoms and only survived by ventilating the room and switching to ether.

6.8 Local Anaesthesia

Ancient civilizations prepared plant extracts for topical use that contained poppy juice, Indian hemp, mandrake, and/or alcohol. Ball and Westhorpe also mention lizard fat, pulverised crocodile skin used by the Chinese, and stone of Memphis rubbed with vinegar by the Egyptians.

Early attempts to create local anaesthesia and/or numbness were limited to local compression or cooling. In Naples, Marcus Aurelius Servino (1580–1656) performed tracheostomies and mastectomies in the early sixteenth century, with the help of snow cracked ice applied to the operation site. A Danish professor of surgery, Thomas Bartholin (1616–1680) learned Servino's technique while visiting Naples and was the first to document the technique of refrigeration anaesthesia in chapter 22 of his book, *De nivis usu medico observationes variae.* Bartholin was also the first to describe the lymphatic system.

In 1812, Dominique Jean, (later Baron) Larrey (1766–1842), chief surgeon to Napoleon, performed amputations on the war wounded during the Russian winter and noted, when the outside temperature got as cold as -30C, that they were almost painless. At the battle of Borodino he performed 200 amputations in a day. During his military career Larrey developed the concept of ambulances to transport the injured rapidly from the battlefield, and also a system of triage.

James Arnott promoted refrigeration anaesthesia using frozen ice and salt though the methodology to produce this "congelation" was difficult to reproduce. Benjamin Ward Richardson (1828–1896) designed a pumping method with ether spray, later replaced by ethyl chloride which was easier to use as it does not require pumping [75, 76].

6.8.1 Cocaine

Cocaine is toxic, addictive, has a short duration of action and is expensive to manufacture. It was first used as a local anaesthetic in 1884, by an Austrian ophthalmologist, Karl Köller (1857–1944). Köller moved to New York in 1888. Although Sigmund Freud (1856–1959) was aware of the pathophysiological effects of cocaine and provided small samples of the drug to his Viennese colleagues including Köller, it was Köller who was experimenting on animals, himself, and colleagues and who discovered the local anaesthetic properties of cocaine and used it to operate on the eye.

In 1880, in the Department of Pharmacology, a young researcher, Vassily von Anrep working under the supervision of Joseph Rossbach, published a paper in which he recommended to "*try cocaine as a local anaesthetic in persons of melancholy disposition*." Köller and colleagues noted the numbing effect of cocaine on his tongue; on the cornea of a frog, rabbit and dog, before trying it on themselves and then operating on the eye of a patient.

It was only in 1895, that Willstätter and others established that the LA properties were due to esterification of basic alcohol with benzoic acid, enabling a whole range of chemical variations to be developed and trialed. One of these, Stovaine, was manufactured in Paris in 1904, and was less toxic and more stable than cocaine. It was used also for spinal anaesthesia, though by the 1920s was considered unsuitable for local infiltration.

Procaine (Novocaine) was the next local anaesthetic to be introduced to clinical practice in 1905 by Professor Heinrich Braun (1862–1934). It is soluble in water, less irritating to the tissues, stable to allow boiling (and thus sterilization) and could be combined with adrenaline. It was to become the preferred local anaesthetic until lignocaine (lidocaine or xylocaine) which was only released in 1948. It was discovered somewhat by accident Swedish researchers, Nils Löfgren and Bengt Lundqvist who tested a series of anilides with anaesthetic properties. Initially, they tested their properties by topical application on their tongues, until they decided to study the properties of an anilide, LL30, when injected in animals. It proved less irritant to tissues, more effective, had a longer duration of action and could have adrenaline added to achieve vasoconstriction. Löfgren and Lundqvist sold their patent to Astra but despite gaining wealth, Löfgren was excluded from subsequent research grants and opportunities and became depressed, taking his own life aged 53. Lundqvist died at the age of 30 from a cerebral hemorrhage after a day of diving under his yacht to clean it [75–77].

The potential for spinal anaesthesia was discovered by accident in 1885 when Leonard Corning injected some cocaine into a dog and accidentally paralysed its hindquarters. His attempts at a true spinal injection of cocaine were probably limited by his knowledge of anatomy. The technique of lumbar puncture was described on five adults and five children in 1891 by Heinrich Irenäus Quincke (1842–1922) in Berlin. He acknowledged the earlier work of an English physician, Walter Essex Winter (1860–1945), who, while a registrar, had performed lumbar puncture on four children with meningitis, all of whom died. The first spinal anaesthetic was administered following Quinke's technique by German surgeon, August Bier (1861–1949), in 1898. In 1908 he also pioneered intravenous regional anaesthesia (Bier's block). In the USA, Babcock was one of the early adopters of spinal anaesthesia between 1910 and 1920, utilizing a solution of Stovaine with strychnine, lactic acid and alcohol. *"The strychnine was to fortify the nerves, the lactic acid to keep Stovaine in solution and alcohol to reduce the specific gavity and ensure a sterile solution."* [78–80]

In England, Arthur Barker, Professor of Surgery at University College Hospital, London, used 5% Stovaine with 5% glucose and distilled water for spinal anaesthesia. He published a report of over 2500 cases between 1907 and 1912.

> *In arranging our own collection of 2,354 cases in the same way .... it will be seen that there were 13 (0.5%) failures to enter the dura in 2,354 cases, of which 3 belong to my own first 100 cases; there were 6 (0.2%) of absence of any analgesia on injection, of which 4 occurred in my own first 100 cases, 2 in the next 200, none since. Then there were100 cases in which after injection the analgesia was insufficient for the completion of the operation (4.2%). So that the technical drawbacks in our 2,354 cases which required the administration of a general anaesthetic (often only a drachm or two), and including failures to enter the dural sac, were in the gross 100=4.2 per cent.* [81, 82]

The first epidural block was performed in 1921 by Fidel Pagés (1886–1923), a Spanish military surgeon. His 1921 article, *Anestesia Metamérica* described the anatomy and technique of access to the thoracolumbar epidural space. Pagés acknowledged the work of the French physicians Fernand Cathelin and Jean-Athanse Sicard, who, in 1901, independently developed the caudal injection as a method for accessing the sacral epidural space. Tragically he died in a car crash at the age of 37. The benefit of epidurals is primarily perioperative pain relief and obstetric analgesia. Initially, Pagés' technique did not attract much attention until 1933, when Argentinian surgeon, Alberto Guttierez (1892–1945), developed the hanging drop technique and gave credit to Pagés earlier pioneering work. An Italian surgeon, Achille Dogliotti (1897–1966), who had, in 1933, described the reproducible loss of resistance sign of entering the epidural space but only belatedly (in 1939) acknowledged Pagés primacy in response to Guttierez's writings on epidurals [83–86].

6.9 Airway Management and Protection

Although Benjamin Pugh, an English obstetrician, described an air-pipe for neonatal resuscitation in 1754, the first endotracheal intubations were utilized for resuscitation of drowning victims and for those suffering from laryngeal diphtheria [13]. Great advances in resuscitation were made by societies created in Amsterdam, Paris, London, Venice, and Philadelphia to rescue drowning victims from the water.

6.9.1 William McEwen (1878)

In 1878, William McEwen (1848–1924), a Scottish surgeon based at Glasgow Royal Infirmary, performed the first endotracheal intubation through the mouth as an alternative to tracheotomy, allowing the patient to breathe despite glottic oedema while receiving general anaesthesia with chloroform.

McEwen was also a pioneer in neurosurgery, successfully resecting a frontal meningioma based on focal clinical signs and for his treatment of brain abscess, mastoiditis, and sinus infections. In the decades before X-rays, he had to localize the site of a brain lesion based on clinical presentation alone [87].

6.9.2 Sir Ivan Magill (1888–1986)

Ivan Magill was born in Ireland, graduated from Queen's University, Belfast in 1913, and served as a Captain in the Royal Army Medical Corps during World War I. At qualification Magill was issued a certificate confirming he had given one anaesthetic. At the time the only gaseous anaesthetics available were ether, chloroform, ethyl chloride, and nitrous oxide. In 1919, after the war he was posted to Sidcup hospital in Kent, where the New Zealand surgeon, Harold Gillies, was reconstructing horrendous facial injuries. The best available method for general anaesthesia was endotracheal insufflation through the mouth or nose using a single gum elastic catheter, with air driven by a motorized pump and vaporized ether. One day, Gilles said to Magill:

> *Maggi – you seem to get this anaesthetic into the patient alright, don't you think you could devise some method of getting it out, so that I am not anaesthetized?*

A solution was found in 1922, when Magill passed a second tube through a patient's nose to counter expiratory obstruction and labored breathing. This two-tube technique also allowed the pharynx to be packed. In Europe a double channeled catheter was used. Magill then explored the use of nasotracheal intubation as it provided better surgical access to the mouth and in 1928, he described the technique of blind nasal intubation with a curved tube, lubricated with paraffin and aided by cocainization to numb the larynx and fauces to aid the process. Magill then introduced a wide bore tube which allowed to and from breathing [87].

Magill published a description of his forceps in 1920, their grasp causing no injury to the end of the insufflation catheter then used. Magill's forceps are still in use today, particularly for the removal of foreign bodies in the pharynx and larynx. In 1921, he described an apparatus that delivered warm ether in air by insufflation and in 1923, a second apparatus for the administration of nitrous oxide, oxygen, and ether. The Magill attachment combines a breathing tube, reservoir bag, and expiratory valve for spontaneous respiration. Magill published a description of an improved laryngoscope in 1926. Once the work at Sidcup reduced Magill moved to the Westminster and Brompton hospitals and made important contributions to anesthesia for thoracic surgery. For thoracoplasty (performed for tuberculosis) he initially preferred the use of nitrous oxide and oxygen by face-piece administration. In the 1930s he added cyclopropane if diathermy was required but maintained that endotracheal intubation was only necessary if suction was required in lobectomy or pneumonectomy for bronchiectasis. Collapse of the relevant lung was achieved by endotracheal anesthesia plus a catheter passed into the bronchus of the affected side for suction when required, or passage of the tube into the non-operated side and inflation of a cuff at the carina, or a suction catheter with a balloon to close off the bronchus could also be passed into the affected side.

Magill practiced throughout World War II, and in the early years of the National Health Service (NHS) until 1955. He gave his last anaesthetic at the age of 84 [87, 88].

6.10 The Development of Anaesthesia as a Specialty

Although a Section of Anaesthetics had been established at the Royal Society of Medicine in 1908, this was not a training, nor examining body as were the Universities and Royal Colleges. In 1912, only 8 out of 22 authorities in the UK providing medical training required instruction in anaesthesia. Once qualified, a doctor could give anaesthesia for any procedure. Surgeons also dictated what sort of anaesthesia they wanted, sometimes favouring their own comfort over the condition of the patient. In 1934, Magill proposed there should be a diploma of Anaesthetics, which was favorably received by the Royal College of Surgeons of England. In 1935, 46 candidates successfully passed their diploma. A Faculty of Anaesthetics was established at RCS in 1948.

In the United States the first Endowed Chair of Anaesthesia was established at Harvard in the name of Henry Isaiah Dorr (1844–1927), a dentist who had graduated from Philadelphia Dental College in 1876. He joined the faculty and was appointed to the Chair of Clinical Dentistry in 1878. While a faculty member he obtained his MD from Jefferson Medical College in 1884. In 1889, his title was changed to Chair of Practical Dentistry, Anaesthetics, and Anaesthesia.

This is the first operation with nitrous oxide gas in combination with oxygen for an anesthetic in short surgery operations and was performed before the entire school. This new method is a long step in the improvement of the use of anesthetics and adds new levels to those which have been won before. The patients under this combination of gases do not exhibit the excitement or groaning as when under the influence of nitrous oxide or ether administration, the lips retain their usual color and the patients experience but little acceleration of the pulse. The duration of the anaesthetic is longer and the operation for the administration is quite simple. It is a very recent importation from England ….

Philadelphia Dental College became part of Temple University in 1905. In 1926, Dorr was elected Emeritus Professor of Anaesthesia and Anaesthetics. Between 1910 and 1917 he negotiated a full chair of Research and Teaching in Anaesthesia and Anaesthetics with Harvard to be established after his death. Initially, the endowment was used to support Dr. Howard Bradshaw and then Dr. Henry Knowles Beecher who were appointed Chiefs of Anaesthesia at Massachusett's General Hospital in Boston and undertook research. Beecher's research led to his being appointed the first Henry Isaiah Dorr Chair at Harvard in 1941. Beecher was succeeded by Richard John Kitz in 1970, and he by Edward Lowenstein in 1998. By the year 2000, there were seven endowed Professorships of Anesthesia at Harvard [87, 88].

6.11 Intravenous Anaesthesia

In the twentieth century intravenous anaesthesia became established both for induction and maintenance of anaesthesia. A range of drugs were developed and trialed for their safety, effectiveness, and lack of side-effects. Avertin, a bromine derivative of alcohol, was found to have narcotic effects but could be administered rectally. The early trials were carried out by German surgeon, Otto Butzengeiger (1885–1968), in 1920s. Sir Francis Shipway reported their initial findings in the Lancet of 1929.

The preparation of the solution was difficult and took about 45 minutes, and it was used particularly for anxious patients and those undergoing thyroid surgery for hyperthyroidism. Robert Macintosh in Oxford was another advocate for Avertin. It's intravenous use was accompanied by some cases of apnoea and drops in blood pressure, and also by thrombophlebitis. Avertin was used for about 40 years [89, 90].

Hexobarbitone was widely used in Europe but not in North America. Ronal Jarman, who passed the first DA examination in 1935, introduced hexobarbitone to the UK in 1934. Thiopentone (Abbot) was given to John Lundy at the Mayo Clinic in 1935, who reported his favourable experience in peacetime. Ronal Jarman and Lawrence Abel introduced thiopentone in Britain [91]. Thiopentone was then widely used but when used on war wounds by non-anaesthetists, as in the Pearl Harbour attack on Honolulu in 1941, it resulted in a number of deaths due to respiratory depression and worsening of shock where the means of resuscitation are not available. Ketamine today is a widely used means of providing short-acting anaesthesia by either the intramuscular or intravenous route. It received FDA approval in 1970 and was used as a field anaesthetic in the Vietnam war. Because it preserves airway reflexes and BP, and its hallucinogenic effects can be countered with diazepam, it is widely used in LMICs [92, 93]. Recommendations to ban its use because it can be abused as a party drug have been opposed to preserve its availability (it is cheap and effective) in low- and middle-income countries, and safe where skilled anaesthetists are not available. The Benzodiazepines, particularly diazepam (valium) and now, Midazolam, have been used as sedation and induction agents although sensitivity varies and they, as the barbiturates, can cause respiratory depression. Propofol was introduced in the 1980s for short stay anesthesia. When the laryngeal mask was released in the 1990s it was appreciated that propofol provided the best conditions for insertion. Today it is commonly used for endoscopic and other short day-stay procedures [94] (Table 6.1).

Table 6.1 Key intravenous anaesthesia drugs of twentieth century [90, 91]

Agent	Clinical use	Comments
Avertin 1922	Mainly rectal some intravenous Trialed by Butzengeiger in 1926–27	Used for about 40 years in UK and Europe Difficult to prepare solution
Hexobarbitone (Evipan) (Short acting) 1932	By 1944, had been used on more than 2 m patients.	Used in Europe but not North America
Sodium Amytal 1929	Used for about 4 years in 1930s	Mainly in North America
Thiopentone 1935	1936 Lundy reports research with 2207 patients; Jarman and Abel used in UK	Mayo clinic for trial Became universally accepted
Methohexitone 1956	Used for short procedures esp. dental	Avoided "hangover" of thiopentone and quicker recovery
Fentanyl (Jansen Pharmaceutica) 1963 in Europe 1968 in USA	Short onset of action, minimal CVS effects, does not release histamine	Intravenous opioid analgesic Inexpensive Used for chronic pain Also nasal, buccal and sublingual applicability
Ketamine 1965	Preserves airway reflexes and BP released in UK in 1970s	Hallucinogenic and therefore greater use in LMICs
Diazepam Synthesized 1961	Stovner and Endresen (Norway) used it in tetanus and then anesthesia (1965)	Irritant to veins thus Diazemuls developed in 1990s but replaced by midazolam
Midazolam 1975	Introduced in 1980s and 1990s	Less likely to cause thrombophlebitis
Propofol ICI (now Astra Zeneca)	FDA approval 1989 released in Europe in late 1980s	1986 AZN released Diprifusor infusion device for total intravenous anesthesia

6.12 Muscle Relaxants

As anaesthesia developed and surgery became more and more developed, it became clear that muscle tone and reflexes limited the scope of surgery, particularly for the abdominal wall, hence the benefit of introducing neuromuscular blocking drugs that would paralyse the patient to allow intubation, and/or ventilation.

South American Indians had used curare as a paralysing poison on darts for blow pipes, arrowheads and spear tips for centuries. Early European explorers to South America in the sixteenth century including Peter Martyr d/Anghera (in 1516) and Sir Walter Raleigh (in 1594), described the poisoned arrows. However, further research awaited the early nineteenth century when an adventurer, Chalres Waterton (1762–1865), managing his family's sugar estates in Demerara, South America, obtained samples and experimented with it on large animals. Later, a demonstration of curare's effects to an audience that included surgeon, Sir Benjamin Brodie (1783–1862) was made on three asses:

> *The first ass was injected with wourali in the shoulder and died. The second had a tourniquet tied around its foreleg and wourali was injected below the tourniquet; the ass was alive and active as long as the tourniquet was in place but died soon after the tourniquet was removed. The third ass appeared to die after having wourali injected but was resuscitated by means of a bellows and lived on in in peace as Wouralia.* [95–98]

In 1846, French Physiologist, Claude Bernard (1813–1878), reported that curare injected into a frog's leg prevented muscle contraction in response to nerve stimulation. However the muscle would contract if stimulated directly. This was the first evidence that curare worked at the neuromuscular junction. In Great Britain, Sir Henry Dale (1875–1968), an MD graduate of Cambridge (1909) and colleagues first identified acetylcholine. The Austrian, Otto Loewi (1873-1961), established the role of acetylcholine in neuromuscular transmission. Together Dale and Loewi shared the 1936 Nobel prize in medicine. In 1938, Loewi, a Jew, and his two sons were arrested and brutalised by the Gestapo. Only an uproar from the international scientific community saved him and he was allowed to leave Austria for Britain where he stayed with Dale until offered a position in Oxford. He later emigrated to the USA where he spent the rest of his life [99–102].

In 1942, Harold Randall Griffith (1894–1985), a Canadian anaesthetist from Montreal, introduced curare into anaesthesia as a paralysing agent "the south American arrow poison." The introduction of curare significantly reduced the amount of anaesthetic required, increased the scope of surgery, improved working conditions for the surgeon and reduced morbidity and mortality [103, 104].

From then on through the 1940s, curare and its various forms such as d-tubocurarine were being used in anaesthetics but there was still a need to develop a synthetic product rather than sourcing the natural product from the Amazon. In 1946, an Italian Chemist, Daniel Bovet, synthesized a product that led to the development of gallamine, the first synthetic non-depolarising muscle relaxant. Gallamine was first used in anaesthesia in 1948 in France, and the following year into Britain. It was able to be mixed with thiopentone which facilitated administration of both agents through a single line. Gallamine was used for many decades before being superceded by other agents with less side effects such as tachycardia and given it is excreted in the urine, its activity is prolonged in patients with kidney impairment. Suxamethonium, a short acting, rapid onset depolarizing neuromuscular relaxant, was originally studied in 1906, but not used in anaesthesia until 1951. Many side effects have been reported including, myalgia, bradycardia, histamine release, and hyperkalaemia. However, no better rapid onset, short acting agent to allow intubation has been developed and suxamethonium is still widely used [104–106] (Table 6.2).

> *In spite of its many disadvantages and some potential lethal dangers, it remains the only drug presently available that will produce a rapid, complete block of about 5–10 minutes duration.* [Stanley Feldman, 1984 cited by Ball and Westhorpe] [105, 106].

Table 6.2 Muscle relaxant approval [99, 100, 103]

Agent	Year and first place of anesthesia use	Comments
Tubocurarine	1942 (Canada)	Releases histamine Hypotension
Gallamine	1948 (France)	Tachycardia, no histamine release
Pancuronium	1967 (Scotland)	Tachycardia, more potent than Tubocurarine, no hypotension or histamine changes,
Vecuronium	1984 FDA approval	Developed as a result of scientific consensus on the ideal muscle relaxant in 1975
Atracurium	1983 FDA approval	1981 synthesized by Strathclyde Uni and Wellcome Some histamine release
Mivacurium	1984 US (Boston)	Slow onset, short duration of action
Rocuronium	1994 (USA)	Deacetoxy analogue of vercuronium Rapid onset, only slightly slower than suxamethonium

6.12.1 Non-depolarizing Muscle Relaxants (Fig. 6.9)

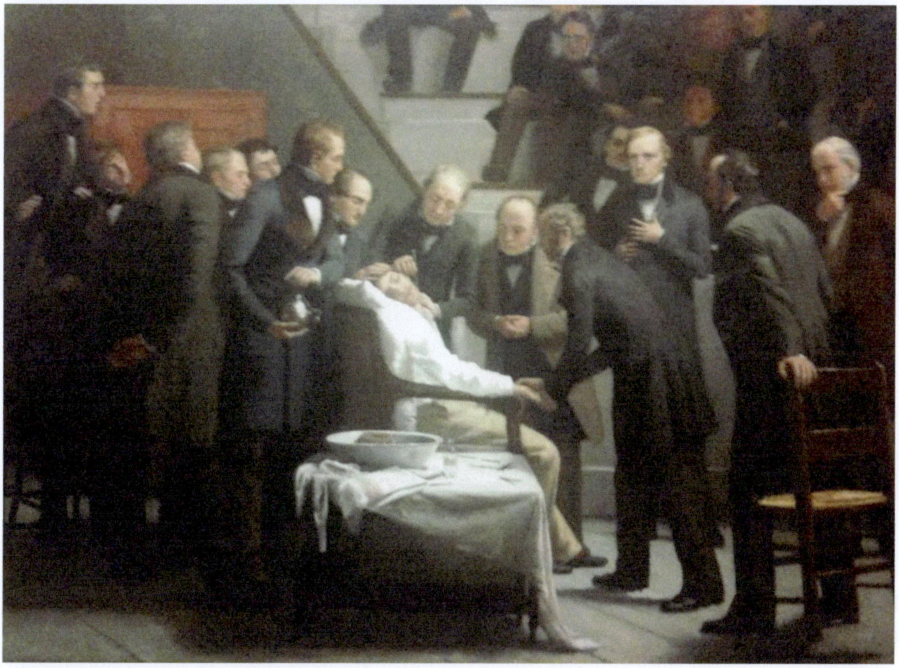

Fig. 6.9 16th Oct. 1846 *"On that historical day Dr. John Warren (surgeon at the Massachusetts General Hospital), was invited to operate before a large audience, Morton administered ether vapour to the patient before Warren removed a tumor from his neck without any pain."* https://en.wikipedia.org/wiki/John_Collins_Warren_(surgeon,_born_1778)#/media/File:Southworth_&_Hawes_-_First_etherized_operation_(re-enactment).jpg

6.13 Modern Regional Anaesthesia

With increasing experience of anaesthesia, knowledge about its complications was accumulating, which led people to think about local or regional anaesthesia that keeps the patient awake and could avoid general side effects and respiratory issues. The development of regional anaesthesia required the knowledge in the nerve anatomy and physiology of the nervous system and pharmacology of local anaesthetic agents.

In 1784, James Moore London, published a description of nerve compression in producing numbness for limb surgery similar to the effect after falling asleep while lying on an arm. The method was used successfully for an amputation performed painlessly by John Hunter, the 'father' of modern surgery, but the experience was not repeated for unknown reason [107].

Pharmacological 'numbing' effects of the South American alkaloid, cocaine, was first discovered in 1860. Carl Koller, a friend of Sigmund Freud, discovered the local anesthetic properties of cocaine in 1884 and used it to perform the first local anesthesia in eye surgery. The results of his trial were read (by a friend, Koller could not afford the trip) at a conference in Heidelberg on 15 September 1884, the news spread throw ought the world in days facilitated by the recent discovery of the electric telegraph.

This discovery revolutionized the field of surgery and allowed for the development of more local agents which helped the development of numerous surgical procedures that were previously impossible or too painful to perform.

Regional anesthesia, also known as peripheral nerve blockade or nerve block, is a technique that uses local anesthetics to produce a loss of sensation in a specific area of the body. This can be used to provide pain relief during and after surgery, as well as for the management of acute and chronic pain [107–109].

Regional anesthesia has been used since the nineteenth century but it has developed significantly in the last decades. William Halsted (1852–1922) was an American surgeon, a father of modern surgery, who is credited with introducing the use of cocaine for nerve block during surgery. Halsted began experimenting with cocaine in the late 1880s and found that it could be used to produce local anaesthesia during certain surgical procedures. However, Halsted also became addicted to cocaine and struggled with addiction throughout his life. Despite this, his contributions to surgery and the development of local anaesthesia are still recognized today [108].

Modern regional anaesthesia techniques have several advantages over general anaesthesia, such as faster recovery time, less nausea and vomiting, and reduced risk of complications.

One of the most widely used forms of regional anaesthesia is spinal anesthesia, which involves injecting a local anaesthetic into the spinal fluid to produce a loss of sensation in the lower half of the body. This technique is commonly used for surgery on the lower extremities, such as knee or hip replacement.

Cerebrospinal fluid has been known since the days of Hippocrates who called it "*brain water*" and treated hydrocephalus by a ventricular puncture. The origin of the first lumbar dural puncture was attributed to Heinrich Quincke of Cologne, Germany, in 1890 [107, 109, 110].

August Bier is credited with performing the first successful spinal anaesthesia in 1898 by puncturing the dura mater. This was a significant advancement in the field of anaesthesia as it allowed for surgical procedures to be performed on the lower body without the need for general anaesthesia, the patients remain awake. The technique involved injecting cocaine into the spinal canal, which temporarily blocked nerve impulses and provided pain relief. Bier, in 1898, made an experiment on his assistant August Hildebrandt by giving him intrathecal cocaine then he hammered his legs with iron hammer, twisted his testicles, and demonstrated that he had no pain. He also demonstrated that lunar puncture leads to headache afterward. However, the use of cocaine was later replaced by other local anesthetics due to its addictive properties and potential for adverse effects.

A year later, in 1899, the first spinal anaesthesia in the United States was performed by Rudolph Matas, a vascular surgeon from New Orleans.

Novocaine (procaine) is a local anaesthetic drug that was first synthesised in 1905 by German chemist Alfred Einhorn (1856-1917). It was one of the first synthetic local anaesthetics developed and was widely used in dentistry and surgery in the early twentieth century [107, 109].

Epidural anesthesia is another widely used form of regional anaesthesia. This technique involves injecting a local anaesthetic into the epidural space, which surrounds the spinal cord, to produce a loss of sensation in the lower half of the body. This technique is commonly used for childbirth, surgical procedures on the lower extremities, and for the management of chronic pain.

Nerve blocks are also a commonly used form of regional anaesthesia [107, 109].

In 1855, James Leonard Corning, a neurologist, punctured dura mater while investigating the effect of cocaine on the spinal nerves of dogs. American neurologist James Leonard Corning of Acorn Hall, Morristown, NJ. is officially considered the founding father of modern epidural analgesia, he was the first to perform neuroaxial block by injecting cocaine into the dog's epidural space and of ten volunteers. He published this experiment in 1885 in the New York Medical Journal. The lumbar approach to the epidural space would be applied only in 1921 after the caudal approach, being first performed by the Spanish surgeon from Madrid, Fidel Pagés Miravé, in 1921, he reported on his work on lumbar epidural anaesthesia for surgery on groin hernias and lower limbs operations. That had marked the birth of the modern epidural analgesia.

With the development of ultrasound technology, nerve blocks have become more accurate and efficient. Ultrasound-guided nerve blocks use the visualization of the nerves by an ultrasound to make the procedure more accurate and safer. The first modern local anaesthetic lidocaine (lignocaine) was introduced in 1948 [110, 111]. The longer acting, bupivacaine (marcaine), was discovered in 1957.

In recent years, there have been many advancements in the field of regional anesthesia. New techniques and technologies, such as continuous nerve blocks, have been developed to improve patient outcomes and provide more effective pain management. Additionally, research is ongoing to develop new local anaesthetics and adjuvants to improve the efficacy and safety of nerve blocks [109–111].

6.14 Tracheostomy

Tracheostomy, a surgical procedure in which an incision is made in the windpipe to establish a direct passage for air, has a long and significant history. It can help with breathing problems, provide a route to clear the airways, and help with long-term breathing support. Its origins can be traced back to ancient civilizations such as the Egyptians, Greeks, and Romans. However, the exact origin of the first tracheostomy remains unknown. Over time, the techniques and instruments used in tracheostomy have been developed and improved, making it an essential and proven surgery. Despite its ancient roots, tracheostomy did not become a commonly performed operation until the 1800s, despite being known for about 4,000 years [112].

Tracheostomy was only recognized as a treatment for longer term mechanical ventilation after World War II. Before this, it was primarily used to address upper airway obstruction [112, 113].

6.14.1 Tracheostomy in Ancient Times

Tracheostomy, a surgical procedure involving the creation of an opening in the windpipe, has a long and storied history. One of the earliest descriptions of surgical tracheostomy can be found in the Rig Veda, an ancient Indian medical text written around 2000 BCE. This text describes how a throat incision is healed.

Choosing between a tracheostomy and a tracheal intubation is very important. Both require a lot of skill to perform correctly. The ancient Egyptians were known to perform tracheostomies. Hippocrates (460–380 BCE) also described intubation of the trachea of humans to support ventilation. In the fourth century BCE, there was a story about Alexander the Great saving a soldier's life. A soldier was choking on a bone stuck in their throat. Alexander acted quickly. He used the tip of his sword to make a small opening in the soldier's trachea. This allowed the soldier to breathe again.

A Greek doctor, Asclepiades (124-40 BCE), described it in the first century BCE), and may have been the first one to write about the operation. He used it to manage airway obstruction from inflammation/infection in the upper airways.

Tracheostomy was documented in medical texts written by Galen, a Greek physician who lived from 129–216 AD. Galen inflated the lungs of dead animals via the trachea and concluded that air movement caused chest "arises." The full significance of that finding was not appreciated for centuries [113, 114].

The ancient physicians believed that cartilage could not heal if severed, which significantly hindered further experimentation and development of the procedure. Caelius Aurelianus, a fifth century physician, stated, "*Laryngotomia is a futile and irresponsible idea set forth by Asclepiades.*"

Paulus Aegineta (620-690 CE), a seventh-century Byzantine physician, performed the procedure with the patient in a sitting position with an extended neck. The outcomes of these operations are unknown, but given the ongoing practice, some are likely to have been successful. The Babylonian Talmud records someone from a village saying, *"There was a sheep in our village that hurt its windpipe. Hollow reeds were introduced into the windpipe and the sheep lived"* [112–114].

Muslim philosopher and physician Avicenna (980–1037 AD) described intubation of the trachea using "a cannula of gold or silver." Albucasis (1013–1116) showed that the cartilage of the trachea could heal. He told the story of a servant girl who tried to kill herself by cutting her throat. He sewed up the cut, and it eventually healed [114].

During the Middle Ages, tracheostomy was primarily applied to address respiratory blockages caused by illnesses or injuries [113].

Further medical progress was largely undocumented until the Renaissance, when the procedure re-emerged as a possible surgical option. In 1543, while Copernicus challenged the Church by claiming that the Earth revolved around the Sun, Andreas Vesalius, a physician anatomist in Padua, published *De Humani Corporis Fabrica* (On the Fabric of the Human Body). This book revolutionized human anatomical knowledge [113, 114].

Italian physician, Antonio Brasavola (1500–1555) performed a documented and successful tracheostomy in a human in 1546. He saved a patient who was near death due to suffocation, likely caused by a peritonsillar abscess rather than an abscess around the windpipe. He was personal physician to a number of European monarchs including Charles V and Henry VIII. He was also physician to four Popes.

In 1617, Hieronymus Fabricius (1533–1619), a renowned anatomist at the University of Padua, described the technical details of the operation, writing, "*The operation is the opening of the aspera arteria ['artery of air'], by which patients, from a condition of almost suffocating obstruction to respiration suddenly regain consciousness, and draw that vital ether, the air, so necessary to life, and again resume an existence which had been all but annihilated.*" It is likely Fabricius never performed the procedure himself.

French Naval surgeon, Nicolas Habicot (1550–1624) reported on four patients who recovered after tracheostomies in 1620. He published the first book on tracheostomy, in which he described the case of a 14-year-old patient who swallowed a bag of gold coins to prevent their theft on the *Mayflower*, a ship carrying over a hundred Protestant pilgrims to the New World. The bag caused upper airway obstruction, which was resolved by a prompt tracheotomy [112–114].

Although positive pressure ventilation using bellows was first used for drowning victims in the 1700s, concerns arose that this therapy could harm the lungs. Forceful bellows ventilation of drowned dogs could cause fatal pneumothorax. As a result, the French Academy and the Royal Humane Society in London abandoned bellows ventilation. Positive pressure ventilation was thus avoided and would not re-surface for over a hundred years.

In Virginia, December 1799, George Washington, the first American president, a few years after his retirement was dying from bacterial epiglottitis. Three physicians gathered around him. He kept shifting his position, gasping for air. It was obvious the patient's airway was severely compromised. One of the physicians present at the scene was aware of tracheostomy but was not willing to do it on such an important man, particularly as he thought the procedure to be futile. George Washington duly died from fully preventable suffocation due to an upper airway obstruction [114–116].

In the first half of the nineteenth century, John Snow (1813–1858) of England resuscitated a baby with a tracheal catheter. Snow was the first to employ tracheostomy to give anaesthesia to a rabbit. Before the advent of antibiotics, diphtheria was a fatal disease. In 1833, Armand Trousseau (1801–1867) reported that he performed the operation on 200 patients, 50 out of them were children who suffered from laryngeal diphtheria; he also invented tracheal dilators that are still in use. This report convinced the doubters and detractors of the operation, and tracheostomy became widely acceptable to the medical profession. At that time, tracheostomy was otherwise done in emergency settings only [113, 115, 117].

In view of Trousseau's achievements 170 years ago, it is remarkable that patients still die today because of the failure to take steps to open an obstructed airway before the patient asphyxsiates. In the twentieth century, the procedure was widely adopted to remove secretions from the airway to improve lung oxygenation. Galloway (1943) is credited for the use of tracheostomy to facilitate aspiration of secretions from the bronchial tree in cases of bulbar poliomyelitis. This major contribution marked the end of a 2000-year-long era in which tracheostomy was used exclusively for the relief of upper respiratory obstruction and ushered in a new concept of the value of tracheostomy as part of the treatment for obstruction of the lower airway enabling suction and evacuation of inflammatory secretions.

In 1730, George Martin in Scotland was the first Briton to carry out the procedure successfully. He was also the first to recommend a double-lumen tube, and also reported that the wound closed spontaneously following removal of the cannula [116, 117].

The German physician Friedrich Trendelenburg (1844–1924) manufactured the first cuffed tracheostomy tube in 1869, and administered the first endotracheal anaesthesia in man in early 1871.

The work of Jackson is an important milestone in the long history of tracheostomy. He standardized the technique and indications of the operation and later recommended that high tracheostomy should be abandoned as it was the chief cause of laryngeal stenosis (Jackson, 1921).

In 1885, after witnessing the mutilating effect of hasty tracheostomies, Joseph O'Dwyer, an American paediatrician developed a series of metal tracheal tubes he inserted orally between the vocal cords in patients who had diphtheria. The tubes were also used in stenosis of the larynx caused by other diseases, such as syphilis, and strictures of the larynx. His method was published in the New York Medical Journal as "Intubation of the Larynx" in 1888. At the end of the nineteenth century, the German surgeon Franz Kuhn constructed metal tubes that he inserted orally Kuhn described the use of a curved tube introducer. He preferred packing the hypopharynx with gauze instead of using cuffed tubes for prevention of aspiration. He also used cocaine to prevent laryngeal spasm [114, 118, 119].

This technique was further developed by Magill in England. Kuhn's efforts were probably the first historical steps toward awake tracheal intubation under topical anaesthesia, a technique frequently used today in patients with difficult airways. During the First World War, Sir Ivan Whiteside Magill (1888–1986), mentioned above, realized that reconstructive surgeries performed on mutilated soldiers were more successful under general anaesthesia with the airway secured by endotracheal tubes [116, 119, 120].

The next giant step in the progress of airway management was the discovery of the importance of lung isolation. It was not until 1930—a year that saw the completion of New York's Empire State Building – that techniques and devices for lung isolation emerged. American Ralph Waters is credited with developing one-lung intubation to facilitate thoracic surgery. Initially it was performed with double-cuffed, single-lumen tubes [120–123].

The most significant factors contributing to the success of endotracheal intubation were the development of laryngoscopy and the ongoing advancements in laryngoscopes. In 1895, Alfred Kirstein first performed direct laryngoscopy, and the discovery is thus attributed to him. A major advancement in the field of tracheal intubation occurred with the introduction of flexible fiberoptic bronchoscopy to medicine by Kensuke Ikeda (Japan) in 1968. Since then, fiberoptic bronchoscopy has become an essential tool in managing difficult endotracheal intubations [124].

The modern era of tracheostomy began in Scandinavia during the poliomyelitis epidemic of 1952–53. This epidemic caused severe respiratory distress, leading to the use of tracheostomy in treating respiratory insufficiency resulting from causes other than airway obstruction. In such cases, tracheostomy facilitates the application of intermittent positive pressure ventilation, whether administered manually or mechanically, and allows for the removal of respiratory secretions since the patient's cough is ineffective.

Today, tracheostomy is commonly used in critically ill patients who have been on a ventilator for an extended period and would otherwise be at risk of tracheal stenosis. It is employed for positive pressure ventilation and the removal of respiratory secretions.

Over the course of human history, the concept of airway management has evolved over nearly 4000 years. This progress has been fueled by the improvement of airway devices and a deeper understanding of respiratory system functioning. The techniques of tracheostomy and tracheal intubation have been refined through centuries of experimentation and refinement. These advancements have played a crucial role in reducing the risk of anaesthesia-related deaths and serve as the basis for contemporary airway treatment methods.

6.15 Intensive Care

6.15.1 The Polio Epidemic of 1952

The polio epidemic in Copenhagen occurred in 1952, and was one of the worst outbreaks of the disease in Denmark's history. Poliomyelitis is a highly contagious viral disease that attacks the nervous system and can cause paralysis, muscle weakness, and even death [125, 126].

During the epidemic, over 1000 people in Copenhagen were infected with the virus, and 200 people died. Most of the victims were children under the age of five, and many were left permanently disabled. Many patients developed respiratory muscle paralysis and/or bulbar palsy as a result of the virus. This led to respiratory failure and pooling of secretions, which could cause further complications. That resulted in 316 patients requiring mechanical ventilation, some of whom required tracheostomy. The outbreak led to widespread panic and a sense of national crisis. The government implemented emergency measures, including closing schools and public spaces, and setting up temporary hospitals to care for the sick. Professor Lassen, chief physician at the Blegdam Hospital, had thought of providing positive pressure ventilation for such patients, after consulting with anaesthetist, Dr. Bjorn Ibsen (1915-2007). The medical team on Copenhagen was then able to treat these patients. During the epidemic, 300 patients were admitted each week. Ten percent of them either choked or drowned in their own fluids.

There were 70 patients needing respiratory support. Medical students were drafted in and paid £1.50 per shift to manually provide ventilation using a bag. Two hundred fifty medical students came in daily and worked shifts with 35–40 doctors. By using such a strategy, mortality from polio in Copenhagen decreased from over 80% to approximately 40%.

Ibsen thought the idea that every patient who needs ventilation should have their own nurse, so in December 1953, the concept of 1:1 nursing and intensive care was born.

6.15.1.1 Blood Gas Analysis

Wilhelm Ostwald (1853-1932) discovered the measurement of hydrogen ion concentration in Leipzig about 1890. He was later awarded the Nobel Prize in Chemistry in 1909. Danish physician, Karl Albert Hasselbalch (1874-1962), adapted Sorensen's pH nomenclature to the Lawrence Henderson (1878 -1942) equation. He then made the first blood pH measurements and proposed that metabolic acid-base imbalance be quantification as the "reduced" pH of blood after equilibration to a carbon dioxide tension (PCO_2) of 40 mm Hg. Van Slyke developed a way to measure plasma CO_2 content with his manometric apparatus. This good idea was never adopted until the 1960s.

Many patients did not get better and needed to be kept alive with respirators. The first pH, pCO_2, and pO_2 electrodes made it possible to adjust ventilation by using blood gas analysis (Astrup) [127].

In the 1960s and 1970s, the development of new technologies, such as cardiac monitoring and dialysis, further expanded the range of conditions that could be treated in the ICU. Max Weil (1927-2011) is known as the "father of modern intensive care." He started a "shock ward" at Los Angeles County/University of Southern California Medical Center in the 1960s. Early ICUs were scary, secretive, and isolated. Staff and visitors often wore shoe covers, masks, and gloves to add to the patient's anxiety [128].

Many initial critical care units were staffed by anaesthetists or medical doctors. Some hospitals had separate surgical and medical ICUs, particularly in the USA and some developed specialty respiratory, cardiac, and neurosurgical ICUs. It turned out that ICU patients all had similar system issues, regardless of the cause of their illness. During the 1970s and 1980s the development of intensive care units required specially trained physicians (intensivists) and nurses to care for critically ill patients. With a multisystem approach to supporting compromised organ systems, patients received better care and had better outcomes [128].

In the UK, the first intensive care professor was Professor Ron Bradley (1929-2023), who ran the ICU at St Thomas' Hospital, London. Prior to that, clinicians would often work part-time or on-call, which led to less continuity of care. Margaret Branthwaite was his senior registrar. They together developed the first pulmonary artery catheter at the Royal Brompton Hospital. With time technology continued to improve, and life-support and monitoring techniques became more sophisticated. Intensive care patients often had invasive monitoring systems, like the pulmonary artery catheter, parenteral fluids, blood products oxygen administration, and vasopressors became a routine therapeutic tool for the intensivists [129].

Today, ICUs are an essential component of modern healthcare, providing specialized care for critically ill patients with a wide range of conditions, including cardiac arrest, respiratory failure, sepsis, and trauma. ICUs are staffed by a team of specialised healthcare professionals, including intensivists (doctors who are specially trained in intensive care medicine), nurses, and respiratory therapists, who work together to provide the highest level of care for critically ill patients. With the advancement of technology, monitoring and diagnostic devices have become more precise and sophisticated, and new protocols have been developed to improve the outcome of critically ill patients.

It's worth noting that ICUs continue to evolve with the integration of emerging technologies and research, with procedures and protocols constantly being updated to improve the care provided to critically ill patients. Today, ICUs are an important component of care for the highest risk patients and those with complications. The last forty years has witnessed critical care being a rapidly developing specialty that continues to save lives and improve the quality of life for critically ill patients. There has been a shift in healthcare towards improved communication with patients and their families, as well as a greater emphasis on patient-centered care, and, when appropriate, end of life decision-making. This shift has been driven by a growing recognition of the importance of involving patients and their families in decision-making about their own care and a move away from more paternalistic approaches to medicine.

One of the key drivers of this shift has been the recognition of the importance of patient autonomy and the need for healthcare providers to respect and support patients' individual values, preferences, and goals. This has led to a greater focus on shared decision-making and informed consent, as well as efforts to improve patient education and communication. At the end of life, in particular, there has been a growing recognition of the importance of involving patients and their families in decision-making and providing support for end-of-life care [130].

The renewed interest in evidence-based medicine in the early 1990s sparked a re-evaluation of many accepted practices within the ICU. The lack of solid, high-level evidence for many interventions was recognized, leading to a greater emphasis on the use of evidence-based guidelines and protocols to guide clinical practice.

This shift towards evidence-based medicine was driven by a growing recognition of the importance of using the best available evidence to guide clinical decision-making, as well as a recognition of the limitations of expert opinion and anecdotal evidence. This has led to a greater emphasis on rigorous research methods, such as randomized controlled trials and systematic reviews, to generate high-quality evidence on the efficacy and safety of different interventions [131].

References

1. Segre JA. What does it take to satisfy Koch's postulates two centuries later? Microbial genomics and Propionibacteria acnes. J Invest Dermatol. 2013;133(9):2141–2. https://doi.org/10.1038/jid.2013.260. Epub 2013 Jul 11. PMID: 23842116; PMCID: PMC3775492
2. Haas LF. Girolamo Fracastoro 1484–1553. J Neurol Neurosurg Psychiatry. 1991;54(10):855. https://doi.org/10.1136/jnnp.54.10.855. PMID: 1744637; PMCID: PMC1014566
3. Gest H. The discovery of microorganisms by Robert Hooke and Antoni Van Leeuwenhoek, fellows of the Royal Society. Notes Rec R Soc Lond. 2004;58(2):187–201. https://doi.org/10.1098/rsnr.2004.0055. PMID: 15209075.
4. Simpson J. Our existing system of hospitalisation, its effect on the results of surgical operations. Edin Med J. 1869;14:816–30.
5. Labarraque A. Method of using the chloride of soda, either for dressing ill-conditioned sores, or as a means of purifying unhealthy places, and of disinfecting animal substances. Translated by Jacob Porter 1830. Available from https://collections.nlm.nih.gov/?f%5Bdrep2.authorAggregate%5D%5B%5D=Labarraque%2C+A.+G.+%28Antoine+Germain%29%2C+1777-1850.
6. Ref Rutala WA, Weber DJ. Uses of inorganic hypochlorite (bleach) in health-care facilities. Clin Microbiol Rev. 1997;10:597–610. https://doi.org/10.1128/cmr.10.4.597.
7. Gould IM. Alexander Gordon, puerperal sepsis, and modern theories of infection control--Semmelweis in perspective. Lancet Infect Dis. 2010;10(4):275–8. https://doi.org/10.1016/S1473-3099(09)70304-4. PMID: 20334850.
8. Smith L. Dr Alexander Gordon of Aberdeen. J Fam Plan Reprod Health Care. 2010;36(4):253. https://doi.org/10.1783/147118910793048854.

9. Bennett P. Alexander Gordon (1752–99) and his writing: insights into medical thinking in the late eighteenth century. J R Coll Phys Edinburgh. 2012;42(2):165–71. https://doi.org/10.4997/JRCPE.2012.217.
10. Ref Rutala WA, Weber DJ. Uses of inorganic hypochlorite (bleach) in health-care facilities. Clin Microbiol Rev. 1997;10:597–610. https://doi.org/10.1128/cmr.10.4.59.
11. De Costa CM. The contagiousness of childbed fever: a short history of puerperal sepsis and its treatment. MJA. 2002;177:668–71.
12. Carter KC, Tate GS. The earliest-known account of Semmelweis's initiation of disinfection at Vienna's Allgemeines Krankenhaus. Bull Hist Med. 1991;65:252–7.
13. Nuland SB. The enigma of Semmelweis—an interpretation. J Hist Med Allied Sci. 1979;34:255–72.
14. Simpson JY. Lancet 1867. http://resource.nlm.nih.gov/101502846.
15. Ehrhardt JD Jr, Nakayama DK, O'Leary JP. Carbolic acid before Joseph Lister: rail ties, sewage, manure, and the great stink. Am Surg. 2020;86(3):176–83. PMID: 32223794.
16. Martini M, Bragazzi NL. Enrico Bottini (1835–1903), medico e politico Italiano: Maestro dell'anti-sepsi e pioniere della chirurgia moderna [Enrico Bottini (1835–1903), Italian Physician and Politician: A Master of Antisepsis and a Pioneer of Modern Surgery]. Acta Med Hist Adriat. 2018;16(2):293–302. Italian. https://doi.org/10.31952/amha.16.2.7. PMID: 30488707.
17. Dronsfield A, Ellis P. Solving an infection problem. R Soc Chem. 2009. Ok. https://edu.rsc.org/feature/solving-an-infectious-problem/2020229.article
18. De l'acide phénique. https://gallica.bnf.fr/ark:/12148/bpt6k6133699d.r=Jules%20lemaire
19. Lister JL. On the antiseptic principle in the practice of surgery. Lancet. 1867;90:353–6. https://doi.org/10.1016/s0140-6736(02)51827-4.
20. Mazzarello P, Garbarino C, Cani V. Bassi, Agostino. In: eLS. Chichester: John Wiley & Sons, Ltd; 2013. https://doi.org/10.1002/9780470015902.a0025074
21. Porter JR. Agostino Bassi bicentennial (1773-1973). Bacteriol Rev. 1973;37(3):284–8. https://doi.org/10.1128/br.37.3.284-288.1973. PMID: 4585794; PMCID: PMC413819.
22. Sabbatani S, Catena F, Neri F, et al. The Bolognese surgeon Giuseppe Ruggi: how and why the aseptic surgery was introduced in Bologna in the middle half of the XIX century. J Surg Res. 2014;192(2):555–63. https://doi.org/10.1016/j.jss.2014.04.018. Epub 2014 Aug 17. PMID: 25240285.
23. Kyle RA, Shampo MA. Agostino Bassi. JAMA. 1979;241(15):1584. https://doi.org/10.1001/jama.241.15.1584. PMID: 372592.
24. Rai L, Ghufran MA, Samo KA, Mangi MH, Babar J, Abbasi MR. A comparative study between use of topical honey and Edinburgh University's Solution of Lime (EUSOL) dressing in necrotizing Fascitis wounds. Cureus. 2023;15(1):e33825. https://doi.org/10.7759/cureus.33825. PMID: 36819392; PMCID: PMC9930691. [Note Honey as good as EUSOL and shorter hospital stay – Murray Drennan produced EUSOL in 1916 (chlorinated lime and boric acid)]
25. Magath TB. The history of steam sterilization. Ann Med Hist. 1937. https://www.ncbi.nlm.nih.gov/pmc/articles/PMC7942947/pdf/annmedhist147410-0048.pdf.
26. Runge F. Ueber einige Produkte der Steinkohlendestillation. Poggendorffs Annalen der Physik und Chemie. 1834, pp. 65–78
27. The history of germ theory by Jemima Hodkinson, in Big Picture. (e-article)
28. Lister J. The antiseptic principle in the practise of surgery. BMJ. 1867;ii:246–8.
29. Lister J. 1827–1912 by Richard B Fisher. 1977 (biography).
30. Loudon I. Commentary on Semelweiss I (1818–1865). The James Lind Library. www.jameslindlibrary.org.
31. Caplan CE. The childbed fever mystery and the meaning of medical journalism. www.med.mcgill.ca/mjm/issues/v01n01/fever.html.

32. Volkmann R. Die Behandlung der complicirten Fracturen. In: Sammlung klinischer Vorträge nos 117 and 118, Volkmann R, editor. Chirurgie II, pp. 923–76 (Breitkopf & Härtel, Leipzig, [1875]), at p. 924.
33. Langenbuch C. Aus den Sectionssitzungen des VII. internationalen medicinischen Congresses zu London. Die Section für Chirurgie. Berl Med Wschr. 1882;19:31–2.
34. Worboys M. Spreading germs. Disease theories and medical practice in Britain, 1865–1900. Cambridge University Press; 2000. p. 98–9.
35. Godlee RJ. Lord Lister. London: Macmillan; 1917. p. 358.
36. Rutala WA, Weber DJ. Uses of inorganic hypochlorite (bleach) in health-care facilities. Clin Microbiol Rev. 1997;10:597–610.
37. Bulloch W. The history of bacteriology. New York: Dover; 1938. p. 198; Gradmann, ibid., 59–83
38. Nightingale F. Florence Nightingale. Cassandra: an essay. 1979. Am J Public Health. 2010;100(9):1586–7.
39. Worboys M. Spreading germs. Disease theories and medical practice in Britain, 1865–1900. Cambridge University Press; 2000. pp. 98–9. The History of Germ Theory by Jemima Hodkinson, in Big Picture. (e-article)
40. Joseph Lister, 1827–1912 by Richard B Fisher, 1977 (biography).
41. Randers-Pehrson J. The surgeon's glove. 1960.
42. Germain MA. L'epopee des gants chirurgicaux. Ann Chir. 2003;128:475–80.
43. Proskauer C.. https://www.jstor.org/stable/24619258
44. Hernigou P. The strange history of surgical gloves in orthopaedic surgery (part I): from no gloves and no hand washing to the introduction of cotton gloves in orthopaedic surgery. Int Orthop 2022;46(11):2705–2714. https://doi.org/10.1007/s00264-022-05537-4. Epub 2022 Aug 17. PMID: 35974184. 5
45. Hernigou P, Boceno A, Potage D. Rubber gloves in orthopaedic surgery (part II).
46. Cooke and Goodyear; Halsted and Caroline's gloves of love; from cotton to rubber after Perthes' experiments; double glove technique with Urist. Int Orthop. 2023;47(4):1115–23. https://doi.org/10.1007/s00264-022-05666-w. Epub 2022 Dec 24. PMID: 36565354.
47. Asepsie et antisepsie chirurgicales, 1893 (with Octave Terrillon)
48. Keyes K, Lee MD, Maurer JJ. Antibiotics: mode of action, mechanisms of resistance and transfer. In: Torrance ME, Isaacson RE, editors. Microbial food safety in animal agriculture current topics. Ames: Iowa State Press; 2003. p. 45–56.
49. Bassett EJ, Keith MS, Armelagos GJ, Martin DL, Villanueva AR. Tetracycline-labeled human bone from ancient Sudanese Nubia (a.D.350). Science. 1980;209:1532–4. https://doi.org/10.1126/science.7001623.
50. Cook M, Molto E, Anderson C. Fluorochrome labelling in Roman period skeletons from Dakhleh Oasis, Egypt. Am J Phys Anthropol. 1989;80:137–43. https://doi.org/10.1002/ajpa.1330800202.
51. Falkinham JO 3rd, Wall TE, Tanner JR, Tawaha K, Alali F, Oberlies NH. Proliferation of antibiotic-producing bacteria. Appl Environ Microbiol. 2009;75:2735–41. https://doi.org/10.1128/AEM.00104-09.
52. Wong RW, Hägg U, Samaranayake L, Yuen MK, Seneviratne CJ, Kao R. Antimicrobial activity of Chinese medicine herbs against common bacteria in oral biofilm. A pilot study. Int J Oral Maxillofac Surg. 2010;39:599–605. https://doi.org/10.1016/j.ijom.2010.02.024.
53. Ehrlich P, Hata S. Die Experimentelle Chemotherapie der Spirilosen. Berlin: Julius Springe; 1910.
54. Pruitt RD. William Osler and his Gulstonian lectures on malignant endocarditis. Mayo Clin Proc. 1982;57:4–9.
55. Porter R. The greatest benefit to mankind. Waukegan: Fontana Press; 1999.
56. Saga T, Yamaguchi K. History of antimicrobial agents and resistant bacteria. Japan Med Assoc J. 2009;52:103–8.
57. Levine DP. Vancomycin: a history. Clin Infect Dis. 2006;42:S5–12.

58. Papp-Wallace KM, Edimiani A, Taracila MA, et al. Carbapenems: past, present and future. Antimicrob Agents Chemother. 2011;55:4943–60.
59. Drawz SM, Bonomo RA. Three decades of β-lactamase inhibitors. Clin Microbiol Rev. 2010;23:60–201.
60. Russell AD. The antibacterial activity of a new cephalosporin, cefamandole. J Antimicrob Chemother. 1975;1:97–101.
61. Gould FK. Linezolid: safety and efficacy in special populations. J Antimicrob Chemother. 2011;66(Suppl 4):3–6.
62. Gould K. Antibiotics: from prehistory to the present day. J Antimicrob Chemother. 2016;71(3):572–5.
63. Dunn PM. Sir James Young Simpson (1811-1870) and obstetric anaesthesia. Arch Dis Child. 2002;86:F207–9.
64. Wawersik J. History of Chloroform anaesthesia. Anaestheliol Reanim. 1997;22:144–52. (German)
65. Ashton TA. Noteworthy chemistry of chloroform. J Anaesth Hist. 2016;2:85–8.
66. Winslow K. Poisoning during chloroform anaesthesia in the presence of a naked flame. BMSJ. 1899;140:443–5.
67. Defalque RJ, Wright AJ. The short, tragic life of Robert M Glover. Anaesthesia. 2004;59:394–400.
68. Brandt L, Artmeier-Brandt U. Sieg über den Operationsschmerz : [Victory over surgical pain : 170 years ago the era of modern anesthesia began - but what happened in the operating theater in the time before?]. Anaesthesist. 2016;65(10):727–45. German. https://doi.org/10.1007/s00101-016-0195-y. PMID: 27421850.
69. Petermann H. Crawford Williamson Long - Der eigentliche Entdecker der Anästhesie? [Crawford Williamson Long - The true discoverer of anesthesia?]. Anasthesiol Intensivmed Notfallmed Schmerzther. 2016;51(10):636–9. German. https://doi.org/10.1055/s-0042-117817. Epub 2016 Oct 20. PMID: 27764872.
70. Stone ME, Meyer MR, Alston TA. Elton Romeo Smilie, the not-quite discoverer of ether anesthesia. Anesth Analg. 2010;110(1):195–7. https://doi.org/10.1213/ane.0b013e3181af7f9a. Epub 2009 Aug 27. PMID: 19713261.
71. Stoller SN, Minehart RD, Alston TA. Obstetric and other uses of ether before ether day, according to the Boston Medical and Surgical Journal of 1828-1846. J Anesth Hist. 2016;2(2):57–61. https://doi.org/10.1016/j.janh.2015.11.003. Epub 2015 Nov 28. PMID: 27080505.
72. 90(1):31–4. https://doi.org/10.1177/0022034510385239. Epub 2010 Oct 12. PMID: 20940364.
73. Makris EM, Makhoul KG, Lee TB, Desai MS. Henry Jacob Bigelow (1818-1890). A champion for anesthesia and catalyst for the advancement of surgery. Ann Surg Open. 2022;1:e118.
74. Ramsay MA. John snow, MD: anaesthetist to the Queen of England and Pioneer epidemiologist. Proc (Bayl Univ Med Cent). 2006;19(1):24–8. https://doi.org/10.1080/08998280.2006.11928120. PMID: 16424928; PMCID: PMC1325279.
75. Ball C, Westhorpe R. Local anaesthesia—before Cocaine. Anaesth Intensive Care. 2003;31:3.
76. Ball C, Westhorpe R. Local Anaesthesia after cocaine. Anaesth Intensive Care. 2004;32:157.
77. Ball C, Westhrope R. Local Anaesthetics—procaine (Novocaine, Ethocaine). Anaesth Intensive Care. 2004;32:303.
78. Ball C, Westhrope R. Local Anaesthetics—the origins of lignocaine. Anaesth Intensive Care. 2004;32:611.
79. Dominique Jean Baron Larrey. Warfare history network 2023. https://warfarehistorynetwork.com/article/dominique-jean-baron-larrey/
80. Goerig M, Bacon D, van Zundert A. Carl Koller, cocaine, and local anesthesia: some less known and forgotten facts. Reg Anesth Pain Med 2012;37(3):318–324. doi: https://doi.org/10.1097/AAP.0b013e31825051f3. PMID: 22531385.

81. dos Reis A Jr. Sigmund Freud (1856-1939) and Karl Köller (1857-1944) and the discovery of local anesthesia. Rev Bras Anestesiol. 2009;59(2):244–57. English, Portuguese. https://doi.org/10.1590/s0034-70942009000200013. PMID: 19488537.
82. Barker AE. A fourth report on experiences with spinal analgesia in reference to 2,354 cases. Br Med J. 1912;1(2672):597–602. https://doi.org/10.1136/bmj.1.2672.597. PMID: 20766058; PMCID: PMC2344916.
83. Pearce JM. Walter Essex Wynter, Quincke, and lumbar puncture. J Neurol Neurosurg Psychiatry. 1994;57(2):179. https://doi.org/10.1136/jnnp.57.2.179. PMID: 8126500; PMCID: PMC1072445.
84. Chinn GA, Gray AT, Larson MD. Overcoming Obstacles: The legacy of Fidel Pagés, founder of the epidural, 100 years after his passing. Anesth Analg. 2024;138(2):475–9. https://doi.org/10.1213/ANE.0000000000006706
85. Frederiks JA, Koehler PJ. The first lumbar puncture. J Hist Neurosci. 1997;6(2):147–53. https://doi.org/10.1080/09647049709525699. PMID: 11619518.
86. van Zundert A, Helmstädter A, Goerig M, Mortier E. Centennial of intravenous. Regional anesthesia. Bier's Block (1908-2008). Reg Anesth Pain Med. 2008;33(5):483–9. https://doi.org/10.1016/j.rapm.2008.04.011. PMID: 18774520.
87. McLachlan G. Sir Ivan Magill KCVO, DSc, MB BCh, BAO, FRCS, FFRACS (Hon), FFARCSI (Hon), (1888–1986). Ulster Med J. 2008;77:146–52.
88. Kitz RJ, Lowenstein E. The Henry Isaiah Dorr Professorship at Harvard University. Bull Anaesth History. 2000;18:1-11 and 22-23.
89. Halford FJ. A critique of intravenous anaesthesia in war surgery. Anaesthesiology. 1943;4:70–3.
90. Ball C, Westhorpe R. The history of intravenous anaesthesia: the barbiturates. Part 1. Anaesth Intensive Care. 2001;29:3.
91. Ball C, Westhorpe R. The history of intravenous anaesthesia: the barbiturates. Part 2. Anaesth Intensive Care. 2001;29:219.
92. Organe G. Ronald Jarman DSC, FRCS, FFARCS, FFARCSI (Hon). Anaesthesia. 1973;28:197.
93. Mion G. History of anaesthesia. The ketamine story—past, present and future. EJA. 2017;34:571–5.
94. Stanley TH. The fentanyl story. J Pain. 2014;15:1215–26.
95. Raghavendra T. Neuromuscular blocking drugs: discovery and development. J R Soc Med. 2002;95:363–7.
96. Brodie BC. Further experiments and observations on the action of poisons on the animal system. Philos Trans R Soc Lond. 1812;102:205–27.
97. Smith WDA. Waterton and Wouralia. Br J Anaesthesia. 1983;55:221–5.
98. Ball C, Westhorpe R. Muscle relaxants—the early history. Anaesth Intensive Care. 2005;33:155.
99. Ball C, Westhorpe R. The first synthetic nondepolarizing muscle relaxant. Anaesth Intensive Care. 2005;33:557.
100. Ball C, Westhorpe R. Muscle relaxants—Suxamethonium and THA.
101. McCoy AN, Tan SY. Otto Loewi (1873-1961): Dreamer and Nobel laureate. Singapore Med J. 2014;55(1):3–4. https://doi.org/10.11622/smedj.2014002. PMID: 24452970; PMCID: PMC4291908.
102. Pernick MS. A calculus of suffering: pain, professionalism and anesthesia in nineteenth-century America. New York: Columbia University Press; 1985. p. 421.
103. Miller RD, Eriksson L, Fleisher L, Wiener-Kronish J, Young W. Miller's anesthesia, vol. 1. 7th ed. Philadelphia: Churchill Livingstone; 2009. p. 24.
104. Macewen W. Clinical observations on the introduction of tracheal tubes by the mouth instead of performing tracheotomy or laryngotomy. Br Med J. 1880;2(1022):163–5.
105. Gillies D, Wynands JE, Griffith HR. The pioneer of the use of muscle relaxants in anaesthesia. Br J Anaesth. 1986;58:943–5.

106. Armstrong Davison MH. The history of anaesthesia. In: Evans FT, Gray TC, editors. General anaesthesia. 2nd ed. London: Butterworths; 1965. p. 1–17.
107. Ball C, Westhorpe R. Local anaesthesia - Freud, Koller and Cocaine. Anaesth Intensive Care. 2003;31(3):249.
108. Gerald E. Genius on the Edge: the bizarre double life of Dr William Stewart Halsted. Anesthesiology. 2011;114(6):1496–7.
109. Bier A. Versuche uber Cocainisirung des Rückenmark- es. [Experiments on the cocainization of the spinal cord]. Deutsche Ztschr f Chir. 1899;51:361–9.
110. Corning JL. Spinal anaesthesia and local medication of the cord. N Y Med J. 1885;42:483–5.
111. Pages F. Anestesia metamerica. Rev de San Mil. 1921;11:351–65, 385–9.
112. Albucasis (1013–1116). Chirurgiae, Pars Secunda (translation by Gerardus Cremonensis, 1532), Cap XLIII (cited by Goodall, E. W.: The story of Tracheotomy, Br J Child Dis. 1934;31:253).
113. Fabricius H. (First published 1617). Opera Chirurgica, cap. XLIV (cited by Goodall); 1723.
114. Galen (2nd century). Introductio Seu Medicus (Kuhn's Latin translation), XIV, p. 734 (cited by Goodall).
115. Galloway TC. Tracheotomy in bulbar poliomyelitis. J Am Med Assoc. 1943;123:1096.
116. Goodall EW. The story of tracheotomy—III. Br J Child Dis. 1934a;31:253.
117. Von Leden H. Newer indications for tracheo- tomy. Trans Am Acad Ophthal Otolaryng. 1952:52–6.
118. Watkinson JJ, Gaz MN, Wilson JA. Tracheostomy. In: Stell and Maran's head and neck surgery. 4th ed. Butterworth Heinemann; 2000. p. 153–68.
119. Mushin WW, Rendell-Baker L. Thoracic anesthesia, past and present (reprinted by the Wood Library Museum, 1991). Springfield: Charles C Thomas; 1953. p. 44.
120. Thomas KB. Sir Ivan Whiteside Magill: a review of his publications and other references of his life and work. Anaesthesia. 1978;33:628–34.
121. Gillespie NA. The history of endotracheal anaesthesia. In: Gillespie NA, editor. Endotracheal anaesthesia. 2nd ed. Madison: University of Wisconsin Press; 1948. p. 67–84.
122. Baker A. Artificial respiration: the history of an idea. Med Hist. 1971;15:336–51.
123. Burkle CM, Zapeda FA, Bacon DR, Rose SH. A historical perspective on use of the laryngoscope as a tool in anesthesiology. Anesthesiology. 2004;100:1003–6.
124. Ikeda S, Yanai N, Ishikawa S. Flexible bronchofiberscope. Keio J Med. 1968;17:1–16.
125. Lassen HCA. A preliminary report on the 1952 epidemic of -poliomyelitis in Copenhagen with special reference to the treatment of acute respiratory insufficiency. Lancet. 1953;1:37–41. https://doi.org/10.1016/S0140-6736(53)92530-6.
126. Reisner-Sénélar. The birth of intensive care medicine: Bjorn Ibsen's records. Intensive Care Med. 2011;37:1084–6. https://doi.org/10.1007/s00134-011-2235-z.
127. Severinghaus JW, Astrup PB. History of blood gas analysis. II. pH and acid-base balance measurements. J Clin Monit Comput. 1985;1:259–77. https://doi.org/10.1007/BF02832819.
128. Tang W, Sun S. Max Harry (Hal) Weil—a leader, mentor, friend, and wonderful colleague. Resuscitation. 2011;82:1481–2. https://doi.org/10.1016/j.resuscitation.2011.09.002.
129. Reynolds LA, Tansey EM, editors. History of British intensive care, c.1950–c.2000. Wellcome Witnesses to Twentieth Century Medicine, vol. 42. London: Queen Mary, University of London; 2011.
130. Carson SS, Stocking C, Podsadecki TA, et al. Effects of organizational change in the medical intensive care unit of a teaching hospital: a comparison of 'open' and 'closed' formats. JAMA. 1996;276:322–8. https://doi.org/10.1001/jama.1996.03540040066035.
131. Curtis JR, Patrick DL, Shannon SE, Treece PD, Engelberg RA, Rubenfeld GD. The family conference as a focus to improve communication about end of-life care in the intensive care unit: opportunities for improvement. Crit Care Med. 2001;29:N26–33. https://doi.org/10.1097/00003246-200102001-00006.

Chapter 7
Radiographs, Radiotherapy and the Battle with Cancer

This chapter covers the introduction of imaging to medicine, first by X-rays, then the introduction of contrast to highlight the renal and biliary tracts and the vascular and gastrointestinal systems. Better modalities of imaging were introduced throughout the second half of the twentieth century involving the use of ultrasound (US), radioisotopes, computerized tomography (CT), magnetic resonance imaging (MRI), and positron emission tomography (PET). Modern imaging enables not only anatomical/pathological views of body structures but also their functional/metabolic activity as well.

7.1 The Discovery of X-Rays

In 1895, Wilhelm Conrad Röntgen (1845–1923) (Fig.7.1), a German physicist, was experimenting with cathode rays that are ionized particles produced by an electrical current passed through various vacuum tubes, including a tube developed by Philipp von Lenard (1862–1947). He noticed that a fluorescent screen (a cardboard screen coated with barium platinocyanide), located several feet away from the vacuum tube through which the current was being passed, began to glow even though the tube was not aimed directly at it. A subsequent experiment produced a shadow of his wife's hand on a photographic plate. When she saw her hand, she was so alarmed she exclaimed, "I have seen my death!" He found that the invisible rays could penetrate many substances, including body tissues, leaving shadows that could be recorded on a photographic plate. His first paper, *Ueber eine neue Art von Strahlen* (*On A New Kind of Rays*), was published on December 28, 1895.

The current order of the chapter is correct with radiographs, radiotherapy and Cancer in that order. The battle with cancer covers the nineteenth to twenty-first centuries and should follow radiotherapy.
Most of this chapter focuses on neoadjuvant and adjuvant cancer therapy. The first version has references 1–30 and the second version has references 31–60. We need to check which is the most updated version.

S. Abbas, D. Watters, *The Road to Modern Surgery*,
https://doi.org/10.1007/978-981-96-4337-0_7

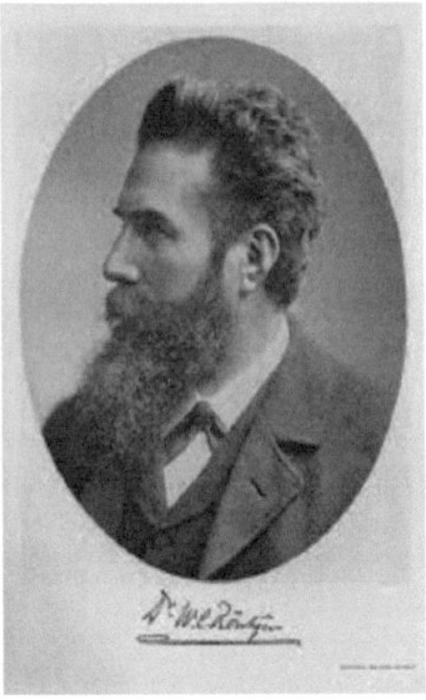

Fig. 7.1 Röntgen. https://upload.wikimedia.org/wikipedia/commons/4/4a/WilhelmRöntgen.JPG. (Images from Wikicommons, public domain)

These rays were called X-rays or Röntgen rays, with the images being called radiograms or röntgenograms. He was awarded, jointly with Philipp Lenard, the British Royal Society's Rumford medal for his discovery. He refused to take out any patents, ethically believing X-rays and radiographs should belong to the public domain. In 1901, he was awarded the first Nobel Prize in physics. Despite a generous inheritance after his father's death, the hyperinflation in Germany after World War I led to his impoverishment, so he lived his final years in his country home in Weilheim, near Munich. He died of colorectal cancer in 1923 [1]. Philipp Lenard was born in Pressburg, Hungary (now Bratislava, Slovakia) was later awarded the Nobel Prize for Physics in 1905. This was for his work on cathode rays, particularly that the energy (speed) of the rays depended on the light's frequency, not its intensity.

Within a year of their discovery, X-rays were being used to identify bullets and shrapnel during the war between Italy and Abyssinia (1896). The technology was then used in several British colonial wars, the Greco-Turkish war, and the Spanish-American war in 1898.

7.2 X-Ray Tubes and Fluoroscopes

In 1896, Thomas Edison (1847–1931), a businessman and inventor, began working on X-ray imaging and developed an improved X-ray machine, a fluoroscope, which was more practical and easier to use than Röntgen's original device. Unfortunately, his worker, Clarence Dally, died of radiation-induced cancer after 8 years of irradiating his hands and arms in 1904.

In 1913, William Coolidge (1873–1975), an American electrical engineer at General Electric, developed the first X-ray tube with a heated cathode, which produced a more stable and predictable X-ray beam than previous designs. This innovation revolutionized the field of X-ray technology, making X-ray machines safer and more reliable [2–4].

7.3 Radiation Therapy

In 1896, the year after Wilhelm Röntgen discovered X-rays, Henri Becquerel (Fig. 7.2) (1852–1908), studying fluorescence, exposed uranium (potassium uranyl sulfate) to sunlight and then wrapped and placed it on a photographic film in order to develop the resulting photograph. He thought his experiment "failed" because it turned out to be a dark cloudy day in Paris but decided to develop the photographic plates anyway. To his great surprise, the images were very clear, proving that the uranium emitted radiation without even being exposed to sunlight. Becquerel had had accidentally discovered radioactivity.

7.3.1 Marie Curie

> *We must not forget that when radium was discovered no one knew that it would prove useful in hospitals. The work was one of pure science. And this is a proof that scientific work must not be considered from the point of view of the direct usefulness of it. It must be done for itself, for the beauty of science, and then there is always the chance that a scientific discovery may become like the radium, a benefit for mankind.* —Marie Curie

Marie Curie (1867–1934) (Fig. 7.3), born Maria Sklodowski in Warsaw, Poland, then part of the Russian Empire, moved to Paris in 1891. She had earlier worked to support her sister, Bronislawa (1865–1939), to study medicine at the Sorbonne (University of Paris). She graduated as an obstetrician and gynecologist in 1890, marrying a Polish-born physician but political exile, Kazimierz Dluski, the same year. Marie moved to Paris in 1891, to live with them and commence her studies at the Sorbonne. She always hoped to return to study in Poland but was refused the opportunity to study in Krakow on the grounds of being female so she returned

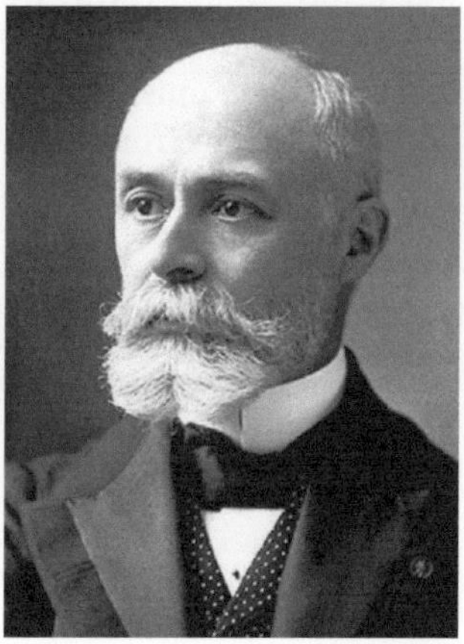

Fig. 7.2 Henri Becquerel. https://commons.wikimedia.org/w/index.php?search=Henri+Becquerel&title=Special:MediaSearch&go=Go&type=image. (Images from Wikicommons, public domain)

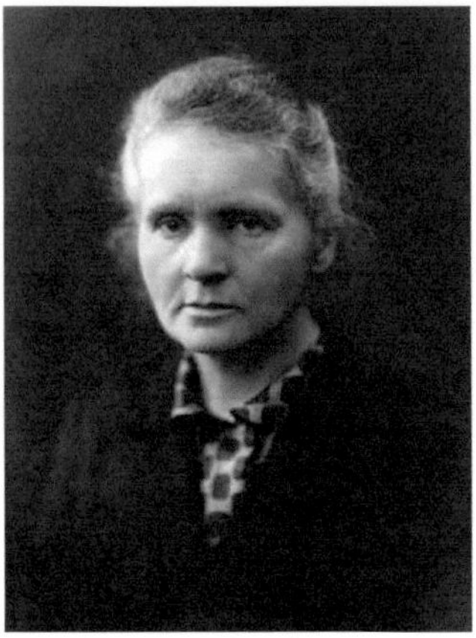

Fig. 7.3 Marie Curie. https://simple.wikipedia.org/wiki/Marie_Curie#/media/File:Marie_Curie_c1920.jpg. (Images from Wikicommons, public domain)

to Paris. She gained degrees in Physics in 1893 and 1894 and married fellow scientist, Pierre Curie (1859–1906), in 1895.

In 1900, she became the first woman faculty member at the École Normale Supérieure and, with her husband, joined the faculty of the University of Paris. She was awarded her doctorate from the University of Paris in 1903, the year she also became the first woman to be awarded a Nobel Prize.

She was awarded the Nobel Prize in Physics (1903), with Henri Becquerel and her husband, Pierre, for their discoveries on radioactivity, which they also named after radium. Their work paved the way for radiation and radiotherapy in medicine. Between 1898 and 1902, Marie and Pierre Curie published papers that showed that radium killed tumor cells faster than normal cells. Her and Pierre's discovery of radium (named after the Latin word ray) and polonium (named after her native Poland) earned her the 1911 Nobel Prize in chemistry [5, 6].

In 1914–1918, during World War I, X-ray machines were used to support the war effort. Marie Curie was active in establishing mobile and stationary X-ray facilities for the Red Cross in France. The films were mainly used to help localize bullets and shrapnel and were taken without any regard to protecting the patient or the physician from radiation exposure. After the war, radiographers and radiologists who suffered were compensated, at least in Britain, from a Compassionate fund.

> *After three German bombs fell on Paris in September 1914, she [Marie Curie] evacuated her research staff and moved her radiation institutes to Bordeaux for her research and teaching about radiation and x-rays. She was named by the French government as Director of the Red Cross Radiology Service. Begging funds from donors and manufacturers, by October of 1914 she funded the building of 20 vehicles equipped with x-ray equipment to be used in the war; the electricity needed for generating their x-rays was from the trucks' engines. Previously, x-ray service was not used near front lines because of a lack of a consistent electricity source. In addition, Madam Curie helped establish 200 stationary x-ray facilities, with consistent electricity sources, to the rear of the battlefields* [7–9].

A radium institute was set up in Paris in 1914, on a street now named Pierre et Marie Curie. In 1932, the Warsaw Radium Institute was opened with funds raised by Marie, and with her sister, Bronislawa Dluska, as the director.

The dangers of radiation were unknown in 1900. Marie Curie (1867–1934) would eventually die from aplastic anemia as a result of radiation exposure from her experimenting with radioactive materials. Also, there were female factory workers in the early twentieth century who painted watch dials with radium-based paint to enable them to glow in the dark. The practice of lip-pointing also led to ingestion of small amounts of radium. At the time, radium was considered a wonder new material, used in consumer products such as paints and cosmetics. As the dangers of radium were not well understood, the women who worked with it were not protected. Many developed radiation sickness, aplastic anemias, and bone cancer. The "Radium Girls" case would lead to major changes in occupational health and safety regulations, as well as increased public awareness of the dangers of radiation.

7.4 Computerized Tomography (CT) Scanning

CT is one of the most important medical innovations with regard to imaging in human history, and since its introduction in 1971, it has revolutionized the way doctors diagnose and treat patients. Overall, CT scans provide doctors with a powerful diagnostic tool that can help them identify a wide range of medical conditions, from cancer and heart disease to bone fractures and internal injuries. By providing multiple detailed axial, coronal, and sagittal 2D views of the body, now with three-dimensional reconstruction, CT scans facilitate unprecedented anatomical and pathological imaging accuracy.

7.4.1 Godfrey Hounsfield and Allan Cormack

The history of computed tomography (CT) scan can be traced back to the early twentieth century, when scientists first began exploring the potential of X-ray technology for creating detailed images of the soft tissues inside the body. In the 1920s and 1930s, British engineer, Sir Godfrey Hounsfield (1919–2004) (Fig. 7.4), and South African engineer, Allan Cormack, each independently, began working on the development of techniques for creating detailed cross-sectional images of the body using X-rays. In Hounsfield's workshop at the Electrical and Musical Industries laboratories, in Middlesex, Hounsfield developed a computer device that could process hundreds of X-ray beams to form a 2D image of soft tissues inside a living organism. He took images on a sensor, not on a film. They were taken with a rotating X-ray source. He could show the different tissue densities, with three-dimensional volumes when the images were taken at short intervals. In 1971, he was

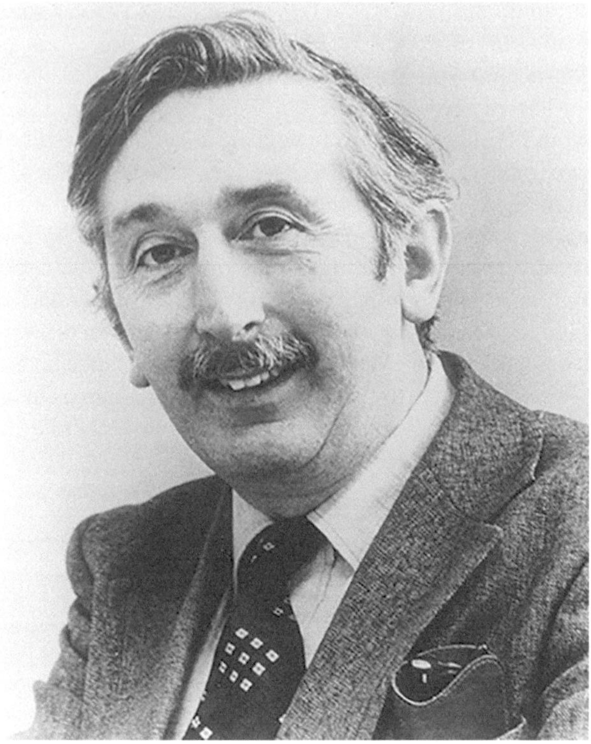

Fig. 7.4 Sir Godfrey Hounsfield. (Images from Wikipedia. license type: no restrictions, public domain. https://en.wikipedia.org/wiki/Godfrey_Hounsfield#/media/File:Godfrey_Hounsfield.jpg)

tasked with testing this new CT methodology using the head of a cow from a slaughterhouse before moving onto his first human patient. In the early 1970s, Hounsfield developed the first CT scanner, which was able to produce detailed images of the brain by taking multiple X-ray images from different angles and then using a computer to combine them into a single cross-sectional image.

Allan Cormack (1924–1998) was a South African, American physicist who independently developed the mathematical algorithms necessary to reconstruct CT images from X-ray data. In fact, Cormack's original motivation in the "discovery" was to image and quantify the electron density within the body. The purpose of using calibrated radiation sources is to more accurately calculate radiation dose during radiation therapy. He was awarded the 1979 Nobel Prize in Medicine jointly with Hounsfield.

The first CT scanner was installed at Atkinson Morley Hospital in London in 1971, and soon after, CT was being used to diagnose a wide range of conditions, including tumors, and internal traumatic injuries.

CT technology has continued to evolve over the years, with improvements in scanner design and computer processing leading to faster scans, higher resolution images, and the ability to acquire multiplanar images and 3D reconstructions. Today, CT is an essential tool in many areas of medicine, including radiology, emergency medicine, and oncology, and has saved countless lives by helping to diagnose and treat a wide range of conditions.

Cardiac CT with coronary CTA (angiography) is a promising new frontier in cardiac imaging, offering doctors a noninvasive way to diagnose and monitor coronary heart disease and potentially improve patient outcomes.

However, CT scans use ionizing radiation, and the overuse and misuse of CT scans has raised concerns about the potential health risks associated with exposure to ionizing radiation. Thus, it is important to use CT scans only when the benefits outweigh the risks. Radiology is transforming with transformative technology, so we can expect AI to play a major role in the future. Medical imaging informatics already gathers, analyzes, and communicates essential imaging information [10, 11].

7.5 Magnetic Resonance Imaging

The history of magnetic resonance imaging (MRI) can be traced back to the early twentieth century, when scientists first began exploring the potential of nuclear magnetic resonance (NMR) for creating detailed images of the inside of the body. Felix Bloch (1905–1983), a Swiss physicist, and Edward Purcell (1912–1997) (Fig. 7.5), an American physicist, independently discovered the phenomenon of nuclear magnetic resonance (NMR) in 1946 while working at different universities. Bloch and Purcell were jointly awarded the Nobel Prize in Physics in 1952 for their work on NMR.

NMR is a technique that allows scientists to study the magnetic properties of atomic nuclei in molecules. By applying a strong magnetic field and a radiofrequency pulse to a sample, scientists can cause the nuclei to align with the magnetic field and emit radio waves that can be detected and analyzed. During the 1970s and

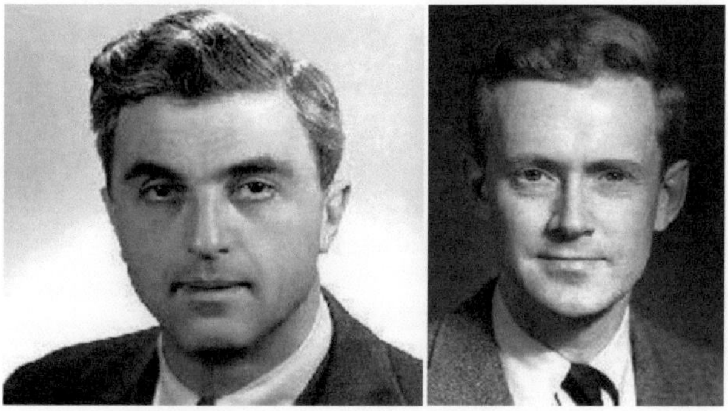

Fig. 7.5 Felix Bloch, Edward Purcell. (**a**) (Photograph by Willy Pragher), Wikimedia. https://commons.wikimedia.org/w/index.php?search=Felix+Bloch&title=Special:MediaSearch&go=Go&type=image. (**b**) Edward Purcell. https://commons.wikimedia.org/w/index.php?search=Edward+Purcell&title=Special:MediaSearch&go=Go&type=image

1980s, significant progress was made in the development of MRI technology. In 1971, an American-Armenian doctor, Raymond Damadian (1936–2022), published a paper in the journal *Science* reporting that NMR can detect tumours in the living body, as it can differentiate tumours from normal tissue by how long it takes for MR to relax. He also invented an "apparatus" to scan the body for tumours. He did this by having the NMR beams go to specific parts of the body. In 1977, he named the focusing NMR concept (FONAR). He and other scientists did the first human full-body scan using the FONAR scan in 1977. The imaging took 5 hours to acquire.

In the following years, improvements in scanner design and computer processing led to faster scans and higher resolution images, making MRI increasingly useful for a wide range of diagnostic applications [12, 13].

In 1973, American chemist Paul Christian Lauterbur (1929–2007) and British physicist Sir Peter Mansfield (1933–2017) worked on producing MR images at faster speeds by varying the magnetic field and developing mathematical process. This earned them a 2003 Nobel Prize in Physiology or Medicine. Their work led to modern MRI scanners with high quality images, that have provided noninvasive ways to diagnose a variety of conditions.

It's worth noting that MRI is now an essential tool for many branches of medicine, including radiology, neurology, and orthopedics, revolutionising the way doctors visualise pathology. Unlike X-ray and CT, MRI doesn't use ionizing radiation so it is considered a safe imaging modality for persons that don't have implanted metal that could move under the force of the magnetic field. It is not suitable for people with claustrophobia as it takes some time of being enclosed within the machine to generate the images. MRI images are detailed and precise and provide a lot of information about the state of soft tissues, particularly the brain and spinal cord, as well as the articular surfaces of joints. MRI is the crown jewel of medical imaging due to its superior soft tissue contrast and anatomic detail. It is used for preoperative staging (e.g., staging rectal cancer).

7.5.1 Functional MRI

The introduction of functional MRI (fMRI) which measures the brain's activity by detecting changes in blood flow can be used to study brain function and response to stimuli. fMRI is used to image central nervous system diseases including vascular mapping for glioma diagnosis and grading [14, 15].

7.6 Ultrasound

Ultrasound uses high-frequency, inaudible, sound waves that are transmitted into the body to map the amplitude of the echoes and time delay to produce images of body structures. It is noninvasive and allows percutaneous biopsies to be performed under imaging control.

Ultrasound (the generation and reception of sound waves in the frequency range of millions of cycles per second or megahertz) is emitted by a piezoelectric process (electricity arising from pressure and latent heat). There are A, B, and M modes of transmission. Initial studies involved only transmission of ultrasonic waves through a specimen to a receiver placed on the opposite site that recorded the amount of sound not absorbed. The pulsed reflection method places both transmitter and receiver on the same side. A (Amplitude)-mode ultrasound provides a one-dimensional image of the amplitude of the wave on a vertical axis with time on the horizontal axis. B (Brightness) mode relates the brightness of the image to the amplitude of the ultrasound wave. M (Motion) mode relates the amplitude of the ultrasound wave to the imaging of moving structures such as cardiac muscle [16].

7.6.1 The Discovery of Ultrasound

7.6.1.1 Lazzaro Spallanzani's Experiments on Bats

The use of echolocation (sound waves) for navigation by bats was first hypothesized in the late 1700s by Lazzaro Spallanzani (1729–1799), an Italian catholic priest who was also a biologist and physiologist. He did experiments on bats showing they did not need light or sight to fly safely in the dark. However, his hypotheses were not generally accepted given at the time he was unaware of the actual scientific basis of sound waves and their echos (Fig. 7.6).

7.6.1.2 Underwater Speed of Sound in Lake Geneva

In 1826, Swiss physicist, Jean-Daniel Colladon, and Charles Sturm conducted studies on the underwater speed of sound in Lake Geneva. In 1877, John William Strutt (Lord Rayleigh) published *The Theory of Sound* and Strutt was appointed to Great Britain's Board of Invention and Research that would later supervise the development of Sound Navigation and Ranging (SONAR) during World War I.

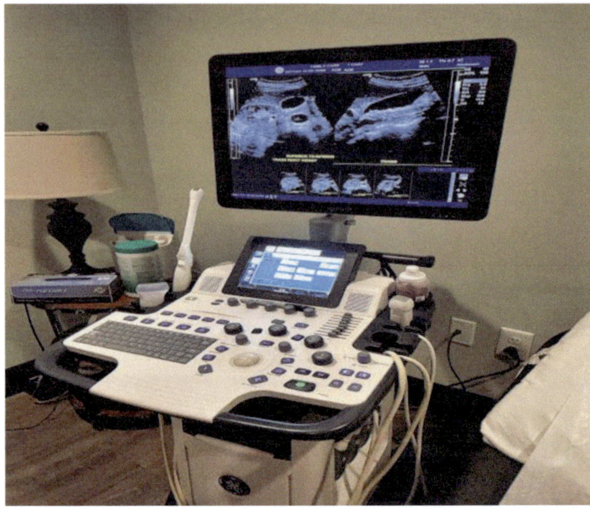

Fig. 7.6 A modern ultrasound scanner. Wikipedia, Public Domain, no restrictions. https://commons.wikimedia.org/w/index.php?search=ultrasound+machine&title=Special:MediaSearch&go=Go&type=image

7.6.1.3 Measuring Ultrasound

In 1877, Jacques and Pierre Curie observed the emission of an electrical potential when mechanical pressure was applied to a quartz crystal. They used Rochelle salt (sodium potassium tartrate tetrahydrate). In 1881, Gabriel Lippman (1845–1921) recognized the reverse effect of a mechanical stress in response to a voltage difference and the underlying mathematics involved. Thus, it was possible to measure the generation and reception of ultrasound waves [16, 17].

7.6.1.4 SONAR and Piezoceramics

Further research and development in piezoelectricity soon followed. Their use of piezoelectricity, a property of certain materials that convert mechanical energy into electrical energy, led to the invention of devices like microphones, speakers, and capacitors. They also led to the development of SONAR which relies upon a pulse echo principle. The initial devices relied upon kilohertz transmission, but ultrasound requires a reduced wavelength for the megahertz range. In 1941, technology was developed in Michigan during World War II that would enable ultrasonic examination of ships' hulls to identify metal defects. With regard to piezoceramics, the original crystals were replaced in the 1940s by barium titanate and later, by lead zirconate titanate in 1954 [16–18].

7.6.1.5 The First Use of Ultrasound for Therapy

Initially, ultrasound was studied as a therapy with University of Illinois' William J Fry (−1968), a physicist who, following animal studies, used high-intensity-focused ultrasound to destroy basal ganglia in patients with Parkinson's disease. He is also credited with improving the imaging of ultrasound by the use of computers. Peter Lindstrom (1907–2000), a Swedish-born American neurosurgeon (married to actress Ingrid Bergman from 1937 to 1950), used high-intensity ultrasound for a number of neurological conditions, including to ablate the frontal lobe in moribund patients with disseminated carcinomatosis. By the 1950s, ultrasound was being used extensively in physical and rehabilitation medicine, and there were reports from the United States of its use in rheumatoid arthritis, whilst in Europe, it was being trialed in the treatment of Menière's disease. It was seen by some as a wonder treatment worth trying for a wide range of conditions which only led to concern over its harmful effects.

7.6.1.6 The First Congress of Ultrasound (1948)

Karl Theodore Dussik (1908–1968) was an Austrian neurologist who, in 1942, used ultrasound to examine the brain. His images (sonograms) were later shown to be generated by echoes from the skull, and today, US is best used diagnostically for the brain with an intact skull when performed through the anterior fontanelle prior to its closure around 9–12 months. The first Congress of Ultrasound in medicine was held in Erlangen, Germany, in May 1948. At this congress, only two papers on diagnostic ultrasound were presented, one by Dussik and the other by Wolf-Dieter Keidel (1907–2011), a pioneer in echocardiology from the University of Erlangen, who relied upon the transmission technique at 60 Khz. At the time, he was only able to generate clear images of cardiac pulsations [17–19].

7.6.1.7 Diagnostic Ultrasound and Echocardiography (1950s)

In the early 1950s, Dr. George Ludwig (1922–1973), a German American physician based in Bethesda, Maryland, and Dr. Inge Edler (1911–2001), a Swedish cardiologist, independently developed techniques to utilize ultrasound diagnostically. Ludwig was interested in imaging gallstones, while Edler was an early developer of echocardiography. Ludwig studied ultrasound in various animal tissues and established that the velocity of sound in soft tissues was an average of 1540 m/sec.

7.6.1.8 "A"-Mode Ultrasound with 15 Khz Transducer

John Julian Wild (1914–2009), born in Kent, England, and a Cambridge graduate (MD 1942), emigrated to the United States after WWII in 1946 to study the use of ultrasound at the University of Minnesota. He used A-mode scanning and a 15 Khz transducer to study the intestines, hoping to distinguish between paralytic ileus and obstruction. They also studied malignant specimens in a water tank, noting that gastrointestinal cancer was more echogenic than normal tissue. He identified a recurrent thigh tumor and a breast cancer, publishing his results in 1952. In 1991, he received the Japan Prize (1m Yen = US$370,000) for his contributions to ultrasound [19, 20].

7.6.1.9 Japan's First A-Mode Ultrasound Scanner (1949)

In Japan, ultrasound was also being simultaneously studied and developed by surgeons, Kenji Tanaka and Toshio Wagai, at Juntendo University. They were interested in imaging intracranial disease. Shigeru Nakajima, Director of the Japan Radio Company, and Rokuro Uchida, physicist and chief engineer, built Japan's first ultrasonic scanner operating in A mode in 1949, modified from a metal flaw detector. The ALOKA company was then founded in 1950, headed by Uchida. By 1955, they were experimenting with B-mode scanning and then water-bag scanners. Tanaka wrote a book, published in 1969, on the *Diagnosis of Brain Disease by Ultrasound.* Michio Ishihara from Tokyo and Hajime Murooka from Saitama delivered a paper in Japanese on the ultrasound diagnosis of gynecological masses in 1958, based on the Ascan.

7.6.1.10 Ian Donald, Tom Brown, and Obstetric Ultrasound

In the mid-1950s, Ian Donald (1910–1987), professor of obstetrics at Glasgow University from 1954, pioneered the application of ultrasound in obstetrics and gynaecology. During the war, in the Royal Air Force, he developed an interest in radar and sonar. At the Western Infirmary in Glasgow, Donald met Tom Brown (1933–20), a technician employed by Kelvin and Hughes. Brown was changing a bulb in the theater while Donald was experimenting with a metal flaw detector on pathological specimens. Brown then worked with Donald building him the first B-mode scanner in 1957. They then published an article titled "Investigation of Abdominal Masses by Pulsed Ultrasound" in 1958 in the Lancet. The case involved a 64-year-old woman with a mucinous ovarian cyst, which was later proven to be benign on resection. Her initial clinical diagnosis had been gastric cancer with ascites! In 1963, Tom Brown presented Ian Donald with the diasonograph. Donald discovered that the full urinary bladder allowed transmission of ultrasound through the pelvis with clearer images, and he was able to identify pelvic tumors, ectopic pregnancy, and the location of the placenta. He also measured the biparietal diameter of the fetus to use as an index of fetal growth.

7.6.1.11 Gray-Scale Scanning

In the early 1960s, ultrasound was limited by the slow and tedious acquisition of images which were also limited in their picture resolution. The images were a binary, black and white, until gray scale allowed compression of the echo amplitudes to allow their full range to be displayed on screen [17, 19, 21].

7.6.1.12 George Kossoff and the Australian Commonwealth Acoustic Laboratory (1960s)

Australian unit that made the technological advances led to the wider availability and use of gray scale. In 1959, a Commonwealth Acoustic Laboratory (CAL) was established in Sydney. By 1968, George Kossoff, a physicist, with his team achieved displaying the gray scale mode following the development of the television scanner converter tube. Digital scanners were introduced onto the market in 1976 and these produced reliable, readable, and reproducible images. David Robinson, a physicist, worked on a water-bath ultrasonic scanner with Dr. William Garrett (1927–1915; an obstetrician) for use in obstetrics. Their work allowed the ultrasonic identification of fetal abnormalities. They also published an early textbook on *Ultrasound in Clinical Obstetrics*. In conjunction with Sydney surgeon, Tom Reeve (1923–2023), a breast ultrasound machine, was installed at Sydney's Royal North Shore Hospital in 1966, while cardiac ultrasound was studied by Dr. David Wilcken (1927–2020) at the Royal Prince Henry Hospital. Kossoff went on to become the president of the World Ultrasound in Medicine and Biology Association (1982–1985) [22].

7.6.1.13 Real-Time Imaging (1968)

In 1968, Siemens released the Vidoson which had real-time imaging, a technique originally introduced by Wild in the 1950s but on inferior equipment. The Vidoson allowed the acquisition and display of higher resolution images so rapidly they were effectively simultaneous. This made ultrasound imaging less operator dependent. Transducers and ultrasound machines were further improved, and in general surgery, ultrasound was being used to diagnose breast, biliary tract, and thyroid pathology. In 1971, it was used to investigate blunt abdominal trauma by Danish surgeon, JK Kirstensen [20, 21].

7.6.2 *Doppler*

In the 1970s, the development of high-frequency ultrasound probes and the use of Doppler techniques made it possible to visualize blood vessels, which led to the application of ultrasound in vascular surgery.

7.6.2.1 Christian Andreas Doppler (1841)

In 1841, an Austrian physicist, Christian Andreas Doppler (1803–1843), studying the colors emitted by stars, published a treatise proposing that the relative motion of a star relative to the earth resulted in a spectral shift of the white light emitted. This became known as the Doppler effect, which although later disproven in relation to stars, the changes in frequency of sound waves when there is relative motion between the source of the wave and the observer were correct.

7.6.2.2 Continuous Wave Emission (1956)

The Doppler effect was used to study the flow of blood by Kalmus in 1954, and Shigeo Satomura (1919–1960) on cardiac valvular motion in Osaka in 1956. The latter's work was published in Japanese so was unrecognized in most Western countries including the United States. The early Doppler imaging relied upon continuous wave emission but could not distinguish different moving structures within the beam path [20, 21].

7.6.2.3 Pulsed Doppler (1970)

Pulsed Doppler did permit this differentiation and a Seattle team produced an instrument to do so in 1970. By the end of the decade, they were able to couple a real-time mechanical sector scanner to a pulsed Doppler machine. This was used in the 1980s to evaluate carotid artery disease. Improvements in the microprocessors allowed Doppler color flow mapping which facilitated the identification of plaques and their hemodynamic effects. Ultrasound was soon being used for a wide range of conditions including midline encephalography for traumatic brain injury, as well as for echocardiography and urology.

Kazunori Baba, University of Tokyo, first reported on obtaining a 3D fetal image. He achieved this through processing 2D images on a mini computer in 1986. Baba collaborated with ALOKA to further develop 3D ultrasound in Japan. A group led by Donald King at Columbia University described different computer algorithms to achieve 3D spatial display in 1990 while HC Kuo, FM Chang, and Ch Wu in Taiwan 3D developed visualization of the fetal face, cerebellum, and cervical vertebral. They used an Austrian machine, the Combison 330 produced in 1989. In 1992,

Thomas Nelson and Dolores Pretorius at University of California, San Diego, produced 3D images of the carotid arteries. A 4D ultrasound, adding motion, was first described at the University College Hospital in London in 1996. This enabled fetal echocardiography to identify congenital heart defects. Between 1995 and 1997, Eberhard Merz in Mainz, Germany, utilized surface and transparent views to diagnose surface and skeletal abnormalities and then demonstrated how intravaginal 3D ultrasound could be used to identify cleft lips and other malformations of the face [21–23].

7.6.2.4 Ultrasound Dissectors in Laparoscopic Surgery (1990s)

From the 1990s, the therapeutic use of ultrasound in surgery was further expanded with the development of laparoscopic surgery, which is a type of minimally invasive surgery that uses small incisions and specialized instruments, including an ultrasound dissector, to perform procedures. In addition to ultrasonic dissectors, during a procedure, ultrasound probes can also be inserted through a port to more accurately image tissue anatomy and pathology and assess for resectability.

7.7 Interventional Radiology

Interventional radiology (IR) involves performing less invasive procedures under the guidance of imaging. The ability to perform such procedures requires the structures and/or pathology to be treated to be first identified, then accessed, whilst the intervention is delivered under guidance. IR encompasses a wide range of minimally invasive procedures, including angiography and embolization (to control bleeding or to downstage a tumor), obtain a biopsy, drain fluid collections, dilate and/or stent a stricture).

Today, interventional radiology (IR) is no longer only the domain of radiologists. Cardiologists replace heart valves, neurologists treat cerebral aneurysms, vascular surgeons stent aortic aneurysms with endovascular grafts, and urologists destroy renal calculi with lithotripsy via the ureter.

7.7.1 Egas Moniz—Cerebral Angiography

Egas Moniz (1874–1955) (Fig. 7.7), a Portuguese neurologist and psychiatrist, developed the technique of cerebral angiography in 1927. He was professor of neurology in Lisbon from 1926 to 1944. This involved injecting radio-opaque contrast directly into the common carotid artery and then taking multiple X-ray images to visualize the cerebral vasculature. He initially experimented on three patients (suspected brain tumor, epilepsy, and parkinsonism) with strontium and lithium

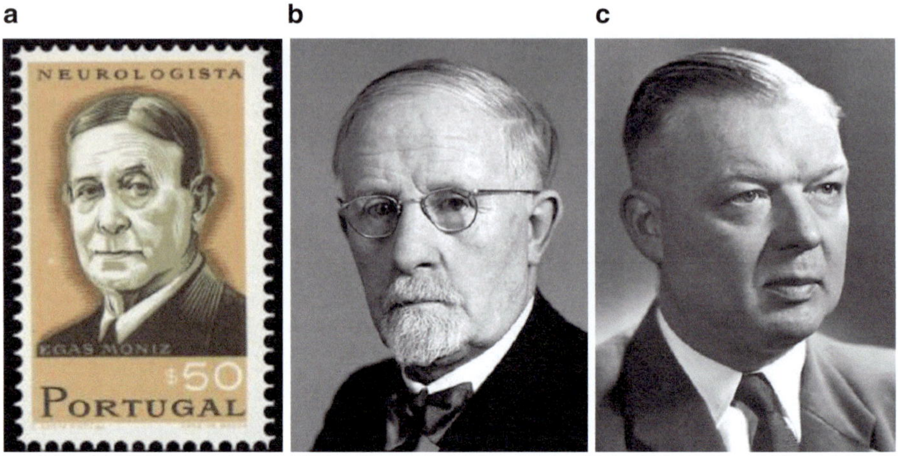

Fig. 7.7 (**a**) Egas Moniz. https://commons.wikimedia.org/wiki/File:Egas-Moniz-neurosurgeon-Nobel-prize_laureed.jpg. (**b**) Rudolph Hess. https://commons.wikimedia.org/w/index.php?search=Walter+Rudolf+Hess+&title=Special:MediaSearch&go=Go&type=image. (**c**) Werner Forssmann. https://commons.wikimedia.org/w/index.php?search=Werner+Forssmann&title=Special:MediaSearch&go=Go&type=image. Moniz, Middle: Rudolph Hess (Image: Wikipedia). Werner Forssmann (right—Wikipedia)

bromide but was unsuccessful and one patient died. He then tried 25% sodium iodide on a further three patients, this time achieving a clear and safe angiogram of the cerebral vasculature. He published over 110 papers on cerebral angiography between 1927 and 1934. Moniz did not give the injections himself as he suffered from gouty arthritis. These were given by Dr. Almeida Lima, a young neurosurgeon. He was twice nominated for the Nobel Prize for this work but his Nobel Prize in Physiology or Medicine was awarded in 1949 for his pioneering work on frontal lobotomy which he called leukotomy. This was jointly awarded with Walter Rudolf Hess (1881–1973) (Fig. 7.7), a Swiss ophthalmologist (1906–1912) turned physiologist (professor of Physiology in Zurich 1917–1951) who also discovered the role of the medulla oblongata, diencephalon, and hypothalamus [24–26].

7.7.2 Cardiac Angiography

Werner Forssmann (1904–1979) (Fig. 7.8), in Germany, performed the first cardiac angiography in 1929 when he inserted a catheter into his arm and into his heart.

> *Using a mirror he advanced the catheter under fluoroscopic control and then climbed the stairs to the x ray department where a chest film was taken. Forssmann had two objects in mind. Firstly to use this technique in emergencies to administer drugs directly into the heart, and secondly 'to study the heart and for diagnosis'. Later he catheterised his own heart on six more occasions. He also injected contrast material, Uroselectan, in 1931 in an attempt to produce an angiocardiogram.*

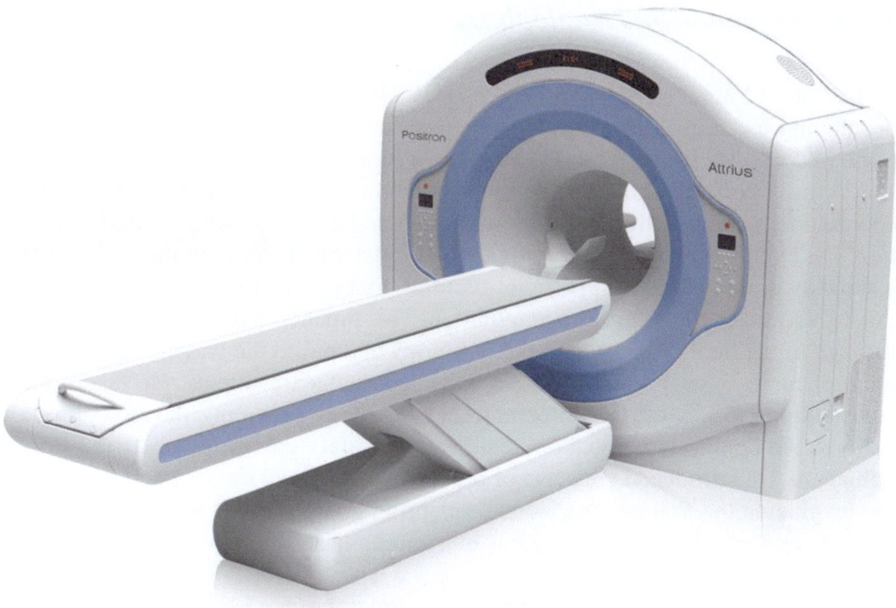

Fig. 7.8 Modern PET scanner. Wikipedia, public domain. https://upload.wikimedia.org/wikipedia/commons/2/29/PET_recortada.jpg

Forssmann's work was initially met with skepticism and criticism from the medical community, but it eventually gained wider recognition and paved the way for the development of cardiac catheterization and interventional cardiology. By 1932, pulmonary angiography using a catheter in the right atrium had been performed in Lisbon, Paris, and Buenos Aires.

André Cournand (1895–1988) was a graduate of the University of Paris whose studies were interrupted by WWI in which he was awarded a Croix de Guerre (bronze). He moved to New York and was appointed to the Bellevue Hospital (Columbia University). He was tasked with establishing a cardiac physiology laboratory under supervision of W. Dickinson Richards (1895–1973). They catheterized the right atrium, right ventricle, and pulmonary artery to measure the pressures in these chambers, in patients with pulmonary and cardiac disease. Their work, begun in 1932, and led in the 1940s, to successful catheterization in humans. In 1953, Cournand chaired a committee on the safety of cardiac catheterization, reviewing four deaths in 5700 catheterizations from 8 laboratories and 1325 venous angiograms from 2 laboratories with no deaths. Forssmann, Cournand, and Dickinson Richards were jointly awarded the Nobel Prize in Physiology or Medicine in 1956 for their pioneering work in cardiac catheterization and cardiac physiology [27, 28].

7.7.3 Percutaneous Angioplasty

In the late 1960s, Charles Dotter (1920–1985), an American radiologist, began developing techniques for percutaneous transluminal angioplasty (PTA), a procedure used to open blocked blood vessels. On January 16, 1964, Dr. Charles Dotter successfully performed the first percutaneous transluminal angioplasty (PTA) procedure on a patient with painful leg ischemia and gangrene who refused amputation. Dr. Dotter used a catheter with a small inflatable balloon on the end to dilate a stenosis in the patient's superficial femoral artery, which restored blood flow to the leg and saved the limb from amputation. This procedure marked a major breakthrough in the field of interventional radiology and paved the way for the development of many other minimally invasive endovascular treatments. He made many contributions to devices for interventional radiology including the flow-directed balloon, the double-lumen balloon catheter, the safety guidewire, and the J-tipped guidewire. He introduced concepts of percutaneous arterial stenting and stent grafting by placing the first percutaneous "coilspring graft" into the femoral artery of a dog, as well as pioneering injection of streptokinase directly into an occluding thrombus.

Andreas Grüntzig (1939–1985), a German-born radiologist, trained in Heidelberg and London before working in Zurich, was the first to perform a femoral artery angioplasty using a balloon-tipped catheter. He had already written up his experience of the Dotter technique but in order to perform an angioplasty, he had to make his own balloons. He successfully performed "percutaneous luminal dilatation" in 1974 and then the first percutaneous coronary angioplasty (PTCA) in 1975. The patient had unstable angina but was not fit for coronary artery bypass surgery. His paper in the Lancet on the first five cases was published in 1978. He ran four live demonstration angioplasty courses in Zurich between 1978 and 1980 for interventional radiologists and cardiologists from around the world. However, Grüntzig was subsequently only able to do two patients a week in Zurich, particularly because his professor (Siegenthaler, known locally in his clinic as the little Napoleon) was afraid something would go wrong. He was never offered a chair or tenure, and so in 1980, he accepted a position at Emory University, Atlanta, Georgia, USA. There he was able to treat two patients a day. He treated over 3000 patients without a death and was able to run 10 educational courses between 1980 and 1985.

Charles Dotter wrote on August 22, 1980 to thank him for a ring given to him by Grüntzig:

> *"You proved to be one of the most skilled catheterizers I have ever seen; not only that but a superb teacher and a doctor who Andreas Grüntzig [over] 40 years of balloon angioplasty never forgot his patient. We will be happy to have you in this country. [...]. In view of your accomplishments and competency it seems inconceivable that Zürich has not given you a full professorship with tenure. Our gain will be their loss."*
>
> *Dotter continues: "I will admit that in the past I have been at times jealous, especially when I heard people talking about the Grüntzig procedure. I find no jealousy now, only admiration at the thorough and innovative job you have done" [...] "The ring is on my desk*

and I will continue to prize it. In an effort to give you something, I am forwarding you a print of our 1968 film on transluminal angioplasty. It's long out of date, but has certain historical significance". [28]

Charles Dotter and Andreas Grüntzig were nominated for the Nobel Prize in 1978. Their nomination did not succeed despite developing the concepts and first tools to perform percutaneous endovascular and coronary interventions. Perhaps the nomination was too early because they were the foremost pioneers in interventional cardiovascular procedures. Those who attended the Grüntzig courses went on to change the practice of cardiovascular medicine in their countries all around the world. Tragically, Andreas Grüntzig and his second wife died in a plane crash in 1985.

7.7.3.1 Interventional Procedures Under Ultrasound Guidance

In the 1970s, ultrasound-guided techniques for minimally invasive procedures were also developed, including percutaneous nephrostomy (insertion of a tube through the skin to drain the pelvis of the kidney), percutaneous liver biopsy, and fine needle aspiration of thyroid nodules.

During the 1980s and 1990s with the introduction of more advanced imaging technology, such as computed tomography (CT) and magnetic resonance imaging (MRI), the development of new devices and catheters further expanded the range of therapeutic options that could be safely performed using IR.

When feasible and successful, IR diagnostic and therapeutic procedures cause less pain, a lower risk of complications, a shorter hospital stay, and lower costs. IR is often performed in the radiology department but may sometimes require anesthesia support. This so-called "off the floor" anaesthesia being provided in a part of the hospital remote from the operating theater does sometimes compromise the ability to provide a safe anesthetic. The radiology department is often some distance from the operating theater which means when surgical rescue is required, this needs to be promptly recognized as it takes time to transfer a patient to the operating theater where a body cavity can be safely opened to stop bleeding or control contamination. For this reason, hybrid theaters are being introduced where the patient can be treated in an operating theater with the best imaging facilities but also undergo surgery if this is also required. Hybrid theaters in the mid-2020s are still limited to larger specialist hospitals of high-income countries [28–30].

7.8 Positron Emission Tomography (PET)

A PET scan is a type of nuclear medicine imaging based on emissions reflecting the metabolic or biochemical activity of tissues (Fig. 7.8). The technique involves a radioactive tracer and produces three-dimensional images of the body's internal structures and functions. The tracer used in PET scans is a radioactive substance that is injected into the body, swallowed, or inhaled. Once inside the body, the tracer accumulates in those tissues that metabolize it, such as the brain, heart, or cancerous tissue. As the tracer undergoes radioactive decay, it emits positrons, which are positively charged particles similar to electrons but with the opposite charge. When a positron collides with an electron in the body, they annihilate each other, releasing two high-energy gamma rays that travel in opposite directions. These gamma rays are detected by a PET scanner, which uses special detectors to measure the radiation and create a three-dimensional image of the area being examined [31, 32].

Gamma rays were discovered by Frenchman, Paul Villard, in 1900. Rutherford classified these types of radiation based on their ability to penetrate matter, with alpha particles being the least penetrating and gamma rays being the most penetrating. He also was the first to propose (correctly) the nuclear model of the atom. Later while bombarding nitrogen with alpha rays, he converted them into hydrogen, becoming the first person to achieve nuclear fission.

Based on these nuclear concepts, the PET scan was developed by David Edmund Kuhl (1945–2008) who was a Canadian neurologist and functional brain imaging pioneer. In the 1970s, Kuhl developed PET scanning, which tracks radioactive tracers in the brain to create detailed images. PET allows more accurate diagnosis, staging, and restaging of tumors [33, 34].

The Warburg effect is a well-established phenomenon in cancer cells, where they convert glucose into lactate even in the presence of oxygen, which is known as aerobic glycolysis. This altered metabolism is thought to provide cancer cells with the energy and building blocks they need to support their rapid growth and proliferation. In the pioneering research conducted during the 1920s, the esteemed scientist Otto Warburg astutely discerned a remarkable characteristic of cancer cells. These insidious cells exhibited a voracious appetite for glucose, even in the presence of ample oxygen, resulting in a striking elevation in the production of lactate. This intriguing phenomenon, aptly termed the Warburg effect, has since been meticulously documented and observed in a diverse array of other tumor types, further solidifying its significance in cancer biology. He was awarded the Noble Prize in 1945 [35].

The first PET scanner was introduced in 1974 at the Mallinckrodt Institute of Radiology, Washington University, St Louis, Missouri. PET scans use a radioactive tracer that is taken up by cancer cells because of their increased glucose metabolism (fluorodeoxyglucose – FDG). This tracer emits positrons, which can be detected by the PET scanner and used to create detailed whole-body images in which the cancer lights up brightly.

7.9 The Battle with Cancer

Over the last 250 years, we have observed several significant breakthroughs in our pursuit to combat cancer, which has plagued humanity for millennia. This chronology presents some significant accomplishments in the field of cancer research.

In 1775, Percival Pott (1714-1778) showed that being exposed to chimney soot increased the risk of developing squamous cell carcinoma of the scrotum. Squamous cell carcinoma is a type of skin cancer that develops in the squamous cells, which are flat cells located in the outer layer of the skin.

At that time, it was noticed that chimney sweeps, who were regularly exposed to the soot and smoke generated by chimneys, were more likely to develop SCC than the general population. Although the carcinogenic properties of soot and smoke were not well understood at the time, this observation marked an early recognition of the link between environmental exposure and cancer [36].

In modern times, we now understand that chimney soot contains a variety of harmful substances, such as polycyclic aromatic hydrocarbons (PAHs) and particulate matter, that can contribute to the development of cancer. Exposure to these substances can occur through various means, such as through air pollution, occupational exposure, or even cooking food over open flames.

This historical observation highlighted the importance of identifying and understanding the environmental factors that contribute to the development of cancer and the need for measures to reduce exposure to harmful substances (Fig. 7.9).

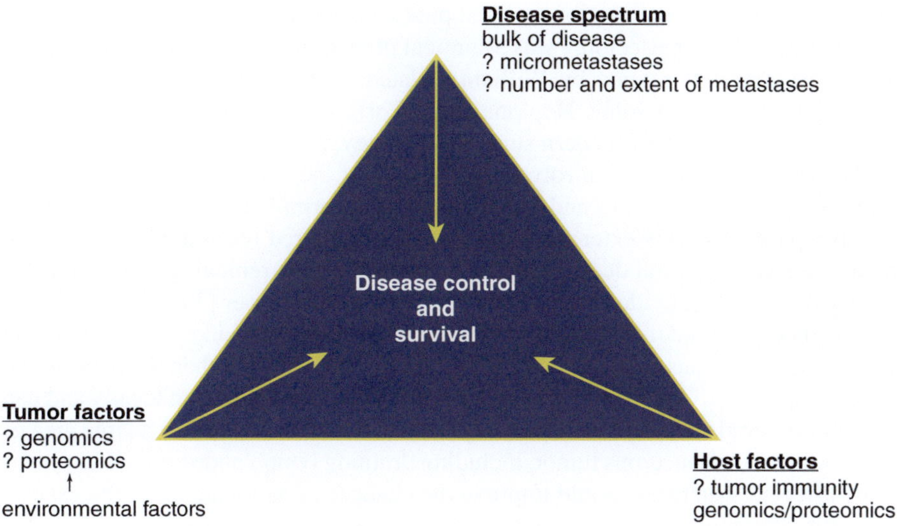

Fig. 7.9 Current theory of carcinogenesis with a flow chart illustrating diseaase control and survival

Rudolf Virchow (1821–1902), a Prussian born, German pathologist, is credited with identifying white blood cells (leukocytes) within cancerous tissue in the mid-nineteenth century. This discovery was a significant step in understanding the relationship between inflammation and cancer.

Virchow noted that the presence of leukocytes in cancerous tissue was not coincidental but rather indicative of a connection between the immune system and cancer. He proposed that inflammation, caused by various factors such as infection or injury, played a crucial role in the development of cancer.

Virchow's findings paved the way for further research into the link between inflammation and cancer, which has since been extensively studied. Today, it is well established that chronic inflammation can contribute to the development and progression of cancer. Moreover, the identification of leukocytes in cancerous tissue has also led to the development of immunotherapy, a type of cancer treatment that harnesses the power of the immune system to fight cancer. This highlights the significance of Virchow's discovery in the history of cancer research and its ongoing impact on cancer treatment today [37].

In 1907, the first epidemiological study linking sunlight exposure to skin cancer was reported. This study built upon earlier observations that chronic skin conditions, common among sailors, were linked to exposure to the radiation effects of the sun. The study provided evidence that sunlight exposure was a risk factor for skin cancer, and later research using animal models confirmed that both ultraviolet light and sunlight can induce skin cancer.

This landmark discovery emphasized the importance of protecting the skin from harmful ultraviolet radiation, leading to the development of measures such as sunscreens and protective clothing to reduce the risk of skin cancer. The link between sunlight exposure and skin cancer has since been well established, and the importance of sun protection remains a critical public health message today [38].

The first radical mastectomy was a surgical procedure used to treat breast cancer. The procedure was refined by William Halsted (1852–1922), an American surgeon and professor at Johns Hopkins, New York, and who is widely considered as one of the founders of modern surgical oncology, in the early twentieth century.

The radical mastectomy involves the removal of the entire breast, including the underlying pectoral muscles and lymph nodes in the armpit area, known as the axillary lymph nodes. This extensive surgery was considered the standard of care for breast cancer for several decades, based on the belief that removing as much tissue as possible would provide the best chance of curing the cancer [39].

The theory behind radical surgery for cancer is based on the idea that the removal of as much cancerous tissue as possible would provide the best chance of curing the cancer. The underlying assumption is that cancer cells tend to spread locally and can potentially invade adjacent tissues or organs, and therefore, removing a large area of tissue around the cancerous tumor, including draining lymph nodes and other potentially affected structures, would improve the chances of removing all of the cancerous cells. The goal of radical surgery is to remove not only the visible tumor but also the surrounding marginal or drainage tissue that may contain cancer cells that are not yet detectable. This approach is particularly important in cases where the cancer has not yet spread beyond the primary site, and surgical removal can potentially provide a cure.

Hilário de Gouvêa (1843–1929) was a Brazilian ophthalmologist who provided the first documented evidence that a susceptibility to cancer can be passed on from a parent to a child. He made this discovery in the early 1900s while studying retinoblastoma, a rare form of eye cancer that affects children. Hilario de Gouvêa reported that two out of seven children born to a father who had been successfully treated for retinoblastoma also developed the disease. This observation suggested that there was a hereditary component to the development of retinoblastoma, and possibly other types of cancer. Gouvêa's findings laid the groundwork for the study of cancer genetics and the identification of specific genes associated with an increased risk of developing certain types of cancer [40].

In 1898, Marie and Pierre Curie's discovery of the radioactive elements radium and polonium had a significant impact on the field of cancer treatment. Prior to their discovery, cancer treatment options were limited and often involved painful and invasive procedures. With the discovery of radium, a new era of cancer treatment began. Radium emits alpha, beta, and gamma rays, which can destroy cancer cells while sparing healthy tissue. Within a few years of the discovery of radium, it was being used in cancer treatment, initially in the form of external radiation therapy and later in the form of brachytherapy, a type of radiation therapy in which a small amount of radioactive material is implanted directly into the tumor [41].

In 1901, two Swedish physicians named Tor Stenbeck and Tage Sjogren made a significant discovery in the field of cancer treatment. They described the first cases of basal cell carcinoma of the skin and squamous cell carcinoma of the skin being cured by X-ray therapy. This was a groundbreaking discovery because, until then, surgery was the only known effective treatment for skin cancer. Stenbeck and Sjogren's discovery showed that external radiation therapy using deep X-ray could also be used to treat skin cancer, which opened up a new avenue of treatment for cancer patients.

Another observation made in 1924, that tumors exhibit anaerobic respiration, now known as the Warburg effect, was named after the German biochemist Otto Warburg (1883–1970). Warburg's hypothesis was that cancer cells have a dysfunctional respiratory system and rely primarily on glycolysis, the process of breaking down glucose into energy, even when oxygen is present. This metabolic shift in cancer cells allows them to generate energy and other metabolites that support their rapid growth and proliferation.

Although the Warburg effect was observed in the 1920s, it was largely ignored until the 1990s, when renewed interest in the topic led to a better understanding of the molecular mechanisms involved. Today, the Warburg effect is recognized as a hallmark of cancer, and researchers are exploring ways to exploit this metabolic difference between cancer and normal cells for cancer diagnosis and treatment. Also, the Warburg effect was used as a working baseline for the development of the positron emission tomography (PET) using FDG (see above) which is heavily applied now for cancer staging.

During the 1950's and 60's radiotherapy was given using gamma rays from Cobalt-60 machines. Whilst representing an advance in the post World War II period, they have largely been replaced by linear accelerators.

In 1943, the first electron linear accelerator designed for radiation therapy was developed, representing a significant advancemilestone in the field of cancerradiation treatment. The linear accelerator is a type of medical device that uses provides high-energy radiation beams tothat aim to destroy cancerous cells in the body. It has allowed for more precise and targeted radiation therapy, with higher doses of radiation delivered to the tumour while sparing nearby healthy tissue. This made radiation therapy a more effective treatment option for many types of cancer, including those that had previously been difficult to treat.

Since its inception, the linear accelerator has undergone many improvements and advancements, including the development of computer-controlled systems that allow for even greater precision and accuracy in radiation delivery. Today, the linear accelerator is the most widely used treatment device in the Western world, and it plays a crucial role in the treatment of many types of cancer.

The development of the linear accelerator for radiation therapy has significantly improved the prognosis and quality of life for many cancer patients. Its continued refinement and advancement remain a major focus of cancer research and innovation, as scientists and clinicians strive to improve cancer treatment outcomes and reduce side effects.

In 1949, Swedish neurosurgeon Lars Leksell (1907–1986) invented a stereotactic apparatus exclusively for human functional neurosurgery. This device allowed for precise and accurate targeting of specific areas of the brain, which has revolutionized the field of neurosurgery and will be increasingly used in the future.

In the late 1960s, Leksell developed the Gamma Knife, a radiosurgical tool that uses multiple beams of high-energy radiation to destroy cancerous tissue with a single, high dose of radiation. The Gamma Knife built upon the precision and accuracy of Leksell's earlier work, and it has become a popular tool in the treatment of many types of cancer [42].

In 1909, the German physician and immunologist Paul Ehrlich (1854–1915) proposed a new concept in the field of cancer research. He hypothesized that the immune system has the ability to recognize and eliminate cancer cells as they develop in the body, thus preventing the formation of tumours. He called this concept "immune surveillance." Ehrlich's hypothesis was a significant departure from the prevailing view at the time, which held that cancer was caused by a single cellular defect and could not be influenced by the immune system.

Ehrlich's proposal sparked a new interest in the relationship between the immune system and cancer and prompted research into the ways in which the immune system could be harnessed to fight cancer. This line of research has continued to this day and has led to the development of new immunotherapies for cancer treatment. These therapies work by boosting the immune system's ability to recognize and attack cancer cells and have shown great promise in treating a range of different cancers.

Ehrlich's "immune surveillance" hypothesis was a seminal moment in the history of cancer research, as it helped to establish the idea that the immune system plays a critical role in preventing cancer [43].

In 1911, Peyton Rous (1879–1970), an American pathologist, discovered a virus that caused cancer in chickens, known as Rous sarcoma virus (RSV). This groundbreaking discovery provided the first evidence that some forms of cancer can be caused by infectious agents. Rous made this discovery while studying a common chicken tumour called sarcoma. He found that the tumour could be transmitted from chicken to chicken through a cell-free filtrate, which suggested the presence of a virus. Rous's discovery of the RSV was met with initial skepticism which took several decades to overcome and be accepted by peers. However, his work eventually led to the identification of many other cancer-causing viruses and paved the way for the development of vaccines and treatments for virus-induced cancers [44].

George Papanicolaou (1883–1962), a Greek-American physician and researcher, made a significant contribution to cancer screening when he discovered that cervical cancer could be detected by examining cells from the cervix under a microscope. He first published his findings in 1928, and the cervical screening test became known as the Pap smear. Prior to Papanicolaou's discovery, cervical cancer was often not diagnosed (because it usually painless) until it had already progressed to an advanced stage, making it much harder to treat. Papanicolaou's method allowed for earlier detection of the disease, leading to better outcomes for patients [44]. The Pap smear involves collecting a small sample of cells from the cervix using a swab or brush, which is then examined under a microscope for any abnormalities. The test has become a routine part of women's healthcare and is recommended as a screening tool for cervical cancer.

In 1937, President Franklin D. Roosevelt signed legislation that established the National Cancer Institute (NCI). The NCI is one of the 27 institutes and centers that make up the National Institutes of Health (NIH) in the United States. The establishment of the NCI marked a significant milestone in the fight against cancer, as it was the first government agency solely dedicated to cancer research. Its mission is to conduct and support research, training, health information dissemination, and other programs with the goal of reducing the burden of cancer. The NCI has played a crucial role in many important discoveries and advancements in cancer research, including the development of new cancer treatments, the identification of cancer risk factors, and the implementation of cancer prevention and screening programs. Today, the NCI remains a leading authority in cancer research and continues to work toward the ultimate goal of finding a cure for cancer.

Charles Huggins (1901–1997) was a Canadian-American physician and physiologist who was awarded the Nobel Prize in Physiology or Medicine in 1966 for his work on the hormonal treatment of prostate cancer [45].

In 1941, Huggins published a landmark study in the Journal of the American Medical Association, which demonstrated the effectiveness of hormonal therapy for advanced prostate cancer. Huggins and his colleagues discovered that the growth of prostate cancer cells was stimulated by the male hormone testosterone and that by removing or reducing the amount of testosterone in a patient's body, the growth of the cancer could be slowed or even stopped [45].

Huggins used a variety of methods to reduce testosterone levels in his patients, including surgical castration and the use of estrogen and other drugs. Although these treatments were not without side effects, they represented a significant breakthrough in the treatment of prostate cancer and paved the way for further research into hormonal therapy and other forms of cancer treatment. Huggins' work has had a lasting impact on the field of oncology and continues to influence the development of new cancer treatments today [45].

Sidney Farber (1903–1973), an American pediatric pathologist, born in Buffalo, New York, and received his medical degree from Harvard Medical School in 1927. In 1947, whilst Assistant Professor (Senior Lecturer) in Pathology at Harvard and the Boston Children's Hospital he made a breakthrough discovery in the treatment of childhood leukemia. Farber had been searching for a way to treat this devastating disease, which was almost universally fatal at the time, when he decided to try using a new type of drug called an antimetabolite.

Antimetabolites are drugs that interfere with the metabolism of cancer cells, preventing them from growing and dividing. Farber chose to use a drug called aminopterin, which is a derivative of folic acid, a nutrient that is essential for the growth and division of cells [46].

Farber's initial experiments with aminopterin showed promising results, with some children experiencing a temporary remission of their leukemia. Over the next few years, Farber and his colleagues refined the use of aminopterin and other antimetabolites, developing new combinations of drugs and refining the dosages and administration methods.

Farber's work with antimetabolites revolutionized the treatment of childhood leukemia and opened the door to the development of new chemotherapy drugs that could be used to treat a wide range of cancers. Today, antimetabolites continue to be an important component of many cancer treatment regimens, saving countless lives each year.

In 1946, two American pharmacologists, Louis Goodman (1906–2000) and Alfred Gilman (1908–1994), began studying the effects of nitrogen mustard, a chemical agent derived from a deadly gas used during the war, on cancer cells after seeing the effect of the poison on war casualties in the form of bone marrow suppression and leukopaenia. Dr. Alfred Gilman, a pharmacologist, and Dr. Louis Goodman, a physician and pharmacologist, led the research team. They confirmed the earlier findings of leukopaenia by showing that lymphomas in animals decreased in size significantly after exposure to mustard gas.

Goodman and Gilman discovered that nitrogen mustard was effective in killing cancer cells in laboratory experiments, and they went on to conduct the first clinical trial of chemotherapy in a patient with non-Hodgkin's lymphoma. The patient experienced a significant reduction in tumor size after treatment with nitrogen mustard, marking a major breakthrough in the treatment of cancer.

The discovery of nitrogen mustard as a cancer treatment paved the way for the development of other chemotherapy drugs, which are now widely used in the treatment of many types of cancer. While chemotherapy can cause significant side effects and is not always effective, it remains an important tool in the fight against cancer.

The use of chemical agents derived from warfare as cancer treatments highlights the important role that scientific innovation can play in addressing major health challenges. While the origins of chemotherapy may be rooted in wartime experimentation, its impact on cancer treatment has been transformative [47].

In 1953, Roy Hertz (1909–2002), an endocrinologist and researcher at the National Cancer Institute, with Min Chiu Li (1919–1980), a Chinese born American oncologist, achieved a major breakthrough in cancer treatment by using the drug methotrexate to achieve the first complete cure of a human solid tumor by chemotherapy. The patient they treated had choriocarcinoma, a rare cancer that affects the reproductive tissue and is often fatal. Hertz and Li had been studying the use of methotrexate, a drug that interferes with the growth and division of cancer cells, for the treatment of choriocarcinoma. They had previously achieved partial remission in some patients but had not yet achieved a complete cure [48].

The patient they treated in 1953, was a young woman who had already undergone surgery to remove the tumor, but the cancer had spread to other parts of her body. Hertz and Li administered high doses of methotrexate over a period of several months, and the patient went into remission. She remained cancer-free for the rest of her life. This landmark achievement demonstrated the potential of chemotherapy as a viable treatment for cancer and opened the door to further research into the development of new chemotherapy drugs and treatment regimens [48].

In the early 1950s, several studies were published that linked cigarette smoking to the development of lung cancer. Three researchers, Ernst Wynder, Evarts Graham, and Richard Doll, played key roles in this landmark discovery.

In 1950, Ernest Wynder (1922–1999) and Evarts Graham (1883–1957) published a study in the Journal of the American Medical Association that showed a strong correlation between cigarette smoking and lung cancer. They studied patients with lung cancer and compared them to a control group of patients without lung cancer. They found that the lung cancer patients were much more likely to be smokers than the control group and that the risk of developing lung cancer increased with the amount of cigarettes smoked.

Around the same time, Richard Doll (1912–2005), a British epidemiologist, was conducting similar studies in the United Kingdom. He published a paper in the British Medical Journal in 1950 that showed a strong association between smoking and lung cancer. Doll continued to study the issue over the next few years, and his research provided some of the most convincing evidence to date linking smoking and lung cancer [49, 50]. He was knighted in 1971 and received many other honours.

Together, these studies helped to establish cigarette smoking as a major risk factor for lung cancer and other forms of cancer. The findings sparked a public health campaign to discourage smoking and led to the development of laws and regulations to limit smoking in public spaces.

In 1953, James Watson (b1928) and Francis Crick (1916–2004) published a groundbreaking paper in Nature (1953) on the structure of DNA, the molecule that carries genetic information and serves as the "information archive" of all cell activity. Their discovery of the double helix structure of DNA was a major breakthrough in the field of molecular biology and ushered in the era of genomics. Watson, Crick and Maruice Williams (1916–2004) were jointly awarded the Nobel prize in physiology or medicine in 1962. There was some controversy over this discovery as the critical photograph from Maurice Williams' lab had been taken by Rosalind Franklin (d1958) and Raymond Gosling, (1926–2015) a PhD student at Kings, who was instructed without Franklin's knowledge to hand over the x-ray diffraction photo of DNA to Maurice Wilkins who showed it to the American, James Watson. This photo enabled Watson and Crick to devise their double helix model and publish their 1953 paper. Franklin had died before the Nobel prize was awarded but there has been considerable ethical debate over the credits for DNA's double helix!

Following the DNA structure discovery, techniques were rapidly developed to sequence DNA and study its inherent genetic material. Today, researchers are using gene-analyzing techniques to examine everything about cancer cells, including the individual genes and the DNA that regulates their activity.

By studying the genetic mutations and alterations that occur in cancer cells, researchers can gain a better understanding of the mechanisms that drive cancer growth and identify potential targets for therapy. This approach, known as precision medicine, involves tailoring treatment to the specific genetic profile of a patient's cancer, with the goal of improving outcomes and reducing side effects.

The discovery of the structure of DNA and the subsequent development of genomic technologies have had a profound impact on cancer research and treatment, providing new insights into the underlying biology of the disease and opening up new avenues for therapy [51].

In 1960, Peter Nowell (1928–2016) and David Hungerford (1927–1993) made a groundbreaking discovery in cancer research when they identified an unusual chromosome in the cancer cells of patients with chronic myelogenous leukemia (CML). The chromosome, later known as the Philadelphia chromosome, was smaller than normal and had a distinctive abnormality.

Nowell and Hungerford used a special staining technique to visualize the chromosomes in cells taken from CML patients. They noticed that one of the chromosomes appeared smaller than usual and had a small piece missing. This abnormal chromosome was present in nearly all of the cells from the CML patients, but not in cells from healthy individuals.

Further research showed that the missing piece of the chromosome had become fused to another chromosome, creating a new, abnormal chromosome. This abnormality was found to be a hallmark of CML and provided a new understanding of the genetic basis of cancer. The discovery of the Philadelphia chromosome paved the way for the development of targeted therapies for CML. In the early 2000s, a drug called imatinib was introduced that specifically targets the abnormal protein produced by the Philadelphia chromosome. This drug has been highly effective in treating CML and has significantly improved the prognosis for patients with this type of leukemia [52].

The Knudson hypothesis, proposed by Alfred G. Knudson Jr (1922–2016). in 1971, suggested that a "two-hit" mechanism of mutation is responsible for the development of certain types of cancer. The first hit is usually a genetic mutation inherited from a parent or acquired during an individual's lifetime, which increases the risk of developing cancer. However, the second hit, which is usually a somatic mutation that occurs in the same gene as the first mutation, is required to actually cause the cancer to develop.

The hypothesis was based on Knudson's study of retinoblastoma, a rare eye cancer that often affects young children. Knudson found that some cases of retinoblastoma were caused by a genetic mutation that was inherited from a parent, while other cases were caused by two separate somatic mutations that occurred during the individual's lifetime. This led him to propose that cancer development may require two separate mutations in the same gene and that the risk of developing cancer increases with the number of mutations acquired over time.

Today, the Knudson hypothesis has been refined and expanded upon and is widely accepted as a general model for the development of many types of cancer. It highlights the importance of genetic mutations in the development of cancer and has helped to guide the development of targeted therapies that focus on specific genetic mutations found in tumors [53].

In 1971, President Richard Nixon declared a "War on Cancer" in his State of the Union Address.

In 1976, Michael Bishop (b1936) and Harold Varmus (b1939) made a groundbreaking discovery when they identified oncogenes, which are genes that control normal cell growth and division but can become mutated and transform a normal cell into a cancer cell. The discovery of oncogenes provided a new understanding of the genetic basis of cancer, demonstrating that cancer is not solely caused by external factors such as environmental toxins but also by internal genetic mutations.

The work of Bishop and Varmus paved the way for further research into the mechanisms underlying cancer development and led to the identification of many other oncogenes. Their discovery also spurred the development of targeted cancer therapies that aim to inhibit the activity of specific oncogenes, such as the drug Gleevec (imatinib) which is used to treat chronic myeloid leukemia (CML) by blocking the activity of the BCR-ABL oncogene. The pair were awarded the Noble Prize in 1989 for their discovery of the cellular origin of oncogenes [54].

In 1979, the TP53 gene, also known as p53, was discovered by a team of researchers led by Arnold Levine (b1939). The TP53 gene is the most commonly mutated gene in human cancer and is a critical component of the body's system for preventing the development of cancer.

The p53 protein, which is produced by the TP53 gene, acts as a tumor suppressor by regulating the cell cycle and preventing the growth and proliferation of abnormal cells. When the TP53 gene is mutated, the resulting p53 protein is unable to function properly, leading to uncontrolled cell growth and the development of cancer.

Mutations in the TP53 gene have been found in a wide range of cancers, including breast cancer, lung cancer, and colon cancer. Studies have shown that up to 50% of all human cancers involve mutations in the TP53 gene.

The discovery of the TP53 gene has had a significant impact on cancer research and has led to the development of new diagnostic tools and targeted therapies for cancer based on human oncogenes. Researchers continue to study the TP53 gene and its role in cancer development, with the goal of developing new treatments that can target this critical pathway in cancer cells [55].

In 1984, a team of researchers led by Robert Weinberg (b 1942) discovered a new oncogene in rat cells that they named "neu." This oncogene was found to promote the growth and proliferation of cells and was later identified as a member of the ErbB family of receptor tyrosine kinases.

Further research showed that the human version of the neu oncogene, which was named HER2 (also known as ErbB2), was overexpressed in approximately 20–25% of breast cancers. This overexpression of HER2 was found to be associated with more aggressive tumor growth and poorer prognosis.

The discovery of HER2 and its role in breast cancer was a major breakthrough in cancer research and led to the development of targeted therapies for HER2-positive breast cancer. In the late 1990s, a monoclonal antibody called trastuzumab (brand name Herceptin) was developed that specifically targets HER2-positive breast cancer cells.

Trastuzumab, approved in 1998, has been highly effective in treating HER2-positive breast cancer and has significantly improved the prognosis for patients with this type of breast cancer. Today, HER2 testing is routinely performed in breast cancer patients to determine if they are HER2-positive and would benefit from targeted therapy. The discovery of the HER2 oncogene has also had implications for the development of targeted therapies for other types of cancer that involve overexpression of the ErbB family of receptor tyrosine kinases [56].

BRCA1 and BRCA2 are human genes that belong to a class of genes known as tumor suppressor genes. Mutations in these genes increase the risk of developing breast and ovarian cancer, as well as several other types of cancer.

In 1990, researchers led by Mary-Claire King (b1947) identified and named the BRCA1 gene, which is located on chromosome 17, and found that mutations in this gene were associated with a significantly increased risk of breast and ovarian cancer. In 1994, the BRCA2 gene was identified, which is located on chromosome 13, and was also found to be associated with an increased risk of breast and ovarian cancer [57].

Mutations in the BRCA1 and BRCA2 genes are relatively rare in the general population, but individuals who inherit a mutation in one of these genes have a significantly increased risk of developing breast and ovarian cancer. Women with a BRCA1 or BRCA2 mutation have a lifetime risk of developing breast cancer that is estimated to be between 60% and 80%, compared to a lifetime risk of approximately 12% in the general population. Additionally, these women have a lifetime risk of ovarian cancer that is estimated to be between 15% and 40%, compared to a lifetime risk of approximately 1% in the general population.

The discovery of the BRCA1 and BRCA2 genes has had important implications for cancer prevention and treatment. Women with a family history of breast or ovarian cancer are often advised to undergo genetic testing for BRCA1 and BRCA2 mutations. For women who test positive for a mutation, options for risk reduction include increased surveillance (such as more frequent mammograms and ovarian cancer screenings) or preventive measures, such as prophylactic surgery (such as a mastectomy or oophorectomy).

Additionally, the discovery of the BRCA1 and BRCA2 genes has led to the development of targeted therapies for breast and ovarian cancer. For example, Poly (ADP-ribose) polymerase (PARP) inhibitors have been developed that are particularly effective in treating tumors with BRCA1 or BRCA2 mutations [58].

In 1984, a team of researchers led by Harald zur Hausen (1936–2023) identified DNA from human papillomavirus (HPV) types 16 and 18 in a large percentage of cervical cancer samples. This discovery established a clear link between infection with these HPV types and the development of cervical cancer.

HPV is a common sexually transmitted infection that can cause a range of health problems, including genital warts and some types of cancer. The HPV types 16 and 18 are high-risk types that are particularly associated with the development of cervical cancer.

The discovery of HPV 16 and 18's link to cervical cancer led to the development of screening tests, such as the Pap test and HPV DNA testing, that can detect early signs of cervical cancer or precancerous changes in the cervix. Additionally, vaccines were developed by Scottish Australian Ian Frazer's (b1953) team to protect against HPV infections and prevent HPV-related cancers, including cervical cancer.

Today, the HPV vaccine is routinely recommended for both males and females in many countries as part of routine immunization schedules [59].

In 1962, Stanley Cohen (1922–2020), an American biochemist, discovered the epidermal growth factor (EGF), a protein that stimulates cell growth and division. EGF is a crucial factor in the regulation of cell growth and plays a role in the development of many types of cancer.

More than a decade later, in 1978, the receptor for EGF was identified, leading to the development of a class of agents known as EGFR inhibitors. These drugs, including cetuximab (Erbitux), are used to treat colorectal cancer and other cancers that overexpress the EGFR protein. Stanley Cohen and Rita Levi-Montalcini (1909–2012) shared the 1986 Nobel prize for physiology or medicine for their discovery of growth factors. Rita Levi-Montalcini, an Italian neurobiologist, discovered nerve growth factor.

EGFR inhibitors work by blocking the activity of the EGFR protein, preventing it from stimulating cell growth and division. This approach has proven to be effective in treating some types of cancer [60].

In 1997, the US Food and Drug Administration (FDA) approved rituximab for the treatment of patients with treatment-resistant, low-grade, or follicular B-cell non-Hodgkin lymphoma (NHL). Rituximab is a monoclonal antibody that targets the CD20 protein, which is expressed on the surface of B cells.

Rituximab was the first monoclonal antibody approved for use in cancer therapy, and its approval represented a major breakthrough in the treatment of NHL. Prior to rituximab, treatment options for NHL were limited, and many patients did not respond well to existing therapies.

Rituximab is now used in the treatment of a variety of B-cell lymphomas, including diffuse large B-cell lymphoma, mantle cell lymphoma, and chronic lymphocytic leukemia. It is often used in combination with chemotherapy or other targeted therapies and has been shown to significantly improve patient outcomes [60, 61].

The success of rituximab has paved the way for the development of other monoclonal antibody therapies for cancer, including trastuzumab (Herceptin) for HER2-positive breast cancer and cetuximab (Erbitux) for colorectal cancer and head and neck cancer. Monoclonal antibodies have become an important class of drugs in cancer therapy and continue to be an active area of research and development [62].

In 2001, the US Food and Drug Administration (FDA) approved imatinib for the treatment of chronic myeloid leukemia (CML). Imatinib, also known as Gleevec or Glivec, is a targeted therapy that works by inhibiting the activity of a specific protein called BCR-ABL, which is responsible for the abnormal growth and proliferation of CML cells. Imatinib was a significant breakthrough in the treatment of CML, as it offered a highly effective and well-tolerated therapy for a disease that had previously been difficult to manage. Imatinib has since become the standard of care for CML and has dramatically improved patient outcomes [62].

Later, it was also shown to be effective in the treatment of gastrointestinal stromal tumors (GIST), a rare type of cancer that arises in the digestive tract. Imatinib works in GIST by inhibiting the activity of a protein called KIT, which is mutated in many cases of GIST and drives the growth of tumor cells.

The success of imatinib has spurred the development of other targeted therapies for cancer, which work by specifically targeting the molecular pathways that are altered in cancer cells. These therapies offer the promise of more effective and less toxic treatments for cancer and have revolutionized the field of oncology over the past two decades [63].

Ipilimumab, also known as Yervoy, is a monoclonal antibody that targets a protein called CTLA-4 on the surface of T cells, which are immune cells that play a key role in fighting cancer. CTLA-4 normally acts as a "brake" on T-cell activity, preventing them from attacking healthy cells in the body. However, in cancer, CTLA-4 can also inhibit the immune response against tumor cells, allowing them to grow and spread.

Ipilimumab works by blocking the activity of CTLA-4, which helps to activate T cells and enhance the immune response against cancer cells. The approval of ipilimumab in 2011 represented a major advance in the treatment of melanoma, which had previously been a challenging cancer to treat. That was also followed in 2014, with the approval of pembrolizumab as Programmed Cell Death Protein 1 (PD1) inhibitor for advanced melanoma [64].

Ipilimumab has since been used in combination with other immune checkpoint inhibitors, such as nivolumab, to further enhance the immune response against cancer cells. These combination therapies have shown promising results in the treatment of melanoma, as well as other types of cancer such as lung cancer and kidney cancer.

The NCI-sponsored PLCO Cancer Screening Trial (Prostate, Lung, Colorectal, and Ovarian Cancer Screening Trial) was a large randomized clinical trial designed to evaluate the effectiveness of different cancer screening tests for reducing mortality. The trial included over 150,000 men and women between the ages of 55 and 74 who were randomly assigned to either screening with flexible sigmoidoscopy, screening with other tests (such as fecal occult blood testing or PSA testing), or usual care.

The results of the trial, which were published in 2012, showed that screening with flexible sigmoidoscopy significantly reduced the incidence of colorectal cancer and mortality from the disease. Participants who were screened with sigmoidoscopy had a 21% lower risk of developing colorectal cancer and a 26% lower risk of dying from the disease than those in the control group who received usual care. These findings provided strong evidence in support of the use of sigmoidoscopy as a screening test for colorectal cancer and led to changes in clinical practice guidelines for colorectal cancer screening.

The NCI-MATCH (Molecular Analysis for Therapy Choice) trial was launched in 2015 by the National Cancer Institute (NCI) and the ECOG-ACRIN Cancer Research Group. The trial was designed to investigate whether targeted therapies that are selected based on the genetic abnormalities of a patient's tumor can be more effective than traditional treatments for a wide range of cancer types.

The NCI-MATCH trial enrolled patients with advanced solid tumors or lymphomas that had progressed despite standard treatment options. Patients underwent genetic testing of their tumor samples to identify specific mutations or other genetic abnormalities that could be targeted with available drugs. Based on the results of the genetic testing, patients were assigned to one of several treatment arms, each of which tested a different targeted therapy.

The goal of the trial was to determine whether these targeted therapies could be effective in a broader range of cancer types than they were originally developed for, and whether genetic testing could help guide treatment decisions for patients with advanced cancers. The trial enrolled more than 6000 patients and represented a major effort to move toward more personalized cancer treatment based on the genetic characteristics of individual tumors.

In 2011, the FDA approved the BRAF inhibitor vemurafenib (sold under the brand name Zelboraf) for the treatment of late-stage melanoma tumors that express the BRAF V600E mutation. BRAF is a kinase enzyme in the mitogen-activated protein kinase (MAPK) signaling pathway, that cell growth and survival. When there is a BRAF mutation this signalling pathway is constantly switched "on". Such a mutation is found in approximately 50% of late-stage melanoma cases. Vemurafenib was approved alongside its companion diagnostic test, the cobas 4800 BRAF V600 Mutation Test, which is used to determine whether a patient's tumor expresses the BRAF V600E mutation. This personalized approach to cancer treatment, based on the genetic makeup of the tumor, is an example of precision medicine [63, 64].

In 2017, the US Food and Drug Administration (FDA) cleared two products to test tumors for genetic changes that may make the tumors susceptible to treatment with FDA-approved molecularly targeted drugs. These tests were designed to help identify patients who may benefit from targeted therapies that are selected based on the genetic abnormalities of their tumors.

One of the products that received FDA clearance was the FoundationOne CDx test, developed by Foundation Medicine. This test analyzes solid tumor samples for alterations in genes and two genomic signatures that are associated with response to targeted therapies. The test is designed to help guide treatment decisions for patients with advanced cancers who have exhausted standard treatment options.

In November of 2017, the FDA also authorized the MSK-IMPACT test developed and used by Memorial Sloan Kettering Cancer Center to analyze tumors for potentially actionable changes in cancer-related genes. Like the Foundation One CDx test, the MSK-IMPACT test is designed to help identify patients who may benefit from targeted therapies based on the genetic characteristics of their tumors.

These tests represent an important step toward more personalized cancer treatment based on the genomic profiling of individual tumors. By analyzing tumors for specific genetic changes, these tests can help guide treatment decisions and identify patients who may benefit from targeted therapies that are designed to exploit the vulnerabilities of cancer cells with specific genetic alterations.

A consortium of international researchers analyzes more than 2600 whole genomes from 38 types of cancer and matching normal tissues to identify common patterns of molecular changes.

The Pan-Cancer Analysis of Whole Genomes study released in 2020, which used data collected by the International Cancer Genome Consortium and TCGA, uncovers the complex role that changes throughout the genome play in cancer development, growth, and spread. The study also extends genomic analyses of cancer beyond the protein-coding regions to the complete genetic composition of cells.

This study has identified new potential therapeutic targets for cancer treatment and highlighted the importance of studying the noncoding regions of the genome. It also reveals the vast complexity and heterogeneity of cancer, which presents challenges for developing effective treatments. However, the insights gained from this study may lead to the development of more personalized and targeted therapies for cancer patients.

Radiotherapy, also known as radiation therapy, is a treatment modality that uses high-energy radiation to kill cancer cells and shrink tumors. The history of radiotherapy in the treatment of cancer dates back to the late nineteenth century, when scientists first discovered that radiation could be used to treat cancer.

In the 1890s, French physicist, Antoine Becquerel, discovered that certain elements, such as uranium, emitted a type of radiation that could penetrate matter. Around the same time, another Frenchman, Marie Curie, discovered that the element radium also emitted this type of penetrating radiation.

In the early twentieth century, scientists began to experiment with using these radioactive elements to treat cancer. In 1896, a German physician, Carl G. G. Gossler, used radium to treat a patient with skin cancer, making it the first recorded use of radiotherapy in the treatment of cancer.

In the following decades, new technologies such as X-ray machines and linear accelerators were developed, which allowed for more precise delivery of radiation to the tumor while minimizing exposure to surrounding healthy tissue.

In recent years, advances in imaging technology have allowed for even more precise delivery of radiation to the tumor, such as 3D conformal radiotherapy, intensity-modulated radiotherapy (IMRT), and image-guided radiotherapy (IGRT). Additionally, newer forms of radiation therapy such as proton therapy, and particle therapy, have been developed which further enhance the precision of radiotherapy.

It's worth noting that radiotherapy is a crucial component of cancer treatment and it can be used alone or in combination with other treatments such as surgery and chemotherapy. The type of radiotherapy and the dose used depend on the type and stage of the cancer, as well as the patient's overall health and medical history. The goal of radiotherapy is to destroy cancer cells while minimizing the damage to surrounding healthy tissue and improving the patient's quality of life.

Image guided radiotherapy, stereotactic radiotherapy, and intensity modulated radiotherapy have been developed which further enhance the precision of radiotherapy.

Even in the 21st century radiotherapy has continued to be one of the most important modalities of cancer treatment, and it's continuously evolving with the incorporation of new technologies and techniques. It has grown from a single method of treatment to a multidisciplinary approach that is used in combination with other forms of treatment to achieve optimal results.

7.9.1 History of Chemotherapy for Cancers

The history of chemotherapy for cancer can be traced back to the early twentieth century, when scientists and doctors first began experimenting with chemical compounds as a way to treat cancer.

In the early 1900s, scientists discovered that certain chemical compounds, such as mustard gas, had the ability to kill cancer cells. However, these early attempts at chemotherapy were not very effective and had significant side effects.

In the 1940s, new drugs, such as nitrogen mustard, were developed and found to be more effective in treating certain types of cancer, such as lymphoma. These early chemotherapy drugs were still highly toxic and had significant side effects.

In the 1950s and 1960s, new chemotherapy drugs, such as methotrexate, were developed and found to be more effective and less toxic than earlier drugs. Additionally, the use of combination chemotherapy, which involves the use of multiple drugs in a single treatment, was found to be more effective than using a single drug.

In the 1970s and 1980s, the development of new drugs such as cisplatin and doxorubicin, and the use of targeted therapy, which uses drugs that specifically target certain molecules involved in the growth and spread of cancer cells, improved the efficacy and safety of chemotherapy.

In the twenty-first century, advances in genomics, precision medicine, and immunotherapy have led to the development of new, highly effective chemotherapy drugs that target specific genetic mutations in cancer cells. Additionally, the use of nanoparticle-based drug delivery systems, and the use of new techniques such as hyperthermia, have improved the effectiveness of chemotherapy by allowing for more precise targeting of cancer cells and minimizing the damage to healthy cells.

It's worth noting that chemotherapy is a complex treatment that involves the use of drugs to kill cancer cells. It is typically administered by oncologists and medical oncologists. The field of chemotherapy continues to evolve with the integration of new technologies, drugs, and techniques which aim to improve the safety and outcomes of these treatments.

References

1. Chodos A, editor. This month in physics history: November 8, 1865: Rontgen's discovery of X-Rays. American Physical Society. Web; 2015. http://www.aps.org/publications/apsnews/200111/history.cfm.
2. "Wilhelm Conrad Röntgen Biographical." Nobelprize.org. Nobel Media AB 2014. Web. 4 Jan 2015. Obituaries, Sir Godfrey Hounsfield. BMJ. 2004:329. https://doi.org/10.1136/bmj.329.7467.687.
3. Wilhelm TM, Röntgen C, et al. découverte des rayons X [Wilhelm Conrad Röntgen and the discovery of X-rays]. Bull Acad Natl Med. 1996;180(1):97–108. French.
4. Nüsslin F. Wilhelm Conrad Röntgen: the scientist and his discovery. Phys Med. 2020;79:65–8. https://doi.org/10.1016/j.ejmp.2020.10.010. Epub 2020 Nov 3.
5. https://www.kumc.edu/school-of-medicine/academics/departments/history-andphilosophy-of-medicine/archives/wwi/base-hospital-28/clinical-services/ radiology.html. Last accessed 1/5/24.
6. https://blog.nationalarchives.gov.uk/x-rays-front/. Last accessed 1/5/24.
7. http://broughttolife.sciencemuseum.org.uk/broughttolife/techniques/mr.
8. All Nobel Prizes in Physics. Nobelprize.org. Nobel Media AB. 2014. Accessed 27 April 2018. Available at: http://bit.ly/2A4rgbY.
9. Gasinska A. The contribution of women to radiobiology: Marie Curie and beyond. Rep Pract Oncol Radiother. 2016;21(3):250–8. https://doi.org/10.1016/j.rpor.2015.11.006. Epub 2015 Dec 29. PMID: 27601958; PMCID: PMC5002019.
10. Isherwood I. In memoriam: sir Godfrey Hounsfield. Radiology. 2005;234:268–70.
11. Obituaries. Sir Godfrey Hounsfield. BMJ. 2004:329. https://doi.org/10.1136/bmj.329.7467.687.
12. Oransky I. Sir Godfrey N Hounsfield. Lancet. 2004;364:1032.
13. Damadian R. Tumour detection by nuclear magnetic resonance. Science. 1971;171(3976):1151–3. https://doi.org/10.1126/science.171.3976.1151.
14. Lauterbur PC. Image formation by induced local interactions: examples of employing nuclear magnetic resonance. Nature. 1973;242:190–1. https://doi.org/10.1038/242190a0.

15. Burt JR, Zimmerman SL, Kamel IR, Halushka M, Bluemke DA. Myocardial T1 mapping: techniques and potential applications. Radiographics. 2014;34:377–95. https://doi.org/10.1148/rg.342125121.
16. Shampo MA, Kyle RA. Karl Theodore Dussik--pioneer in ultrasound. Mayo Clin Proc. 1995;70(12):1136. https://doi.org/10.4065/70.12.1136.
17. Wild JJ, Reid JM. Further pilot echographic studies of the histologic structure of tumors of the living intact human breast. Am J Pathol. 1952;23:389.
18. Willocks J. Medical ultrasound: a Glasgow development which swept the world. Avenue. 1996;19:5–7.
19. Newman PG, Rozycki G. The history of ultrasound. Surg Clin N Am. 1998;78:179–95.
20. Wells PN. Ultrasonic opportunities. 1992 William J. Fry memorial lecture. J Ultrasound Med. 1993;12(1):1–9. https://doi.org/10.7863/jum.1993.12.1.1.
21. Wang JB, Di Ianni T, Vyas DB, Huang Z, Park S, Hosseini-Nassab N, Aryal M, Airan RD. Focused ultrasound for noninvasive, focal pharmacologic neurointervention. Front Neurosci. 2020;14:675. https://doi.org/10.3389/fnins.2020.00675. PMID: 32760238; PMCID: PMC7372945.
22. Gill R. Medical ultrasound in Australia: a short history. Australas J Ultrasound Med. 2018;21(1):3–8. https://doi.org/10.1002/ajum.12085. PMID: 34760495; PMCID: PMC8409875.
23. Woo J. A short history of the development of ultrasound in obstetrics and gynaecology. Parts 1, 2 and 3. Available at http://www.obst-ultrasound.net/ history1.html. Last accessed 1st May 2024.
24. Tan SY, Yip A. António Egas Moniz (1874-1955): lobotomy pioneer and Nobel laureate. Singapore Med J. 2014;55(4):175–6. https://doi.org/10.11622/smedj.2014048. PMID: 24763831; PMCID: PMC4291941.
25. Ligon BL. The mystery of angiography and the "unawarded" Nobel Prize: Egas Moniz and Hans Christian Jacobaeus. Neurosurgery. 1998;43:602–11.
26. Davies MK, Hollman A. Werner Forssmann. Heart. 2002;87(5):409. PMCID: PMC1767093.
27. Braunwald E. André Cournand, Bellevue's cardiopulmonary laboratory, and research on heart failure. Ann Am Thorac Soc. 2018;15(Suppl 1):S12–4. https://doi.org/10.1513/AnnalsATS.201706-433KV.
28. Barton M, Grüntzig J, Husmann M, Rösch J. Balloon angioplasty - the legacy of Andreas Grüntzig, M.D. (1939–1985). Front Cardiovasc Med. 2014;1:15. https://doi.org/10.3389/fcvm.2014.00015. PMID: 26664865; PMCID: PMC4671350.
29. Josef R, et al. The birth, early years, and future of interventional radiology. J Vasc Interv Radiol. 2003;14(7):841–53.
30. Sabharwal T, Fotiadis N, Adam A. Modern trends in interventional radiology. Br Med Bull. 2007;81–82:167–82. https://doi.org/10.1093/bmb/ldm006.
31. Jones T. The role of positron emission tomography within the spectrum of medical imaging. Euro J Nucl Med Mol Imag. 1996;23(7):807–13. https://doi.org/10.1007/BF00843711.
32. Burnham CA, Aronow S, Brownell GL. A hybrid positron scanner. Phys Med Biol. 1970;15:517–28. https://doi.org/10.1088/0031-9155/15/3/012.
33. Kuhl DE, Edwards RQ. Image separation radioisotope scanning. Radiology. 1963;80(4):653–62. https://doi.org/10.1148/80.4.653.
34. Kuhl DE, et al. Quantitative section scanning using orthogonal tangent correction. J Nucl Med. 1973;14(4):196–200.
35. Warburg O, Wind F, Negelein E. The metabolism of tumors in the body. J Gen Physiol. 1927;8:519–30. https://doi.org/10.1085/jgp.8.6.519.
36. Brown JR, Thornton JL. Percivall Pott (1714-1788) and chimney sweepers' cancer of the scrotum. Br J Ind Med. 1957;14(1):68–70. https://doi.org/10.1136/oem.14.1.68.

37. Parkin DM, Pisani P, Ferlay MN, Newton R, Beral V, Weiss R. Infections and human cancer. Cold Spring Harbor: Cold Spring Harbor Laboratory Press; 1999.
38. Ghossain A, Ghossain MA. History of mastectomy before and after Halsted. J Med Liban. 2009;57(2):65–71.
39. Monteiro AN, Waizbort R. The accidental cancer geneticist: hilário de gouvêa and hereditary retinoblastoma. Cancer Biol Ther. 2007;6(5):811–3. https://doi.org/10.4161/cbt.6.5.4420. Epub 2007 May 10.
40. Gasinska A. The contribution of women to radiobiology: Marie Curie and beyond. Rep Pract Oncol Radiother. 2016;21(3):250–8.
41. Bhatnagar JP, Novotny J, Niranjan A, Kondziolka D, Flickinger J, Lunsford D, Huq MS. First year experience with newly developed Leksell Gamma Knife Perfexion. J Med Phys. 2009;34(3):141–8.
42. Valent P, Groner B, Schumacher U. Paul Ehrlich (1854-1915) and his contributions to the foundation and birth of translational medicine. J Innate Immun. 2016;8:111–20.
43. Kidd JG, Rous P. The carcinogenic effect of a papilloma virus on the tarred skin of rabbits: II. Major factors determining the phenomenon: the manifold effects of tarring. J Exp Med. 1938;68:529–62.
44. Berenblum I. The mechanism of carcinogenesis. A study of the significance of cocarcinogenic action and related phenomena. Cancer Res. 1941;1:807.
45. Huggins C, Hodges CV. Studies on prostate cancer. I, the effect of castration, of estrogen and of androgen injection on serum phosphatases in metastatic carcinoma of the prostate. Cancer Res. 1941;1:293.
46. Farber S, Diamond LK, Mercer RD, et al. Temporary remissions in acute leukemia in children produced by folic acid antagonist, 4-aminopteroyl-glutamic acid (aminopterin). N Engl J Med. 1948;238(23):787–93.
47. Goodman L, Wintrobe M, Dameshek W, Goodman M, Gilman A, McLennan M. Nitrogen mustard therapy: use of methyl-bis (beta-chloroethyl)amine hydrochloride and tris (beta-chloroethyl) amine hydrochloride for Hodgkin's disease, lymphosarcoma, leukemia and certain allied and miscellaneous disorder [landmark article]. JAMA. 1946;132:126–32.
48. Yarris JP, Hunter AJ. Roy hertz, M.D. (1909-2002): the cure of choriocarcinoma and its impact on the development of chemotherapy for cancer. Gynecol Oncol. 2003;89(2):193–8.
49. Doll R, Hill AB. Smoking and carcinoma of the lung: preliminary report. Br Med J. 1950;221:739–48.
50. Wynder EL, Graham EA. Tobacco smoking as a possible etiologic factor in bronchiogenic carcinoma. JAMA. 1950;143:329–36.
51. Watson JD, Crick FH. Molecular structure of nucleic acids: a structure for deoxyribose nucleic acid. Nature. 1953;171(4356):737–8.
52. Nowell P, Hungerford D. A minute chromosome in human chronic granulocytic leukemia [abstract]. Science. 1960;132:1497.
53. Knudson AG Jr. Mutation and cancer: statistical study of retinoblastoma. Proc Natl Acad Sci USA. 1971;68(4):820–3.
54. Bister K. Discovery of oncogenes: the advent of molecular cancer research. Proc Natl Acad Sci USA. 2015;112(50):15259–60.
55. Tabin CJ, Bradley SM, Bargmann CI, et al. Mechanism of activation of a human oncogene. Nature. 1982;300(5888):143–9.
56. Slamon DJ, Clark GM, Wong SG, et al. Human breast cancer: correlation of relapse and survival with amplification of the HER-2/neu oncogene. Science. 1987;235(4785):177–8.
57. Hall JM, Lee MK, Newman B, et al. Linkage of early onset familial breast cancer to chromosome 17q21. Science. 1990;250(4988):1684–9.
58. Wooster R, Neuhausen SL, Mangion J, et al. Localization of a breast cancer susceptibility gene, BRCA2, to chromosome 13q12-13. Science. 1994;265(5181):2088–90.

59. Durst M, Gissmann L, Ikenberg H, zur Hausen H. A papillomavirus DNA from a cervical carcinoma and its prevalence in cancer biopsy samples from different geographic regions. Proc Natl Acad Sci USA. 1983;80(12):3812–5.
60. Cohen S. Isolation of a mouse submaxillary gland protein accelerating incisor eruption and eyelid opening in the new-born animal. J Biol Chem. 1962;237:1555–62.
61. Maloney DG, Liles TM, Czerwinski DK, Waldichuk C, Rosenberg J, Grillo-Lopez A, et al. Phase I clinical trial using escalating single-dose infusion of chimeric anti-CD20 monoclonal antibody (IDEC-C2B8) in patients with recurrent B-cell lymphoma. Blood. 1994;84:2457–66.
62. Pegram MD, Lipton A, Hayes DF, et al. Phase II study of receptor-enhanced chemosensitivity using recombinant humanized anti-p185 HER2/neu monoclonal antibody plus cisplatin in patients with HER2/neu-overexpressing metastatic breast cancer refractory to chemotherapy treatment. J Clin Oncol. 1998;16(8):2659–71.
63. Reichardt P. The story of Imatinib in GIST - a journey through the development of a targeted therapy. Oncol Res Treat. 2018;41:472–7. https://doi.org/10.1159/000487511.
64. Leach DR, Krummel MF, Allison JP. Enhancement of anti-tumor immunity by CTLA-4 blockade. Science. 1996;271(5256):1734–6.

Chapter 8
The History of Abdominal Surgery

8.1 Intestinal Surgery

All diseases begin in the gut. Hippocrates

Surgery for abdominal organs, particularly the intestines, was very limited as it represented a risky and often deadly procedure. In Europe, until the nineteenth century, surgery was primarily performed by barber-surgeons, who were not usually university graduates and were often not recognized as physicians. During the Middle Ages, the most common surgical procedures for bowel conditions were the treatment of anal fistulas and hemorrhoids and the removal of anal tumors (probably skin tags or warts). These procedures were performed with crude instruments and without anesthesia, which made them extremely painful and dangerous.

8.1.1 Ambroise Paré (1510–1590)

Ambroise Paré was a French barber-surgeon whose father was a barber, but not a surgeon. His sister married a barber-surgeon, his elder brother was a master barber-surgeon, and after an apprenticeship with his brother, at the age of 22, he secured an appointment at the Hotel Dieu in Paris, where he gained considerable surgical experience. At the age of 26, he became a military surgeon and was appointed colonel-general to Mareschal de Montejan. The standard management of gunshot wounds of his day was based on the work of Giovanni da Vigo (1460–1525) who advised gunshot wounds should be treated with "*boiling oil of elders mixed with a little theriac*."

S. Abbas, D. Watters, *The Road to Modern Surgery*,
https://doi.org/10.1007/978-981-96-4337-0_8

However, his early observations in the field taught him that boiling oil and cautery did more harm than good and so he introduced wound management with egg yolk, rose oil, and turpentine, a treatment that caused less pain and produced better outcomes. His discovery was somewhat fortuitous in that he only adopted this management because his oil ran out, but he then rightly observed that the egg yolk, rose oil, and turpentine caused less pain and inflammation than the oil! He also treated bleeding vessels by ligation rather than cautery, publishing his 1552 technique adopted during the siege of Danvillier, 12 years later, in 1564 [1–3].

Another notable contribution by Paré was for repair of intestinal injuries. His method, which represented a significant surgical advance, involved suturing the damaged area of the intestine rather than just sealing it with a hot iron as was common practice at the time. Paré also introduced other techniques for treating intestinal injuries, such as the use of ligatures to tie off mesenteric vessels to prevent bleeding during surgery.

In *An Apology and Treatise*, he also described a method of treating a sigmoid volvulus conservatively which may not necessarily have been very safe! One assumes that some volvuli must have untwisted and/or deflated as the bellows inflated:

> *...cause the belly to bee blowne with a pair of Bellowes, putting the nosell of them into the rectum and then blow there until the belly be much stretch, afterwards to give an emollient glister...* [1].

8.1.1.1 Louis XIV'S Perianal Abscess and Anal Fistula (1686)

King Louis XIV (1638–1715) had severe pain and swelling in the anal region that kept him from getting out of bed for a week. The skin became inflamed, and an abscess formed, whereupon the physicians placed a feather broom coated with a suppurative and drew out the infection with Manus Dei (Hand of God). The king suffered from obesity, diabetes, and lack of hygiene as the church prohibited public baths while it was thought that diseases spread from water in contact with human skin. It has been reported that the king had only two baths in his entire lifetime! Charles-François Felix, the royal physician, was called upon. On May 21, 1686, the faculty of physicians officially recognized that the king had developed an anal fistula. From the Middle Ages, fistulas had been operated on by a "syringotome," a sharp, almost circular knife developed by Galen in the second century [2].

Felix was advised to perfect his operation on impoverished patients and prisoners. About 75 such operations were performed. His experience led him to devise a new instrument and a retractor to be used during the king's operation.

In the king's palace of Versailles, November 18, 1686, Felix performed the operation with no anaesthesia. The king never uttered a sound of pain, and an hour later, he submitted to bloodletting by his physicians. A month later, Felix had to perform further surgeries for complications. However, in early January 1687, Louis XIV's fistula had healed. He was able to ride a horse again. His 2-month ordeal was over.

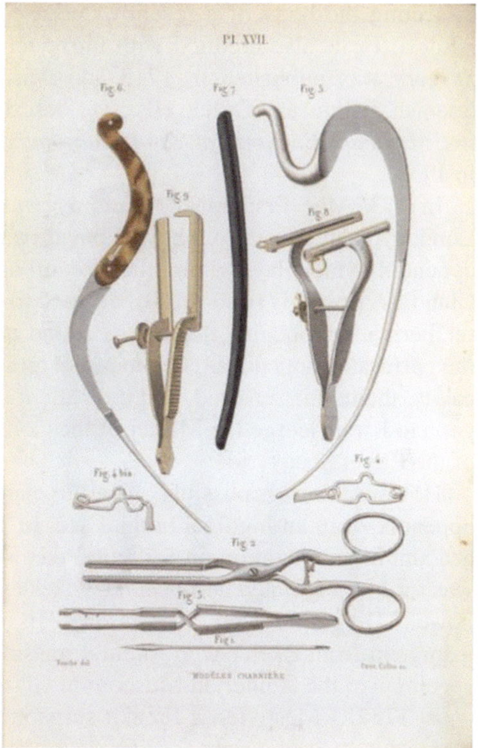

Fig. 8.1 Felix's anal instruments (The Wellcome collection, license: public domain, no restrictions). https://wellcomecollection.org/works/ynxtkxps/images?id=tu3hxdms

Under King Louis XV, the right of surgeons to teach was upheld, and in 1731, French surgeons were allowed to establish what became the Royal Academy of Surgery, the leading surgical organization in Europe, and one which marked the end of the era of the barber-surgeon [3] (Fig. 8.1).

8.1.2 The Appendix and Appendicectomy

Galen (130–201 AD) did his anatomical dissections on monkeys who, unfortunately for Galen, do not have an appendix. The first surviving anatomical drawing of the appendix was made by Leonardo da Vinci (1452–1519) around 1508. The first written account was by Jacopo Berengario de Carpi (1460–1530) in 1522. *"Its shape appeareth strictly compacted, but within it is empty, and is less in breadth than the least finger of the hand, and it is of length of three inches (7.6cm) or thereabouts."*

It was also described by Andreas Vesalius in 1543 in *De Humani Corporis Fabrica Libri Septem*. Giovanni Battista Morgagni also included drawings of the appendix in 1719, showing it had a lumen and was in continuity with the caecum [1, 3].

The first postmortem section of appendicitis (gangrenous, not perforated) was made by a German surgeon, Lorenz Heister (1683–1758), in 1711. He was publicly dissecting the body of a recently deceased criminal in the anatomical theater at Altdorf. He is also credited with introducing the term *tracheotomy*. His textbook *Surgery* was published in 1718 and was soon translated into English, French, Spanish, Italian, and Dutch. His 1711 description of the above autopsy findings is in his *Medical, Chirurgical, and Anatomical Cases and Observations* published in 1753.

In 1735, the first appendicectomy was performed at St. George's Hospital, London, on an 11-year-old boy who had swallowed a pin. The pin had perforated his appendix which lay within the sac of an inguinoscrotal hernia. The surgeon, Claudius Amyand (1680–1740), decided to operate on account of symptoms within the hernia. On opening the sac, he found omentum, gut, and the pin in addition to the perforated appendix. The omentum and caecum were returned to the peritoneal cavity, the hernia repaired, and the patient survived. Amyand was, at the time, surgeon to King George I, a Master of the Company of Barber-Surgeons, and a Fellow of the Royal Society [4].

However, there is possibly an earlier claim to have accidentally removed the first appendix from an inguinal hernial sac. In 1742, William Cookesley published his account of an operation on William Pike, a chimney sweep in 1731. The operation was for a strangulated hernia and Cookesley excised what he called "necrotic small bowel." The patient died 31 years later. His autopsy was performed by John Symons, a surgeon from Exeter who found a missing appendix and caecal pole so sent the specimen to the Hunterian Museum in Glasgow.

In 1757, J Mestivier, a French surgeon working at the St. Andrew Hospital in Bordeaux, incised a right iliac fossa abscess that yielded a pint of pus. The patient died soon after and an autopsy showed the cause to be a pin which was perforating the appendix (Fig. 8.2).

London surgeon, Henry Hancock (1809–1880), was the first to successfully drain an appendix abscess almost a century later in 1848 but he later specialized in ophthalmology [4, 5]!

Willard Parker (1800–1884), Professor of Surgery at the New York College of Physicians and Surgeons from 1839 to 1869, independently described the successful drainage of an appendix abscess on a physician in 1843. However, his description of the case and procedure was only published in 1867. He also believed that alcohol is a poison, only to be taken when prescribed by physicians under exceptional circumstances [5].

It was not until 1880, that Robert Lawson Tait (1845–1899), a Scottish surgeon working in Birmingham, made the first correct preoperative diagnosis of appendicitis in a 17-year-old woman. She had a 3-month history of pain and a mass in the right iliac fossa. Tait made an abdominal incision expecting to find peritonitis but instead found an abscess cavity enclosing a gangrenous appendix.

The actual term appendicitis was only introduced in 1886 by Reginald Heber Fitz (1843–1913) in Boston. Previously, it had been called "typhlitis" and/or "perityphlitis." McBurney's point was named after New York surgeon Charles McBurney (1845–1913) [5, 6].

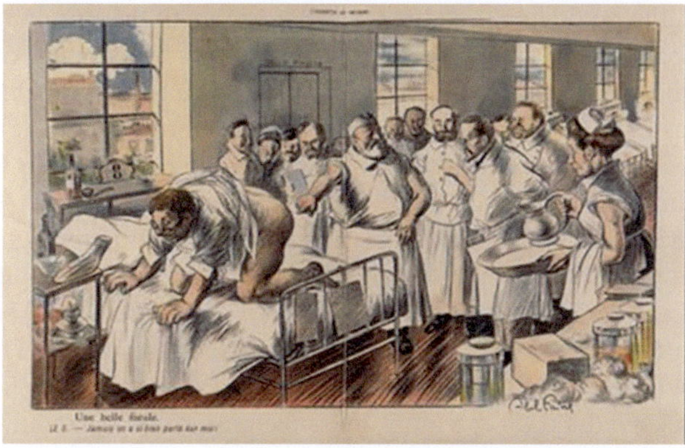

Fig. 8.2 Instruments designed by Felix to do the king's surgery. The patient happily thinks to himself that he has never before been the object of such attention. Color process print after J-A. Faivre, 1902. Faivre, Abel, 1867–1945.Date: 22 March 1902, Public Domain. https://www.google.com/search?vsrid=CI3Bk68DEAIYASIkNzFjYjRhMjEtODk5ZC00YWE2LWFjYjAtM2E0MTEzZWY5MzQ3&gsessionid=cO_AFvv-SQ6HTqhtDA3YovF93mTNWKpu3s9SAitXCiTMLSLh2TLKmg&lsessionid=EaKk5mG7xAFDVwRWgoX3Gvzb2_vh8xORfKVWnsIZtvCUnGX30Y3K7Q&vsdim=760,496&vsint=CAIqDAoCCAcSAggKGAEgATojChYNAAAAPxUAAAA_HQAAgD8lAACAPzABEPgFGPADJQAAgD8&lns_mode=un&source=lns.web.iosbcm&udm=26&qsubts=1733451161594&biw=428&bih=751

8.1.3 Laparotomy

It is likely that laparotomy had been attempted on a number of occasions prior to the introduction of anaesthesia, most of which would have been fatal.

The first reliable record of a successful Caesarean is by Jacob Nüfer, a Swiss farmer, in 1500, who used his own instruments to save his wife and deliver a live child by Caesarean. She not only survived but went on to have several more children. Nüfer operated only because 13 midwives and several stonecutters (lithotomists) were unable to help her [7].

The term Caesarean comes from the Latin word *caedere* "to cut." From the eighth century BCE, the law gave the right to remove a live baby from a mother who had died or was dying in childbirth. This was continued in the Roman legal code or *lex Caesare*. Julius Caesar's mother, Aurelia, outlived her son to bury him 55 years later so Julius Caesar was certainly not born by Caesarean. Even in the late nineteenth century, Caesarean section carried a mortality of 56% in 1878 [8].

In 1550, Mathias Cornax (b 1520) illustrated a procedure performed by a Viennese surgeon, in Dirlewang, of a laparotomy for a woman, Marguerite Walezer, to remove a retained, dead fetus from a tubal pregnancy that had ended 4 years earlier.

In 1694, Abraham Cyprianius (c1660–1718) in Amsterdam removed a dead baby that was a full-term ectopic tubular pregnancy. The woman survived and went on to have three further children (second and third were twins). A surgeon, N Simonides, who assisted at the procedure, and the Court Physician of the Prince van Oranje, Dr. Portius, managed the postoperative care. There was a fair amount of discharge of fluid through the lower end of the wound and between the sutures until the wound healed. She was out of bed and fully mobile after 3 months [1, 9].

The first documented successful laparotomy is credited to Ephraim McDowell (1771–1830). In 1809, in Danville, Kentucky, McDowell operated on Jane Crawford, draining and then removing a 10.2 kg ovarian tumor with the pedicle secured by a ligature tied around the fallopian tube near the uterus. The procedure took 25 minutes and Jane Crawford lived another 32 years. Although McDowell had undertaken medical education for 3 years under Dr. Alexander Humphreys (1752–1802) in Virginia, and at the University of Edinburgh (1793–4) under John Bell (1763–1820), he had never received a diploma until the University of Maryland awarded him an honorary one in 1825 [1, 9]!

8.1.3.1 Intestinal Suturing

In 1826, Antoine Lembert (1802–1851) published a paper describing a new technique for intestinal suturing that became known as the "Lembert suture." The Lembert suture involved sewing the edges of the intestinal wound together using a seromuscular stitch that included both the muscular layer and the outer serosal layer of the intestine. He used interrupted sutures of silk to approximate the serosa of the two inverted edges of the bowel wound. This was a significant improvement over previous techniques that had previously only involved suturing the mucosal layer of the intestine. Lembert tested his technique on a cadaver pumping air into the sutured bowel and holding it under water. He then performed it on five dogs who all survived [4].

Since his original description, there are other modifications of Lembert's seromuscular technique. Early reports were from Antoine Jobert de Lamballe (1799–1867) who used full-thickness sutures (including the mucosa), Breidenbech who tied the knot inside the lumen, and Dupuytren (1777–1835) who used a continuous suture. In France, there was some controversy as to whom the honour of introducing the seromuscular technique should go. Two senior French surgeons, Philibert-Joseph Roux (1780–1854) and Jules Cloquet (1790–1883), adjudicated on the matter, concluding that Jobert had introduced the idea of serosal apposition while Lembert applied it to both longitudinal and transverse incisions and for deliberate transection of the bowel. They denied Denans of Marseille's claim also published in 1826 using silver or zinc rings in each bowel end stump, connecting the two rings with a third intraluminal ring and allowing the inverted part of the bowel to necrose with the rings and then passing in the stool. The bowel remained intact, thanks to the serosal to serosal apposition. Fauvre also made a competing claim that he had done the experimental work in 1821 while an intern at St. Louis Hospital, but also only published his method in 1826 [10].

William Stewart Halsted (1852–1922) modified the suturing technique of the bowel. Halsted's technique involved suturing the bowel by taking a bite of the full thickness of the intestinal wall, including the submucosal layer. This was based on his observations that the submucosa was the most important layer for the healing of bowel anastomosis, as it contained important blood vessels that were essential for proper healing. [It is also the strongest layer made up of crisscross fibers of collagen in a viscoelastic matrix] [4, 10–12].

8.1.3.2 The Stoma

Ancient physicians such as Hippocrates, Celsus, and Galenus described that sometimes the only possibility to survive after a penetrating bowel injury was the spontaneous formation of a fistula (natural stoma).

In 1710, Alexis Littré (1654–1726), a French surgeon, speaking at the Royal Academy in Paris, described a dead neonate with imperforate anus and proposed that a stoma might deal with this condition. The procedure involved creating an opening in the abdomen and bringing a loop of the distended colon through the opening to form a stoma, which would allow faecal matter to pass out of the body. He also suggested that a lumbar stoma might help for adults with a large bowel obstruction. Littré's name is associated with the name of the condition in which a Meckel's diverticulum is contained within an inguinal hernia (Littré's hernia) [13, 14].

Lorenz Heister (1683–1758) regarded the adherence of open bowel to the abdominal wall as a "hint of nature" of which the surgeon should take heed. He advised "*stitch it to the external wound either by the continued or interrupted suture....the same method of cure may conveniently enough be put in practice where any part of the intestine is mortified by being forced out of the abdomen....*" [13].

In 1750, William Cheselden (1688–1752) operated on a Mrs. Margaret White aged 73, and removed 55 cm of ischaemic bowel due to a volvulus or strangulated hernia. The end of the healthy bowel was left hanging out of the abdominal wall for drainage and she survived many years. However, Cheselden's greatest contribution to surgery was his advocacy for the separation of surgeons from the Company of Barber-Surgeons. The Corporation of Surgeons, the forerunner of the Royal College of Surgeons, was founded by Act of Parliament in 1745.

The first true stoma was performed in 1776 by French surgeon, Henri Pillore in Rouen. This was a caecostomy for an obstructing rectal cancer, diagnosed by digital examination. The patient died 20 days later, not from his surgery but from a large dose of quicksilver (mercury) he had been prescribed by his physicians.

In 1781, Henri Le Dran, a French military surgeon noticed that soldiers in great pain would lance apparent boils arising from wounds on their abdomen that were in fact colocutaneous fistulae. The resulting wound might then heal forming a permanent stoma and with relief of pain. Then in 1793, Duret, a French Naval Surgeon performed a stoma on a newborn with imperforate anus. That child went on to live for 43 years with a stoma in the left iliac fossa.

Jean Amussat (1796–1856) collected 27 previously reported stomas performed between 1716 and 1839. Only six had been successful [12–14].

Samuel Gross (1805–1994) from Philadelphia regarded the operation of stoma formation to be immoral:

> *...that anyone possessed of the proper feeling of humanity should seriously advocate a procedure so fraught with danger and followed, if successful, by such disgusting consequences... I cannot, I must confess, appreciate the benevolence which prompts a surgeon to form an artificial outlet for the discharge of faeces, in case of imperforate anus* [15].

In his book *The Science and Art of Surgery*, published in 1853, Jon Eric Erichsen (1818–1896), a Danish-born British surgeon based at University College Hospital in London, described four indications for colostomy: imperforate anus, intractable constipation, cancer of the rectum, and stricture of the rectum or colon. The stomas formed were generally loop colostomies performed in two steps where the loop was exteriorized usually over a glass rod, and once the skin and bowel were sealed, the stoma (which had no sensation) could be opened on the ward. Immediate opening of the stoma was not performed until first introduced by Patey in 1951 [14, 15].

8.1.4 Colonic Resections

In 1823, a French surgeon, Reybard (1795–1863), performed the first documented segmental colonic resection for a tumour of the sigmoid colon. The patient survived their operation but died of cancer recurrence one year later [17].

Until 1880, only 10 colonic resections had been recorded in medical literature, with 7 deaths reported. The procedure was still considered very risky at this time due to the lack of aseptic technique and effective anesthaesia. However, with the introduction of antiseptic techniques by Joseph Lister and the development of safer anaesthesia in the late nineteenth century, the number of colonic resections performed increased significantly. Between 1880 and 1890, 48 colonic resections were recorded, with a mortality rate of around 45% [9]. Despite an alarmingly high mortality rate in cases mainly presenting with large bowel obstruction, these early colonic resections offered the patients their only hope of relief, even if temporary, and also informed the development and evolution of colorectal surgery [16, 17].

8.1.5 Rectal Resection

Jean Fajet performed a posterior approach to rectal resection in 1793, but the patient did not survive. The first successful rectal resection was in 1826, performed by Jacques Lisfranc (1787–1847) in Paris. In 1833, he reported nine cases of rectal resection through a posterior approach with the resection remaining below the peritoneal reflection. All patients died within 2 years as this was not a radical resection. The introduction of general anaesthesia, first with ether and also with chloroform, played a significant role in the development of colorectal resection [18].

Theodor Billroth (1812–1894) in Vienna performed 45 rectal resections between 1860 and 1872 using the posterior approach of Lisfranc [8]. Aristide Auguste Stanislas Verneuil (1823–1895), a French surgeon and pupil of Lisfranc at the Pitié Hospital in Paris, then modified the Lisfranc resection, by excising the coccyx, gaining better access to allow a more radical resection [19].

Carl Gussenbauer (1842–1903), an Austrian working under Billroth, was the first to excise the rectum through an anterior approach in 1879. In 1884, Vincent Czerny (1842–1916), Professor of Surgery in Heidelberg and a former pupil of Billroth, used a combined posterior/anterior approach. After starting with a planned posterior approach, in response to complications during the procedure, he repositioned his patient supine to complete the operation via an anterior approach. This patient did not survive.

In 1885, Paul Kraske (1851–1930) was Professor of Surgery at the University of Freiberg in Germany. He had trained earlier in his career under Richard von Volkmann (1830–1889) in Halle, the same Volkmann who had named Volkmann's ischemic contracture (due to vascular injury associated with a supracondylar fracture of the elbow) in 1881. Volkmann had also excised a rectal cancer in 1878. However, Kraske was able to perform a perineal excision by making an incision from the sacrum to the anus and disarticulating the left side of the coccyx and sacrum so allowing the rectum to be freed of its attachments and removed. The technique was rapidly adopted and utilized into the twentieth century. A review of 1500 rectal resection cases from 12 surgical centers reported a 20.9% perioperative mortality but, unfortunately for the surviving patients, an 80% recurrence [20–22].

William Ernest Miles (1869–1947) was an 1891 graduate of St. Bartholomew's Hospital and London University, worked as house surgeon under David Goodsall (1843–1906) who described Goodsall's rule in 1900 at St. Marks Hospital. Miles also worked under Harrison Cripps (1850–1923), a pathologist who was the first to describe metastases as arising from the primary tumor and spreading through blood vessels and/or lymphatics. Prior to Cripps' work, metastatic disease was thought to be due to multifocal de novo developing cancers. Miles performed 57 perineal resections of the rectum between 1899 and 1906. Of his patients, 95% had a recurrence, often within 6 months. He performed autopsies on these patients and, from the pattern of recurrent and metastatic disease, worked out that approaching from below alone would not normally be curative. Miles added an anterior approach to the procedure to address the upward route of metastatic spread. In 1908, he reported a perioperative mortality of 5 from his first 12 abdominoperineal resections (APR). In 1923, he reported a reduced recurrence rate of 29.5%, and by the end of his career, the perioperative mortality had reduced to 15% [13]. It should be remembered that these rates were obtained at a time when cancer presented late. Most tumors were diagnosed by digital examination, contrast (barium) enemas, and rigid sigmoidoscopy that enabled the distal 20–25 cm of the anus, rectum, and sigmoid colon to be visualized [22].

John Percy Lockhart-Mummery (1875–1957) was a British surgeon who worked at St. Mark's Hospital in London during the early twentieth century. He is best known for his work on the surgical treatment of rectal cancer, and in 1907, he proposed a two-stage abdomino-perineal resection (APR) technique for the treatment of rectal cancer [16].

In 1912, William James Mayo (1861–1939) in Rochester, Minnesota, USA, adopted the APR approach as a two-stage procedure. Initially, he performed a colostomy and only mobilized the rectum, to be followed after some weeks by resection of the rectum through a perineal approach. In 1921, Henri Hartmann (1860–1952), Chief of Surgery at the Hotel Dieu in Paris, advocated an anterior approach with stoma for high rectal tumors. His first report was of two patients, both of whom had recovered well [21, 22].

The APR approach was the most popular until 1948 when Claude Dixon (1893–1968), Chair of Surgery at the Mayo Clinic, presented a series of anterior resections and restoration of large bowel continuity for tumors of the upper rectum and sigmoid colon using a two-layered sutured anastomosis. This began an era of sphincter-saving surgery for cancer resections when adequate distal margin clearance could be obtained. The ease of performing the anastomosis deep in the pelvis was considerably improved by the development of the mechanical circular stapler during the 1980s [21–23].

The concept of Total Mesenteric Excision (TME) was introduced by Bill Heald (b 1936) in 1982 [15]. This significantly reduced local pelvic recurrence and enabled surgeons to better dissect in the safest plane of dissection above the autonomic nerves, thereby preserving function. Heald demonstrated that the complete removal of the mesorectum, which is the fatty tissue surrounding the rectum that contains lymph nodes and blood vessels, significantly reduces the risk of tumor recurrence and improves long-term survival rates for patients with rectal cancer. Heald also defined the concept of the "holy plane," which refers to the surgical dissection plane that separates the mesorectum from the pelvic nerves and the sacral plane. He and his pathologists also introduced the concept of the completeness of the TME resection, and reporting clearance of the circumferential resection margin around the primary tumor, not just the distal and proximal margins [24–27].

With the advent of laparoscopic abdominal surgery in the 1990s, colorectal resections began to be performed laparoscopically without compromising cancer outcomes compared with open surgery. However, many emergency operations, particularly where there are adhesions from previous surgery or very distended bowel, are still done by open, anterior, laparotomy approaches. This has led to less pain and more rapid recovery after the surgery with discharge from hospital often achieved within 2–3 days for cases that are not complicated. Robotic colorectal surgery also offers some advantages over laparoscopic surgery when operating deep the pelvis because its instruments have better versatility (degrees of freedom) than laparoscopic ones [28, 29].

The introduction of preoperative chemoradiotherapy for pT3 rectal cancers prior to rectal resection has not only led to better outcomes and lower local recurrence rates but also resulted in some patients undergoing complete remission of their tumor such that no residual cancer can be found on the resected rectum where the original tumor was found. This has led to a "watch-and-wait" approach for selected patients for whom no sign of residual cancer can be found on rectal examination and imaging over the past 20 years. This strategy was originally proposed by Brazilian surgeon Angelita Habr-Gama (b1933).

Another recent major improvement in early rectal cancer treatment is transanal minimally invasive surgery (TAMIS), a surgical technique that was first reported in 2010 as an alternative to transanal endoscopic microsurgery (TEM) for the resection of rectal polyps and early-stage rectal cancers. Like TEM, TAMIS is a minimally invasive technique that allows for the removal of tumors through the anus, without the need for abdominal surgery [20].

TAMIS had its origins with Sir Alan Parks (1920–1982). In the 1970s, Parks and his team reported transanal local resection as a surgical technique for the removal of villous tumors of the anal canal. This technique involves the following steps: The patient is placed in the prone jackknife position and a self-retaining anal retractor is inserted to expose the anal canal. The tumor is identified and marked with a suture. A circumferential incision is made around the base of the tumor using a scalpel or electrocautery. The tumor is then carefully dissected away from the surrounding tissue, using sharp dissection and electrocautery as needed. Hemostasis is achieved and the wound is closed with sutures [30, 31].

In 2013, a transanal endoscopic approach to resection of low rectal cancers (TaTME) was proposed by Antonio de Lacy, a Spanish surgeon based in Barcelona. The rectal cancer including mesorectum is excised from a bottom-up approach, and to date in well-selected cases, the results are comparable with the laparoscopic anterior resection approach in terms of cancer outcomes.

8.1.5.1 Robotic Colorectal Surgery

In the 1980s, the da Vinci® surgical robot was developed by Intuitive Surgical, Inc. in the 1990s, with initial funding from the US Army's Telemedicine and Advanced Technology Research Center (TATRC). The idea was to develop a robot that could be controlled by a surgeon from a remote location, allowing for surgical procedures to be performed on soldiers injured in combat zones without the need for the surgeon to be physically present. However, as the technology developed, it became clear that the da Vinci® robot's true potential was in assisting surgeons in performing minimally invasive surgeries in a wide range of specialties, including urology, gynecology, and general surgery, and was approved by the FDA in 2000. Today, the da Vinci® surgical robot is used in thousands of hospitals around the world for a variety of surgical procedures. The first reported use of the da Vinci® surgical robot for colorectal cancer surgery was in Japan by Dr. Masahiko Hashizume and his team at the University of Tokyo in 2002. The team performed a laparoscopic-assisted low anterior resection using the da Vinci® robot on a patient with rectal cancer [32].

8.1.5.2 Colorectal Resection Outcomes in 2024

Today, at the time of writing, in the mid-2020s, planned (elective) colorectal resections have a mortality risk of around 1% in patients without significant added risks from their comorbidities or age. Emergency colorectal resections requiring an emergency laparotomy carry a mortality risk that can be as low as 4–8%, depending on

the condition of the patient and their pathology. However, the standard mortality rate, particularly in countries or places where emergency laparotomies are not part of a quality improvement registry such as NELA in the United Kingdom, is likely to still be above 10% for laparotomies for colorectal pathology.
Although surgeons are able to perform lower sphincter-saving operations and even form ileoanal or coloanal J pouches, the outcome is dependent on the patient, their age, state of their pelvic floor, and their goals. Low anterior resection syndrome (LARS) that results in social incapacitation due to stool or gas leakage and urgency of defecation is becoming increasingly recognized. The pendulum may have swung too far toward restoring gastrointestinal continuity, and wherever there is a reasonable and affordable supply of stoma bags and support, some patients will always be better treated by stoma than a low or ultralow anastomosis. However, stomas are also, by definition, a hernia and parastomal hernias are common following APR or Hartmann procedures. These may also incapacitate the patient, never mind inevitably carrying a their own risk of complications. Therefore, the choice of operation to perform for a patient with a colorectal cancer always needs to be carefully considered and matched to delivering the best outcomes aligned with the goals of the individual patient [31–34].

8.1.5.3 St Mark's Hospital

St. Mark's Hospital, founded by Frederick Salmon, was initially established in 1835 as a small infirmary in London, to provide treatment for poor patients suffering from rectal diseases such as fistula. In 1851, a new site was purchased in City Road, and the hospital was moved there in 1854. The new hospital was officially named "St. Mark's Hospital for Fistula and Other Diseases of the Rectum" in honor of the patron saint of Venice, who was traditionally associated with the treatment of rectal diseases. St. Mark's Hospital quickly became recognized as a center of excellence for the treatment of colorectal disease. In 1871, David Henry Goodsall (1843–1906) was appointed as Consultant Surgeon at the St. Marks Hospital, where he studied the relations of perianal fistulae and became famous for his "rule," the Goodsall rule, described in 1900 and still applicable today. In 1959, Sir Alan Parks (1920–1982) was appointed as surgeon and made significant contributions to the field of pelvic floor surgery during his time at St. Mark's Hospital. Parks developed new surgical techniques for repairing pelvic floor damage, including the use of mesh grafts to support the pelvic organs and the development of new methods for repairing rectal prolapse [10]. He also co-authored the paper reporting the first five patients with ileoanal pouches with John Nicholls (b1943) in 1978 [33, 34].

8.1.5.4 Colorectal Anatomy and Physiology

The anatomical and physiological foundations of modern colorectal surgery were established during the late nineteenth and early twentieth centuries by several key figures in the fields of anatomy and surgery. Dimitrie Gerota (1867–1939)

was a Romanian anatomist. He was also the assistant of Professor Heinrich Wilhelm Gottfried von Waldeyer-Hartz (1836–1921) with whom he studied anatomy of the rectum. Gerota made significant contributions to the understanding of the anatomy of the colon and rectum. He is best known for his work on the peritoneal reflections and mesenteric attachments of the colon and rectum, which helped to establish the surgical anatomy of the gastrointestinal tract. Carl Toldt (1840–1920) was an Austrian anatomist who is known for his detailed descriptions of the blood supply and lymphatic drainage of the colon and rectum. He pointed out how the primary mesocolon of the ascending and descending colon attaches posteriorly. His work on the mesenteric circulation of the colon was particularly influential and helped to lay the groundwork for modern surgical techniques.
John Hilton (1804–1878) was an English surgeon who made significant contributions to the understanding of the nerve supply of the colon and rectum and the lymphatic drainage of the anal canal. His work on the innervation of the gastrointestinal tract helped to establish the principles of sphincter-preserving surgery for rectal cancer [15, 16, 18].

8.1.5.5 Gastrointestinal Staples

Due to the technical challenge of anterior resections, surgeons across the world started to devise a stapling technique. One of the early reports of stapling anastomosis of the gastrointestinal tract was from Hungary in 1908 by Humer Hultl, a surgeon with his brother engineer, but progress came to a halt by the first world war (Fig. 8.3).

In 1951, the Scientific Research and Trial Institute of Medical Engineering in Moscow produced several prototypes of surgical staplers, the so-called "Russian gun."

In 1978, Dr. Michael Ravitch and his colleagues developed a gastrointestinal suturing device that made it possible to perform highly complex end-to-end anastomosis after rectal or esophageal resection. This device, called the Ravitch anastomotic instrument, was a significant advancement in surgical technology and made it easier for surgeons to perform complex anastomosis with greater precision and accuracy [17]. That was followed by Knight et al. in 1980 who reported the double stapling technique, which enhanced the dissemination of anterior resection that remains the basis for circular stapling techniques today [26].

The modern era had seen various modes of progression and changes for rectal cancer treatment such as extended lymph nodes dissection, neoadjuvant chemoradiotherapy, watch and wait after clinical complete response to chemoradiation, local excision followed by chemoradiation for early rectal cancer of early stage, chemoradiation followed by full-thickness local excision, and total neoadjuvant therapy (TNT). Based on that evidence, the NCCN guidelines classify TNT as a viable treatment strategy for rectal cancer. It can also increase the population of patients eligible for the watch-and-wait strategy [31, 35].

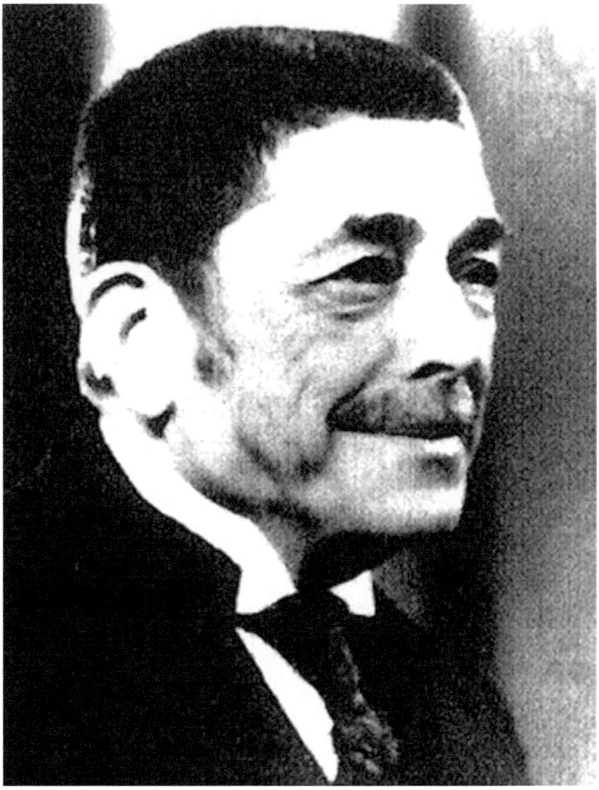

Fig. 8.3 Humer Hultl, Wikipedia, public domain. https://en.wikipedia.org/wiki/Hümér_Hültl#/media/File:Hültl_Hümér.jpg

8.2 Surgery of the Stomach and Duodenum

Indigestion is as old as human existence and various medications have been recommended since the earliest of times. An example of this is the discovery of a male body preserved in 167 BCE, from the time of the Western Han dynasty (China). When the body was discovered and studied in the 1970s, the man was found to have died of peritonitis from a perforated prepyloric ulcer.

It was only with the aid of autopsy that the true pathology of upper gastrointestinal disease could be matched to the presenting symptoms and signs. Not all ulcers cause pain and discomfort and not all epigastric pain is due to ulcers or inflammation. The many causes for epigastric and indigestive-type pains include gastritis (inflammation without ulceration), hepatitis, pancreatitis, and cholecystitis (relatively rare until the twentieth century). Gastric and pancreatic cancers may present with pain but often are quite far advanced when they become symptomatic. Among the common causes of gastric outlet obstruction and persistent vomiting are benign stricture and scarring of the pylorus or duodenum, distal gastric cancer, or a cancer in the pancreatic head encroaching the duodenum. This chapter begins with the history of gastric resection and the management of peptic ulcers. The final section of this chapter will cover the history of pyloric stenosis in infants.

Giovanni Battista Morgagni (1682–1771) was an Italian anatomist who is considered one of the fathers of modern anatomical pathology. He studied medicine at Bologna (graduated with distinction in 1701), became an assistant to Antonio Maria Valsalva (1666–1723), and became Professor of Medicine at the University of Padua in 1711. He systematically correlated clinical symptoms and signs with anatomical findings at autopsy. Morgagni's seminal book, *De Sedibus*, *On the Seats and Causes of Diseases Investigated by Anatomy,* was published in 1761 and was based on the results of more than 700 autopsies he had conducted [36, 37].

8.2.1 Early Gastric Resections in the Late Nineteenth Century

8.2.1.1 Partial Gastrectomy

The first two surgeons to document performing a partial gastrectomy were, in 1879, French surgeon, Jules-Émile Péan (1830–1898), and in 1880, Ludwik Rydygier (1850–1920) in Culm, Poland. Both their patients died within a few days. Rydygier performed a successful antrectomy in November 1881, but this was after the first successful gastric resection by Theodor Billroth (1829–1894) in Vienna.

Jules-Émile Péan (1830–1898) worked in Parisian hospitals. He performed a splenectomy in 1867 and developed a pioneering shoulder arthroplasty made of platinum and cemented with plaster and pumice. It had to be removed after 2 years. He never obtained an appointment as professor and was therefore denied admission to the Society of Surgeons though he was accepted by the Academy of Medicine. He was a keen philanthropist, founding a hospital to treat the poor which was posthumously named after him. In 1892, he became a commander of the French legion of honour.

Ludwik Rydygier (1850–1920), worked in Culm (1879–87) and Krakow (1887–1897) where he succeeded respectively, Johannes Mikulicz-Radecki and Lemberg (1897–1920). He was a strong advocate for antisepsis and the Polish language, publishing his first surgical texts in Polish rather than German. The first meeting of the Polish surgeons was held in Krakow in 1889. He was appointed a Privy Councillor of the Austrian Empire and the Pope made him a Commander of the Order of St. Gregory. He became a radiotherapy pioneer in Lemberg. He was also staunchly opposed to women undertaking a career in medicine and surgery.

Billroth's introduction of partial gastrectomy was based on the knowledge that two assistants, Gussenbauer and Winiwarter, had already, in 1876, demonstrated the feasibility of a partial gastrectomy in the laboratory. The operation was performed at Vienna's Allgemeine Krankenhaus (General Hospital). The patient was a 43-years-old woman who survived 4 months after the operation and died from liver metastases. Her autopsy specimen showed an intact anastomosis. The operative technique used by Billroth still bears his name today as Billroth I, involving a gastroduodenal anastomosis directly narrowing, then connecting the gastric stump to the duodenum. In 1885, Billroth and von Hacker modified the operation for a more radical resection (not out of dissatisfaction with the gastroduodenal anastomosis), known as Billroth II, utilizing a gastrojejunostomy anastomosis. By 1885, there had been 37 Billroth II procedures reported with 10 survivors, 8 of which were from Billroth's team or his pupils. His success in gastric resection was due in part to his extensive training, skill, and diligence, but also to his adoption of antisepsis to minimize the risk of infection [37]. In 1881, he published a textbook on the use of antisepsis to prevent postoperative infection. By 1897, Billroth and his assistants had done 46 gastric resections with a 35% mortality [37–39].

8.2.1.2 Christian Albert Theodor Billroth (1829–1894) (Fig. 8.4)

Billroth was a brilliant pianist and violinist and wanted to be a musician but was persuaded by his mother and two medical uncles to study medicine in Göttingen, Germany (then Prussia). He wrote his MD thesis on the effect of vagotomy on the lungs (1852) and, as an aspiring surgeon, found, "*Observation of the sick bed is so much more favorable than microscopy.*" He went to Berlin where he worked under von Langenbeck, where Rudolf Virchow (1829–1902) was chair of Anatomical Pathology. After refusing chairs in Göttingen and Heidelberg, he was appointed Chair of Clinical Surgery in Zurich from 1860 to 1867, where he trained Theodor Kocher. In Zurich, he was the music critic for the newspaper *Zeitung* and was often asked to conduct for the Zurich Symphony Orchestra. He was appointed to the Chair in Wien (Vienna), Austria (1867–1894), where his tenure proved an outstanding success. There, he performed the first laryngectomy (1873) and first hemilaryngectomy (1878). Both pioneering procedures were successful. However, he was a chain smoker who could never resist a cigar, drank copiously, with a BMI above 35, and who died prematurely at the age of 64.

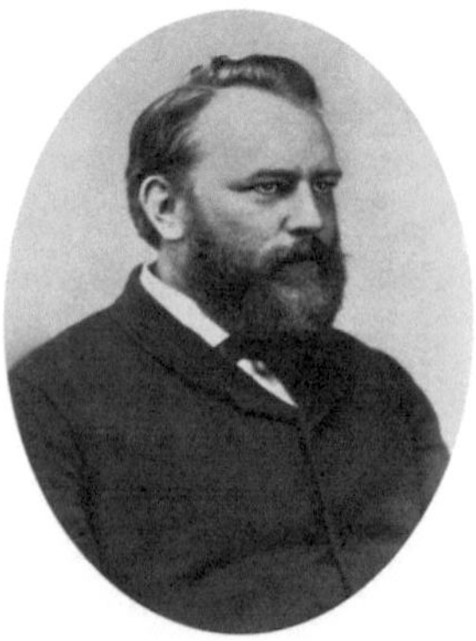

Fig. 8.4 Billroth, Wikipedia, Public Domain. https://nl.wikipedia.org/wiki/Theodor_Billroth#/media/Bestand:Theodor_Billroth_NIH.jpg

8.2.1.3 Billroth's Legacy in Gastric Surgery

During his years in Zurich and Vienna, Billroth trained some of the finest surgical leaders of Europe. In 1881, Woelfler and Nicoladoni, members of his department, performed the first anterior gastrojejunostomy. In 1882, Czerny, also a member of his department, performed a local excision of a gastric ulcer. Although Courvoisier was the first to perform a posterior gastrojejunostomy through the transverse mesocolon, von Hacker of Billroth's department appropriately modified the Courvoisier method to preserve the middle colic vessels. In 1884, Rydygier (not a pupil of Billroth) in Poland performed a gastrojejunostomy for an obstructing duodenal ulcer.

8.2.1.4 Total Gastrectomy

Total gastrectomy is an even more technically demanding procedure with higher risks of complications involving an oesophago-jejunal anastomosis and a jejuno-jejunal anastomosis. The patient undergoing such a procedure is often significantly deconditioned and malnourished so is at high risk of complications such as bleeding, infection, and anastomotic leaks.

There are conflicting accounts regarding credit for the first total gastrectomy for diffuse gastric cancer. While some sources credit Ludwik Rydygier, others claim that Karl Schlatter (1864–1934) performed the first total gastrectomy for diffuse gastric cancer in 1897 in Zurich, Switzerland. Schlatter's patient was a 42-year-old woman with a diffuse, infiltrating gastric cancer. Schlatter removed the entire stomach anastomosing the oesophagus end to side with the jejunum, and the patient survived the surgery for a short period of time before ultimately succumbing to the disease [39, 40].

In 1898, Dr. John Collins Warren Brigham (1842–1927), a surgeon from Boston, Massachusetts, reported the second successful case of total gastrectomy. The patient was a 32-year-old man who presented with gastric cancer, and Brigham was able to remove the entire stomach, anastomosing the esophagus to the mobilized duodenum. Brigham's case helped to establish total gastrectomy as a viable option for the treatment of advanced gastric cancer, thus paving the way for further advances in the field of gastrointestinal surgery [41, 42].

In 1900, Arthur Mayo-Robson (1853–1933) published a report on 188 consecutive gastric operations that had been performed at the Leeds General Infirmary in England. The report showed a mortality rate of 16.4% for these procedures. This was a significant improvement compared to earlier mortality rates, which had been as high as 50% or more for some types of gastric surgeries. The report also highlighted the importance of careful patient selection and meticulous surgical technique [42].

The discovery of X-rays gave surgeons at the start of the twentieth century the opportunity to diagnose malignancy and benign ulcers by using radio-opaque material using oral contrast. It also allowed functional studies of gastric emptying and thus motility to be performed.

8.2.2 Surgery for "Peptic" Ulcer

Although gastric and duodenal ulcers are as old as mankind, their accurate clinical description appears to have waited until the eighteenth and nineteenth centuries. They usually cause pain, though some are painless. There may be associated anorexia and weight loss. They are more common in smokers. If untreated and/or fail to heal, they may perforate causing peritonitis, or that perforation may be contained by the left lobe or the liver or the pancreas (so-called penetrating ulcer). They may also heal with stenosis, causing gastric outlet obstruction, particularly when the original ulcer is in the duodenum, pylorus, or prepyloric area of the stomach. Benign gastric ulcers need to be differentiated from gastric cancer as their prognosis and treatment are different. Prior to the twentieth century, prepyloric and gastric ulcers were more common than duodenal [43, 44].

The first accurate description of gastric ulcer was by Matthew Baillie (1761–1823), a Scottish physician. In 1793, he published a book *The Morbid Anatomy of Some of the Most Important Parts of the Human Body* in which he provided an accurate and detailed description of gastric ulcers and gastric cancer.

Prior to Baillie's work, the understanding of gastric ulcers and cancer was limited, with medical texts often containing vague or incomplete descriptions of these conditions [40].

Duodenal ulceration was described in 1808, by Benjamin Travers (1763–1858), a British surgeon who served on the Council of the Royal College of Surgeons from 1830 until 1858. He observed that these ulcers were different from gastric ulcers in their location and symptoms, establishing duodenal ulceration as a distinct medical condition [37].

Once the techniques of anterior and posterior gastroenterostomy had been developed by Billroth's and Rydygier's teams, the operation rapidly gained popularity in the late nineteenth and early twentieth centuries as a treatment for peptic ulceration complicated by pyloric obstruction or as a palliative bypass for an unresectable distal gastric carcinoma [45, 46].

However, gastroenterostomy is not without its own complications. Gastroenterostomy was initially a challenging procedure with high mortality rates. According to historical records, up until 1884, only 2 out of 7 cases of gastroenterostomy survived. The procedure may also cause morbidity, for example, from biliary regurgitation, which can occur when bile from the small intestine flows back into the stomach, causing irritation and inflammation. The gastroenterostomy may also fail to function for some weeks resulting in ongoing vomiting, and within a year or two, ulceration may recur in the jejunum (so-called stomal ulcer) or the patient might suffer from diarrhea or dumping (see below). Nonetheless, gastroenterostomy, by succeeding in diverting acid from the duodenum directly to the jejunum, did result in some 75% of duodenal ulcers healing.

Surgeons also debated the location (anterior and posterior to the colon) and orientation (prograde or retrograde in relation to motility) of the gastrojejunal anastomosis.

In 1897, a Swiss surgeon and head of the University of Lausanne surgical clinic, César Roux (1857–1934) introduced the "en-y" type of gastroenterostomy, which involved creating a Y-shaped anastomosis that reduced the risk of biliary regurgitation and provided a more secure connection between the stomach and the small intestine but at the risk of needing to perform two extra anastomoses. With time, improvement of surgical anastomotic techniques helped to reduce the mortality. [César Roux was also the first surgeon to lead a team to remove a pheochromocytoma in 1926 [45].

Despite its challenges and potential complications, gastroenterostomy remained an important surgical option for patients with peptic ulceration until the development of the various vagotomy procedures (1940s to 1980s), which were progressively replaced by the introduction of better medical management, first with histamine 2 receptor blockers (1970s, cimetidine/ranitidine), proton pump inhibitors (1989, omeprazole), and anti-helicobacter therapy (1990s) [41]. Today, uncomplicated duodenal and benign gastric ulcer disease is a medical condition with surgery reserved for stenosis, perforation, and uncontrollable hemorrhage [47].

8.2.3 Pyloroplasties for Pyloric Stenosis

The are three main types of pyloroplasty—the Heineke-Mikulicz, Jaboulay, and Finney. Each has their indications and ease of construction.

In 1886, Walter Herman von Heinecke (1834–1901), and in 1887, Johannes Mikulicz-Radecki (1850–1905) independently developed their technique of what is now called the Heinecke-Mikulicz pyloroplasty involving a longitudinal incision in the distal stomach and proximal duodenum with transverse closure [38, 48, 49].

Walter Hermann von Heineke (1834–1901), a Prussian, son of a physician, and graduate of the University of Greifswald (1859), was appointed Chair of Surgery in Erlangen in 1867.

Johannes Mikulicz-Radecki (1850–1905) was a pupil of Billroth's until he went to the Chair in Krakow (1882–87), where he described the repair of a perforated peptic ulcer in 1885. His career progressed to the Chair of Surgery at Konigsberg (1887–1890) and then Breslau (1890–1905). He died of advanced gastric cancer.

The Jaboulay technique (a gastroduodenostomy between separate incisions in the stomach and the second part of the duodenum) was introduced in 1896, and in 1898, von Mikulicz performed, on the advice of his pupil, Henle, after mobilizing the second part of the duodenum, a gastroduodenal side-to-side anastomosis bypassing the pyloric stenosis. Although the Jaboulay pyloroplasty requires the duodenum to be mobilized, it was Kocher whose name was later given to this aspect of the procedure [41, 45, 46].

Mathieu Jaboulay (1860–1913) was a graduate of Lyon (1884) where he ascended to the Chair of Surgery in 1892. In addition to his pyloroplasty technique, he is better known for his operation for hydrocele. He devised an early form of vascular anastomosis, everting the intima, and pioneered xenotransplantation. Among his most famous pupils were René Leriche and Alexis Carrell.

John Miller Turpin Finney (1863–1942) was a Harvard graduate who subsequently trained and spent his whole career at Johns Hopkins under William Halstead. Instead of two separate incisions, the Finney pyloroplasty (1902) involves a longitudinal single incision centered on the pylorus along the distal stomach greater curvature to the second part of the duodenum and performing a gastroduodenal anastomosis. In 1929, he presented his 25-year experience with a 5% mortality. Finney was a founding member of the American College of Surgeons, a brigadier during World War I, and was trusted to perform an appendicectomy on Halstead's wife.

8.2.4 Oesophagoscopy and Gastroduodenal Endoscopy

In 1868, the first oesophagoscopy using a rigid oesophagoscope was described by Adolf Kussmaul (1822–1902), a German physician, managing to visualize something of the interior of the stomach of a living patient. In 1881, Billroth's pupil, Mikulicz-Radecki, improved the instrumentation and view to being able to differentiate between malignant lesions and benign ulcers [43]. He described the pathophysiology of achalasia, calling it cardiospasm, in 1882. Flexible endoscopes were developed in the 1950s, and by the 1970s, oesophageal and gastric pathologies were able to be diagnosed under direct vision with pathological tissue obtained for confirmation by histology.

8.2.4.1 The Complications of Gastric Surgery

In 1899, H Braun described the first case of jejunal ulcer resulting from a gastroenterostomy. Once described, they were frequently reported and recognized as a cause of recurrent pain. It was later noted that these ulcers tended to occur more frequently in cases where a Roux-en-Y-type anastomosis had been performed [43].

Rapid gastric emptying in patients with gastroenterostomy, with or without partial gastrectomy, can lead to debilitating vasomotor and gastrointestinal symptoms. These were first described in France (Denecheau) and Germany (Jonas) in 1907–8, and then by a physician Arthur Hertz of London (1879–1944). In 1922, physician Charles Louis Mix in America published the first article on what he called the "Dumping Syndrome." This is a group of symptoms that can occur after a gastrectomy or gastroenterostomy and includes nausea, vomiting, abdominal pain, diarrhea, and weakness. The term "dumping" refers to the rapid emptying of the stomach contents into the small intestine, which can cause a sudden surge in blood glucose levels, rapid insulin response, and other metabolic changes. Mix's article helped to increase awareness of this syndrome and spurred further research into its causes and treatment [45, 47]. The gastroenterostomy technique was from then on to change little, and further work was focused on improvements in gastric resections. The Billroth I lost its popularity due to the risk of leaks due to the tension on the anastomosis, and which is less in the Billroth II.

Dr. Edward D. Churchill and Dr. Edward W. Connell from Wisconsin introduced the concept of "fundusectomy" in the late 1930s as a way to treat peptic ulcer disease. This procedure involved the removal of the acid-secreting portion of the stomach (the fundus and body), leaving behind only the nonacid-secreting antrum. The idea was that this would reduce the amount of acid produced in the stomach and thus alleviate symptoms of peptic ulcer disease. However, the procedure was eventually abandoned due to high rates of complications and recurrence of ulcer disease [49].

Dragstedt and Owens reported on two cases of duodenal ulcer treated by vagotomy in 1943, which ushered in a new era in the treatment of peptic ulceration. Vagotomy involves cutting the vagus nerve, which controls the production of stomach acid, in order to reduce acid secretion and promote healing of the ulcer. This technique became widely used in the 1950s and 1960s as an alternative to gastrectomy for the treatment of peptic ulcer disease [50]. Exener and Latarjet expressed concerns about delayed gastric emptying after vagotomy which was mitigated by gastroenterostomy or selective vagotomy by denervating the acid-producing area and keeping the vagal branches that supply the antrum and pylorus.

The postoperative complications and poor quality of life for many patients who underwent total gastrectomy for stomach cancer led to a reevaluation of the procedure. In the mid-twentieth century, some surgeons began to consider more limited resections, such as subtotal gastrectomy or even local excision, for certain types of gastric cancer. Dr. Edward A. Hunt of the University of Minnesota first described the procedure of creating a "jejunal pouch" in 1952, which involved removing the stomach and attaching a loop of jejunum to the oesophagus with small intestine serving as a reservoir for food [51].

8.2.4.2 "Peptic" Ulcers in the Stomach and Duodenum

In 1799, Matthew Baillie (1761–1823), the nephew of John Hunter, published a series of engravings that included a patient with a perforated duodenal ulcer. Benjamin Travers (1783–1858), in 1817, described a series of patients who had suffered perforations. In 1843, just prior to the introduction of anaesthesia, Edwards Crisp (1806–1882) published a series of 50 patients concluding that *"once perforation has occurred the case must be considered hopeless."* Crisp suggested that operative closure might be possible, and during the later part of the nineteenth century, a handful of cases of survival after spontaneous closure were reported [40].

Billroth's pupil, von Mikulicz, performed a laparotomy and closure in 1884, but the patient died postoperatively. It was not until 1892 that the first two successful procedures on perforated gastric ulcers were carried out, one by Ludwig Heusner (1843–1916) in Barman, Germany, and the other by Hastings Gilford (1861–1941) in Reading, England. Prepyloric and gastric ulcers were more common than duodenal ulcers in the nineteenth century, and it was only in 1894, that the first duodenal ulcer was treated operatively by Henry Percy Dean (1864–1931) in London. Laparotomy and omental patch repair became the common procedure until, in the second half of the century, some patients, fit enough for a longer procedure, were also treated by definitive surgery involving vagotomy and antrectomy or pyloroplasty/gastroenterostomy depending on the site of the ulcer and the degree of scarring. Since the advent of effective medical treatment for gastric and duodenal ulcers, twenty-first-century best practice is to perform an omental patch repair either by laparotomy or by laparoscopy, the laparoscopic approach being introduced for perforated ulcer in the early 1990s. The mortality for a patch repair has fallen from around 40% prior to World War II to around 5–10% today. In 1935, Wangensteen demonstrated the possibility of treating selected patients conservatively, by nasogastric aspiration of the stomach and relying on spontaneous closure. This technique is seldom used today unless the patient presents late and is not deteriorating, or the patient is not fit for surgery. Self-sealing and absence of ongoing leak from the ulcer can be demonstrated using radiological contrast injected down the nasogastric tube [47, 48].

8.2.4.3 Bleeding Peptic Ulcers

Upper gastrointestinal bleeding presenting with hematemesis and/or melaena may be due to a number of causes including a posterior duodenal ulcer that erodes the gastroduodenal artery behind the first part of the duodenum. Gastric or jejunal ulcers may also cause bleeding as may a Dieu-la-foy lesion from the short gastrics on the greater curve of the proximal stomach. Oesophageal varices complicating portal hypertension may cause life-threatening hemorrhage and require intervention while Mallory-Weiss tears of the lower oesophagus will usually settle with expectant management.

In the early part of the twentieth century, gastrointestinal hemorrhage was treated medically. The use of selective surgical interference for the selection of patients with gastroduodenal hemorrhage was proposed by Gordon-Taylor in 1939. In his article, he suggested various criteria for selecting patients who would benefit from surgical intervention, including the presence of an actively bleeding ulcer, recurrent bleeding despite conservative treatment, and evidence of haemodynamic instability. His approach marked a significant shift from the previous haphazard selection of patients and helped to improve the outcomes of surgical treatment for gastroduodenal haemorrhage [47]. During the second half of the twentieth century, many lives were saved by performing a gastroduodenotomy, underrunning a vessel in the base of an ulcer.

During the 1960s and 1970s, in the absence of effective conservative treatment, and following endoscopic diagnosis, the best management involved early operation for ongoing or recurrent significant hemorrhage, particularly for patients whose age or general condition carried a high risk of mortality should there be a further bleed. With the introduction of endoscopic methods of managing a bleeding ulcer during the 1980s (injection with adrenaline, clips, or other local applications such as use of a heater probe), surgery became reserved for those in whom endoscopic methods failed and/or there was a high risk of recurrence due to a visible vessel in the ulcer base.

The treatment of significant upper gastrointestinal bleeding depends on the cause as varices may need endoscopic banding or sclerosing. In the twenty-first century, interventional radiology is being increasingly used to stop gastrointestinal bleeding although this facility is still only available in major centers in high-income countries. Emergency surgery for haematemesis and melena is now relatively rare but still provides a good option in patients whose life is at risk if the bleeding is not arrested urgently [47, 49, 50].

8.2.4.4 Effective Medical Treatment and Prevention of Ulcer Recurrence

In the mid-1970s, histamine (H) 2 receptor blockers were released, the initial agents being cimetidine and then ranitidine. These cured most ulcers but required ongoing maintenance treatment, and there was a significant recurrence rate when a 1- to 2-year treatment was ceased. Surgery for peptic ulcer (usually some form of vagotomy and/or drainage procedure) continued for recurrent or H2 receptor-resistant ulcers. The reason for the recurrent ulceration was that the role of H. pylori had not been appreciated in the generation of ulcer.

In the early 1980s, Barry J. Marshall (b1951) and Robin Warren (1937–2024) discovered that Helicobacter pylori (H. pylori) was the primary cause of peptic ulcer disease, overturning the long-held belief that stress and diet were the main culprits. This discovery revolutionized the management of peptic ulcer disease and led to the development of effective antibiotic treatments (today combined with proton pump inhibitors) that could cure the infection, leading to better outcomes for patients. The discovery of H pylori's role in causing gastritis, peptic ulcer disease, and gastric cancers was a significant breakthrough in the understanding of these conditions. Prior to their work, it was widely believed that ulcers and other gastrointestinal problems were caused by stress, spicy food, missing meals, or other lifestyle factors. For their discovery, Marshall and Warren were awarded the Nobel Prize in Physiology or Medicine in 2005. Today, peptic ulcer disease surgery is limited to treating complications such as perforation, stenosis, and bleeding. If laparotomy is required, simple closure is sufficient in most cases of peptic ulcer, and elective ulcer surgery is no longer needed in these patients [51].

Proton pump inhibitors (PPIs) are a class of drugs that are used to reduce the production of stomach acid. The first PPI, omeprazole (AstraZeneca), was approved for use in Europe in 1989 and in the United States in 1990. Omeprazole was initially developed as a treatment for duodenal ulcers, but it was soon found to be effective in treating other acid-related conditions such as gastric ulcers, GORD (gastro-oesophageal reflux disease), and Barrett's esophagus. The discovery of the proton pump enzyme (H^+/K^+ ATPase) as the target of these drugs was a major step forward in understanding acid secretion mechanisms in the stomach.

After the success of omeprazole, other PPIs were developed, including lansoprazole, pantoprazole, rabeprazole, and esomeprazole. These drugs have similar mechanisms of action and are used to treat the same acid-related conditions as omeprazole, but they have slightly different chemical structures.

PPIs are now considered first-line therapy for acid-related conditions. [51].

They have greatly improved the quality of life for many people with acid-related conditions from peptic ulcer to stress ulcers and more importantly the treatment of gastro-oesophageal reflux (GORD), which is an extremely common condition that can lead to Barrett's esophagus and eventually to cancer of the gastro-oesophageal junction [58].

8.2.4.5 Further Developments in Gastrectomy for Cancer

Currently, radical gastrectomy with lymphadenectomy is the standard surgical treatment for gastric cancer. However, in recent years, there has been a debate about the extent of lymphadenectomy needed to achieve optimal outcomes. While some studies have shown the benefit of super-extended lymphadenectomy (D3), others have reported an increased risk of morbidity and mortality associated with this approach. The decision to perform an extended lymphadenectomy depends on various factors, including the patient's age, comorbidities, and the stage of the disease. It is typically determined on a case-by-case basis by the surgical team, usually informed by discussions at a multidisciplinary meeting that also includes pathologists, radiologists and oncologists [52].

Groves et al. reported the first case of omentobursectomy in 1910. They addressed the importance of complete removal of the great omentum by cutting through the peritoneum and also emphasized the need for careful preservation of the hepatic artery and the portal vein during the procedure. Omentobursectomy involves the removal of the great omentum along with the lesser omentum, and it is commonly performed as part of a radical gastrectomy procedure for gastric cancer. The procedure is based on the principle that gastric cancer has a high potential for lymphatic spread, and thus, the removal of the lymphatic drainage pathways around the stomach, including the omentum, may help to prevent the spread of the cancer cells to other parts of the body [53]. But that was associated with high operative mortality of 20–30% [53].

Pauchet, in 1920, emphasized the importance of removing the greater omentum in continuity with the stomach for the treatment of carcinoma. He also recommended clearing the pyloric and pancreatic lymphatic field to improve the effectiveness of the surgery [47, 48, 50].

Appleby et al. introduced a procedure in 1953 that involved the resection of the whole stomach and distal pancreas, but not the spleen. The procedure became known as the Appleby operation. It was originally used to treat advanced pancreatic cancer but has also been applied to gastric malignancies. The procedure is also associated with a high rate of morbidity and mortality [54].

The first global RCT comparing total versus subtotal gastrectomy for gastric antrum cancer was conducted in France in 1989. Another RCT by the Italian Gastrointestinal Tumor Study Group in 1999 also found no survival advantages of total gastrectomy over subtotal gastrectomy [55].

The issue of extended lymph nodes clearance had been heavily debated after Japanese reports of survival improvement with extended node dissection combined with splenectomy and possibly dial pancreatectomy (D2). The MRC ST01 trial, which included over 400 patients with resectable gastric cancer, found no survival advantages of D2 over D1 dissection (removal of lymph nodes only around the stomach). Similarly, the Dutch D1/D2 trial also showed that D2 dissection (removal of lymph nodes around the stomach and those further away) was associated with higher rates of postoperative morbidity and mortality, but no difference in overall survival rate compared to D1 dissection. These trials have led to a shift toward more limited lymphadenectomy in the surgical treatment of gastric cancer [56, 57].

8.3 Infantile Hypertrophic Pyloric Stenosis

Pyloric stenosis in infants is characterized by hypertrophy of the pylorus that leads within a few weeks of life to projectile vomiting with consequent emaciation and death if not treated.

In 1717, Patrick Blair (1665–1728) was the first to describe the clinical and autopsy findings in an infant with pyloric stenosis. The vomiting had started when the child was a month old and was violent (projectile). In 1767, George Armstrong (1717–1789) published an essay on the diseases most fatal to infants with a description of the disease. The first report from America was by Hezekiah Beardsley (1748–1790) of New Haven in 1788. One hundred years later, Harald Hirschsprung (1830–1916), a Danish pediatrician, provided a detailed description of the condition in two female infants. In 1882, Petro Loreta, Professor of Surgery in Bologna, performed a laparotomy and digitally dilated the pylorus. The procedure was successful. Between 1898 and 1907, Karl Löbker (1854–1912) in Bochum, Germany, performed a gastroenterostomy which was successful in 4 of 7 cases. By 1907, 134 cases of gastroenterostomy with a 53% death rate had been reported, while those who performed a Heinecke-Mikulicz pyloroplasty (25 cases) reported a 40% mortality [37–39, 48].

In 1906, James Nicoll (1863–1921) in Glasgow performed an intramucosal partial, and transverse, pyloroplasty in six infants, five of whom survived, and combined this with a Loreta's dilatation. In 1907, Pierre Fredet of Paris performed a successful extramucosal pyloroplasty and a gastroenterostomy on a 10-week-old infant, and a year later, Wilhelm Weber of Dresden performed two further successful extramucosal pyloroplasties. Nicoll, Fredet, and Weber all closed their pyloroplasties transversely [38, 39, 49].

In August 1911, Conrad Ramstedt (1867–1963) of Münster unintentionally developed the operation of pyloromyotomy. He was operating on the firstborn son of a nobleman and his intent had been to perform a pyloroplasty. However, when he divided the hypertrophic pyloric muscle down to the submucosa (with a silver teaspoon), he found that the pylorus was open. He decided not to open into the lumen. In attempting to suture transversely, the first sutures cut through so he decided it would do more harm than good if he proceeded. He closed with an omental patch for safety and the operation was a success. The child survived. He performed a second successful pyloromyotomy in June 1912 but did not, this time, use an omental patch. Ramstedt's name is now given to the operation of pyloromyotomy [41, 47, 58].

However, the first longitudinal pyloromyotomy without pyloroplasty was performed 18 months earlier by Sir Harold Stiles (1863–1946) in Edinburgh. He divided the pylorus longitudinally with a tenotomy knife right up to the duodenum. He had been planning to combine the procedure with a Loreta dilatation but this did not seem necessary. Unfortunately, the infant died of chloroform poisoning some 4 days later, so Stiles never published the case, and its record was only published in 1956. Of further interest, Mazurak and Patkowski's history of the surgical correction of pyloric stenosis notes that one of Stiles' pupils was Gertrude Herzfeld (1890–1981), the second female Fellow of the Royal College of Surgeons of Edinburgh. She operated on Graham Fraser with infantile pyloric stenosis in 1932. Graham Fraser, having studied medicine at Aberdeen University and training in pediatric surgery, went on to become Clinical Professor of Pediatric Surgery in Vancouver! He met Gertrude Herzfeld for the second time 38 years later in 1960, then a young surgeon attending the British Society of Pediatric Surgeons [58–61].

8.4 Surgery on the Liver

> *Achilles stabbed with his sword at the liver, the liver was torn from its place, and from it the dark blood drenched the fold of his tunic and Troy's eyes were shrouded in darkness and the light went out.* Homer (8th century BCE)

> If there wasn't bleeding everybody would do surgery. Sir William Osler (1849–1919)

The liver was shrouded in mystery for a long time. However, the organ is formidable and intimidating to surgeons because of the risk of massive bleeding that can accompany attempted resection. The liver is a highly vascular organ, connecting two circulations, portal and systemic. As a result, even minor damage to the liver during surgery can cause significant bleeding. It also holds remarkable regenerative powers, recognized in even ancient times, and also mythically through Prometheus, the God of fire, who was "*chained by Zeus to a rock in the Caucasus by Hephaestus where an eagle fed by day on his liver which regenerated each night.*"

The liver does indeed regenerate when part of it is removed, albeit not as swiftly in humans as for a god such as Prometheus (Fig. 8.5)!

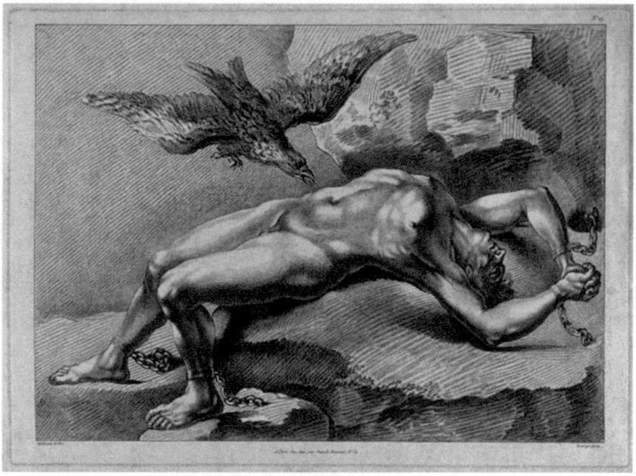

Fig. 8.5 Prometheus bound to a rock. His liver eaten by an eagle. Crayon manner print by Lucien after P.T. Leclerc. Le Clerc, Pierre Thomas, approximately 1740-approximately 1796. License: Public Domain Mark. https://commons.wikimedia.org/w/index.php?search=Prometheus+liver&title=Special:MediaSearch&go=Go&type=image

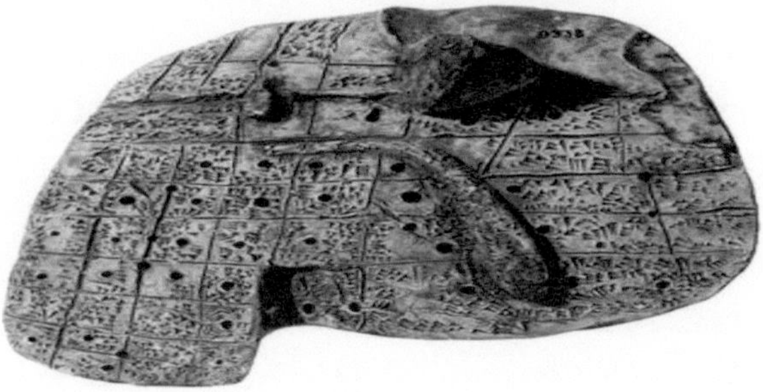

Fig. 8.6 Sheep's liver with Latin and Babylonian-Assyrian designations, public domain. License: Clay model of a sheep's liver, Babylonian Temple School. https://commons.wikimedia.org/w/index.php?search=Sheep%27s+liver+with+Latin+and+Babylonian-Assyrian+designation&title=Special:MediaSearch&go=Go&type=image

8.4.1 Understanding of the Liver in Ancient Civilizations

In Ancient Babylonia (2000 BC), fortune tellers determined the future based on the shape of a sacrificed animal's liver (as shown by the sheep liver models at the British Museum). This understandably promoted a religious and superstitious interest in the liver's anatomy (Fig. 8.6).

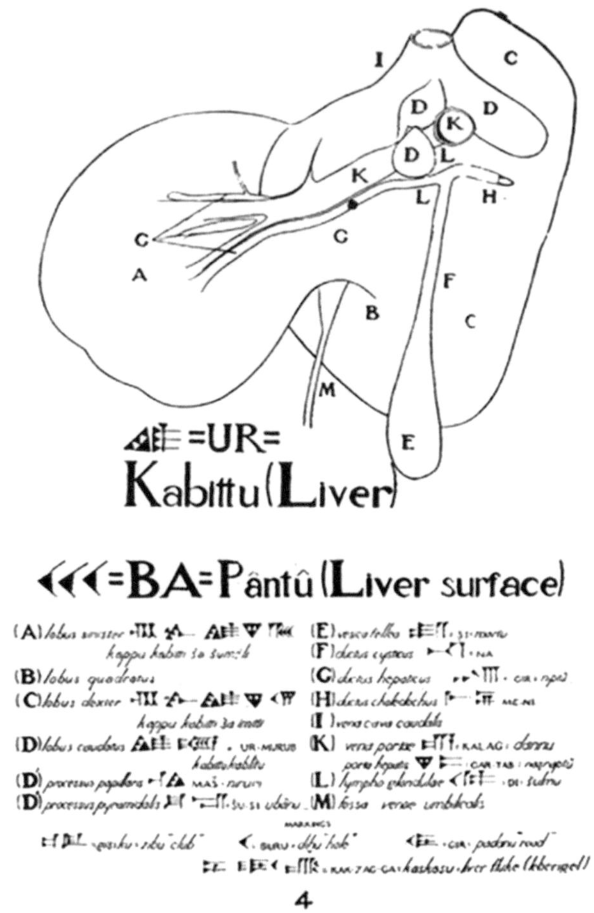

https://wellcomecollection.org/works/jvf4zhtb/images?id=n7364by2

Hippocrates recommended the incision and drainage of liver abscesses with cautery or a knife. The abscesses may have been pyogenic or amoebic and are likely only to have been evident when presenting as a mass below the costal margin or between the ribs posterolaterally. This technique may still be used today for abscesses not responding to antibiotic therapy.

Celsus and Galen described debridement of exposed or protruding liver from penetrating trauma. Galen understood the central role of the liver in digestion but thought that the liver was the source of the blood. The Byzantine surgeon, Paulus of Aegina also recommended debriding exposed liver in traumatic wounds. However, these writers did not provide any results of the treatments they recommended [62, 63].

8.4.2 Understanding the Anatomy of the Liver

8.4.2.1 Francis Glisson (1654)

Francis Glisson (1597–1677) examined cast specimens of the liver in 1654, and published *Anatomia Hepatis* which described the liver's triple vascular anatomy involving the portal venous system and systemic circulation through hepatic arteries and hepatic veins eventually draining into the vena cava [62]. His casts were created by boiling the human liver for 1 hour and then picking off the parenchyma to obtain a cast of the vessels which he also infused.

8.4.3 Early Liver Surgery in the Nineteenth Century

8.4.3.1 John Thomson at Waterloo (1815)

There are various reports of liver debridements as a result of traumatic wounds sustained during the seventeenth and eighteenth centuries. For example, British surgeon, John Thomson (1765–1846), Regius Professor of Military Surgery in Edinburgh from 1806–1822, (FRCSEd 1793), was at Waterloo (1815) and described 12 liver wounds, some of whom survived. Later in the 19th century, during the Franco-Prussian War (1870–1871) Victor von Bruns of Breslau (1818–1883) removed a piece of prolapsed liver through a wound and the soldier was back on the battlefield 2 months later [64].

8.4.3.2 Lawson Tait (1880): Echinococcus

In 1880, Lawson Tait (1845–1899) of Birmingham, England, drained an Echinococcus cyst of the liver, suturing the cyst wall to the abdominal wall, without resecting any liver or cyst.

8.4.3.3 Antonio Lius: Partial Hepatectomy (1886)

In 1886, Antonio Lius attempted the world's first partial hepatectomy on a 67-year-old patient with a hepatic adenoma. The case involved an "adenoma" on a pedicle 15.5 × 13 × 11 cm. Lius' attempts to suture the stump to the abdominal wall failed and the stump was left in the abdomen. Sadly the patient died 6 h later due to hemorrhage.

8.4.3.4 The First Successful Hepatic Resections (1888)

Carl Langenbuch (1846–1901) is credited with performing the first successful hepatic resection in 1888. He was also the first to perform cholecystectomy in 1882. This was again a tumour on a pedicle which, despite being sutured several times before closure, required a return to the operating room for postoperative hemorrhage. This was also at a time where there was no blood transfusion. The patient endured a long postoperative recovery but survived.

The first successful liver resection in the United States was done by William Williams Keen (1837–1932) of Philadelphia in 1892. Keen became much better known for his contributions to surgery on the brain, having already successfully removed a brain tumor in 1887. His patient was a 31-year-old woman who had an 8.75 cm cystadenoma hanging from the right lobe. He found cautery was not successful in dealing with the bleeding and reverted to using his thumbnail (this was probably the finger fracture technique). The patient was kept in bed for 3 weeks, stayed in the hospital for 42 days, but was alive 7 years after her operation. In 1897, Keen removed a pedunculated haemangioma by looping a rubber tube around the pedicle and bringing the whole mass out of the abdomen. He waited 6 days until the tumor was necrotic and then removed it, *without the loss of a drop of blood.* Keen's third liver resection was in 1899 for a patient with primary cancer of the left lobe which was removed without incident using 5 catgut sutures and cautery. She survived, but only to die 5 months later of metastatic disease.

In his paper reporting his third case, Keen also presented the results of 76 liver resections that had been done until 1899. The mortality was an impressive 14.1%. This was much better than the 30–45% mortality of those who suffered major trauma to the liver and underwent laparotomy (see below).

There was a spate of liver resections in the period up to World War I, but after the war, there was little further progress. Surgeons tended to avoid liver resection because of the ongoing high mortality. Major advances in liver surgery would only occur after World War II and were awaiting advances in imaging, blood storage, and intensive care including metabolic support.

However, several surgeons began to report outcomes of liver trauma surgery up to, and including, World War I. In 1887, Edler reported a 66% mortality, Louis Félix Terrier (1837–1908) in France reported 31% mortality for liver trauma, and Benjamin Tilton (1868–1945) in the United States reported a 44% mortality in 1905 (Table 8.1).

Table 8.1 Liver trauma outcomes 1880s to 1905

Paper and author	Country	Blunt trauma	Stab	Gunshot
Edler 1887 (66%)	Germany	78.1%	39.0%	37.5%
Terrier 1896 (31%)	France [44]	5/11 (45.5%)	5/20 (25%)	4/14 (28.3%)
Tilton 1905 (44%)	New York [26]	7/11 (63%)	1/4 (25%)	2/7 (28.5

Table footnote: Result cited in or reported in Tilton [64]

Not all cases [43] recorded by Tilton at New York Hospitals with Major Emergency Services were operated. The figures given are for the operated cases [64]

8.4.3.5 Pringle's Manoeuver (1908)

In 1908, J. Hogarth Pringle (1863–1941), an Australian-born surgeon who worked in Glasgow, Scotland, reported eight patients with liver trauma. Three died before operation, one refused operation, and all four of those undergoing laparotomy died, two of them on table. However, during the surgery, Pringle conceived of applying digital pressure to the porta hepatis via finger and thumb on either side and inserted through the foramen of Winslow. It reduced the hemorrhage but not enough to be successful. He conducted experiments on rabbits to show his manoeuver worked and clamping to the hilar region even allowed a lobe to be resected without bleeding. He clamped the hilum for an hour in one of his experiments without detriment to the rabbit. It was only in 1978 that it was shown that the human liver can survive up to an hour of hilar clamping.

8.4.3.6 Hepatic Artery Ligation (1909)

In 1909, Hans von Haberer (1875–1959), then Professor of Surgery in Innsbruck, ligated the left hepatic artery before resecting the left lobe in a boy with a large cystic tumor. Von Haberer was also to become a pioneer in vascular surgery. In 1910, Wendel tied off the right hepatic artery and right hepatic duct before removing a large adenoma from a 44-year-old woman. This was the first anatomical right lobectomy.

8.4.4 Defining Liver Anatomy: The Rex-Cantlie Line

8.4.4.1 Rex

The traditional concept of dividing the liver into right and left lobes was based on the falciform ligament. However, this view was anatomically false. Rex in 1888, based on the anatomy of the portal system, divided the liver into right and left lobes based on an imaginary line drawn connecting the gallbladder fossa to the inferior vena cava.

8.4.4.2 James Cantlie

Cantlie also independently identified this line in 1897 [63] (Fig. 8.7), which is today referred to as the Rex-Cantlie or Cantlie line. Scottish surgeon, Sir James Cantlie (1851–1926), observed this demarcation in a patient with atrophy of the right lobe and hypertrophy of the left lobe in 1887. He injected dye into the left and right side of the portal system to confirm his observation. Cantlie worked at Charing Cross Hospital in London and was a pioneer of first aid (first responder) which was unknown at the time. He took a position in Hong Kong where he founded the Hong

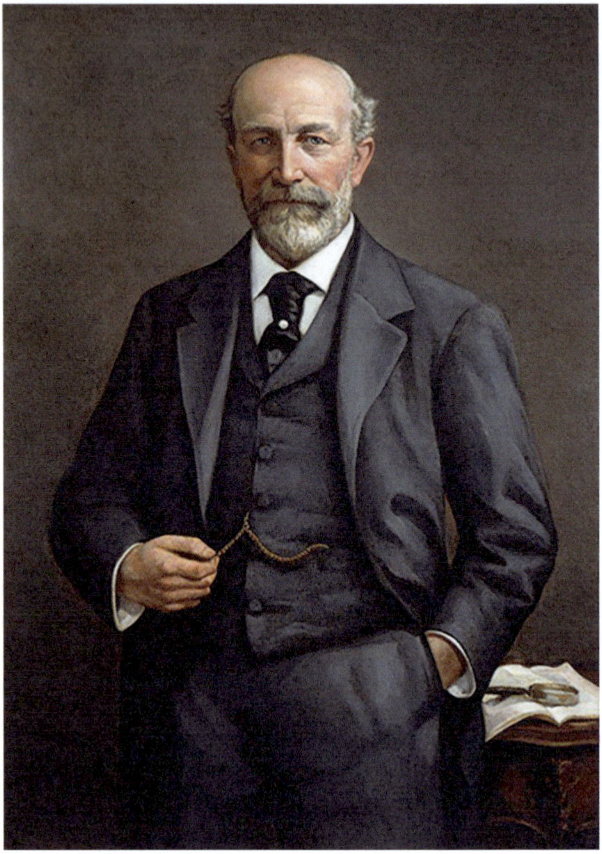

Fig. 8.7 Sir James Cantlie (by Herman Solomon) 1925. Portrait of Sir James Cantlie by H. Salomon. License no restrictions. https://en.m.wikipedia.org/wiki/File:James_Cantlie_by_Solomon.jpg

Kong College of Medicine for Chinese students, which later became the University of Hong Kong. One of his notable pupils was the future Chinese leader Sun Yat-sen. He returned to London in 1896 and his experience of leprosy and other tropical diseases from the Far East resulted in his being a founder of the Journal of Tropical Medicine. His youngest son, born in Hong Kong, was Sir Neil Cantlie (1892–1975), who became Director General of the British Army Medical Services (1948–52). Neil wrote a book about his father, *A Romance in Medicine* (1939) [64–66].

8.4.5 Liver Surgery: Progress Since the 1950s

Enormous progress was made in understanding the liver's anatomy and operative approaches to the organ from the 1950's onward. Safety and accuracy improved dramatically, particularly with advances in imaging and the development of specialist units. Further progress required hepatic functional evaluation to determine the safety limit of liver resections, intraoperative ultrasonography to define the extent of

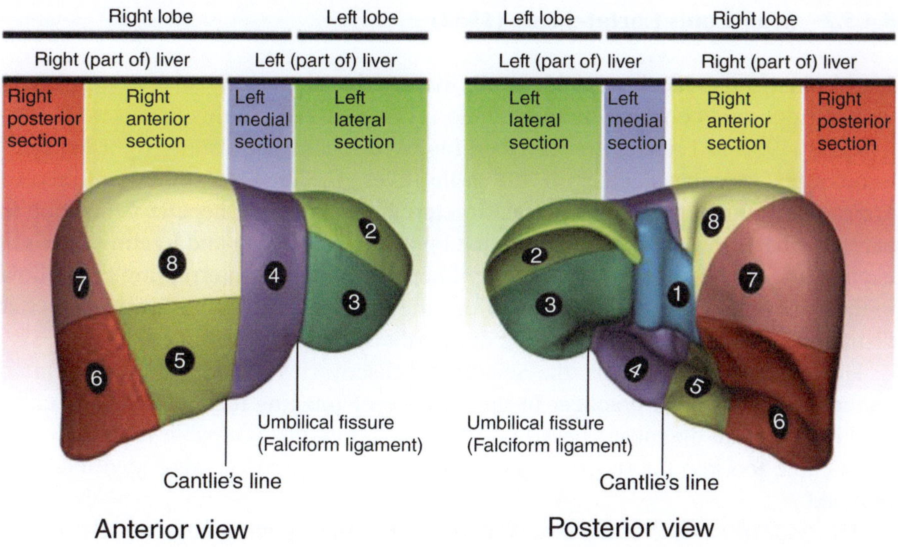

Fig. 8.8 Liver segments. Creative Commons, Polygon data is generated by Database Center for Life Science (DBCLS), no restrictions. https://commons.wikimedia.org/wiki/File:Liver_04_Couinaud_classification.svg-ar.png

pathology, and portal vein embolization to increase remnant liver volume and staged liver resections [62] (Fig. 8.8).

8.4.5.1 Claude Couinaud and Henry Bismuth (1954)

The rediscovery that the liver has a remarkable ability to regenerate itself was a major milestone in the history of liver surgery. The first experiments to demonstrate this were carried out by two French surgeons, Claude Couinaud (1922–2008) and Henri Bismuth (b 1934), in the 1950s and 1960s. Couinaud and Bismuth showed that it was possible to remove up to three quarters of the liver in experimental animals without causing fatal liver failure. They also observed that the remaining liver tissue would regenerate, and within a few weeks, the liver would be close to its original weight [67].

The year 1954 marks the establishment of the current concept of the segmental anatomy of the liver by French surgeon, Claude Couinaud. He divided the liver into eight independent functional units, called Couinaud segments, based on the distribution of portal and hepatic veins. Couinaud used 120 cast models of the liver's inner structure to explore fissures, pedicles, and basic surgical segments. He then confirmed his findings through the dissection of 50 fresh organs. Couinaud found that there was no intercommunication between the pedicles (blood vessels and bile ducts) of the eight different segments [64–66].

8.4.5.2 Jean-Louis Lortat-Jacob (1952)

Jean-Louis Lortat-Jacob's (1908–1992) manuscript on anatomical liver resections was an important contribution to the field of liver surgery. In this manuscript, published in 1952 in France, he described his experiences performing right hepatectomy after vascular control of the right liver, the first procedure to involve extrahepatic ligation of right portal structures and the right hepatic vein prior to parenchymal transection. This technique involved identifying and ligating the right hepatic artery, right portal vein, and right hepatic vein, thus interrupting blood flow to the right lobe of the liver before performing the resection. This allowed for better visualization and control of bleeding during the surgery [63–65] (Fig. 8.9).

However, until the 1980s, the anatomical discoveries of the 1950s had limited application in surgical practice. In the absence of imaging technology, physicians could only make diagnoses based on physical symptoms (palpable tumor), which often came too late for surgery. Thus, only large liver lesions were identified and resected.

The widespread use of ultrasound in the early 1980s greatly improved the ability to diagnose and locate small liver tumors, making it possible to detect them earlier which paved the way to the rapid development of liver surgery. This enabled surgeons to perform smaller, more precise resections and to treat liver tumors with a greater chance of success.

Additionally, the development of advanced imaging techniques, such as CT and MRI, further improved the accuracy of tumor detection and localization, allowing for more precise surgical planning and execution. MRI demonstrated its utility in the diagnosis of benign simple cysts, hemangioma, and focal nodular hyperplasia. Consequently, with more use of MRI, it became unusual to remove liver lesions without a correct preoperative diagnosis [68, 69].

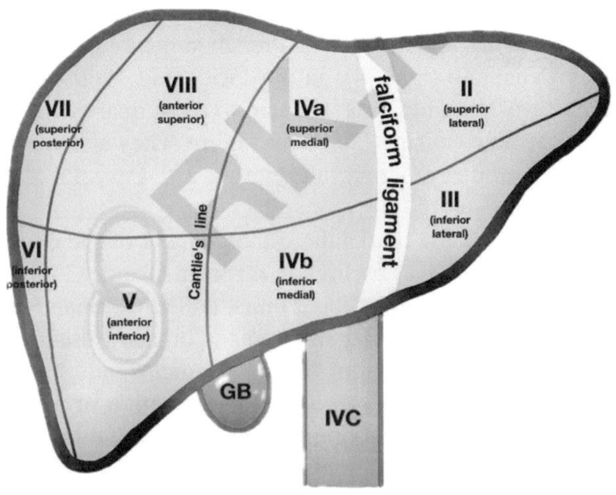

Fig. 8.9 Illustration of anatomical resection. Rishi https://rk.md/wp-content/uploads/2020/06/anatomic-liver-segments-rk.webp Kumar, MD—https://rk.md, September 15, 2024 At 07:11. Hey Saleh! Absolutely, just please leave the reference to my website: Rishi Kumar, MD—https://rk.md

Henri Bismuth's paper in 1982 was a turning point in the practice of liver surgery. The popularity of liver resections based on anatomy increased over time and evolved into bloodless surgery that removed independent segments or groups of two or more segments [70].

8.4.5.3 Masatoshi Makuuchi (1987)

In 1987, a Japanese Professor of Surgery, Masatoshi Makuuchi (b1946), developed a method of hemi-hepatic vascular intermittent occlusion which improved the safety of liver resection. The method avoids ischaemia of the remnant liver, reduces intraoperative blood loss, lessens postoperative hyperbilirubinemia, prevents splanchnic congestion, and maintains haemodynamic stability during the resection. Makuuchi also pioneered subsegmental resections (defined in 2021 as "*removal of liver parenchyma within the portal territory or territories of less than a Couinaud segment")* [69, 70].

Intraoperative Ultrasound

Intraoperative ultrasound (IOUS) was first introduced into the practice of liver surgery in 1984, which allowed for more precise and accurate mapping of the liver anatomy and localization of tumors during surgery. This has greatly improved the success rates and outcomes of liver surgeries. The technique allowed the surgeon to map liver vasculature and biliary duct anatomy during the operation. The liver was then rendered transparent, which allowed for a better understanding of the various structures within the organ. The introduction of IOUS into liver surgery had the same impact as the inclusion of intraoperative cholangiography in biliary surgery in the early part of the twentieth century. By using IOUS to find the liver's lines of division and locating the tumor, the surgeon could determine the relations among the portal elements, hepatic veins, hepatic parenchyma, and tumor and choose the appropriate type of anatomical resection to be performed [71].

Liver Resection and the Control of Hemorrhage

Controlling bleeding during liver resection is a major challenge for the surgeon. The liver is a highly vascular organ, and any surgical procedure on the liver involves a risk of bleeding. In addition, as mentioned earlier, the liver has a complex blood supply that makes controlling bleeding during liver resection even more challenging. Prior to the 1950s, most surgery relied upon mattress sutures, cautery, and vascular occlusion techniques, such as Pringle maneuver, portal triad (hilar) clamping, and selective vascular occlusion. Hemostatic agents such as fibrin glue (developed in the 1980s and 1990s), hemostatic sponges, and absorbable hemostats now provide additional and sometimes better methods to control hemorrhage.

The technique and accuracy of resection also influences bleeding as Keen and others had already discovered early in the twentieth century. The finger fracture technique was reintroduced by Dr. TY Lin in 1958 but had already been formally described by Anschutz in 1903. The technique involves fracturing the liver parenchyma manually with the surgeon's fingers to identify and control bleeding vessels and bile ducts. By using this technique, the surgeon can achieve better control of bleeding during liver resection, even in the absence of modern surgical instruments such as vascular staplers and energy devices [69, 72, 73].

Cavitron Ultrasonic Surgical Aspirator (CUSA)

Currently, ultrasonic dissection using the Cavitron Ultrasonic Surgical Aspirator (CUSA) has become the standard technique for liver parenchyma dissection. The history of the Cavitron Ultrasonic Surgical Aspirator (CUSA) goes back to the 1960s when Dr. John Reid developed the first prototype of an ultrasonic surgical device in collaboration with the Jet Propulsion Laboratory. The device used ultrasonic energy to break up and aspirate tissue during surgery. In the 1970s, Valleylab, a medical equipment company, acquired the rights to the technology and developed the first commercial ultrasonic surgical device, the CUSA. It was initially used for neurosurgery but then expanded to other surgical specialties, including liver surgery. The CUSA was first used in liver surgery in the 1980s and quickly gained popularity due to its ability to dissect liver tissue without causing excessive bleeding [73]. Today, the CUSA remains a commonly used tool in liver surgery and has undergone several advancements and improvements to enhance its safety and efficacy.

Although the Pringle manoeuver has proved to be effective to reduce bleeding during liver parenchymal dissection, prolonged inflow occlusion (over 120 min) may have deleterious effects on liver functions. Techniques were developed to selectively occlude hepatic inflow to one side, or to a single segment, by clamping the Glissonean pedicle at the hilum or inside the liver parenchyma for the part of the liver to be removed [74].

The main indication for liver resection today is liver metastasis resulting from cancers of the colon and rectum or primary liver cancers. Modern anaesthesia practice to support a patient during surgery includes maintaining low central venous pressure during resection combined with autologous blood donation, limited intravenous fluids, and cardiovascular support.

As late as 1963, Alexander Brunschwig (1901–1969) reported 50% mortality after 8 right lobectomies and 18% mortality after 16 left lobectomies performed in New York [76]. However, the mortality rate for liver resection decreased in the second half of the twentieth century to less than 1% in specialized centers. However, liver resection still represents high-risk surgery from a patient perspective, particularly where there is underlying liver disease (cirrhosis) or a complex liver tumor. Therefore, careful patient selection and meticulous preoperative planning, taking into account the patient's comorbidities, values, and goals of care, are crucial to achieving optimal outcomes in liver surgery [75].

Even if we were to take a closer look at this high mortality rate [of resection] and criticise it, we cannot help but admire the incredible persistence and dedication of the early resectionists.... We might not have developed operations on the heart, brain, or liver without some bold, brash, or ethically questionable efforts. Courage may come with wisdom, but maybe wisdom takes courage away. Let's not think too much about that, or we might stop operating [76].

By the end of the twentieth century, patients with metastases from colorectal cancer, well selected on the basis of site and number of metastases (less than four), could expect a 5-year survival of 25%, with control of the cancer in the liver in 50%. Liver resection also became an alternative option to washout drainage for patients with hydatid disease [77–82].

8.4.6 Liver Transplantation

8.4.6.1 Thomas Starzl (1963–1968)

Dr. Thomas E. Starzl (1926–2017), in Denver, Colorado, was the first to attempt orthotopic liver transplantation in 1963 on a 3-year-old child with biliary atresia. Starzl's team performed four further liver transplantations that year, while FD Moore's group in Boston did another. None of those patients survived longer than 23 days. Starzl's first successful procedure was in 1968. Starzl later moved to Pittsburg.

8.4.6.2 Roy Calne (1968)

Roy Calne (1930–2024) began a liver transplantation program in Cambridge, England, performing the first British transplant in 1968. The early days of transplantation were beset by organ rejection. Calne had initially experimented with 6-mercaptopurine and then with its derivative, azathioprine, but these agents had significant toxic effects and so their effectiveness was limited [83, 84].

In January 1971, the American College of Surgeons/NIH organ transplant registry had recorded 102 orthotopic liver transplants. Only 12 patients were still alive, with the longest survival being 29 months [84].

8.4.6.3 Cyclosporin to Prevent Rejection

Cyclosporin, the game changer, was developed by Jean-François Borel (b 1933), a Belgian immunologist with the Swiss Sandoz company. The company were about to abandon it as an antifungal agent, when Calne was told about its immunosuppressant actions and asked for a supply of the drug. He studied it in animal transplants before the drug was finally introduced in humans in 1978. This led to rapid and dramatic improvements in kidney and liver transplantation outcomes. and its use became a standard practice in the ensuing decades [85].

8.4.6.4 Reduced Size Liver Transplantation (1984)

Further advances in liver transplantation were made during the 1980s. For example, in France, Dr. Henri Bismuth (b 1934) and Dr. Daniel Houssin performed the first reduced size liver transplantation in 1984 [80]. In Hanover, Germany, Dr. Rudolf Pichlmayr (1932–1997) and his team performed the first split liver transplantation in 1988. In 1989, Russell Strong (b1938) in Brisbane, Australia, performed the first live donor liver transplant from a Japanese mother to her child. In 1993, Makuuchi and others from Shinshu University performed a live donor transplant between adults. These procedures allowed for more efficient use of donor organs and expanded the pool of potential donors [83].

8.5 Surgery on the Biliary System and Pancreas

> *God placed the pancreas in the back as he does not want surgeons messing with it.*
> Theodore Billroth

Pancreatic and duodenal resection is one of the most challenging surgical procedures not only for surgeons but also for their patients. Pancreatic cancer is often asymptomatic and tends to present late, often by then with obstructive jaundice when in the head, or may present with back pain in the body or tail. Patients with ampullary or periampullary cancers will develop jaundice much earlier in the progression of disease and are therefore much more likely to be resectable when they present. It wasn't until very late in the nineteenth and into the twentieth centuries that there had been significant advances in anaesthesia, sterilization, and surgical techniques to make it possible to perform the first pioneering operations on the duodenum and pancreas [86]. Even then, it would be another 50–60 years before pancreaticoduodenectomy could be regarded as feasible and safe, with its complications manageable. First, there needed to be an understanding of pancreatic physiology and pathology. Physiologically, the pancreas has both endocrine and exocrine functions.

However, in order to understand the development of pancreatic surgery, it is also important to review the introduction of surgery for gallstones. The techniques devised laid the foundations for ameliorating the obstructive jaundice associated with pancreatic cancer and the ability to perform a safe pancreatic resection.

8.5.1 The Early Surgical History of Gallstones

Gallstones were found in a skeleton from Greece around 1500 BCE and also in mummified bodies from Ancient Egypt. A concretion in the bile duct was described by Byzantine physician, Alexander of Tralles (525–605 CE), in his 12 books on medicine [86, 87].

During the Renaissance period, Antonio Benivieni (1443–1502) in Florence provided the first account of gallstones in a woman who had died of abdominal pain. His anatomical and pathological work, *Abditis morborum causis* (The hidden causes of disease), based on clinical observations and autopsy findings, was published more than two centuries before Morgagni's *De Sedibus*. Benivieni also compiled the first, at least European, descriptions of intestinal perforation, and gastric cancer [88]. In 1658, Francis Glisson (1597–1677) described his own biliary colic as a condition *"from which there is no release except by death."* There was a great need to treat gallbladder disease definitively, as the various medical treatments were ineffective (though acute cholecystitis may settle spontaneously), and aspiration of a distended gallbladder was prone to complications, including peritonitis and death [87, 88].

Wilhelm Fabricius von Hilden (1560–1634) was the first to remove a human gallstone in 1618. In 1676, Joenisius, removed a gallstone from a spontaneous biliary fistula, while in 1687, Stalpaert von der Wiel opened a purulent upper abdominal abscess and, to his surprise, extracted gallstones. Parisian surgeon, Jean-Louis Petit (1674–1750), in 1733, advised that if the anterior abdominal wall became inflamed over the gallbladder in a patient with biliary colic, the area should be lanced to leave a "gall fistula." In 1859, Tudichum proposed a two-stage cholecystostomy, suturing the inflamed gallbladder to the anterior abdominal wall and then a few days later extracting the stones without contaminating the peritoneal cavity.

8.5.1.1 The First Cholecystostomy (1867)

Cholecystostomy (opening the gallbladder) was first performed accidentally by John Stough Bobbs (1809–1870) in 1867 in Indiana. He was searching for an ovarian cyst in a patient who actually had a 4-year history of biliary colic. He removed the gallstones and closed the cholecystostomy incision placing the gallbladder under the wound. The patient survived and recovered. Marion Sims (1813–1883) performed a cholecystostomy in Paris in April 1878, but the patient died of a hemorrhage on day eight. Theodor Kocher (1841–1921) performed the first successful planned cholecystostomy in June 1878 [87, 88].

8.5.1.2 The First Cholecystectomy (1882)

The first cholecystectomy (removing the gallbladder) was performed by Carl Langenbuch (1846–1901) at the Lazarus Hospital in Berlin in 1882. His patient was a 43-year-old man who had suffered from biliary colic for 16 years. The incision was a subcostal transverse with vertical T through the lateral rectus. There were two cholesterol stones and a chronically thickened gallbladder. Cholecystectomy soon proved to be a much safer operation than cholecystostomy. By 1886, the mortality of cholecystostomy was 27% versus one of eight cholecystectomies (12%). Unfortunately, Langenbuch was to die in his prime in 1901 of a ruptured appendix [87, 88].

8.5.2 Stones in Bile Duct

The problem of bile duct stones then had to be tackled. Robert Lawson Tait (1845–1899) advocated crushing them with forceps while Kocher recommended crushing them with the fingers.

Both approaches relied upon the small fragments passing spontaneously into the duodenum rather than acting as a nidus for a larger stone to form. Common duct exploration followed in 1889. Robert Abbe (1851–1928) at St. Lukes, New York, removed an impacted stone in a strictured common duct of a 36-year-old woman. Three weeks later, J. Knowsley Thornton (1845–1904) in London removed two impacted stones [88].

8.5.2.1 Mayo-Robson's Book *on Gallstones and Their Treatment* (1892)

In 1892, Arthur Mayo-Robson (1853–1933) from Leeds published a book of almost 300 pages *On Gallstones and Their Treatment*. In chapter 10, he described his personal series of 41 cases.

> Case 41 was a 51-year-old man with deep jaundice and multiple septic attacks, and this case is indicative of best practice in the early 1890s. "*In deference to medical opinion olive oil was given for three weeks without the slightest amelioration of the symptoms in any way.*" So medical treatment having failed, he underwent cholecystostomy,
>
> "*the gall bladder was thick, small and shrunken, and the ducts thick and full of concretions; both bladder and ducts being completely enveloped by adhesions of omentum and other viscera. After the adhesions had been separated the gall bladder was incised, the walls being thickened and cavity reduced to a mere tube, through which a few fragments of gall stones were removed, those in the ducts being crushed by the finger and thumb and by padded forceps.*" The patient was closed with the gallbladder sutured to the parietal peritoneum, and despite an attack of "bronchitis" delaying recovery, the jaundice completely disappeared within a fortnight and bile passed in the motions within a week.

In 1903, Mayo-Robson reported in BMJ that he had never lost a patient after an operation for gallstones in the absence of malignant disease or deep jaundice of cholangitis. When operating for cholangitis, his mortality was 1.7%.

8.5.2.2 Transduodenal Sphincterotomy (1919)

The operation of transduodenal sphincterotomy was first performed by Edward Archibald (1872–1945) in Montreal in 1919.

Cholecystectomy became one of the most common surgical operations in the twentieth century with many small modifications to manage different clinical scenarios [86, 92, 93].

8.5.2.3 The First Laparoscopic Cholecystectomy (1985)

During the 1980s, a laparoscopic approach was introduced. German surgeon, Erich Mühe (1938–2005), performed the first in 1985, followed by Philippe Mouret (b 1938) in Lyon in 1987. Mouret was a private surgeon but had access to a laparoscope through sharing a practice with a gynecologist. News of his operation reached Professor François Dubois in Paris, who practiced the technique on animals and performed his first laparoscopic cholecystectomy in 1988. Jacques Perissat (b 1933) in Bordeaux commenced laparoscopic surgery in 1989. In 1990, the laparoscopic approach to cholecystectomy, and later to many other abdominal surgical procedures, spread around the world. Today, the commonly practiced approach for both emergency and planned cholecystectomies is laparoscopic [86–88].

8.5.3 Understanding Pancreatic Pathophysiology

8.5.3.1 Scirrhus of the Pancreas

Giovanni Battista Morgagni (1682–1771), an Italian anatomist, and inspired by Benivielli, is credited with making several important observations about the pancreas and its diseases. His book, *De sedibus et causis morborum per anatomen indagates (The Seats and Causes of Diseases Investigated by Anatomy),* was published in 1761. Morgagni reported on several cases of what he called "scirrhus" of the pancreas. Scirrhus is likely used to have been used to describe a pancreatic adenocarcinoma, but with the lack of microscopic studies, it was not known then whether he was referring to cancer or scarring due to chronic pancreatitis. Morgagni described three cases, Bonetus had five, and Lieutaud amassed 36. There was also an early description of pancreatic diseases in general from Matthew Baillie in 1818 [89, 90].

8.5.3.2 Jacob Mendes Da Costa (1858)

The first reliable account of the symptoms and pathology of pancreatic ductal adenocarcinoma (PDAC) was published by Jacob Mendes Da Costa (1833–1900) in 1858. At the time of writing, Da Costa noted that William Heberden (1810–1901) had also described the condition but the reports were likely to have included inflammatory and malignant pathologies [91].

Da Costa collected a series of 37 cases, some with histological confirmation [88]. There were 22 males and 15 females, ranging from age 14 to 76. The cases in the series had been reported in the literature or by personal communication since 1827. He noted the frequency of late presentation, lymph node spread and distortion/ involvement of adjacent organs.

In several cases, no marked symptoms occurred until 4–5 months before death [91].

Patients undergoing pancreatic surgery are at high risk of anastomotic leak, kidney impairment, dehydration, malnutrition, and electrolyte imbalances, all of which contributed to early poor outcomes. In addition, bleeding (obstructive jaundice carried a high risk of bleeding prior to the discovery of vitamin K) while also asepsis and infection control were also major challenging in the early days of pancreatic surgery. The first successful pancreatic and duodenal resections were developed during the pre-antibiotic era.

8.5.4 Bilioenteric Bypass

However, following the advent of surgical anaesthesia and antisepsis in the mid-nineteenth century, abdominal surgery became more frequent, and surgeons were suddenly able to intervene upon previously nonsurgical diseases. Relevant to pancreatic surgery is the bilioenteric bypass, which had its origins in the management of benign biliary disease before its application to malignant obstructive processes.

Bilioenteric bypass involves creating an artificial connection, or anastomosis, between the biliary system and the small intestine, bypassing the blockage caused by a tumor in the ampulla of Vater or pancreatic head. This procedure can relieve the distressing symptoms such as pruritus associated with jaundice and improve quality of life for patients with advanced pancreatic cancer.

8.5.4.1 Alexander von Winiwarter (1880)

In 1880, Alexander von Winiwarter (1848–1917), an Austrian surgeon and former pupil of Billroth, was Professor of Surgery in Liege, Belgium. He was treating a 34-year-old man with obstructive jaundice, so exteriorized the gallbladder and adjacent ascending colon with the intent of, at a second stage, creating a fistula between the two once they had adhered. In short, a series of procedures occurred in which the patient was left with biliary fistulae, and some weeks later, a subsequent cholecystojejunostomy resulted in two enterotomies that formed external fistulae. The patient disappeared for some months but then returned with the fistulae almost healed and a further operation closed them. This led Winiwarter to recommend a two-stage cholecystoenterostomy for obstructive jaundice. However, no one else attempted the procedure for 5 years.

Meanwhile, in Florence, Italy, Francesco Colzi (1855-1903), ligated the common bile duct in five dogs and performed a cholecystojejunostomy in 1883. All the animals survived without a change in digestive function. He also advocated for jejunal rather than colonic anastomosis to reduce the risk of ascending infection. JM Gaston in Atlanta, USA, also experimented on dogs with a cholecystoduodenostomy, showing that it was feasible. Unfortunately, Colzi died of tetanus following an accident with his rifle on a hunting trip when he sustained a gunshot wound to the axilla.

8.5.4.2 Nestor-Dimitrievich Monastyrski and Cholecystoenterostomy (1887)

The first successful cholecystoenterostomy was performed by a Russian surgeon, Professor Nestor-Dimitrievich Monastyrski (1847–1888), in 1887. Monastyrski had studied and trained in Vienna under Billroth. He had previously performed the first gastroenterostomy in Russia. The cholecystoenterostomy was on a 50-year-old with a periampullary cancer. When the patient died of metastases, the autopsy confirmed an intact anastomosis [87, 88, 93].

A second successful procedure was performed soon after for a pancreatic cancer causing obstructive jaundice by Swiss surgeon, Alexander Otto Kappeler (1841–1909), another pupil of Billroth. His patient also died later of metastases with another autopsy confirming a patent anastomosis.

8.5.4.3 Cholecystoduodenostomy (1889)

Louis Félix Terrier (1837–1908), a French surgeon working in Paris, performed the first successful cholecystoduodenostomy in 1889. He splinted the anastomosis with a 4 cm rubber tube in a 54-year-old woman with an impacted gallstone.

8.5.4.4 Cholecysto-Colonic Anastomosis (1889)

Also, in 1889, A W Mayo-Robson (1853–1933), Professor of Surgery in Leeds, treated a patient with an external biliary fistula by bilioenteric anastomosis. The patient had originally undergone a cholecystostomy for empyema of the gallbladder. Mayo-Robson, because of dense adhesions, used the hepatic flexure to perform enteric side of the anastomosis. However, using the colon carries a high risk of backflow cholangitis and this anastomosis proved unpopular [93].

8.5.4.5 Ludwig Georg Courvoisier (1890)

Ludwig Georg Courvoisier (1843–1918) in his *Pathology and Surgery of the Biliary Tract*, published in 1890, presented 109 cases of gallbladder dilatation in which 92 were the result of malignancy or stricture and only 17 related to impacted gallstones. His eponymous sign is a sign, not a law, and highlights the likelihood of malignancy when Courvoisier's sign (a distended gallbladder in the presence of obstructive jaundice) is palpable or present. Courvoisier also summarized the first 10 reported cholecystoenterostomies in 1890 for which the mortality was two (20%) and concluded that the operation was as effective as cholecystostomy [94].

In 1892, Robert Gersuny (1844–1924), better known for his injection of Vaseline and Paraffin fillers, anastomosed the gallbladder to the lesser curve of the gastric antrum. This was necessitated by dense adhesions encasing the duodenum and small intestine in a 45-year-old woman with episodic biliary colic and jaundice [88, 92, 93, 95].

A significant evolution of pancreatic surgery occurred when, in 1904, Ambroise Monprofit (1857–1922) of Angers, France, performed the first Roux-en-Y cholecystojejunostomy to bypass a pancreatic tumor. The origins of the Roux-en-Y technique are actually somewhat unclear. The Roux-en-Y procedure is named after César Roux (1857–1934), a Swiss surgeon based in Lausanne, who described use of a jejunal loop in 1893 for the treatment of gastric outlet obstruction. However, Roux's original procedure did not involve the gallbladder or the pancreas. The advantage of employing a Roux loop is to prevent ascending cholangitis from bacteria in the intestinal tract entering the biliary tract. In 1909, Robert Dahl of Stockholm, Sweden, successfully treated a hepatic duct fistula using a Roux-en-Y limb [93].

8.5.5 Pancreatic Resection

Nicolas Senn (1844–1908), a preeminent American surgeon of the late nineteenth and early twentieth centuries, wrote extensively on the surgical treatment of pancreatic disease, including an 1886 monograph *The Surgery of the Pancreas*. In this monograph, Senn noted that "*the most favourable conditions for extirpation are presented if the disease is primarily located in the tail of the pancreas.*" Senn recognized that compared to the head of the pancreas, the body and tail were easily accessible to resection without the need for gastrointestinal reconstructions [96, 97].

Friedrich Trendelenburg (1844–1924), a German surgeon, is credited with performing the first anatomical resection for a solid tumor of the pancreas in 1882. Trendelenburg's procedure involved removing the body and tail of the pancreas, along with the spleen (due to a concomitant splenic artery injury), in a patient with a pancreatic tumor. The case demonstrated that surgical removal of a portion of the pancreas was possible and represented a technical advance [93]. This was despite the patient developing a leak, but insisting on discharge and dying at home from likely infective complications. Over the next two decades, surgeons, including

Trendelenburg, only slowly started to perform this operation with 24 procedures between 1882 and 1905, and by 21 different surgeons [97]!

The question of how to drain the pancreatic secretions has been a source of considerable debate since the early days of pancreatic surgery. It was initially believed that the flow of pancreatic juice was essential for survival, so attempts were made to preserve as much of the pancreatic tissue as possible. However, surgeons soon realized that leaving the pancreatic duct intact during surgery could lead to postoperative complications, including leakage of pancreatic juice into the abdominal cavity. To avoid these complications, surgeons began to explore different methods for draining these pancreatic secretions after surgery. One early approach was to create an external fistula, or drainage tube, through the abdominal wall to allow them to drain directly into a collection bag outside the body. While this approach was effective at preventing early postoperative complications, it was associated with a number of drawbacks, including protein, fluid and electrolyte loss as well as skin and stoma excoriation.

In the late nineteenth century, many surgeons experimented with removing parts of the duodenum or parts of the head of the pancreas and preserving the duodenum or enucleating pancreatic tumors. Most of these attempts resulted in pancreatic leaks and other complications. For example, Giuseppe Ruggi (1844–1925) in Italy enucleated a pancreatic head tumor in 1889, and Domenico Biondi performed a partial pancreatic head resection, sparing the duodenum in 1894.

In 1898, Alessandro Codivilla (1861–1912) in Bologna resected part of the head of the pancreas, distal stomach, proximal duodenum, and distal common bile duct, reconstructing with a Roux-en-Y gastrojejunostomy and cholecystojejunostomy. There is no description of what was done about the pancreatic stump which was probably tied off. The patient developed a pancreatic fistula and intractable diarrhea and died on the 5th postoperative day.

8.5.5.1 Halsted's Successful Resection of a Periampullary Tumor

Five days after Codivilla's procedure, William Halsted (1852–1922) (Fig. 8.10) reported a successful resection of a periampullary tumor at Johns Hopkins in Baltimore. He opened the duodenum, resecting en bloc a large portion of duodenum surrounding the growth with short segments of the adjacent pancreatic and common bile ducts. The ducts were then reimplanted into the duodenum. The patient survived for 12 months and died from cancer recurrence.

In 1907, Abel Desjardins (1814–1886) published his experimental work with duodenectomies on cadavers, in which he described his techniques and the results of his experiments. He eventually proved that dogs could survive after removing the entire duodenum. But it would be some more decades before any real success with pancreaticoduodenectomy [95].

The question of how to drain the pancreatic secretions was answered in 1909, by Robert Coffey, an American surgeon, who also did experimental pancreatico-enterostomies on dogs [95]. He invaginated the pancreatic stump into a draining limb of jejunum, surrounding the cut edge of the pancreas with a protective collar by peritoneum-covered bowel [95, 96, 98].

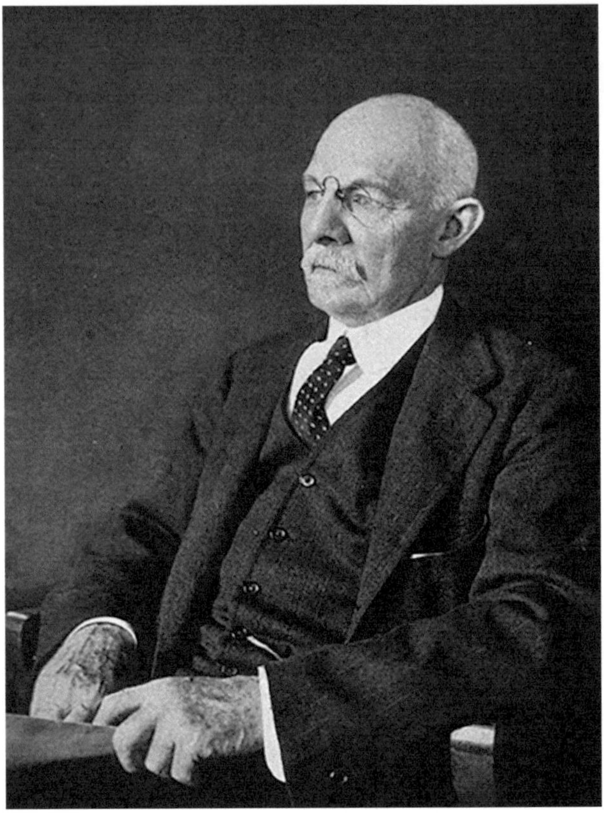

Fig. 8.10 William Halsted. Public domain. https://commons.wikimedia.org/w/index.php?search=William+halsted&title=Special:MediaSearch&go=Go&type=image

8.5.5.2 Walther Kausch: The First Successful Two-Stage Pancreaticoduodenectomy (1912)

Walther Kausch (1867–1928) was a pupil of Mikulicz in Breslau and had married Mikulicz's daughter in 1903. In 1906, he was appointed to head the surgical department at Auguste-Viktoria-Krankenhaus in Berlin. In 1912, he performed a two-stage resection of the majority of the duodenum en bloc with a significant portion of the pancreas for a patient with obstructive jaundice due to ampullary cancer. The first stage was a cholecystojejunostomy. The second, 2 months later, was the partial resection of the head of the pancreas, the duodenum, and part of the stomach, followed by reconstruction of the digestive tract with a gastrojejunostomy and end-to-end pancreticoduodenostomy similar to R C Coffey's experiments in dogs. The patient lived 9 months before dying of cholangitis.

Despite this relatively successful outcome, there were only two further reports of other successful pancreaticoduodenectomies for two decades. One was performed in Heidelberg, Germany, by George Hirschel in 1912 and the patient lived a year [100, 102].

Kausch suffered many personal setbacks in his life and career, including the death of his son, Wolfi. Kausch died of a pulmonary embolus while recovering at home from surgery for a perforated appendix. He would have deserved to be recognized along with Whipple (who eventually did 37 procedures and made many improvements to the original)—at least as the one who did in fact complete the first two-stage pancreaticoduodenectomy. Surgical history is littered with many such stories where the first pioneer is overlooked in favor of a better connected and more influential follower who, in this case, was Allen Oldfather Whipple [101–103].

During this period and even in subsequent decades, surgeons were indeed limited by the advanced stage of disease at presentation. It would only be with the development of modern imaging techniques such as computed tomography (CT) and magnetic resonance imaging (MRI) that clinicians developed the ability to diagnose pancreatic cancer at an earlier stage. Eleven weeks was the average time of survival when presenting with obstructive jaundice due to unresectable pancreatic cancer, even in the 1970s. Patients with periampullary cancers were more fortunate in that their jaundice developed earlier when their tumor was less advanced. In many cases, palliative procedures such as bypass to relieve obstructive jaundice offered a limited, but at least some palliation from the terrible itch associated with jaundice, and a few weeks of survival rather than dying from attempts at curative resection. The absence of parenteral nutrition support in the event of complications was another major limiting factor until the 1970's.

8.5.5.3 Roscoe Reid: Enucleation of an Insulinoma (1927)

The next landmark in pancreatic surgery after Kausch came in 1927, just 5 years after the discovery of insulin by Frederick Banting (1891–1941) and Charles Best (1899–1978) [97]. That led to being able to diagnose insulin-secreting tumors and removing them, eventually resulting in the categorization of a specific group of hormone-secreting tumors of the pancreas (pancreatic neuroendocrine tumors). In 1927, Roscoe Reid Graham (1890–1948) in Toronto successfully cured a patient with an insulinoma by enucleation and this sparked renewed interest in pancreatic surgery and its potential success.

8.5.5.4 Allen Oldfather Whipple

Allen Oldfather Whipple (1881–1963) (Fig. 8.11) was born on the second of September 1881 to Christian missionaries in Azerbaijan, Persia (now Iran). This was a formative upbringing as his three older siblings died in childhood, two from diphtheria and one from scarlet fever. He developed typhoid at the age of 4 and was bedridden for 2 months. This probably allowed him to survive a further typhoid outbreak. He and his family lived in Tabriz (1892) but returned to the United States in 1896 where he studied at Princeton (1901–4), and then medical school at Columbia University, graduating third in his class in 1908. His surgical training was undertaken at the Presbyterian Hospital where he established a detailed data

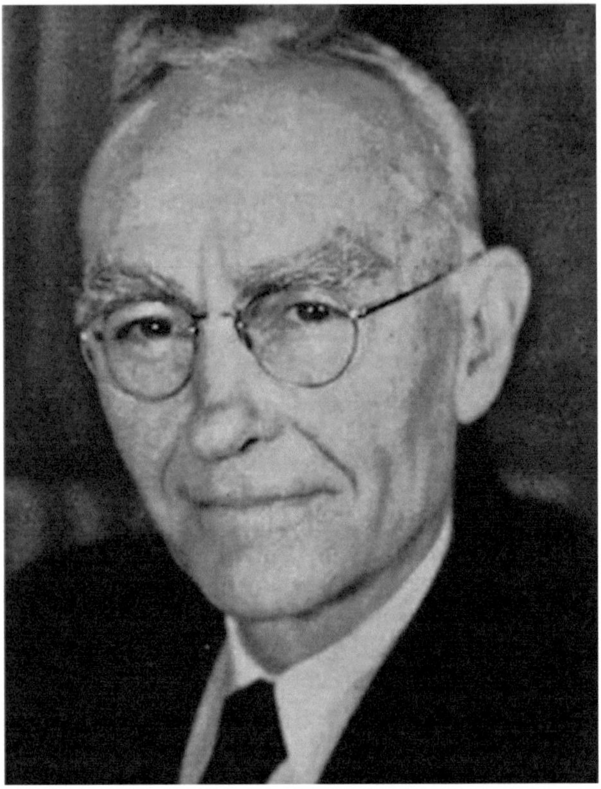

Fig. 8.11 Allen Oldfather Whipple, Wikimedia public domain. https://litfl.com/wp-content/uploads/2018/11/Allen-Oldfather-Whipple-1881-1963.jpg

collection protocol for biliary and pancreatic diseases. Whipple became Professor and Chief of Surgery at the Columbia-Presbyterian Medical Center in New York in 1921 at the age of 39 and held this post until retiring in 1946.

The success with neuroendocrine tumors provided an opportunity to revive interest in more radical pancreatic resection [98].

Whipple described the pancreaticoduodenectomy in his landmark manuscript entitled "*The Radical Operation for Carcinoma of the Ampulla of Vater*" published in 1935 and presented that same year to the American Surgical Association meeting in Boston. He presented a two-stage technique for the radical resection of periampullary cancers consisting of cholecystogastrostomy and posterior loop gastrojejunostomy (1st stage of bypass) followed by partial duodenectomy, partial pancreatic head resection, and pancreaticojejunostomy (resection stage). The procedure was later named the "Whipple procedure" in his honor although he was not the first to perform a successful pancreaticoduodenectomy. He later revised the first stage to a Roux-en-Y cholecystojejunostomy and then choledochojejunostomy to minimize the risk of cholangitis and anastomotic structure at the bilioenteric anastomosis.

Alexander Brunschwig (1901–1969) in Chicago became the first to apply the procedure successfully to PDAC in 1937. Brunschwig did make important contributions to the development of the procedure, including the use of a pylorus preserving modification that is still widely used today [99].

His major contributions to medicine however were in gynecological surgery when he was Chief of Gynecology in New York at the Memorial Hospital for Cancer and Allied Diseases. However, he did write a book on the surgery of pancreatic tumors, inspired by his father's death from pancreatic cancer [104, 105].

8.5.5.5 The First One-Stage Pancreaticoduodenectomy (1940)

In 1940, Whipple performed the first successful one-stage PD as unplanned on a patient believed to have gastric cancer. After transecting the midportion of the stomach, Whipple was surprised to discover that the tumor originated from the pancreatic head. The patient was not jaundiced, so Whipple decided to proceed with conversion to a one-stage PD. To accomplish this, he expanded the usual en bloc resection to include the distal stomach, the entire duodenum, and the pancreatic head, followed by reconstruction with a loop gastrojejunostomy and end-to-side pancreaticojejunostomy. The pathology showed a nonfunctioning islet cell tumor and the patient survived for 9 years until dying of metastatic disease. Other surgeons were then convinced so the operation established itself in surgery [106].

Vitamin K became widely available for clinical use in 1940, the same year that Whipple performed the first successful one-stage pancreaticoduodenectomy. This was a fortunate coincidence as vitamin K plays a critical role in blood clotting, and pancreaticoduodenectomy is a highly invasive surgery that can result in significant bleeding. When combined with bile salts, it effectively reversed the coagulopathy caused by prolonged biliary obstruction and lack of intestinal absorption of Vitamin K. The availability of vitamin K helped improve the outcomes of this surgery by reducing the risk of bleeding complications [106, 107].

Whipple believed that the pancreatic anastomosis was a source of potential complications and he sought to avoid it whenever possible. Instead, he preferred to occlude the pancreatic duct stump to prevent leakage of pancreatic juice, which could lead to fistula formation and other complications. However, by the early 1940s, several surgeons were successfully employing pancreatico-enterostomies. Animal studies were also demonstrating that rapid epithelialization of pancreatic anastomoses could be achieved within 24–48 h. Whipple started to incorporate an end-to-side pancreaticojejunostomy using the duct-to-mucosa technique. Whipple described his procedure thus:

> (I) At least two days of vitamin K and bile salts therapy; (II) the distal half of the stomach, the entire duodenum, the terminal portion of the common duct and the head of the pancreas were removed en masse; (III) a vertical limb of the jejunum, starting at the duodenojejunal junction, was brought up through a rent in the mesocolon, behind the colon, with the following anastomoses in sequence: (i) a choledochojejunostomy, end-to-end; (ii) an anastomosis between the pancreatic duct and the wall of the jejunal opening the size of the pancreatic duct, followed by the tacking of the stump of the resected pancreas to the wall of the jejunum; (iii) an end-to-side gastrojejunostomy. A sump drain in the bed of the duodenum was used. Silk technic was employed throughout [101–103].

Whipple went on to perform 37 pancreaticoduodenectomies with a mortality of 33%. The mortality rate remained 20–40% for some 30 years after Whipple.

Even in the 1960s and 1970s, the high mortality and poor long-term survival rates associated with pancreaticoduodenectomy (PD) led some surgeons to question whether the procedure should be abandoned altogether. However, improvements in surgical techniques, availability of antibiotics, anaesthesia, perioperative intensive care, nutritional support, diagnostic and interventional radiology led to better case selection, outcomes, and wider acceptance of PD as a viable treatment option for certain pancreatic diseases.

At the same time, pathological data were emerging to suggest that PDAC was often a multifocal disease arising from field changes in the ductal mucosa. Because it eliminated the pancreatic anastomosis and tumor multicentricity, total pancreatectomy (TP) was, for a time, advocated over PD on the grounds that standard partial resections likely left disease behind in the pancreatic remnant. However clever this was in theory, the benefits of TP were not borne out in practice, with no survival advantage at the cost of brittle diabetes that was hard to control [104].

Prior to the 1980s, the mortality rate associated with PD for PDAC was high, typically ranging from 10% to 20%. However, beginning in the 1980s, several institutions reported significant improvements in outcomes, with mortality rates of less than 5%. These improvements were attributed to the growing trend of centralization of care at high-volume centers, where surgeons specialized in pancreatic surgery. Today, units performing pancreaticoduodenectomy would be expected to have a 30-day/in-hospital mortality under 2%.

The centralization of care allowed for the concentration of multidisciplinary expertise and resources and led to better patient outcomes. Surgeons who specialized in pancreatic surgery were able to perform the procedure more efficiently and with fewer complications. Additionally, these centers were often equipped with the latest technology and had access to multidisciplinary teams that could provide comprehensive care for patients, including interventional radiology, intensive care, and nutritional support [107–110].

Due to the wide availability of imaging modalities, incidental lesions became a common theme, and asymptomatic lesions of the pancreas and other organs were increasingly reported. Intraductal papillary mucinous neoplasm (IPMN) of the pancreas was first described by Japanese pathologist Dr. Masayuki Ohashi and his colleagues in a paper published in the American Journal of Gastroenterology in 1982. The paper reported on a series of six cases of a new type of pancreatic tumor that they called "*mucin-producing pancreatic tumors with intraductal growth*." Since then, IPMN has been recognized as a distinct clinical entity and has become an area of active research and clinical interest. IPMN is now known to be a relatively common pancreatic lesion, accounting for 10–15% of all cystic pancreatic tumors. It is typically slow growing and may not cause any symptoms but may progress to invasive pancreatic cancer if left untreated. IPMN can be detected using various imaging modalities, including CT scan, MRI, and endoscopic ultrasound (EUS) [111].

In the twenty-first century, these lesions often undergo further investigation and if deemed high risk, they will undergo surgical resection. This has taken pancreatic surgery a further step forward into cancer prevention [106]. Endoscopic ultrasound proved to be crucial for investigating these lesions since its development. By combining ultrasonography and endoscopy, EUS opened an entirely new dimension in imaging. EUS was designed in the early 1980s in an attempt to improve US imaging of the pancreaticobiliary system [111, 112].

8.5.6 Pancreatitis and Pancreatic Cysts and Pseudocysts

Patients with acute pancreatitis are usually admitted under a surgeon because they have acute abdominal pain that may be due to another cause. The role of surgery in acute pancreatitis has traditionally been one of excluding other diagnoses or managing its complications such as pseudocysts and abscesses, but also sometimes performing a necrosectomy, when required, in the second or third week when there is severe, necrotic pancreatitis. A risk of surgery is that it converts a closed, less likely to become infected, inflamed bed into one that has been potentially exposed to microorganisms and which provides a rich nutrient environment for their growth.

Abscesses complicating acute pancreatitis should be externally drained. For most of the twentieth century, this meant open surgery but these can now be drained effectively radiologically or even sometimes laparoscopically depending on their location. In 1979, Stephen Gerzof (b1942), working at Tufts University School of Medicine in Boston, first demonstrated the utility of draining these abscesses under imaging control.

The management of acute pancreatitis without pseudocyst formation or necrosis is based on observation, conservative management, monitoring for organ dysfunction, and organ support whenever there is respiratory, kidney, or circulatory failure.

Pancreatic cysts may cause extrinsic compression to adjacent structures and result in persistent vomiting. Pseudocysts following pancreatitis tend to develop over a few weeks after the acute attack. When expanding or becoming infected, they may erode vessels in the lesser sac, resulting to significant hemorrhage that, without interventional radiology or immediate surgery and packing, is likely to prove fatal. Pseudocysts not causing significant compressive problems can be observed and may recede. Those in whom the cyst is expanding or the patient is deteriorating require prompt intervention [97].

Friedrich Wilhelm Wandesleben (1800–1863) in Stromberg, Germany, externally drained a pancreatic pseudocyst caused by blunt trauma in a 28-year-old man in 1841. The patient only survived 5 months.

Auguste Le Dentu (1841–1926) performed a percutaneous drainage of a large cyst in Paris in 1862.

It was in 1881 that Carl Thiersch (1822–1895) published a cyst drainage on a longer-term a survivor. The patient was a 38-year-old man from whom three liters of chocolate-colored fluid was drained with a persistent fistula from the pancreatic tail.

Nathan Bozeman (1825–1903) in New York (1881) removed a 5 L cyst hanging from the pancreatic tail but originally thought it was an ovarian cyst. The patient was discharged healthy.

Carl Gussenbauer (1842–1903), Billroth's assistant, marsupialized a pancreatic cyst of the abdominal wall with the patient surviving 8 years. Gussenbauer's success led to 149 cases being operated from around the world in 1900 with a 19% mortality for resection and 3% for marsupialization. He performed three further operations for pancreatic cysts during his career.

Pancreatic cysts and pseudocysts were first differentiated in 1898 by German surgeon Werner Körte in 1898.

8.5.6.1 Internal Drainage of a Pancreatic Pseudocyst (1911)

It was being recognized that external drainage led to enzymatic damage to the patient's skin, and this led to Louis Ombrédanne (1871–1956) in Paris performing, in 1911, the first internal drainage [97–99] (pancreaticoduodenostomy) of a pseudocyst. The patient died 11 days after the procedure. In 1921, Rudolf Jedlicka (1869–1936) in Prague performed the first cystogastrostomy. Adolf Henle (1864–1936), a German surgeon, performed the first cystojejunostomy in 1923. However, he resected most of the cyst rather than just internally draining it.

8.5.6.2 Further developments in Internal Drainage

In 1931, Antoni Jurasz (1882–1961), Professor of Surgery in Poznan, Poland, performed the first successful cystogastrostomy through the stomach. This technique is virtually complication free for suitably located cysts.

In 1946, Köning performed a cystojejunostomy using a Roux loop to minimize the risk of infection of the cyst contents.

Endoscopic approaches to internal drainage were introduced in the 1980s. Endoscopic stents were used in 1989, by Cremer in Brussels. Imaging support for accurate placement of stents using endoscopic ultrasound was introduced by Grimm from Hamburg in 1992 [99].

8.5.7 Pancreatic Surgery in the Twenty-First Century

The majority of pancreatic cancers remain advanced at presentation though the proportion that are resectable is improving. Pancreatic surgery in the twenty-first century is generally and appropriately concentrated in specialist centers with the full complement of resources. There, mortality rates for PDAC resections are in the range of 1–2%, although despite these low mortality rates, the morbidity is still considerable, being in the range of 20–40%. Resection and grafting of the portal vein have become an option even for tumors, previously considered unresectable due to their having invaded the portal venous vasculature behind the head and neck of the pancreas.

The modern treatment of obstructive jaundice due to an unresectable cancer is transhepatic stenting by interventional radiology, supported by palliative chemotherapy. Bypass procedures are reserved for those for whom interventional radiology is not available or not possible.

Even the procedure of cholecystostomy in patients not fit enough for an emergency cholecystectomy is performed today transhepatically, usually by a radiologist under imaging control rather than a surgeon. This reduces the risk of leakage from the cholecystostomy site and subsequent peritonitis.

Pancreatic necrosectomies for necrotizing pancreatitis may be performed minimally invasively, laparoscopically, or endoscopically. Pancreatic pseudocysts can be internally drained into the stomach endoscopically also averting the need for open surgery.

Endoscopic retrograde choledochopancreatography (ERCP) offers an endoscopic route to manage bile duct and/or pancreatic duct stones and to urgently drain cholangitis. The operation of transduodenal sphincterotomy, first performed as an open procedure by Edward Archibald (1872–1945) in Montreal in 1919 is now performed endoscopically.

8.6 Minimally Invasive Abdominal Surgery—The Surgical Revolution of the 1990s

There is nothing so difficult or so dangerous as to change the order of things. – Machiavelli

In the ancient world, there were instruments developed to inspect body orifices such as the nose and throat, urethra, rectum, and vagina. These were little more than specula but nonetheless show there was an understanding of the need to inspect, to remove foreign bodies, and to treat pathology. Susruta (8–6 century BCE) described throat, anal, and vaginal specula with a hole at one or both ends and/or in the side. A different speculum was developed for treating anal fistula from that for treating hemorrhoids. In the time of Hippocrates (460 BCE), specula were used, as were various catheters using hollow tubes of bamboo or similar tubes made of metal. Erasistratus (310–250 BCE) described an S-shaped catheter for the urethra.

There were rectal and vaginal specula uncovered in the ruins at Pompei, a Roman city destroyed by Mt. Vesuvius' eruption in 79 CE. However, the ancients' efforts to perform endoscopy were always limited by lack of illumination.

During the Renaissance, Giulio Cesare Aranzio (1530–1589) developed an early light source in 1587, in order to inspect the nasal cavity and remove polyps. He used a water-filled spherical bottle with a hole in a shutter to concentrate the light source. He is better known for describing the foramen ovale, ductus arteriosus, and the hippocampus.

George Arnaud de Ronsil (1698–1774), a French physician, used a covered lantern inside a silver-painted box to focus the light through a convex lens and inspect the vagina through a speculum.

In 1806, Philipp Bozzini (1773–1809), in Frankfurt, introduced an instrument with two channels, one to conduct light and the other to view the images. The light source was a candle with concave mirrors behind it to reflect the light into the relevant body cavity. Although Der Lichtleiter (the light conductor) was weak and the field of vision too small, developments in the next 70 years were based on Bozzini's principle of illumination. There is no record of Bozzini's device being used in clinical practice [113]. Bozzini was censured by the Medical Faculty of the University of Vienna for his "undue curiosity!" In 1826, a similar cystoscope developed by Pierre Ségalas (1792–1874) was also ignored by the medical community [113–116].

8.6.1 French Pioneers in Endoscopy

In the early nineteenth century, there were several French surgeons in Paris developing their field of endourology. Endoscopic lithotripsy was first introduced by Leroy d'Etiolles (1798–1860) in 1822. Cornay de Rochefort introduced an aspirator. In 1823, Jean Civiale (1792–1867) reported a series of endoscopic lithotripsies based on d'Etiolle's experiments. He introduced a double-channel irrigation system, a device for crushing bladder stones, a wire basket and cutter, and a retractable blade for urethral strictures. Civiale founded the first urology service in the world at the Necker Hospital in Paris.

In 1843, Antonin Jean Desormeaux (1815–1894) developed a portable cystoscope and was able to perform diagnostic and therapeutic cystoscopies and is credited with introducing the term endoscopy. He modified Bozzini's mirrors and reflectors and used a spirit lamp fueled by alcohol and turpentine as a light source. The heat of the lamp caused some patients' legs and operators' hands to be burned, though in the urinary tract, the urine cooled the cystoscope, and so was safe.

Another Parisien, Jean Pierre Bonnafont (1805–1891), invented the first otoscope and presented his device to the Parisian Medical Academy in 1834. His lens system was based on the microscope with a conical mirror as introduced by Ségalas [117–119].

8.6.2 Early Development of Urology in the United Kingdom

British developments included John Avery's trial in 1844 of an early endoscope used in the urinary tract and to inspect the larynx. At London's Charing Cross Hospital, he employed a large Palmers lamp reflector (as used by miners) to redirect candlelight onto a speculum's mirror. He didn't get the support of his colleagues as not much could be seen in the bladder and the headlight was regarded as too bulky. In 1855, George Robinson used electricity to crush bladder stones. He used a Leyden jar as the source of electricity attached to two copper wires along which he pulsed electricity. He coined the term electro-lithotripsy.

In 1865, Sir Francis Cruise (1834–1912) in Dublin performed endoscopic urethrotomies through an improved version of Desormeaux's cystourethroscope. Cruise was also President of the Royal College of Physicians of Ireland from 1884 to 1886.

Sir Henry Thompson (1820–1904) learned the technique of lithotripsy from Civiale in 1847. He gained a reputation as an adept proceduralist within the urethra. He was later called upon to manage the stones of King Leopold of Belgium (1863) and Napoleon III of France (1873). The Belgian King fared better than the French. Leopold's stone was successfully treated but Napoleon III died of infected obstructive uropathy after two unsuccessful procedures.

Endoscopes lit by electricity only became possible after the light bulb was invented by Sir Joseph Swan (1828–1914) of Newcastle. Swan's house and street in Newcastle were the first in the United Kingdom to be lit by electricity in 1880. Thomas Alva Edison took out a US patent in America in 1879 and successfully commercialized Swan's invention. They formed the Edison-Swan company with Edison switching from a bamboo filament to Swan's 1881 cellulose filament in 1892 [120, 121].

In Berlin, Maximilian Nitze (1848–1906) developed a variety of endoscopic instruments eventually settling on what would be the Nitze-Leiter cystoscope. Leiter was the instrument maker in Vienna who collaborated with Nitze. The initial device included an irrigation system with an electrically heated incandescent platinum wire as an internal lighting source. They added the electric light bulb after its invention. Henry Thompson introduced the Nitze-Leiter cystoscope to Britain in 1880. This instrument was also adapted for examination of the upper gastrointestinal tract. David Newman (1853–1924) in Glasgow is the first to use a miniature version of the light bulb in 1883. This afforded him sufficient view to endoscopically catheterize the ureters of females [121–123].

8.6.3 Russian Developments in Endoscopy

Alexander Ebermann (1830–1902), Alfred Couriard, and Benjamin Tarnowsky worked in St. Petersburg and developed cystoscopy independently of their Western European peers during the 1860s. Ebermann adapted an electrical device to improve illumination connecting it to the cystoscope or to a headlight. Couriard used a convex lens adjacent to the kerosene lamp to improve illumination and modified the end of the scope to reduce distortion of the image. Couriard and Tarnowsky separated the components of the cystoscope to improve portability and handling, as well as improving image quality by allowing direct visualization rather than a reflected view.

Dimitrij Oscarovic Ott (1855–1929) in St. Petersburg (Petrograd), from 1901, introduced a technique that was the forerunner of natural orifice transluminal endoscopic surgery (NOTES). He placed the patient in Trendelenburg position (head down), incised the vagina, and inserted two specula into the pelvis. He could view the pelvic organs, and in a series of over 1000 ventroscopies, he was able to diagnose 64 ectopic pregnancies, ovarian cysts, 60 cases of pelvic inflammatory disease, and 15 cases with adhesions. He performed three appendicectomies. His mortality was 2.14% as opposed to the laparotomy mortality of 11.11%. He was also a personal physician to Tsarina Alexandra Feodorovna (1874–1918). These were and are remarkable outcomes from a time when abdominal surgery still carried a high morbidity and mortality [124, 125].

8.6.4 First Laparoscopies

Georg Kelling (1866–1945), a German physician from Dresden, is credited with performing the first endoscopy of the abdomen in 1901 using a cystoscope. However, the basic principles of endoscopy of the abdomen were not fully described by Kelling. He called the technique as "coelioscopy." Kelling's doctoral thesis was on the gastrointestinal tract. He developed the method from his discoveries about insufflation of air into the abdomen. He used a cystoscope to study the abdominal cavity of a dog into which he had insufflated filtered air. This may be considered the first instance of diagnostic laparoscopy [114]. In a lecture about the technique, he stated somewhat prophetically:

> *Gentlemen, I conclude this lecture by expressing the hope that endoscopic methods will be used to a greater extent in the digestive tract than has been common practice so far. In fact, in many instances, endoscopic methods are destined to replace laparotomy.*

Kelling along with his second wife were killed in a heavy air attack on Dresden in February 1945 [126, 127]. Nine years later, in 1910, Hans-Christian Jacobaeus (1879–1937), a Swedish internist, performed the first documented laparoscopy in a human. He used a cystoscope to examine the abdominal cavity in 19 patients, 17 of whom had ascites (excessive peritoneal fluid). He then reported a second series with 97 patients, 8 of whom were not ascitic. In 1911, he also performed the first thoracoscopy, using a cystoscope to examine the pleural cavity in collaboration with Ludolph Brauer (1865–1951) in Hamburg, inducing a pneumothorax and dividing adhesions. Brauer was an advocate for therapeutic pneumothorax to collapse a tuberculous lung, which was then, and until the introduction of streptomycin in 1945, a recognized and sometimes effective treatment. In 1948, Brauer was nominated for, but did not receive the Nobel Prize which was awarded instead to Paul Hermann Müller for his discovery of DDT and its toxic effects to insects and thus value in controlling the spread of malaria and typhus [116].

In 1911, Bertram Bernheim (1880–1958), at Johns Hopkins Hospital in Baltimore, performed the first laparoscopy in the United States. He used a proctoscope via an epigastric incision in a patient with jaundice.

Otto Goetze (1886–1957) was a German radiologist and a pioneer in the use of X-rays for diagnostic purposes. In 1918, he published a treatise in the Munich Medical Weekly on the X-ray diagnosis of the abdominal cavity, including the insufflation of the peritoneal cavity with oxygen to outline the intra-abdominal organs through the "principle of solid displacement." He coined the term "pneumoperitoneum." In the United States, Walter Alvarez (1884–1978), in 1921, and Richard Zollikofer (1871–1963), a Swiss gynecologist in 1924, replaced oxygen with carbon dioxide rather than air for radiological and laparoscopic procedures [117, 126, 128].

In 1920, Benjamin Orndoff, an American radiologist, performed diagnostic peritoneoscopies. He used a spinal needle to insufflate oxygen, then performed fluoroscopy, and used a sharp trocar to insert his peritoneoscope. He presented a case series of 42 cases but got little recognition from his peers.

8.6.4.1 Janos Veres

Janos Veres (1903–1979), a Hungarian physician designed his trocar/needle with a spring-loaded tip to minimize the risk of causing injury once in the peritoneal cavity. It was first developed for accessing the thorax to create a pneumothorax to treat tuberculosis. He performed 862 thoracic procedures with his needle in 1933, and published a paper in a Hungarian journal. It was not until 1938 when he published in a German medical journal that his invention became known to the world. The Veress needle was later used in the abdomen. Unfortunately, injuries still occur with a Veress needle, and particularly in patients at risk of having intra-abdominal adhesions, when a cut-down procedure under direct vision in a non-operated part of the abdomen is safest.

8.6.4.2 Harrith Hasson (1971)

The use of the Veress needle in the abdomen for gynaecolological procedures was not popularized until 1971, when open laparoscopy was described by Harrith Hasson (1931–2012). Hasson was born and educated in Egypt, graduating from the University of Cairo before moving to the United States and establishing his career as a gynaecologist in Chicago.

8.6.4.3 Heinz Kalk and Laparoscopic Liver Biopsies

Diagnostic laparoscopy was starting to gain momentum. Heinz Kalk (1895–1973) was a German gastroenterologist who used laparoscopy to take liver biopsies under direct vision. He made several significant contributions to the field, including the development of a 135-degree lens system and a double trocar technique for laparoscopic procedures. The 135-degree lens system allowed for better visualization of the abdominal cavity, while the double trocar technique allowed for improved access and maneuverability, in performing liver biopsy and, where necessary, access after division of adhesions [118]. There was an outbreak of infectious hepatitis (hepatitis A) in the German troops in early 1940, which led to a large clinical practice in the management of liver pathologies. Kalk performed over 2000 liver biopsies under local anesthesia and reported his results in the medical literature which ensured his contributions were well recognized [128–130].

8.6.4.4 John Ruddock and the Staging of Gastric Cancer

John Ruddock (1891–1964) in the 1930s, popularized laparoscopy for the diagnosis and staging of gastric cancer in the United States. He developed a peritoneoscope that enabled him, with the use of urological biopsy forceps, to sample the liver, spleen, stomach, omentum, and peritoneum. He also used monopolar cautery to ensure his biopsy sites did not bleed.

8.6.4.5 Rudolf Schindler (1932)

The first detailed description of the basic principles of abdominal endoscopy is often attributed to another German physician, Rudolf Schindler, who published a paper on the topic in 1932. Schindler described the use of a modified cystoscope for abdominal endoscopy and outlined the technical aspects of the procedure, including the use of insufflation to expand the abdominal cavity and the use of a camera and light source to visualize the internal organs [118]. Following Schindler's pioneering work, the field of abdominal endoscopy continued to slowly develop, with advances in technology and technique allowing for more sophisticated instruments and procedures. The first fallopian tube electrocautery was performed in 1936 by Swiss gynecologist Boesch [118, 119].

8.6.5 Laparoscopy After World War II

In the first few decades after the second world war, the surgical establishment was generally hostile to the progress of minimally invasive surgery in general and abdominal surgery. While minimally invasive surgery was being advanced in urology, the tipping point and scramble for change did not come for general surgeons until the advent of laparoscopic cholecystectomy in the 1980s.

> *It has been said that change is a little like heaven; everyone wants to go there, but no one wants to be there* [120].

8.6.5.1 Harold Hopkins and Fiber-Optic Cables

However, the practice of urology was being transformed by the introduction of flexible fiber-optic cables and lighting systems. British physicist, Harold Hopkins (1918–1994) had a doctorate in optical physics and had already developed the zoom lens which was first used in 1948 to televise a cricket match at Lords in London. Hopkins and his research student (1926–2020) produced a bundle of narrow glass fibers which transmitted light round corners. Their paper was published in Nature in 1954. Hopkins struggled to find further research funding in the United Kingdom, but South African Basil Hirschowitz (1925–2013), a gastroenterologist in Michigan, sought him out to collaborate on developing the flexible gastroscope. Hirschowitz even performed his own gastroscopy before introducing it into clinical practice in 1957! James Gow (1917–2001), a British urologist based in Liverpool, then collaborated with Hopkins and developed a system to photograph the image at the end of the cystoscope (1961).

8.6.5.2 Karl Storz

Karl Storz (1911–1996), who was at that time running a small instrument company in Germany founded in 1946, then contacted Hopkins, and their work led to the combination of Storz's cold light to Hopkins rod lens. They presented their technology to the International Urology meeting in Munich in 1967, and from that time on, urologists were on board. Indeed, since then, all endoscopic and laparoscopic procedures use devices based on the Hopkins' and Storz' technology [129, 130]. During the 1960s and 1970s, urologists and gynaecologists took the lead in the development of endoscopic surgery while most of the general and thoracic surgical community continued to ignore the possibilities of the new technique. Before keyhole surgery, most people thought large problems required large incisions. There was little opportunity afforded by surgical leaders to appreciate the advances of "keyhole" surgery.

Laparoscopic Tubal Ligations in the United States

In 1971, 35 years after Boesch's breakthrough, only 1% of tubal ligations in the United States were being performed laparoscopically. However, by 1976, that figure had surged to 60%. The slow pace of laparoscopic evolution was partly related to limitations in technology. Also, there was often skepticism among surgical communities. Pioneer laparoscopic surgeons were repressed and criticized by the champions of traditional surgery. Progress was hampered by inadvertent injuries when proceduralists were learning the techniques. These included an increase in incidents of bladder and bowel injury during laparoscopy and also some incidents of failure of sterilization in tubal ligation [120, 130].

The movement from diagnostic to operative laparoscopic abdominal surgery is credited to Raoul Palmer and Kurt Semm. Raoul Palmer (1904–1985), a French gynaecologist, is credited with performing the first laparoscopic removal of an oocyte in 1961 and also performed tubal cautery and tubal ligations. He introduced a number of innovations and also promoted the use of CO_2 insufflation in preference to air or oxygen. This procedure marked a major milestone in the development of minimally invasive surgery, as it demonstrated the feasibility of performing complex abdominal surgeries through small incisions [120, 131, 132].

8.6.5.3 The First Laparoscopic Appendicectomy (1983)

Kurt Semm (1927–2003), a German gynaecologist, is known for his pioneering work in the development of operative laparoscopy. In 1983, he introduced the laparoscopic appendectomy, and he went on to develop a wide range of laparoscopic instruments and techniques. He is also credited with coining the term "gynaecologic laparoscopy" to describe the use of laparoscopic techniques in gynecologic surgery [121, 128].

Semm also developed an automated insufflator, which helps maintain the correct level of gas pressure in the abdomen during laparoscopic surgery and a suction-irrigator system to remove fluids and debris from the surgical site. He also improved the electrocoagulation instruments used during laparoscopic surgery, as well as the techniques for intracorporeal and extracorporeal knot tying. Semm also developed an electrical morcellator for myomas, a device used to remove fibroids from the uterus during laparoscopic surgery.

Although Semm and his promotion of laparoscopic surgery revolutionized the future of traditional open surgery, many of his colleagues were initially critical of him. In his words, the medical world reacted strongly, exhibiting hostility and opposition he had never experienced before.

> *Both surgeons and gynecologists were angry with me, they virtually stoned me. All my initial attempts to publish a report on laparoscopic appendectomy were rejected with the comment that such non-sense does not, and will never, belong in general surgery* [122, 128].

In an interview, his close colleague, Liselotte Mettler, said that Semm was once summoned from the operating room and had to undergo a computed tomography investigation of his skull in order to prove that he was in good health! In 1981, the President of the German Society of Surgery urged the German Society of Obstetrics and Gynaecology to revoke his medical license. The fact that a gynaecologist was willing to show surgeons how to do an appendectomy was simply inconceivable! Semm had overstepped a mark that was considered a step too far!

8.6.5.4 Eric Mühe and the First Laparoscopic Cholecystectomy (1985)

Erich Mühe (1938–2005) was a German surgeon who is credited with performing the first laparoscopic cholecystectomy, (removal of the gallbladder), using a 3-cm laparoscope of his own design, which he called the "galloscope." He performed the procedure in 1985 and presented his work at the 1986 Congress of the German Surgical Society. Initially, Mühe also faced skepticism and criticism from other surgeons who believed that laparoscopic surgery was too risky and would never replace traditional open surgery.

Despite the success of his procedure, Mühe faced legal action and censorship from medical authorities in Germany, who were concerned about the safety and ethical implications of laparoscopic surgery. He was ultimately forced to stop performing the procedure and was censured by the courts. The laparoscopic revolution was yet to come [123, 129, 130] and one must feel sorry for Mühe. However, in the 1980s with the development of high-resolution video technology, laparoscopic surgery became a more practical, safer and effective option minimizing postoperative pain. This technology allowed surgeons to view the surgical site in real time, with magnification, and to perform the surgery using minimally invasive technique and less abdominal trauma to the patient [124].

8.6.5.5 Camran Nezhat and Video Endoscopy (1983)

Berci was a gynaecology resident in Buffalo who until 1977, was advocating the video technology for teaching purposes and possibly for documentation. Camran Nezhat (b1947) had graduated MD at Tehran University in Iran, before moving to Buffalo, New York, where he was a gynaecology resident (1974–78). Nezhat saw the potential for using video technology during laparoscopic surgery and operating while looking at the monitor, not into the patient. In 1983, he developed a technique for coupling a video camera to his laparoscopic eyepiece and working from a monitor rather than looking directly through the laparoscope. This technique allowed for real-time visualization of the surgical site by the entire surgical team and paved the way for the widespread use of video technology in laparoscopic surgery [123, 129, 130]. It is not uncommon for innovative medical ideas and techniques to face skepticism and criticism from established medical institutions and publications, especially when they challenge conventional wisdom or long-held beliefs. Dr. Nezhat, like many other pioneers such as Seem and Mühe in the field of minimally invasive surgery, faced significant challenges and resistance to his ideas and research in the early stages. He was rewarded only with criticism. His papers were refused by established journals for years; there was even a formal investigation, following which he was fully exonerated [115, 121, 129].

8.6.5.6 Phillippe Mouret: First Video Laparoscopic Cholecystectomy (1987)

In 1987, French surgeon Phillippe Mouret performed the first video laparoscopic cholecystectomy, which is now standard practice and, like Mühe, Semm, and Nezhat, was strongly criticized by those in the field for not being in accordance with best practices. François Dubois, a young Frenchman, was the second surgeon to perform video laparoscopic cholecystectomy in 1988. He was the first to publish his early experience [125]. Eddie Reddick and Douglas Olsen were among the first surgeons to perform laparoscopic surgery in the United States, and they published a series of cases in the late 1980s that helped to popularize the technique in the country. The technique of intraoperative cholangiography that they established is currently using an instrument called the Reddick-Olsen. With their experiences, the evolution phase was over and the revolution of laparoscopic surgery took off. Laparoscopic cholecystectomy was introduced to the world in the exhibit hall of the American College of Surgeons annual meeting in October 1989. The spread of laparoscopic gallbladder surgery in the 1990s occurred relatively quickly, certainly within 2–3 years, but without strong scientific evidence to support it. It offered some advantages over traditional open surgery, including less pain, shorter hospital stays, and faster recovery times. One of the key drivers of the rapid adoption of laparoscopic gallbladder surgery was patient demand. Many patients were eager to avoid the large incisions and longer recovery times associated with open surgery, so were willing to seek out surgeons who were trained in laparoscopic techniques. In addition, instrument companies saw an opportunity to market their laparoscopic equipment and instruments to surgeons, and they often sponsored courses and training programs to help increase adoption of the new technique despite some lingering doubts about its safety, at least while surgeons were learning to perform the operation from a different view or perspective. Initially, there was a higher risk of bile duct injuries during the introduction of laparoscopic surgery compared to the results of established open cholecystectomy. Some academic surgeons, including the Maltese-born, Alf Cuschieri (b1938) in Dundee, Scotland, called for a more cautious approach to the adoption of laparoscopic surgery in its early days. These surgeons argued that the new technique should be carefully evaluated and validated before it was widely adopted by the surgical community [124, 126, 129, 133, 134]. The media helped spread excitement about the new surgery, and patients wanted it. Now was the right time for the revolution of minimally invasive surgery. It first developed in private hospitals and then migrated to academic centers. The surgical community was enthusiastic about the potential benefits of minimally invasive surgery. Surgeons were eager to learn about new applications, instrumentation, and techniques for laparoscopic procedures, and there was a growing demand for training and education in this area.

8.6.5.7 The Society of Laparoendoscopic Surgeons

The Society of Laparoendoscopic Surgeons (SLS) was incorporated in 1990, as a nonprofit organization dedicated to promoting laparoscopic and minimally invasive surgery. Its mission is to advance the science, education, and technology of minimally invasive surgery. The Society of Laparoscopic Surgeons (SLS) has played an important role in promoting and supporting research and education in laparoscopic and minimally invasive surgery. It has developed a range of educational programs and resources, including conferences, workshops, online courses, and publications, to help train and educate surgeons in the latest techniques and technologies in this field. During the early 1990s, virtually every abdominal operation was performed and perfected by laparoscopic technique. These include appendicectomies, colorectal resections, splenectomies, gastrectomies, oesophagectomies, liver resections, and adrenalectomies. In the thorax, lung resections and decortications/pleural washouts are performed thoracoscopically. Abdominal urological procedures such as nephrectomy, partial nephrectomy, and pyeloplasties are also performed laparoscopically. Although laparoscopic radical prostatectomy was introduced during the

1990s and 2000s, the greater versatility of robotic instruments in the male pelvis has resulted in a safer radical prostatectomy when performed robotically (see below).

8.6.5.8 Endovascular Surgery

Endovascular surgery has become the preferred route of operation for many elective aortic aneurysm repairs, and some emergency ruptured aneurysms too. Whilst minimally invasive, these vascular procedures are not endoscopic or laparoscopic as they are done under imaging control rather than under vision.

8.6.5.9 Robotic Surgery

Robotic surgery is considered as the second evolution of minimally invasive surgery. The first robotic system for laparoscopic surgery, called the "AESOP" (Automated Endoscopic System for Optimal Positioning), was introduced in 1994. This system was designed to hold and control the laparoscope during surgery, allowing the surgeon to focus on operating the instruments. The da Vinci robotic surgical system (Intuitive Surgical, Sunnyvale, CA) was introduced in Europe in 1997. Guy Cadiere performed the first robot-assisted cholecystectomy in Brussels. Da Vinci was the first FDA-approved integrated robotic surgical system in 2000. Robotic surgery has had a significant impact on the field of urology and gynaecology, particularly in the areas of radical prostatectomy and complex gynaecological surgeries. The company Intuitive Surgical was founded by a team of entrepreneurs and engineers with backgrounds in medical technology, robotics, and computer science. The use of robotic technology has allowed less experienced laparoscopic surgeons to perform complex procedures with greater precision and accuracy.

8.6.5.10 Natural Orifice Surgery (1990s)

Natural orifice surgery (NOS) was introduced in the 1990's with endoscopic instruments for treatment of gastro-oesophageal reflux. In 2006, a joint working group of the American Society for Gastrointestinal Endoscopy (ASGE) and the Society of American Gastrointestinal and Endoscopic Surgeons (SAGES) published a position statement on the development and introduction of NOTES (natural orifice transluminal endoscopic surgery). The statement called for a measured, stepwise approach to the introduction of the technology into clinical practice, with careful evaluation of the safety and effectiveness of the procedures. The working group recognized the potential benefits of NOTES but also acknowledged the need for further research and development to address technical challenges and ensure patient safety [115, 128, 135].

8.7 Endoscopy

The earliest exploration of the interior of the human body was attempted in antiquity by Greek, Roman, and Arab physicians.
Rectoscopes were used by Hippocrates (460–377 BCE). Advanced three- and four-pronged dilatation specula were recovered from the ruins of Pompeii.

Albukasim (Khalaf ibn Abbas AL-Zahrawi) (912–1013 CE), an Arabian physician, used reflected light to view the inside of the body. He held a glass mirror in front of the vulva and thus reflected light into the vaginal vault [136]. Philipp Bozzini (see below) is credited with inventing the first practical endoscope, a medical instrument used for examining the inside of the body. His device, called the "Lichtleiter" or "light conductor," was essentially a candlelight source that could illuminate the inside of the body through a tube. Bozzini first demonstrated the Lichtleiter in 1806, and later published a book on the subject in 1807, titled "*Lichtleiter, eine Erfindung zur Ausführung innerer Untersuchungen und Operationen ohne Hilfsmittel der Sonnenstrahlen*" ("Light conductor, an invention for the execution of internal examinations and operations without the aid of sunlight") [116].

8.7.1 *Philipp Bozzini (1773–1809)*

On a tombstone in a Frankfurt cemetery, an epitaph records: "*In memory of the devout deceased soul of Philipp Bozzini, medical doctor. This urologist was the first who tried seriously to look into the hollow cavities of the human body by ingeniously conducted light.*"

Bozzini's (1773–1809) contribution to the field of endoscopy was significant because his device represented a major technological advancement over earlier methods, which relied on mirrors and sunlight to illuminate the inside of the body. The Lichtleiter (light conductor) was created to fit various types of specula that were suitable for different bodily orifices with their varying dimensions and shapes. The intent was that doctors could conduct internal examinations and surgeries with much greater accuracy and precision. Bozzini's invention paved the way for the modern endoscopes that are used in medicine today. The instrument required a candle made of beeswax to produce light and a silver mirror to reflect the light through the speculum. He looked through a small hole in the middle of the mirror to see through the speculum, thus beginning the era of rigid endoscopy [116]. An English soldier, during the coalition wars, took one of the instruments that Bozzini had sent for testing to the Josephinum, which was a surgical military academy located in Vienna. The work of Bozzini had been antagonized by rivalry and was also dismissed as "*but a magic lantern.*" Pierre Salomon Segalas presented a modified version of the Bozzini instrument to the Academie des Sciences in Paris in 1826. This instrument was called a "urethro-cystique" speculum which allowed Segalas to diagnose medical conditions related to the urethra and bladder [137] (Fig. 8.12).

Many years later, the first open tube endoscope was made in 1853 by Desormeaux and was used to examine the urethra and bladder. Because the batteries that could

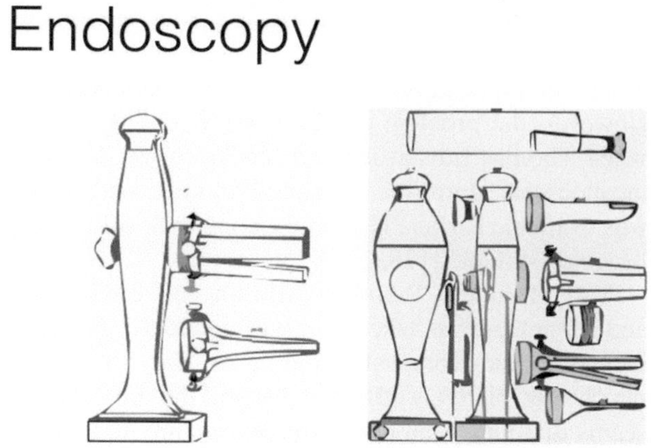

Fig. 8.12 Lichtleiter by Bozzini. Wikicommons, public domain. https://en.wikipedia.org/wiki/Philipp_Bozzini#/media/File:Bozzini_Lichtleiter.jpg

store electricity at the time were too heavy to carry and required an assistant to adjust them, he instead came up with a new idea of using a lamp that burned a combination of alcohol and turpentine. He showcased his rectoscope, which was 12 cm long, to the Academie des Sciences. After that, he also created an angled speculum and longer sigmoidoscopes were produced gradually. Eventually, around 1890, the length of the unyielding steel tube stabilized at 30 cm, and that remained the standard until the fiber-optic endoscope was developed. His instrument stimulated the interest of American medical instruments makers [138].

The history of endoscopy highlights two significant observations. Firstly, innovation in this field emerged as a result of close partnerships between physicians who faced clinical challenges to view pathology, and artisan-engineers who could devise solutions to those problems. Secondly, the advancement of endoscopy was mainly achieved by adapting technology from other domains. In fact, most of the technological innovations used in endoscopy were not originally developed exclusively for this purpose. Looking back, it becomes apparent that the basic components for every significant technological breakthrough were available for quite some time, often for many years. Due to the fact that endoscopy relied heavily on technology from other disciplines, once its practical use was imagined and piloted, it was able to evolve and improve more quickly.

8.7.2 Kussmaul (1898): First Gastroscopy

The pioneers of endoscopy encountered two significant challenges: The gastrointestinal tract is not a straight path, and the interior of the tract is dark. The first gastroscopy is usually attributed to Adolf Kussmaul (1822–1902) in 1868. During a gathering of the Freiburg Society of Naturalists, Adolf Kussmaul, a German Professor of Medicine, demonstrated the first gastroscope by inserting a stiff, hollow metal tube down the esophagus and into the stomach of a professional sword-swallower, which was the first gastroscope. Illumination was provided by a Desormeaux lamp attached proximally, but visibility was poor. Kussmaul's name is associated Kussmaul's breathing, the deep and laboured breathing associated with diabetic ketoacidosis, and with a sign where there is a paradoxical rise in JVP on inhalation in the presence of constrictive pericarditis.

However, the problem of illumination was not solved until approximately 1878, when Thomas Edison made a breakthrough. It took another 25 years before the incandescent lamp was integrated into endoscopes, even though Edison's solution was available earlier. Then endoscopy took off when a convenient electricity lamp became available [138, 139].

Von Mikulicz, Theodore Billroth and Leiter took an interest in gastroscopy and advantage was taken of a willing elderly female patient of von Mikulicz who had an aptitude for swallowing tubes. They shifted the light to the end of the tube which was relatively effective, but still the procedure required general anesthesia. It seems that they used the instrument mainly to investigate the normal stomach and oesophagus. By chance, the International Exhibition of Electricity took place in Vienna in 1885. It was there that Leiter discovered Edison's incandescent electric lamps, which he quickly incorporated into the endoscopes. Von Mikulicz made significant contributions to the field of medicine but passed away at the age of 55 due to stomach carcinoma. He is credited with having 18 medical procedures and pathological conditions named after him. Johann Mikulicz is credited with the design of the first successful and practicable esophagoscope in 1881 [140]. When people used these instruments, the results were mixed and some abandoned them altogether likely due to the occurrence of perforation.

8.7.3 George Kelling's Gastroscope (1898)

In 1898, George Kelling (1866–1945) created a gastroscope with a lower flexible segment that had a tip which could be angled using a system of wires controlled from the proximal end. However, this instrument was not widely accepted due to its clumsiness. In 1911, Elsner made modifications to the instrument by adding a safety device in the form of a rubber tip for insertion. Despite the lens system being prone to obstruction by mucus and stomach contents, it became popular and was used as the standard gastroscope for the next two decades [141].

Hoffmann (optical engineer from Munich) proposed a solution to the challenge posed by the convoluted nature of the gastrointestinal tract. He showed that light, and an image, could be conducted around a bend with a flexible tube containing articulated lenses and prisms. This approach was first introduced in 1911 [142].

It took around 20 years for the idea of using articulated lenses and prisms to be improved and implemented in the form of a semi-flexible gastroscope. *"By this time, the rigid endoscope proved to be too dangerous for regular gastroscopy due to esophageal and gastric perforations."*

This work was the result of collaboration between Schindler, a physician, and Richard Wolf, a manufacturer of medical instruments [143]. While exploring a store in Munich in 1920, Rudolf Schindler (1888–1968), a charismatic doctor, stumbled upon an old Elsner instrument that had been sitting unused for a decade. The idea of utilizing flexible quartz fibers for image transmission was developed in the late 1920s. He improved it with insufflating air which largely overcame the problem of the lens smearing. Schindler used the modified Elsner gastroscope successfully until 1932, at which point he reported his experience with a new semiflexible instrument. This instrument featured a flexible bronze spiral covered in rubber that replaced the lower third of the gastroscope. Schindler collaborated with the well-known Berlin instrument maker, George Wolf, to create this new device. Schindler was an inspiring teacher who meticulously recorded every examination he conducted. He also conducted extensive research into the structure and pathology of the upper alimentary tract, advancing the diagnosis and treatment of gastrointestinal disease.

In 1928, Heinrich Lamm (1908–1974), a medical student in Munich, attended a lecture by Schindler. After the lecture, Lamm approached Schindler with an idea. He suggested that a bundle of glass rods could conduct light and images more effectively than a system of lenses. This conversation between Schindler and Lamm is considered to be the beginning of the development of fiber-optic technology, which has revolutionized the visualisation of internal structures of the body and their pathology. Lamm was probably aware of the work of Daniel Colladon, who was an optical engineer based in Geneva, who in 1841 drew attention to the phenomenon of light being carried around a curve in water. This phenomenon is known as total internal reflection and is the principle that underlies the use of fiber optics. Total internal reflection occurs when light passes through a medium, such as glass or water, and is reflected back at the boundary between that medium and another medium with a lower refractive index, such as air. The reflected light remains trapped within the medium, and this property is harnessed in fiber-optic technology to transmit information via light signals.

Schindler's wife, Gabrielle Winkler, also played a significant role in his work. She was a charming and beautiful nursing attendant who had a calming effect on patients who were about to undergo endoscopy. Her presence and support likely helped to ease the anxiety and discomfort that patients may have felt during the procedure, which could have contributed to the overall success of Schindler's practice. Munich became the mecca of endoscopy.

In 1934, Schindler dismissed a housekeeper from his employ. The woman, unhappy with her dismissal, went to the Gestapo and reported that Schindler held anti-Nazi opinions. Sadly, despite his accomplishments and contributions to the field of medicine, Schindler, who was Jewish, was arrested and sent to the Dachau concentration camp. His non-Jewish German colleagues and colleagues in the United States protested and urged for his release. After 6 months of internment, Schindler was finally released from the camp. He was permitted to leave the country. He settled in Chicago as a visiting professor.

A German endoscopist named Sternberg used an instrument that resembled an elongated cystoscope and inserted it into patients while they were in a knee-elbow position. He claimed to have conducted 20,000 examinations with only six negative incidents, and one patient had been examined 100 times.

However, during a demonstration of his skill at a meeting of surgeons in Munich in 1923, he was unable to pass the instrument and ended up rupturing the patient's oesophagus. Unfortunately, the patient died due to mediastinitis as a result of the incident [143].

Up until 1947, the design of oesophagoscopes remained largely unchanged from those originally used by von Mikulicz in the 1880s. The only significant update during this time was the incorporation of an Edison lamp for illumination, which replaced the earlier gas lighting used in these instruments. This lack of innovation and improvement in oesophagoscope design is likely due to the limitations in technology and materials during this period, as well as the focus of medical research on other areas.

Nevertheless, it took until 1954 for Hopkins to construct a functional prototype of a flexible fiber imaging device [144].

In 1949, a new oesophagoscope was introduced by the Eder Instrument Company, which was designed by A. Ray Hufford. This instrument was significantly improved compared to previous models, especially with the substitution of a magnifying telescopic eyepiece for the previous lens-in-a-tube system. These improvements made the instrument more effective, and it quickly became the standard instrument used by doctors for oesophagoscopy [145]. The same year, a doctor working at the University of Tokyo Medical Center approached Olympus Optical Co., Ltd. (now known as Olympus Corporation) with a request to develop a camera that could be used to photograph and examine the interior of a patient's stomach. This request was prompted by the need for a less invasive and more effective method of diagnosing gastrointestinal diseases, as traditional methods such as oesophagoscopy and gastroscopy were often uncomfortable and produced low-quality images. Olympus responded by developing the first gastrocamera, which used a small camera attached to the end of an endoscope to capture high-quality images of the stomach and other parts of the digestive system. This invention was the next major advance the field of endoscopy and paved the way for further improvements in medical imaging technology.

In 1958, Larry Curtis, who was a physics graduate student at the time, collaborated with South African born Basil Hirschowitz (1925–2013), then a gastroenterology trainee, to develop a flexible fiber-optic endoscope [146, 147].

Further progress in fiber-optic endoscopy can be traced back to three conversations that took place during conversations in 1954. Timothy Counihan, who was working as a cardiology registrar at the Hammersmith Hospital in London, had a series of lunchtime conversations with Keith Henley [144]. During one of his visits to Arbor, Michigan, USA, Timothy Counihan had lunch with Basil Hirschowitz, a gastroenterology fellow who had been trained in the specialty with Avery Jones at the Central Middlesex Hospital in London. Hirschowitz told Henley about his research on creating a miniature camera that could be inserted into the stomach to capture diagnostic images.

During the 1960s, significant advancements occurred in the field of rigid laparoscopy. The work of Harold Hopkins, a British scientist, and Karl Storz, a German instrument engineer, revolutionized the field and laid the groundwork for modern laparoscopic technology and surgery. Specifically, the integration of the rod-lens optical system in 1967 played a crucial role in this transformation. Karl Storz, a German instrument maker, had proposed the idea of using fiber optics for medical applications to Professor Hopkins of Imperial College, London, prior to the lunchtime chats in 1954 that led to the development of the first fiber-optic endoscope. This idea was based on the concept of transmitting light through flexible glass fibers, which had been proposed by Hoffmann in Munich in the early 1900s. The principle they suggested was that light and image could be transmitted through a bent bundle up to 360°, making the lens in endoscopes replaceable [144]. Curtis solved the issue of preventing light leakage from individual fibers by covering them with a blend of glass core with high refractive index and a low refractive index that was melted together. A year later, they had developed a functional fiber bundle with sufficient length, a bright enough light source for color photography, a method for applying torque, and a waterproof coating. The first flexible endoscope that was both fully operational and effective was then developed by Basil Hirschowitz and made available for commercial use by ACMI in the autumn of 1960. Larry Curtis enhancements to prevent signal leakage were integrated into this device. Hirschowitz was then able to use the bundle on himself without the need for medication or surface anesthesia, and 1 week later, he successfully used it on a patient. This marked the birth of fully flexible fiber-optic endoscopy [147]. During a meeting of the American Gastroscopy Society in 1957, Hirschowitz presented a successful demonstration of the prototype for fiber-optic endoscopy. In attendance was Rudolf Schindler, who recalled his experience in 1928 with Heinrich Lamm and noted that the glass rods used at the time were inadequate due to the lack of coating and the absence of physicist input to further develop the design.

In 1969, the charge-coupled device (CCD) was invented. A decade after its invention, this technology was integrated into an endoscope [142]. With the invention of the CCD, electronic images could be produced, which made endoscopy accessible to a larger audience, including television viewers. Additionally, the digital nature of the images allowed for an immediate connection between the endoscope and computer interface [148].

From 1962 to 1972, American and Japanese instrument manufacturers made several improvements to endoscopes. They added separate channels for suction and introducing water and air, tips that could move in four directions, and an elongated model that could enter the duodenum. They also introduced an ultraslim model that could fit through a standard instrument's channel.

In 1966, a gastroenterologist from Glasgow named William Watson used an endoscope that entered the duodenum and observed the papilla of Vater. He suggested that it was possible to explore the ampulla using this method. Additionally, in 1965, two radiologists used a tube introduced through the mouth to cannulate the pancreatic duct and fluoroscopy confirmed its position. In 1968, the ampulla was cannulated endoscopically [149]. Classen and Demling performed a procedure in 1974 in which they used a bowstring wire diathermy to divide the papilla of the Ampulla of Vater, allowing them to remove a gallstone from the biliary tract, which marked the birth of the endoscopic retrograde cholangiopancreatography (ERCP) [150], the techiques for which were further developed and later taught by British gastroenterologist, Peter Cotton (b1939), working in Charleston, North Carolina.

In Sardinia in 1974, Luciano Provencales and Antonio Revignas replicated the procedure, but they made some modifications by adding a basic pulley system. They created a small bend at the end of the 4.5 meter tube that was inserted into the patient, and then threaded another 3 meter tube through it, folded in half. Once the combined system was pulled out from the anus, they attached a Hirschowitz side-viewing gastroscope to the end of it. By manipulating the instrument, they managed to reach the caecum and so colonoscopy was born [151].

ACMI Ltd. and Olympus corporations engaged in a process of continuous improvement resulting in endoscopes with improved angle of view, full-tip steerability, and effective biopsy capabilities along with other features for diagnosis and treatment, especially polypectomy. Wire loop snares passed through flexible endoscopes were a crucial development, allowing for polypectomy. This breakthrough was pioneered by William Wolff and Hiromi Shinya and paved the way for colon cancer surveillance and timely interventions [152].

A fiber-optic transmission-free endoscope was created by Welch Alleyn Incorporated in New York in 1983. Instead of a fiber-optic bundle, it had an electronic sensor at the tip of the instrument. This sensor contained a grid of photocell receptors that electronically transmitted images to a video processor, which then displayed them on a TV monitor. Later, improved versions of this technology were introduced by the Olympus Company and other Japanese manufacturers. Today, endoscopy of the upper and lower gastrointestinal tracts is one of the commonest procedures performed and allows for screening, diagnosis and surveillance of gastrointestinal conditions.

8.8 Thyroid Surgery

There are many reasons for enlargement of the thyroid gland or a goitre. These range from iodine deficiency, more common in mountainous regions, inflammatory causes of hypothyroidism, thyrotoxicosis (excess thyroid hormone) to cancer. The enlargement can be nodular (single or multiple) or diffuse throughout the whole gland. The thyroid secretes thyroid hormones which are essential to life, for without them, death from hypothyroidism (myxoedema) occurs within a few months. Goiter and thyroid nodules have afflicted humans since the earliest times, but in the ancient world, only persons who were being choked by the size of their gland would have contemplated surgery. Even then, a total thyroidectomy would not have been compatible with survival beyond a few weeks or months. The role of the thyroid in causing the myxoedematous symptoms was not appreciated until the end of the nineteenth century. Although thyroid extract then started to be given, thyroxine was not available until the early twentieth century. The parathyroid glands, responsible for calcium balance, were only discovered in the mid-nineteenth century.

Goitres were recognized in antiquity and were described in Chinese literature in 2700 BC. Abu al-Qasim (also known as Al-Zahrawi, 936–1013 CE), Islam's legendary medieval surgeon, is credited with performing the first goitre excision in Andalucia, Spain, during the Islamic Golden Age. In "*Al-Tasrif,*" Abu al-Qasim described his surgical techniques and instruments, including those he used in thyroid surgery. His work was to greatly influence the development of surgery in medieval Europe and beyond [153].

8.8.1 *The Development of Thyroid Surgery in Europe (Nineteenth to Twentieth Centuries)*

The history of modern thyroid surgery can be traced back to the late nineteenth and early twentieth centuries, when scientists and doctors first began developing the techniques and tools necessary to perform surgical procedures on the thyroid gland. The mid-nineteenth century marked a significant period of development, as the procedure became more widely practiced. However, there were still concerns about the considerable risks and challenges associated with the surgery (Fig. 8.13).

8.8.1.1 Dieffenbach

Johann Friedrich Dieffenbach (1792–1847), a prominent German surgeon of the early nineteenth century, was skeptical of thyroid surgery and cautioned against its widespread use. He believed that the surgery was too risky and offered little benefit to patients, dismissing the operation as "*foolhardy performance.*" Thyroid surgery was also banned by the French Academy of Medicine in the early nineteen century [153].

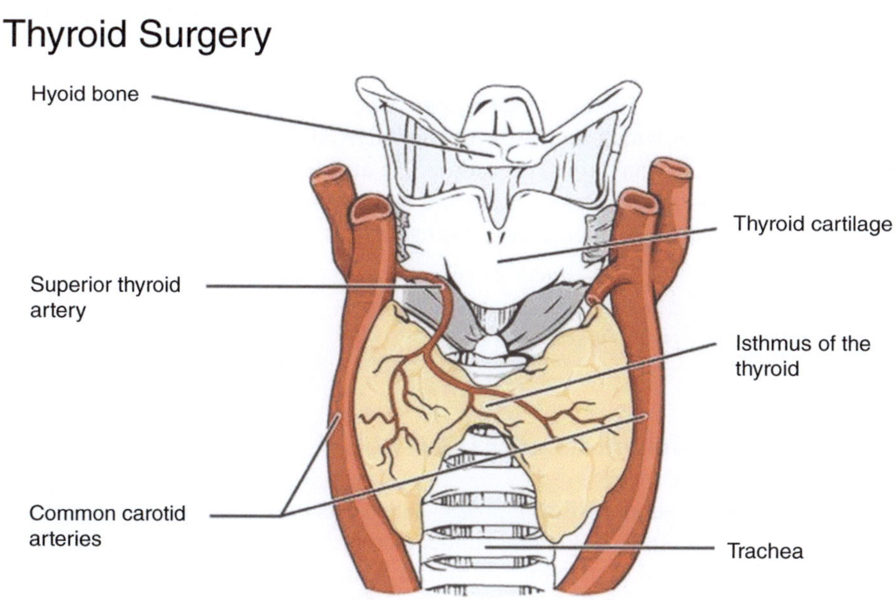

Fig. 8.13 Anterior anatomy of the Thyroid. Creative Commons Attribution-Share Alike. https://en.wikipedia.org/wiki/Thyroid#/media/File:Anterior_thyroid.jpg

8.8.1.2 Liston (1836)

Robert Liston (1794–1847), an Edinburgh University graduate who became Professor of Surgery at the University College Hospital in London, was one of the first surgeons to attempt this "*foolhardy performance*" with thyroidectomy in the 1820s. However, his early attempts were fraught with complications, including excessive bleeding and death. As a result, he became an outspoken critic of thyroid surgery and discouraged its use. In 1836, still before the introduction of anaesthesia, Liston published a paper in which he warned of the dangers of thyroid surgery, stating that it was a risky and potentially fatal procedure. He argued that the gland was too vascular and too closely intertwined with vital structures in the neck, making it nearly impossible to remove without causing serious bleeding or injury as he "*could not cut the thyroid gland out of the living body in its sound condition without risking the death of the patient from haemorrhage. It is a proceeding by no means to be thought of*" [154].

By 1850, some 4 years after the introduction of general anesthesia with ether or chloroform, there were about 70 reports of thyroidectomy having been performed with a mortality of 41%.

8.8.1.3 Samuel Gross in Philadelphia (1854)

Samuel David Gross (1805–1884) was an American surgeon who practiced in the mid-nineteenth century. A Jefferson Medical College graduate, whose early career was in Louisville, Virginia, he returned to Jefferson and Philadelphia as Professor of Surgery in 1856. Like Liston, he was a prominent and influential figure in his field but also shared some of Liston's reservations about thyroid surgery. In 1854, Gross published a paper in which he was critical of thyroid surgery, believing it to be a risky, and potentially dangerous, procedure. He argued that the gland was difficult to remove without causing serious harm and that removal of the gland could lead to a range of complications, including hypothyroidism (myxoedema), so denounced the procedure as

> *horrid butchery .... deserving of rebuke and condemnation ....* [that] *no honest and sensible surgeon would ever engage in* [155].

8.8.1.4 Theodor Billroth in Zurich (1860–67)

In his early career, Theodor Billroth (1829–1894) was Professor of Clinical Surgery in Zurich (1860–1867), having trained under Bernard von Langenbeck (1810–1887) at the Charité Hospital in Berlin. Billroth, a strong proponent of surgical audit, reporting good and bad results, initially recommended thyroid surgery for compressive symptoms but became disappointed when 8 of his 20 patients died postoperatively. This led him to abandon the operation. In Zurich, Billroth did train Theodor

Kocher (1841–1917) who was to be the one who would make the operation of thyroidectomy safe and effective.

8.8.1.5 Theodor Billroth in Vienna (1867–94)

However, with later improvements in general anesthesia and haemostats, he was able to reinstitute the operation, reducing the mortality to less than 10%. He was one of the first surgeons to perform thyroidectomy using a laryngoscope to visualize the vocal cords and avoid injury to the recurrent laryngeal nerves, whose innervation of the vocal cords is so crucial for a normal voice. He also developed a technique for ligating the blood vessels supplying the gland to minimize bleeding during surgery.

Billroth trained an amazing generation of surgeons. One was his assistant Anton Wölfler (1850–1917) who, in Vienna, described the condition of tetany following thyroid surgery. Although this was due to parathyroid damage or removal, the function of the parathyroid glands was not known at this time. Wölfler's career progressed to become Professor of Surgery in Graz in 1886, and then in Prague from 1895.

8.8.1.6 Parathyroid Identification by Ivar Sandström in Sweden (1877)

In 1877, in Uppsala, Sweden, Ivar Sandström (1852–1889), then a medical student, identified the last organ in the human body, "glandulae parathyroideae" [156]. His paper was published in Swedish in 1880 based on the evidence amassed from human cadaver dissections and animals. A parathyroid gland had been previously described from the dissection of an Indian rhinoceros at London Zoo by Sir Richard Owen (1804–1892) in 1852, though his paper was not published until 1862. Owen, also a surgeon and previously Hunterian Professor then Curator at the RCS (1836–1956), was then Curator of the Natural History Museum in London. Sandström was not aware of Owen's previous discovery of the gland.

At the time of discovery of the parathyroid glands by Sandström, their function was not known. Another decade passed before, in 1891, Eugéne Gley (1857–1930), Professor of Physiology in Paris, showed that tetany occurs when the parathyroids were removed with the thyroid, but also, sometimes, even if the thyroid was left in situ [157].

8.8.1.7 Ernst von Eiselsberg

Ernst von Eiselsberg (1860–1939) was a prominent Austrian surgeon and another former assistant of Theodor Billroth. In the late nineteenth and early twentieth centuries, he made significant contributions to the field of endocrine surgery, including pioneering work on the transplantation of parathyroid tissues. Eiselsberg was one of the first surgeons to recognize the importance of the thyroid gland in regulating metabolism and growth. Another of Billroth's assistants, Johann von Mikulicz developed the idea of subtotal resection to preserve thyroid function and to spare the parathyroids from damage.

8.8.1.8 Theodor Kocher in Bern

Theodor Kocher (1841–1917) was a prominent Swiss surgeon and one of the most influential figures in the development of modern thyroid surgery. When he accepted a chair at the University of Bern in 1872, he found himself surrounded by patients suffering from endemic goiter, a condition caused by iodine deficiency, particularly prevalent in mountainous regions of the world.

At the time, thyroid surgery was still considered a risky and dangerous procedure, so many surgeons, including his mentor Billroth, had suspended the practice due to the high risk of complications. However, Kocher was determined to find a safe and effective way to remove the enlarged thyroid gland and alleviate the symptoms of endemic goiter. Through years of experimentation and innovation, Kocher developed a series of better techniques and approaches for thyroid surgery that significantly reduced the risk of complications and improved patient outcomes. He introduced ways of visualizing and protecting the recurrent laryngeal nerve, which is crucial for normal voice function, and for controlling bleeding during surgery.

Kocher's work on thyroid surgery quickly gained acceptance among peers across the world. His greatest contribution to physiology was that he showed that the thyroid gland was essential for human health. He also recognized the risk of recurrent laryngeal nerve injury and tetany as serious postoperative complications, advocating for more cautious dissection during surgery. He went on to become one of the most celebrated surgeons of the early twentieth century, receiving the Nobel Prize in Physiology or Medicine in 1909 for his contributions to the field of thyroid surgery and endocrine physiology. He was the first surgeon to receive a Nobel Prize. Remarkably, Kocher's operative mortality rate had reduced to 0.2% by 1898 [157]. Unsurprisingly, as his fame spread, Bern became the global capital for thyroid surgery, attracting observers from far and wide.

One of his most important contributions was the development of staged thyroid surgery, which involved a series of procedures designed to gradually reduce the size of the thyroid gland and alleviate the symptoms of goitre or thyrotoxicosis, a disease that was first described by Robert Graves. In the first stage of the procedure, Kocher would ligate several named thyroid arteries to reduce the blood supply to the gland and decrease its size. This was followed by a second stage in which one side of the thyroid gland was removed in a procedure known as lobectomy. If the patient continued to experience symptoms of thyrotoxicosis or if the gland continued to grow, a third stage would be considered in which the remaining lobe of the thyroid gland would be removed or reduced in size [159]. Kocher (among others) proposed that surgeons conserve part of the gland to prevent *cachexia strumipriva*, which is hypothyroidism, a "bad condition due to removal of a struma (goitre)." The thyroid hormones and their effect on metabolism were not yet known.

In Kocher's time, thyroid surgery became neither "foolhardy" nor "deserving of rebuke and condemnation." It was also safe, with a low operative mortality, and the complications of postoperative hypothyroidism, tetany and vocal cord paralysis, were understood and minimised.

8.8.1.9 William Halsted

William Halsted (1852–1922) visited the main clinics of Europe, observing Billroth and Kocher in performing their thyroid surgery. Halsted was intrigued by this gland, the surgical techniques employed, and the differences in outcomes between Kocher's and Billroth's procedures. Halsted observed that Kocher's meticulous approach to tissue handling and haemostasis resulted in complete excision of the thyroid gland with minimal damage beyond its capsule with less cases of hypothyroidism and less parathyroid dysfunction. In contrast, Billroth's less meticulous approach may have resulted in incomplete excision of the thyroid gland, leaving residual tissue but potentially also damaging or excising the parathyroid glands resulting in less hypothyroidism but more parathyroid damage. Returning home, Halsted's subtotal thyroidectomy technique proved successful and was subsequently widely adopted around the world.

In the early years of thyroid surgery, postoperative sepsis and operative haemorrhage were major causes of mortality. To combat these issues, European surgeons began adopting principles of asepsis and using multiple haemostats to ensure adequate control of bleeding during surgery. Halsted adopted the new measures of adequate haemostasis and asepsis. This involved using multiple clamps and ligatures to control blood flow to the thyroid gland, as well as carefully dissecting the gland to avoid damage to surrounding blood vessels. These changed the surgical landscape for thyroidectomy in North America. Halsted demonstrated relief from tetany with injection of parathyroid extract. He went on to verify that parathyroid transplants would alleviate hypocalcemia and tetany.

William Halsted is also credited with introducing the use of rubber gloves during surgery which not only protected the hands of surgical personnel but also improved asepsis in the operating room by reducing the risk of contamination from the hands of surgical personnel [160].

8.8.1.10 Charles and William Mayo (1890)

Charles Mayo (1865–1939) undertook urgent thyroid surgery in 1890 when a burly local farmer had a goitre with compressive symptoms that threatened his breathing. In view of the precarious airway, he and his brother William (1861–1939) used a slash-and-grab technique. Hemorrhage was heavy, but control was achieved by packing the cavity and oversewing the skin. Packs were removed days later, and the patient returned to work on his farm soon after.

8.8.2 *Graves Disease*

Graves' disease (thyrotoxicosis), now known to be an autoimmune condition against TSH receptors in the thyroid, and is associated with exophthalmos in about 20–30% of cases.

8.8.2.1 Robert Graves (1796–1853)

The exophthalmic presentation was described on three patients in 1835 by an Irish physician, Robert James Graves (1796–1853). Graves was an outstanding, eloquent, and systematic teacher, fluent in many European languages including French and German, who was to become President of the Royal College of Physicians in Ireland (1843–44) where there is a statue in his honour. His other contributions to medicine include timing the pulse using a watch and describing the pinhole pupil of pontine hemorrhage. He even suggested that his own epitaph should be "*he fed fevers.*"

Graves may not have been the first to describe thyrotoxicosis and exophthalmos despite his name now forever associated with it. Caleb Hillier Parry (1755–1822), a physician in Bath, England, saw a patient with exophthalmic goitre in 1786. He amassed eight patients with the disease but his paper was not published until 1825, 3 years after his death.

Another claimant would be an Italian surgeon and anatomist, Giuseppe Flajani (1741–1808), who described the condition in 1802. Carl von Basedow (1799–1854) in Merseburg, Germany, described a triad of goitre, exophthalmos, and heart palpitations in 1840, five years after Graves.

8.8.2.2 Surgery for Graves' Disease

Mayo's success with thyroid surgery led to offering surgery for Graves' disease. However, it was his physician colleague, Dr. Henry Plummer (1847–1936), who made surgery for Graves' disease safe. Plummer, who also provided the first description of toxic multinodular goiter, recognized the benefit of using iodine in the preoperative preparation of patients with exophthalmic goiters, which helped to reduce the size and vascularity of the thyroid gland, making the surgery safer and more effective. With Plummer's preoperative management, Mayo's operative mortality rate for Graves' disease decreased significantly to less than 1%, and the need for staged surgery was also reduced. The use of iodine in the preoperative preparation of patients with difficult to control thyrotoxicosis remains an important part of modern thyroid surgery practice [161, 162].

Surgery remained challenging and risky on patients with thyrotoxicosis with high mortality rates. George Washington Crile (1864–1943) was caught in a "thyroid storm" during his early career in Cleveland. In 1895, he performed a total thyroidectomy on a patient with Graves' disease, but the patient died 2 days later from postoperative hyperthyroid crisis. This experience led Crile to investigate the physiology of the thyroid gland and ultimately develop the first effective treatment for thyroid storm [163]. Lahey also recognized the importance of proper preoperative preparation and introduced the use of the basal metabolic rate as a marker for hyperthyroidism. He allowed patients to rest in the hospital for several days to stabilize their metabolic rates and then administered iodine to reduce the rates to normal before proceeding with surgery. This approach helped to reduce the risk of postoperative complications in patients with hyperthyroidism [162, 164]. However, many thyroid pathologies are only amenable to adequate treatment with thyroid hormone replacement and this was till not available in the nineteenth century, nor first decade of the twentieth.

8.8.3 Thyroid Hormone Replacement

The key to understanding the physiological role of the thyroid was to make the link between the thyroid and myxoedema.

8.8.3.1 The Discovery of Iodine

Iodine was only discovered by French chemist Bernard Courtois (1777–1838) in 1811. He was working in the saltpetre business but the Napoleonic wars had created a shortage of wood ash from which potassium nitrate is made. He used seaweed as an alternative source of potassium nitrate but also accidentally discovered iodine was emitted after adding sulphuric acid to the seaweed ash. The gas produced was crystallized into iodine flakes and further studied by French chemist Louis Gay-Lussac (1778–1850). British scientist, Humphrey Davy (1778–1829), who proposed the name iodine, assisted by Michael Faraday (1791–1867), worked on the new substance in Paris in 1813, having received special permission to do so from Napoleon. In 1822, Courtois began manufacturing high-quality iodine and its salts and later received the prestigious Montyon Prize from the French Royal Academy of Sciences, awarded on account of its medicinal value. In 1808, Humphrey Davy was also the first to isolate pure calcium and magnesium.

8.8.3.2 Iodine for Endemic Goitre

Swiss physician, Jean-Francois Coindet (1774–1834), in 1820, was perhaps one of the first in Europe to report iodine's efficiency in treating endemic goitre. He also recommended using it preoperatively to reduce the size of the thyroid and its vascularity. However, he may have been preceded by William Prout in London in 1816, who treated one case but did not publish an account until 1834. St. Thomas' Hospital adopted the remedy in 1819 [165].

August Hirsch (1817–1894), a German physician based in Danzig, wrote a three-volume work, *Handbook of Geographical and Historical Pathology*, noting the prevalence of goitre and cretinism in mountainous regions and its absence in costal regions. The three volumes were published between 1883 and 1886. There is mention of the curative power of iodine, but none of iodine being preventative [166].

8.8.3.3 Treatment of Goiter in Ancient China

However, the Chinese had long used seaweed to treat goitre with references to the practice in 1600 BCE. They also recognized that living in the mountains too long was associated with goitre. In the fifth century CE, *the Goitre Prescriptions of Abbot Shen* lists a treatment with powdered shells of mollusks.

There are also accounts of seaweed and algae being imported into South America's Andean Highlands, another endemic goitre area [167, 168].

The Chinese also used animal thyroid extracts to treat hypothyroidism. Air-drying animal thyroids to a powder and drinking with wine was mentioned in *Old and New Tried and Tested Prescriptions* (*Gujin lu yanfang*) about 640 CE. *The Medical Secrets of an Official (Waitai Miyao)* by Wang Tao, recommends steeping sheep's thyroids in wine and afterward roasting them and taking one daily (752 CE). At the end of the sixteenth century, Li Shizen's *Great Pharmacopoeia* published in 1593, mentions treating goitre with thyroid extract.

8.8.3.4 Hypothyroidism and Cretinism

Hypothyroidism was recognized as a clinical condition as a result of a series of cases presented in London. In 1850, Thomas Blizzard Curling (1811–1888), surgeon at the London Hospital, described two children, aged 10 and 6 months, with cretinism and in whom no thyroid tissue was found at autopsy.

8.8.3.5 Hypothyroidism and Myxedema

In 1871, Charles Hinton Fagge (1838–1883), a physician at Guy's Hospital presented four cases aged 8 to 20 without goitre who were cretinous but whose mental development was normal. Further reports followed by Sir William Withey Gull (1816–1890) in 1873, also at Guy's Hospital, who described cretinous signs (thick deep voice, loss of hair, folds of skin around the neck, and weight gain) in those without a goitre. He made the first true clinical description of hypothyroidism. William Miller Ord (1834–1902) described non-pitting "mucous oedema" and called the condition myxoedema and also the practical annihilation of the thyroid at autopsy. Once Ord had published his paper and made the connection of his case with the earlier reports, many other physicians and surgeons realized they had seen cases of hypothyroidism too [169–171].

8.8.3.6 Postoperative Hypothyroidism

In 1882–3, Swiss surgeon, Jacques-Louis Reverdin (1842–1929), and his cousin, Auguste Reverdin (1848–1908), presented and later published a series of 22 cases of thyroidectomy to the Medical Society of Geneva with outcomes similar to Gull and Ord's myxoedematous patients. Reverdin began modifying his technique to perform subtotal thyroidectomies. Kocher, who was to receive the Nobel Prize in 1909, claimed to be the first to note the effect of a total thyroidectomy in these goitrous patients. However, Stefan Slater, in part 2 of his three-part series of the discovery of thyroid replacement therapy, finds Reverdin's account the more convincing, as is claimed in Henri Reverdin's biography of his father! Kocher had the larger series, well researched and verified, but his 1883 paper describing *cachexia strumipriva* was, in fact, myxoedema or hypothyroidism, as described by Ord, but in Kocher's series, the hypothyroidism was caused by surgical removal of the thyroid. Kocher was an amazing surgeon, but he was also described as *"very touchy, he hardly overcame setbacks. Likewise he insisted on the priority of his work and merits, where aggressively defended.... he had only a few close friends"* (Slater, Liebermann-Meffert) [156–159, 166].

Felix Semon (1849–1921) was to become a prominent laryngologist and a knight of the British realm. However, in 1883, as a young surgeon at St. Thomas' Hospital, he proposed, on the basis of a presentation he heard from Theodor Kocher the year before, that myxoedema, *cachexia strumipriva*, and cretinism were all due to thyroid degeneration or deficiency. Semon's (not Kocher's) presentation was said to have evoked some ridicule (officially, "polite skepticism") at the time. We should note in Kocher's presentation of 1882 that Reverdin had presented to the Geneva Medical Society in September 1882, when Kocher was present. Yet Kocher gave Reverdin no acknowledgment in his Nobel lecture in 1909 [167, 168].

8.8.3.7 Experiments with Thyroid Replacement

In 1885, Victor Horsley (1857–1916) reported the effects of thyroidectomy in monkeys, concluding that myxoedema was due to loss of the thyroid. In 1884, Moritz Schiff in Geneva transplanted canine thyroid into thyroidectomized dogs. Kocher had also tried thyroid transplantation in one patient. In 1890, Antonio-Maria Bettencourt-Rodrigues (1854–1933) and J-A Serrano in Lisbon inserted half of a sheep's thyroid subcutaneously into the inframammary region of each side of one of their patients. They found the graft worked immediately, before it could have derived a blood supply. Others injected thyroid extract intravenously into dogs with good temporary effect, so there was a growing recognition of the thyroid's function, though the word "endocrine" was not coined until 1904. A proposal in 1891, by George Murray (1865–1939), to give an extract of sheep's thyroid subcutaneously was ridiculed by the profession, most probably because Murray was only 3 years qualified! However, he proceed to treat a 46-year-old woman with myxoedema, and in 3 months, she was better. In two of Murray's cases, they died while on treatment, probably from myocardial infarction, but it was only years later that he found that for these cases, the butcher had supplied thymus not thyroid [158–160, 169, 170]!

Although Murray was in England, publishing in English, he was not the first to give subcutaneous injections. He duly acknowledged Bettencourt and Serrano (see above) in his 1891 publication.

Thyroid extract was then taken orally with success though it tastes awful and needs to be flavored, similar to what the Chinese had found over 1500 years before. Murray's first patient lived 28 years until her death aged 74 and by then, having switched to oral ingestion, had consumed 5 liters of thyroid extract, from 870 sheep!

8.8.3.8 Thyroid Hormone (1914)

On Christmas day, 1914, Edward Kendall's isolation of thyroid hormone represented a major breakthrough, paving the way for the later synthesis of thyroxine (T4) by Charles Harington and George Barger in 1927. This work revolutionized the diagnosis and treatment of thyroid disorders, and T4 became a mainstay of thyroid hormone replacement therapy. It was not commercially manufactured until 1947 [171].

Radioactive Iodine

As the role of iodine in thyroid hormone synthesis became better understood, on November 12, 1936, at a Harvard Medical School seminar entitled "*What Physics Can Do for Biology and Medicine*," Dr. Karl Compton (1887–1954) mentioned that "the 1938 Nobel prize-winning physicist Enrico Fermi (1901–1954) had successfully produced by neutron bombardment several short half-life radioactive isotopes in his laboratory." In the audience was a group of clinicians interested in iodine metabolism. They included Saul Hertz (1905–1950), then Director of the Massachusetts General Hospital Thyroid Unit, as well as Howard Means (1885–1967), then head of the Department of Medicine at MGH. Hertz asked Compton, "Could iodine be made radioactive artificially?" A few days later, after discussing the question with his collaborator, Dr. Robley Evans, Compton replied to Dr. Hertz by letter and a fruitful collaboration for radioactive iodine treatment began. In 1936, Massachusetts Institute of Technology (MIT) president, Karl Compton, and the Massachusetts General Hospital thyroid group produced small amounts of short-lived radioiodine (iodine 128, 25 min). They demonstrated that it was selectively trapped by the follicles of the thyroid gland. Radioiodine treatment of hyperthyroidism was not widely adopted by the end of the war in 1945, due to a shortage of radioiodine and the invention of antithyroid drugs. However, by 1946, radioiodine became readily available as a by-product of the Manhattan project, begun a decade earlier. Hundreds of patients were soon being treated for hyperthyroidism, and later, adjuvant radioactive iodine treatment of thyroid cancer was introduced based on the iodine 131 radioisotope [172].

Medical Treatment of Thyrotoxicosis

During the 1940s, Edwin Bennett Astwood (1909–1976), an American endocrinologist, discovered thiourea had antithyroid properties, then thiouracil was found to be better. Propylthiouracil received FDA approval in 1947. He also found methimazole (thiamazole), a drug discovered in 1889, had less side effects which led to its publication and widespread use as the antithyroid drug of first choice from the 1950s [173].

8.8.4 Hashimoto's Thyroiditis

Hakaru Hashimoto (1881–1934) was the first to describe an inflammatory condition of the thyroid marked by histological findings in four middle-aged women of lymphoid follicles, changes in thyroid epithelial cells, extensive connective tissue, and diffuse round cell infiltration. All four women had goitres, while two had hypothyroidism. He named the goitrous lymphocytic thyroiditis *struma lymphomatosa*. He described lymphocytic infiltration formation of lymphoid follicles with germinal centers.

He was a third-generation Japanese doctor who graduated from Kyusyu Imperial University in Fukuoka in 1907. He worked in a surgical department for 4 years on thyroid tissue, publishing his work in 1912, in a German Journal. He then worked in Professor Kaufmann's surgical department in Göttingen until World War I (1914–18) broke out and he was forced to return to Japan (which was on the allies side, not Germany's during the war). His 30-page monograph was the only publication he ever wrote on the thyroid because he abandoned his academic career at the age of 35, returning to his birthplace (Midau, Nishi-tsuge in the Mie prefecture, IgaUeno) to take over the family practice, making the career and life choice to financially support his family. He then ran the family practice for two decades until he died of typhoid fever in 1934.

Hashimoto's thyroiditis started to be used in his honour posthumously in Europe and North America in the 1930s, but the eponym was not reintroduced to Japan until 1950.

Riedel's thyroiditis was first described by Bernhard Moritz Carl Ludwig Riedel (1846–1916), a former pupil of Bernhard von Langenbeck (1810–1887), in 1896, although he had first recognized it in 1883 while working in Aachen. The disease is characterized by extensive fibrosis—*struma fibromatosis*.

Riedel's lobe of the liverd (a rare downward projection of tissue from the right lobe) is named after him. Riedel is also renowned for performing the first choledochoduodenostomy and was a pioneer of appendicectomy and cholecystectomy. From 1888, he worked as Director of the Surgical Clinic at the University of Jena, and became President of the German Surgical Society in 1907.

Fritz De Quervain (1868–1940) was a Swiss Surgeon who was Professor of Surgery in Basel (1910–1918), then from 1918, becoming Professor of Surgery in Bern (succeeding Kocher). He gave his name to the transient, self-limiting, but often painful thyroiditis associated with a viral illness. He also named a tenosynovitis of extensor tendons of the thumb. In 1914, he designed an operating table that won the "*grand prize*" at the World Exhibition in Paris. He introduced iodized table salt to treat endemic goitre in Switzerland [174].

8.8.5 Hyperparathyroidism

The discovery of the parathyroids and their role in postthyroidectomy tetany has been described above. Most humans have four parathyroid glands, though a small number will have three or five. They are derived from the third and fourth pharyngeal pouches and descend in development with the third pouch derivatives descending further than the fourth to become the inferior parathyroid glands, usually somewhere lateral to the recurrent laryngeal nerve.

One or more of the parathyroid glands may develop an adenoma or all of them may be subject to hyperplasia. The excess parathyroid hormone secreted demineralizes the bones, with excessive blood calcium that is then excreted in the urine. Patients with hypercalcemia present with a range of symptoms from fatigue, memory loss, poor concentration, polyuria, and thirst to florid bone disease, urinary calculi, confusion, and mental disturbance. Hyperparathyroidism is a rare cause of pancreatitis and from the 1930s was recognized to be also associated with peptic ulcer. *Bones, stones, and abdominal groans* was a description given by Walter T St. Goar in 1957. *Psychic moans* were added by William Mieher, Yvan Thibaudeau, and Boy Frame reporting on the neuropsychiatric impact of primary hyperparathyroidism. These include apathy, agitated depression, psychosis with hallucinations or delusions, paranoia, and dementia.

8.8.5.1 Osteitis Fibrosa Cystica of von Recklinghausen

In 1891, Friedrich Daniel von Recklinghausen (1833–1910) reported a patient who had recurrent fractures, with malformed long bones, showing extensive fibrosis, cysts, and brown tumors. The condition became known as osteitis fibrosa cystica of von Recklinghausen, a severe form of long-standing hyperparathyroidism. However, it was not until 1915, that Friedrich Schlagenhaufer (1866–1930) in Vienna made the connection between the parathyroids and the disease.

Similar cases were described by Max Askanazy in 1904, Schmorl in 1907, Molineus and Poltauf in 1913, and Harbitz in 1915.

Parathyroid hyperplasia was noted by Jakob Erdheim (1874–1937) in Vienna to be associated with osteomalacia in 1906, but in this case, the hyperplasia was secondary to the bone disease.

8.8.5.2 Parathyroids and Calcium Homeostasis

In 1909, William MacCallum (1874–1944) and Carl Voegtlin (1879–1960) recognized that the parathyroids controlled calcium homeostasis and that the tetany complicating thyroidectomy could be managed by intravenous calcium.

William MacCallum was Professor of Pathology at Columbia University/New York Presbyterian Hospital (1908–17) before being appointed to Johns Hopkins in Baltimore from 1917 to 1943. Voegtlin was a Swiss, University of Basle, graduate who emigrated to the United States and worked at Johns Hopkins.

8.8.5.3 Sir John Bland-Sutton and the First Intentional Parathyroidectomy

Sir John Bland-Sutton (1855–1936) performed the first intentional parathyroidectomy at the Middlesex Hospital, London. He had already described a parathyroid tumour found at autopsy in 1886 and had removed a parathyroid cyst in 1909, before carrying out a parathyroidectomy on a young woman prior to 1917. The case is described in the 1917 (sixth) edition of his textbook *Tumours, Innocent, and Malignant,* but was never published in a journal. The patient's left-sided parathyroid tumour was clinically palpable below the thyroid and had earlier presented as a choking attack with dyspnoea. At surgery, the mass removed was the size of a cherry, confirmed to be parathyroid on histology.

Bland-Sutton went on to be President of the Royal College of Surgeons in 1923. One of his most important contributions to clinical surgery was to transform abdominal hysterectomy from a high-risk, disreputable procedure into one that was safe and effective.

8.8.5.4 Felix Mandl Performs Parathyroidectomy in Vienna (1925)

Felix Mandl (1898–1993) is usually credited with having performed the first parathyroidectomy in Vienna in 1925. His 34-year-old patient, Albert Jahne, developed leg pains and fatigue and 2 years later had radiological evidence of osteopaenia and bone cysts, soon followed by a fracture. Mandl found that he had hypercalcaemia and high calcium excretion in the urine. After giving treatments with thyroid and then parathyroid extracts to no avail, Mandl then explored the neck and removed a 21 × 15 × 12 mm parathyroid adenoma. He soon began to improve over the next few weeks. However, Martell developed recurrent disease after 7 years for which he was reexplored but died of renal failure. His autopsy did not show any evidence of parathyroid disease.

8.8.5.5 Charles Martell and His Seven Explorations

The next documented patient who had a parathyroidectomy reminds all parathyroid surgeons as to what can go wrong. Charles Martell was a sea captain with severe bone disease. In May 1926, he was operated on by Edward Richardson at the Massachusetts General Hospital (MGH) but without success.

He ended up having seven procedures in New York and Boston before the tumour was found. At MGH, Edward Churchill (1895–1972), assisted by 1928 Harvard graduate, Oliver Cope (1902–1994), reexplored the neck but no gland was found and they then opened the chest to find the elusive gland. Unfortunately, Martell experienced tetany and died in renal failure. However, not to be deterred, Churchill and Cope went on to perform 30 cases by 1936. In 1951, Cope published an 11-case series of hyperparathyroidism due to parathyroid hyperplasia, the first person to differentiate this condition from parathyroid adenoma. Cope also published a series of 200 cases in 1958, finding a single adenoma in 79%, double adenoma in 5%, and hyperplasia in 7%.

Parathyroid carcinoma was first described by Russell Wilder in 1929. By 1953, there had been 120 cases reported.

Parathyroid hormone was first isolated in 1925, by Canadian James Bertram Collip (1892–1965). He, together with Leitch, treated tetany successfully, that same year. It was first named *parathyrin*. Collip was also a co-discoverer of insulin together with Banting, Best, and McLeod. The parathyroid hormone was isolated and purified by Ramussen and Craig in 1959, with its polypeptide structure defined by them in 1962.

At MGH, endocrinologists Fuller Albright (1900–1969) and Read McLane Ellsworth (1899–1970) and team first described idiopathic primary parathyroidism and also described secondary hyperparathyroidism in 1932. Tertiary hyperparathyroidism was described in the late 1960s being recognized as the development of an adenoma when the secondary hyperparathyroidism has been resolved (e.g., renal transplantation).

8.8.5.6 Preoperative Localization

Attempts at preoperative localization of parathyroid adenomas began in the 1950s. Selective venous sampling, preoperative injections of toluidine blue and methylene blue were then used. Thyroid ultrasound and CT were introduced in the 1970s. In the 1980s, Thallium 201 Tc 99 pertechnetate was introduced, and then Tc 99 sestamibi. Today, 4D (the fourth dimension is time) parathyroid CT scan is also used. Localization of a single gland preoperatively allows a focused approach to surgery resulting in a small scar and earlier recovery. The skill of the surgeon remains the most important method of actual localization of an adenoma, which are, predictably, sometimes elusive and difficult to find. Nonetheless, 95% of persons with primary hyperparathyroidism can expect to be cured by surgery. Where patients are not suitable for surgery or need to wait for their surgery, cinacalcet offers a pharmacological means of lowering serum calcium. It was first approved for use in the United States and Europe in 2004 [175, 176].

References

1. Rutkov IM. Surgery: an illustrated history. St. Louis: Mosby Year Book; 1993.
2. Bodemer CW. France the fundament and the rise of surgery. Dis Colon Rectum. 1983;26:743–50.
3. Hourly History. King Louis XIV: a life from beginning to end. Monee: Hourly History; 2017.
4. Herrod PJJ, Kwok AT, Lobo DN. Three centuries of appendicectomy. WJS. 2023;47:928–36.
5. Hancock H. Disease of the appendix caeci cured by operation. Lond Med Gaz. 1848;7:547–50.
6. Editorial. Lorenz heister (1683–1758) eighteenth century surgeon. JAMA. 1967;202:136–7.
7. Bellis S. Surgery for the acute abdomen—an intriguing history of the laparotomy procedure. Cam Med J. 2018:1–3. https://doi.org/10.7244/cmj.2018.12.002.
8. Todman D. A history of caesarean section: from ancient world to the modern era. Aust N Z J Obstet Gynaecol. 2007;47:357–61.
9. Kompanje EJO. A remarkable case in the history of obstetrical surgery: a laparotomy performed by the Dutch surgeon Abraham Cyprianius in 1694. Eur J Obs Gyn Rep Biol. 2005;118:119–23.
10. Antoine Lembert 1802–1851. Study on intestinal suture with a description of a new procedure for performing this surgical operation. 1826. Dis Colon Rectum. 1988;31(6):489–94.
11. Guivarc'h M. Antoine-Joseph Jobert de Lamballe 1799-1867; ou l'essor de la chirurgie moderne [Antoine-Joseph Jobert de Lamballe 1799-1867; or the impetus of modern surgery]. Hist Sci Med. 2000;34(3):253–70. French. PMID: 11640520.
12. Hardy KJ. A view of the development of intestinal surgery. Part II. Principles and techniques. ANZ J Surg. 1990;60:377–84.
13. Ellis H. Operations that made history. Cambridge University Press; 1996.
14. Wilson E. A place for colostomy in the treatment of ulcerative colitis. Dis Colon Rectum. 1973;16:98–102.
15. Gross SD. A system of surgery. Philadelphia: Blanchard and Lea; 1866.
16. Meade RH. An introduction to the history of general surgery. Philadelphia: WB Saunders; 1968. p. 277–314.
17. Baum W. Resection eines carcinomatoses Dickdarmstuckes. Centralblatt fur Chir. 1879;6:169.
18. Dukes CE. Frederick Salmon. Founder of the St Mark's Hospital, London. Med Hist. 1959;3:312–6.
19. Hilton J. The classic: on rest and pain: lecture XIV. Clin Orthop Relat Res. 2009;467(9):2208–14. https://doi.org/10.1007/s11999-009-0928-1. Epub 2009 Jun 16. PMID: 19529972; PMCID: PMC2717375.
20. Corman ML. John Percy Lockhart-Mummery. Dis Colon Rectum. 1984;27:208–14.
21. Perrin WS. Some landmarks in the history of rectal surgery. Proc R Soc Med. 1931;
22. Dixon CF. Anterior resection for malignant lesions of the upper part of the rectum and lower part of the sigmoid. Ann Surg. 1948;128:425–42.
23. Heald, R. J.; Husband, E. M.; Ryall, R. D. H. (1982). "The mesorectum in rectal cancer surgery—the clue to pelvic recurrence?". Br J Surg 69 (10): 613–616. https://doi.org/10.1002/bjs.1800691019. PMID 6751457. S2CID 6200459.
24. Heald RJ, Ryall RDH. Recurrence and survival after total mesorectal excision for rectal cancer. Lancet. 1986;327:1479–82.
25. Graney MJ, Graney CM. Colorectal surgery from antiquity to the modern era. Dis Colon Rectum. 1980;23:432–41.

26. Ravitch MM. The use of stapling instruments in surgery of the gastrointestinal tract, with a note on a new instrument for end-to-end low rectal and oesophagojejunal anastomoses. Aust N Z J Surg. 1978;48:444–7.
27. Knight CD, Griffen FD. An improved technique for low anterior resection of the rectum using the EEA stapler. Surgery. 1980;88:710–4.
28. Bonjer HJ, Deijen CL, Abis GA, Cuesta MA, van der Pas MH, de Lange-de Klerk ES, et al. A randomized trial of laparoscopic vs open surgery for rectal cancer. N Engl J Med. 2015;372:1324–32.
29. Atallah S, Albert M, Larach S. Transanal minimally invasive surgery: a giant leap forward. Surg Endosc. 2010;24:2200–5.
30. Habr-Gama A, Perez RO, Nadalin W, Sabbaga J, Ribeiro U Jr, Silva e Sousa AH Jr, et al. Operative vs nonoperative treatment for stage 0 distal rectal cancer following chemoradiation therapy: long-term results. Ann Surg. 2004;240:711–7; discussion 717.
31. Petrelli F, Trevisan F, Cabiddu M, et al. Total neoadjuvant therapy in rectal cancer: a systematic review and meta-analysis of treatment outcomes. Ann Surg. 2020;271:440–8.
32. Hashizume M, Konishi K, Tsutsumi N, Yamaguchi S, Shimabukuro R. A new era of robotic surgery assisted by a computer-enhanced surgical system. Surgery. 2002;131:S330–3.
33. Parks AG. A technique for excising extensive villous papillomatous change in the lower rectum. Proc R Soc Med. 1968;61:441–2.
34. Parks AG, Nicholls RJ. Proctocolectomy without ileostomy for ulcerative colitis. BMJ. 1978;2(6130):85–8. https://doi.org/10.1136/bmj.2.6130.85. PMC 1605901. PMID 667572.
35. Nestorovic M, Petrovic D, Stanojevic G, Milijkovic D, et al. One hundred years of miles' operation – what has changed? Acta Med Med. 2008;47:43–6.
36. A tale of two surgeons. Gertrude Herzfeld and Graham Fraser. Ghosh SK. Giovanni Battista Morgagni (1682–1771): Father of pathologic anatomy and pioneer of modern medicine. Anat Sci Int. 2017;92:305–12. https://doi.org/10.1007/s12565-016-0373-7.
37. Lau WY, Leow CK. History of perforated duodenal and gastric ulcers. World J Surg. 1997;21(8):890–6. https://doi.org/10.1007/s002689900323.
38. Lovasik BP, Dodson TF, Srinivasan JK. Heineke, Mikulicz, Jaboulay, and Finney: innovators of surgical pyloroplasty. Am Surg. 2021;87(5):737–40. https://doi.org/10.1177/0003134820952820. Epub 2020 Nov 10
39. Hertz AF. IV. The cause and treatment of certain unfavorable after-effects of gastro-enterostomy. Ann Surg 1913;58(4):466–472. https://doi.org/10.1097/00000658-191310000-00004. PMID: 17863076; PMCID: PMC1407579.10.5958/0976-5506.2018.01521.8.
40. Baillie M. The morbid anatomy of some of the most important parts of human body. London: L Johnson; 1793. p. 87.
41. Balfour DC. JAMA. 1925;84:876.
42. Brigham CB. Boston Med Surg J. 1898;138:415.
43. Weil PH, Buchberger R. From Billroth to PCV: a century of gastric surgery. WJS. 1999;23:736–42.
44. Markatos K, Sardiniari S, Brilakis E, Apostolopoulos I, Tsoucalas G, Chronopoulos E. Jules Pean (1830–1898)-A Pioneer surgeon: his achievements and his Total shoulder arthroplasty. Surg Innov. 2019;26(6):763–5. https://doi.org/10.1177/1553350619875303. Epub 2019 Sep 11
45. Roux JC. Rev Gynae. 1897;I:67.
46. Mayo-Robson A. Lancet. 1904;I:671.
47. Gordon-Taylor G. The present position of surgery in the treatment of bleeding peptic ulcer. Br J Surg. 1946;34:336–45. https://doi.org/10.1002/bjs.18003313207.
48. Pauchet V. Trans. by I. Macdonald (1920). Lancet. 1920;I:308.
49. Connell AM. Fundusectomy: a new approach to surgical treatment of duodenal ulcer. J Int Coll Surg. 1955;24(5 Pt 1):531–47.
50. Dragstedt LR, Owens FM. Proc Soc Exp Biol (NY). 1943;53:152.

51. Watts G. Nobel prize is awarded to doctors who discovered H. Pylori. BMJ. 2005;331:795.
52. Adachi Y, Mimori K, Mori M, et al. Morbidity after D2 and D3 gastrectomy for node-positive gastric carcinoma. J Am Coll Surg. 1997;184:240–4.
53. Groves EW. On the radical operation for cancer of the pylorus: with especial reference to the advantages of the two-stage operation and to the question of removal of the associated lymphatics. Br Med J. 1910;1:366–70. https://doi.org/10.1136/bmj.1.2563.366.
54. Appleby LH. The coeliac axis in the expansion of the operation for gastric carcinoma. Cancer. 1953;6:704–7. https://doi.org/10.1002/1097-0142(195307)6:4<704::AID-CNCR2820060410>3.0.CO;2-P.
55. Gouzi JL, Huguier M, Fagniez PL, et al. Total versus subtotal gastrectomy for adenocarcinoma of the gastric antrum. A French prospective controlled study. Ann Surg. 1989;209:162–6. https://doi.org/10.1097/00000658-198902000-00005.
56. Cuschieri A, Weeden S, Fielding J, et al. Patient survival after D1 and D2 resections for gastric cancer: long-term results of the MRC randomized surgical trial. Surgical Co-operative Group. Br J Cancer. 1999;79:1522–30. https://doi.org/10.1038/sj.bjc.6690243.
57. Huang JQ, Hunt RH. pH, healing rate and symptom relief in acid-related diseases. Yale J Biol Med. 1996;69:159–74.
58. Georgoula C, Gardiner M. Pyloric stenosis a 100 years after Ramstedt. Arch Dis Child. 2012;97(8):741–5. https://doi.org/10.1136/archdischild-2011-301526. Epub 2012 Jun 9
59. Spaner SJ, Warnock GL. A brief history of endoscopy, laparoscopy, and laparoscopic surgery. J Laparoendosc Adv Surg Tech A. 1997;7(6):369–73. https://doi.org/10.1089/lap.1997.7.369.
60. Morgenthal CB, Richards WO, Dunkin BJ, Forde KA, Vitale G, Lin E, SAGES Flexible Endoscopy Committee. The role of the surgeon in the evolution of flexible endoscopy. Surg Endosc. 2007;21(6):838–53. https://doi.org/10.1007/s00464-006-9109-4. Epub 2006 Dec 16. PMID: 17180263.
61. Mazurak M, Patkowski D. A history of the surgical correction of pyloric stenosis. J Pediatr Surg. 2021;56(10):1904–7. https://doi.org/10.1016/j.jpedsurg.2021.05.009. Epub 2021 May 26
62. Foster JH. History of liver surgery. Arch Surg. 1991;126:381–7.
63. Kokudo N, Takemura N, Ito K, Mihara F. The history of liver surgery: achievements over the past 50 years. Ann Gastroenterol Surg. 2020;4:109–17. https://doi.org/10.1002/ags3.12322.
64. Tilton BT. Some considerations regarding wounds of the liver. Ann Surg. 1905;41:20–30.
65. Glisson F. Anatomia hepatis Typ. London: Du-Gardianis; 1654. Available on Google Scholar
66. Cantlie J. On a new arrangement of the right and left lobes of the liver. J Anat Physiol (London) (Section Proc Anat Soc Great Britain & Ireland). 1898;32:4–10.
67. Keen WW. IV. Report of a case of resection of the liver for the removal of a neoplasm, with a table of seventy-six cases of resection of the liver for hepatic tumors. Ann Surg. 1899;30(3):267–83. https://doi.org/10.1097/00000658-189907000-00023.
68. Parks RW, Garden OJ. Liver resection for cancer. World J Gastroenterol. 2001;7:766–71.
69. Pringle JH. Notes on the arrest of hepatic haemorrhage due to trauma. Ann Surg. 1908;48:541.
70. Bismuth H, Eshkenazy R, Arish A. Milestones in the evolution of hepatic surgery. Rambam Maimonides Med J. 2011;2(1):e0021. https://doi.org/10.5041/RMMJ.10021. PMID: 23908793; PMCID: PMC3678786.
71. Fineberg C, Goldburgh WP, Templeton JY 3rd. Right hepatic lobectomy for primary carcinoma of the liver. Ann Surg. 1956;144:881–92. https://doi.org/10.1097/00000658-195611000-00013.
72. Lortat-Jacob JL, Robert HG. Well defined technic for right hepatectomy. Presse Med. 1952;60:549–51. French.
73. Lin TY, Tsu K, Mien C, Chen C. Study on lobectomy of the liver. J Formosa Med Assoc. 1958;57:742–9.
74. Pamecha V, Gurusamy KS, Sharma D, Davidson BR. Techniques for liver parenchymal transection: a meta-analysis of randomized controlled trials. HPB (Oxford). 2009;11:275–81.
75. Brunschwig A. Hepatic lobectomy for metastatic cancer. Cancer. 1963;16:277–82.

76. Felekouras ES, Kaparelos DC, Papalambros E. The history of liver surgery, hepatectomy and haemostasis. Hell J Surg. 2010; https://doi.org/10.1007/s13126-010-0046-2.
77. Gosink BB. Evaluation of hepatic neoplasms. AJR Am J Roentgenol. 1980;134:621.
78. Couinaud C. Lobes et segments hepatiques. Presse Med. 1954;62:709–12.
79. Bismuth H. Surgical anatomy and anatomical surgery of the liver. World J Surg. 1982;6:3–9. https://doi.org/10.1007/BF01656368.
80. Bismuth H, Houssin D, Castaing D. Major and minor segmentectomies "réglées" in liver surgery. World J Surg. 1982;6:10–24. https://doi.org/10.1007/BF01656369.
81. Lazorthes F, Chiotasso P, Chevreau P, Materre JP, Roques J. Hepatectomy with initial suprahilar control of intrahepatic portal pedicles. Surgery. 1993;113:103–8.
82. Asiyanbola B, Chang D, Gleisner AL, et al. Operative mortality after hepatic resection: are literature-based rates broadly applicable? J Gastrointest Surg. 2008;12:842–51. https://doi.org/10.1007/s11605-008-0494-y.
83. Starzl TE. Experience in hepatic transplantation. Philadelphia: W.B. Saunders; 1969.
84. Calne RY. Immunosuppression for organ grafting-observations on cyclosporin A. Immunol Rev. 1979;46:113–24.
85. Hardy KJ. Liver surgery: a revolution. ANZ J Surg. 1989;59:519–21.
86. Gawande A. Two hundred years of surgery. N Engl J Med. 2012;366:1716–23.
87. Ahrendt SA, Pitt HA. A history of bilioenteric anastomosis. Arch Surg. 1990;125:1493–500.
88. Cervantes J. Common Bile duct stones revisited after the first operation 110 years ago. WJS. 2000;24:1278–81.
89. Griffin JF, Poruk KE, Wolfgang CL. Pancreatic cancer surgery: past, present and future. Chin J Cancer Res. 2015;27:332–48.
90. Navarro S. The art of pancreatic surgery. Past, present and future. The history of pancreatic surgery. Gastroenterol Hepatol. 2017;40:648.e1.
91. Da Costa J. On the morbid anatomy and symptoms of cancer of the pancreas [Extracted from the Proceedings of the Pathological Society of Philadelphia]. Philadelphia: J. B. Lippincott & Co.; 1858. Available at https://iiif.wellcomecollection.org/pdf/b21113142
92. Thornton JK. The surgical treatment of diseases of the liver. BMJ. 1886;2:901–3.
93. Monprofit A. On Cholecystenterostomy in the form of a "Y.". Br Med J. 1908;2:991.
94. Witzel O. Aus der Klinik des Herrn Prof. Trendelenburg. Beiträge zur Chirurgie der Bauchorgane. Deutsche Zeitschrift für. Chirurgie. 1886;24:326–54.
95. Halsted WS. Contributions to the surgery of the bile passages, especially of the common bile-duct. Boston Med Surg J. 1899;141:645–54.
96. Howard JM. History of pancreatic head resection—the evaluation of surgical technique. Am J Surg. 2007;194:S6S10.
97. Senn N. Surgery of the pancreas as based upon experiment and clinical researches. Trans Am Surg Assoc. 1886;4:99–123.
98. Desjardins A. Technique de la Pancréatectomie. Rev Chir. 1907;35:945–73.
99. Coffey RC. XVII. Pancreato-enterostomy and pancreatectomy: a preliminary report. Ann Surg. 1909;50:1238–64.
100. Kausch W. Das Carcinom der Papilla duodeni und seine radikale Entfernung. Beitr Klin Chir. 1912;78:439–86.
101. Banting FG, Best CH. The internal secretion of the pancreas. J Lab Clin Med. 1922;7:251–66.
102. Are C, Dhir M, Ravipati L. History of pancreaticoduodenectomy: early misconceptions, initial milestones and the pioneers. HPB. 2011;13:377–84.
103. Whipple AO, Parsons WB, Mullins CR. Treatment of carcinoma of the ampulla of Vater. Ann Surg. 1935;102:763–95.
104. Crile G Jr. The advantages of bypass operations over radical pancreatoduodenectomy in the treatment of pancreatic carcinoma. Surg Gynecol Obstet. 1970;130:1049–53.
105. Collins JJ Jr, Craighead JE, Brooks JR. Rationale for total pancreatectomy for carcinoma of the pancreatic head. N Engl J Med. 1966;274:599–602.

106. Hall AD, Kumar JE, Mazur JP, Bondoc AJ, Griffin BF, Bryant WK. Dr Allen Oldfather Whipple (1881-1963): Namesake of the pancreaticoduodenectomy. J Med Biogr. 2023; https://doi.org/10.1177/09677720231197430.
107. Brunschwig A. Resection of head of pancreas and duodenum for carcinoma–pancreatoduodenectomy. CA Cancer J Clin. 1974;24:363–7.
108. Whipple AO. A reminiscence: pancreatic duodenectomy. Rev Surg. 1963;20:221–5.
109. Whipple AO. Observations on radical surgery for lesions of the pancreas. Surg Gynecol Obstet. 1946;82:623–31.
110. Crist DW, Sitzmann JV, Cameron JL. Improved hospital morbidity, mortality, and survival after the Whipple procedure. Ann Surg. 1987;206:358–65.
111. Ohhashi K, Murakami F, Maruyama M, Takekoshi T, Ohta H, Ohhashi I, Takagi K, Kato Y. Four cases of mucous secreting pancreatic cancer. Prog Dig Endosc. 1982;20:348–35.
112. Dimagno E, Regan P, Wilson D, et al. Ultrasonic endoscope. Lancet. 1980;315:629–31.
113. Hargest R. Five thousand years of minimal access surgery: 3000BC to 1850: early instruments for viewing body cavities. J R Soc Med. 2020;113(12):491–6. https://doi.org/10.1177/0141076820967913. Epub 2020 Nov 2. PMID: 33135953; PMCID: PMC7816654.
114. Hargest R. Five thousand years of minimal access surgery: 1850 to 1990: technological developments. J R Soc Med. 2021;114(1):19–29. https://doi.org/10.1177/0141076820967918. Epub 2020 Nov 2. PMID: 33135950; PMCID: PMC8173353.
115. Hargest R. Five thousand years of minimal access surgery: 1990-present: organisational issues and the rise of the robots. J R Soc Med. 2021;114(2):69–76. https://doi.org/10.1177/0141076820967907. Epub 2020 Nov 2. PMID: 33135951; PMCID: PMC7879007
116. Bozzini P. Der Lichtleiter oder die Beschreibung einer einfachen Vorrichtung und Ihre Anwendung zur Erleuchtung innerer Höhlen und Zwischenräume des lebenden animalischen Körpers. Weimar: Verlag des Landes Industrie Comptoir; 1807.
117. Hatzinger M, Fesenko A, Büger L, Sohn M. Dimitrij Oscarovic Ott (1855–1929) "Die Ventroskopie": Sein Beitrag zur Entwicklung der Laparoskopie [Dimitrij Oscarovic Ott (1855–1929) "Ventroscopy": His contribution to development of laparoscopy]. Urologe A. 2013;52(10):1454–8. https://doi.org/10.1007/s00120-013-3224-3.
118. Hatzinger M, Badawi JK, Häcker A, Langbein S, Honeck P, Alken P. Georg Kelling (1866–1945): the man who introduced modern laparoscopy into medicine. Urologe A. 2006;45:868–71. https://doi.org/10.1007/s00120-006-1068-9.
119. Kelling G. Über Oesophagoskopie, Gastroskopie und Koelioskopie. Münchener Medizinische Wochenschrift. 1902;49:21.
120. Litynski GS. Endoscopic surgery: the history, the pioneers. World J Surg. 1999;23:745–53. https://doi.org/10.1007/s002689900576.
121. Goetze O. Die Röntgendiagnostik bei gasgefüllter Bauchhöhle; eine neue Methode. Munch Med Wochenschr. 1918;65:1275–80.
122. Kalk H. Erfahrungen mit der Laparoskopie (zugleich mit Beschreibung eines neuen Instrumentes). Z Klin Med. 1929;111:304–48.
123. Fiorina C. Presented at: Richmond forum; January 19, 2008; Richmond, VA.
124. Nezhat C, Page B. Let there be light: an historical analysis of endoscopy's ascension since antiquity. Available at: http://laparoscopy.blogs.com/endoscopyhistory. Accessed January 2008
125. Veres J. Neues Instrument zur Ausführung von Brust oder Bauchpunktionen und Pneumothoraxbehandlung. Deut Med Wochenschr. 1938;64:1480–1.
126. Hopkins H, Kapany N. A flexible fibrescope, using static scanning. Nature. 1954;173:39–41.
127. Schollmeyer T, Soyinka AS, Schollmeyer M, Meinhold-Heerlein I. Georg Kelling (1866–1945): the root of modern day minimal invasive surgery. A forgotten legend? Arch Gynecol Obstet. 2007;276:505–9. https://doi.org/10.1007/s00404-007-0372y.

128. Litynski GS. Kurt Semm and the fight against skepticism: endoscopic hemostasis, laparoscopic appendectomy, and Semm's impact on the "laparoscopic revolution". JSLS. 1998;2:309–13.
129. Nezhat F. Triumphs and controversies in laparoscopy: the past, the present, and the future. JSLS. 2003;7:1–5.
130. Berci G, Davids J. Endoscopy and television. BMJ. 1962;1:1610.
131. Kelley WE Jr. The evolution of laparoscopy and the revolution in surgery in the decade of the 1990s. JSLS. 2008;12(4):351–7. PMID: 19275847; PMCID: PMC3016007
132. Dubois F, Icard P, Berthelot G, et al. Coelioscopic cholecystectomy: preliminary report of 36 cases. Ann Surg. 1990;211:60–2.
133. Cuscheri A, Berci G, McSherry CK. Laparoscopic cholecystectomy. Am J Surg. 1990;159:273.
134. Gagner M, Lacroix A, Bolte E. Laparoscopic adrenalectomy in Cushing's syndrome and pheochromocytoma. N Engl J Med. 1992;327(14):1033.
135. Allori A, Leitman M, Heitman E. Natural orifice transluminal endoscopic surgery: lessons learned from the laparoscopic revolution. Arch Surg. 2008;143:333–4.
136. Semm K. Pelviskopie und Hysteroskopie. Farbatlas und Lehrbuch. Stuttgart: F.K. Schattauer Verlag GmbH; 1976. p. 7–14.
137. Segalas PR. Un moyen d'eclairer I'uretre et la vessie de maniere a voir dans I'interieur de ces organes. Revue Medicale Francaise et de L'etrangere. 1827;1:157–8.
138. Desormeaux AJ. De l'Endoscopie, instrument propre a' ec lairer certaines cavities interieures de l'economie. C R Acad Sci. 1855;40:692–3.
139. Kluge F, Seidler E. Zur Erstanwendung der Ösophago- und Gastroskopie: Briefe von Adolf Kussmaul und seinen Mitarbeitern. Med Hist J. 1986;21:288–307.
140. Mikulicz J. Uber Gastroskopie und Oesophagoskopie. Weiner Medizinische Presse. 1881;22:1406–7.
141. Kelling G. Endoskopie fur Spiesrohre und Magen. Munchener MedizinischWochenschrifter. 1898;49:1556–9.
142. Hoffmann M. Optische Instrumente mit beweglicher Achse und ihre Verwendlung für die Gastroskopie. Münch Med Wochenschr. 1911;58:2446–8.
143. Schindler R. Gastroscopy with a flexible gastroscope. Am J Dig Dis Nutr. 1935;2:656.
144. Hopkins HH, Kapany NS. A flexible fiberscope, using static scanning. Nature. 1954;76:864–9.
145. Taylor H. A new gastroscope with controllable flexibility. Lancet. 1941;2:276–7.
146. Hirschowitz BI, Curtiss LE, Peters CW, et al. Demonstration of a new gastroscope, the "fiberscope.". Gastroenterology. 1958;35:50–3.
147. Hirschowitz B, Peters CW, Curtis LE. Preliminary report on a long fibres cope for examination of stomach and duodenum. Med Bull (Ann Arbor). 1957;23:178–80.
148. Sivak MV Jr, Fleischer DE. Colonoscopy with a video endoscope: Preliminary experience with a new type of endoscope. Gastrointest Endosc. 1983:29187.
149. McCune WS, Shorb PE, Muscovitz H. Endoscopic cannulation of the Ampulla of Vater; a preliminary report. Ann Surg. 1968;167:752–6.
150. Classen M, Demling L. Endoskopische Sphinkterotomie der Papilla Vateri and stein-extraction aus dem Ductus Choledochus. Deutsche Mediziner Wochenschrift. 1974;99:496–7.
151. Provenzales L, Revignas A. Metodica originaledi esplorazione strumentale transanale polivalente del colon intero. A Rap Med Sarda. 1966;69:131–40.
152. Wolff I, Shinya H. A new approach to colonic polyps. Ann Surg. 1973;178:367–78.
153. Diffenbach JF. Die Operative Chirurgie II. Leipzig: FA Brockhaus; 1848.
154. Liston R, Mutter TD. Lectures on the operations of surgery and on diseases and accidents requiring operations. Philadelphia: Lea & Blanchard; 1846. p. 318.
155. Gross SD. A system of surgery. 4th ed. Philadelphia: Lea & Febiger; 1866. p. 394.
156. Sandstrom Ueber eine neue druse beim menschen und dei verschiedenen saugethieten. Upsala Lakarfor Forhandl. 1880;14:441.
157. Gley E. Sur les effets de l'estirpation du corps thyroide. C R Soc Biol (Paris). 1891;43:55.
158. Becker WF. Presidential address: pioneers in thyroid surgery. Ann Surg. 1977;185:493–504.

159. McGreevy PS, Miller FA. Biography of Theodor Kocher. Surgery. 1969;65:990.
160. Graves RJ. Newly observed affection of the thyroid gland in females. Lond Med Surg J. 1835;7:516.
161. Halsted WS. The operative story of goiter: the author's operation. Johns Hopkins Hosp Rep. 1920;19:71.
162. Mayo CH. Surgery of the thyroid: observations on 5000 operations. JAMA. 1913;61:10.
163. Crile GW. Graves disease, a new principle of operating, based on a study of 352 operations. JAMA. 1911;56:637.
164. Lahey FH. Exposure of recurrent laryngeal nerves in thyroid operations. Surg Gynecol Obstet. 1944;78:293.
165. Slater S. The discovery of thyroid replacement therapy. Parts I, II and III. J R Soc Med. 2011;104:15-18/59-63/100-106.
166. Reverdin J-L, Reverdin A. Note sur vingt-deux opération de goitre. Rev Med Suisse Romande. 1883;3:169–98.
167. Kocher T. Ueber kropfextirpation unde ihre folge. Archive fur Klinisiche Chirugie. 1883;29:254–337.
168. Liebermann-Meffert D. Short story of Theodor Kocher's life and relationship to the International Society of Surgery. WJS. 2000;24:2–9.
169. Bettencourt R, Serrano J-A. Un cas de myxoedème traité par la greffe hypodermique du corps thyroide d'un mouton. Sem Med. 1890;10:294.
170. Murray GR. Note on treatment of myxoedema by hypodermic injections of an extract of thyroid gland of a sheep. BMJ. 1891;ii:796–7.
171. Kendall EC. The isolation in crystalline form of the compound containing iodine, which occurs in the thyroid: its chemical nature and physiologic activity. JAMA. 1915;64(25):2042–3.
172. Becker DV, Sawin CT. Radioiodine and thyroid disease: the beginning. Semin Nucl Med. 1996;26(3):155–64. https://doi.org/10.1016/s0001-2998(96)80020-1. PMID: 8829276
173. Burch HB, Cooper DS. Anniversary review: Antithyroid drug therapy: 70 years later. Eur J Endocrinol. 2018;179(5):R261–74. https://doi.org/10.1530/EJE-18-0678.
174. Sawin CT. The heritage of Dr. Hakaru Hashimoto (1881-1934). Endocr J. 2002;49:399–403.
175. Delbridge LW, Palazzo FF. First parathyroid surgeon: Sir John Bland-Sutton and the parathyroids. ANZ J Surg. 2007;77:1058–61.
176. Dorairajan N, Pradeep PV. Vignette hyperparathyroidism: glimpse into history. Int Surg. 2014;99:528–33.

Chapter 9
Daring to Dream of Equal Opportunity in Surgery

Female Pioneers in Surgery

9.1 Trotula and the Medical School of Salerno [1]

9.1.1 Salerno, Europe's First Medical School in the Second Millennium CE

Salerno opened the first University in Europe including a Medical Faculty in the eleventh century CE. Remarkably, their courses were open to both genders! The city was a Mediterranean port, South of Naples, which fused influences of Arab and Byzantine-Greek culture. It became a stopover city on the Crusade route. The school had benefited from the teachings of Constantine the African in 1077 and his translation of many texts back from Arabic to Latin. The Medical School of Salerno was initially sanctioned by the church and grew in reputation and size becoming a point of attraction for both the sick and students of medicine from all over Europe. However, recognizing the need for doctors to be properly qualified, in 1231, the authority of the school was sanctioned by Emperor Federico II. By authority of the constitution of Melfi, it was established that the activity of a doctor could only be carried out by doctors holding a diploma issued by the Medical School of Salerno. In 1280, Charles II of Anjou approved the first statute in which the School was recognized for the General Study of Medicine.

Trotula de Ruggiero (1050–1090) was at least a midwife, most probably a gynaecologist, who wrote at least three major works on *Conditions of Women*, *The Treatments for Women*, and *On Women's Cosmetics*. *De Passionibus Mulierum*

This section covers the nineteenth to twenty-first centuries and belongs as a transition to the advances of the twentieth to twenty-first centuries.

S. Abbas, D. Watters, *The Road to Modern Surgery*,
https://doi.org/10.1007/978-981-96-4337-0_9

Curandorum became the textbook of obstetrics and gynecology for four centuries [2]. She wrote the following on inducing menstruation:

The best remedy for producing the menses is to take an equal quantity of flammula, Hemlock, caftorei, myrrh, century and saliva; let a flower be made and let one Dram be given in water in which nettle and myrrh have been cooked. Let her drink this In a bath, one scruple to be taken at a time....

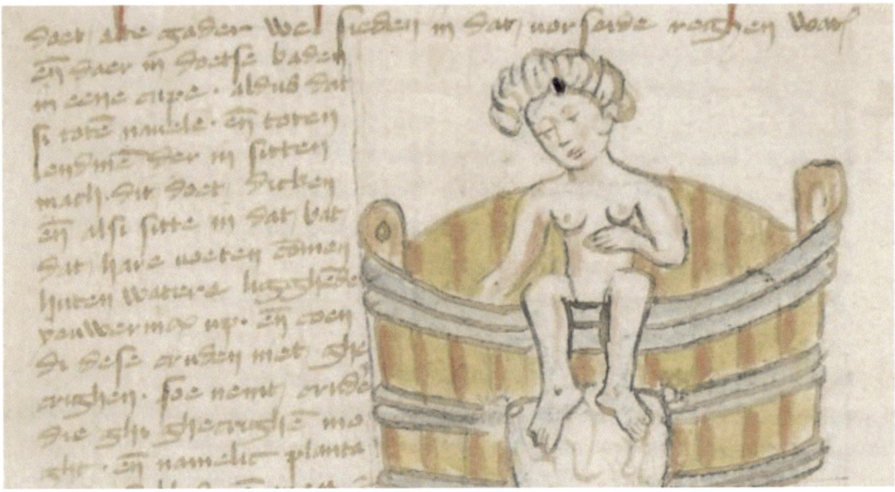

Figure: De Passionibus Mulierum Curandorum

In the book she describes accurately how to repair a third degree tear, and also how to reduce uterine prolapse.

"Likewise to some women harm occurs in childbirth on account of the mistakes of those attending.

There are some for whom vulva and anus become one and the same passage. From these women the womb comes out and becomes hard.

These we aid by putting it back. We apply to the womb hot wine in which butter has been boiled. We carefully foment it until the womb is rendered soft

And then we gently put it back. After this, we sew the break between the anus and the vulva in three or four places with a silk thread; afterwards we apply a

Linen cloth to the vulva... we smear this with a liquid pitch, which on account of its stench makes the womb withdraw.

Although there is also much on herbal remedies that looks strange and off beam today, the recipes and concoctions were then mainstream and state-of-the-art treatments for medieval times. Later, Guy de Chauliac in the fourteenth century, or Symphorien Champier in the sixteenth century, would offer similar treatment recommendations, and some will have been based on those recommended by Trotula whose work was well known and regarded! Some historians have questioned Trotula's credentials, perhaps because she was a woman, and have queried whether Trotula was or became a *nom de plume*. Given that, in every age, women have practiced medicine despite the prejudice shown and obstacles put in their way, one suspects that some male historians may have let their prejudice against women doctors cloud their assessment of Trotula's authorship.

From the eleventh to fifteenth centuries, women were not only able to study medicine but were able to be members of Faculty. At least five other women certainly taught at the Medical School of Salerno during these centuries, one of whom, Constance Calenda, an ophthalmic surgeon, was the daughter of the Dean of the Faculty of Medicine in 1415, with a medical degree from the University of Naples. The others are known for their medical texts. Rebecca de Guarna (circa 1200) was the author of *De Urinis*, *De Febrius*, and *De Embrione*; Abella (circa 1380) wrote *De atrabile (black bile)* and *De natura seminist.* In the fourteenth century, Mercuriade wrote three medical texts (*De Febre Pestilenti, De Curatio*, and *De Ungentis*), and Clarice di Durisio da Foggia (fifteenth century) who treated only women but did surgery and ophthalmology.

However, even the presence of female faculty at a University did not mean that there was equal opportunity for women in Southern Italy. In the first 35 years of the fourteenth century in the city State of Naples, there were only 18 licenses issued to women, while there were over 3000 for men. Those women who were registered tended to come from medical families, often being the wife or daughter of a surgeon. Two examples were Lauretta and Francesca de Romana. In 1309, Lauretta was licensed as competent to treat abscesses and external wounds and to operate for stone. Her medical and surgical expertise was such that she was even forgiven by the authorities for not knowing Latin! She had been examined by Professor Francesco da Piedmonte who declared:

> *She has been examined by our royal physicians and surgeons in the art of surgery, and although she knows no Latin, she has been found competent.*

In 1321, Francesca de Romana, the wife of Matteo, was a surgeon who passed an examination before a commission of doctors and surgeons even although she had not undergone a University Training.

9.1.2 Paris Eleventh to Sixteenth Centuries [3]

In Paris, one could practice medicine or surgery with a license, but it would not be until the 1860s that women were allowed to enter the University of Paris, and during the Renaissance years, physicians made it progressively harder for the mediciennes and chirugiennes, as they were called, to practice. In 1292, there were eight licensed female physicians in Paris. When Jacobina Felice (trained in Florence and with 30 years of experience) faced Court, the Court ruled: "*of course men can understand the subject of medicine better because of their gender.*"

From 1484, there was further restriction of women's right to practice until finally in 1694, even the widows of surgeons were also banned from surgical practice, "*except in cases of dire want.*"

As the power of the universities grew, they became places for the education of men, and, whether deliberate or not, women found themselves excluded and legally exposed, having no alternative but to practice without a certificate – and yet such female practitioners were still desperately needed by their families, by their communities, and especially by the poor!

However, it was still possible for women to train as a midwife in Paris. One of the most famous midwives was Louise Bourgeois (1563–1568), the wife of a Barber Surgeon, who had been examined by a panel of a physician, two surgeons, and two midwives, and so received her certificate to practice. She became the royal midwife, delivering the children of Henry IV and Marie de Medici. She was paid 500 crowns for a boy and 300 for a girl! Her surgical repertoire included operating for stone, excising tumors, and repairing wounds. In 1627 she delivered the Duchess of Orleans who died of puerperal sepsis after the birth. The male doctors who performed the autopsy reported there was a retained placenta, so Bourgeois had to defend her knowledge and standards of practice:

> *By your report [...] you expose your utter ignorance of what constitutes a woman's afterbirth [placenta], whether before or after labor....I have practiced my profession now for fully thirty-four years, faithfully, diligently, and honourably, and acquired not only a good certificate, after various examinations, but have also written books treating on this subject, which have been printed and published in several editions and were translated into foreign languages, for which trouble many noted physicians have rendered me thanks and have gladly confessed that they were of great use to humanity.*

However, health practitioners were a varied lot in the late Middle Ages, and throughout the fifteenth and sixteenth centuries at a time when medical practice was just beginning to distance itself from astrology and occultism.

The City of Worms (1609) warned against a variety of itinerant practitioners peddling drugs. They should not sell internal medicines but stick to their tooth whitening powders and roots. The health peddlers were not only the selling drugs but also bogus health concoctions, while occulists, palm readers, and astrologers sought to derive profitability from their medical offerings. Some of itinerants were clearly women which led the German city of Worms to pronounce:

> *We will tolerate the practice or prescription of medicine by no one in our city regardless of whether they are man or woman, Christian or Jew, or whatever they like to call themselves, who does not hold the higher degree of Doctor of Medicine or some other good certificate from a reputable University.* [Wolfenbuttel HAB 34.3 MED (8), 16]

9.2 Daring to Dream of Equal Opportunity: Women in Medicine in the Nineteenth Century

The professionalization of medicine and growth in medical knowledge throughout the eighteenth century resulted in women being increasingly excluded from licensed practice. The universities only admitted male students, and their professors were male. The University Senates, College Councils, and Regulatory Boards consisted entirely of men who governed the institutions of a profession that admitted only men. Nonetheless women continued to treat the sick in the community either under the supervision of men, or independently but with some risk of being reported to the authorities should there be a bad outcome or jealous male physician.

The nineteenth century was to be the century in which the battle for female entry to medical school would be won. But it was a difficult, protracted, and often disheartening campaign, in which the pioneers faced abuse, harassment, exclusion, ridicule, and misrepresentation. The account contained in this chapter covers some of the early woman doctors who succeeded in a limited number of regions where women won the right to a medical education during the nineteenth century. It is focused on Western Europe, the USA, Great Britain (as it was then called), Russia, China, and India.

By 1900 women in many countries were able to matriculate to study medicine in their universities and become registered as Medical Practitioners. However, they would still face difficulties with obtaining a hospital position outside of a Women and Children's hospital, and have limited academic advancement or leadership opportunities, often only offered in institutions and professional bodies run by women for women. All doctors qualifying in the nineteenth century would have been expected to operate, at least for common general surgical problems. However, many women surgeons concentrated their specialist surgical practice on obstetrics and gynecology.

9.2.1 James Miranda Barry [4] (Margaret Ann Bulkley) 1795–1865 (Fig. 9.1)

One option taken in the first half of the nineteenth century was to pretend to be a man. James Miranda Barry (1799–1865) or rather, Margaret Ann Bulkley, went undetected throughout an entire medical and surgical career. Although some may have suspected, Barry continued to practice until her death, when her corpse revealed the secret of her gender. That a woman should have to deny her gender in exchange for a life in the profession of medicine is grossly unfair, no matter her

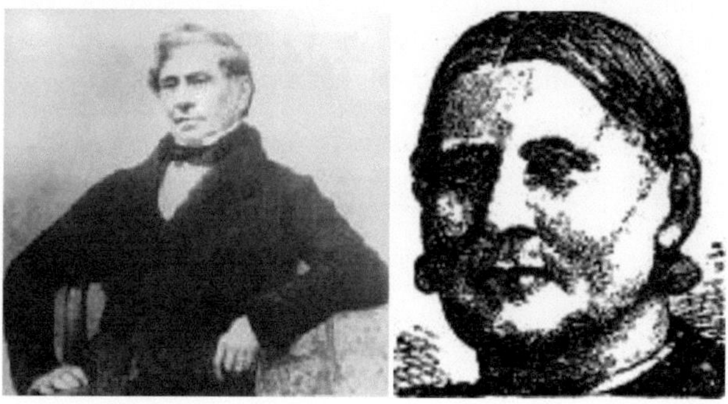

Fig. 9.1 Women doctors of the early nineteenth century: James Miranda Barry (1795–1865) Lovisa Åhrberg (1801–1881) [5] wikimedia. https://upload.wikimedia.org/wikipedia/commons/9/90/Joseph_Barry.jpg

sexual drive and orientation. This would only have been an option for those with the body type that could, dressed in male clothing, pass as a man.

James Barry studied medicine at Edinburgh University from 1809 to 1812 and wrote her (Margaret Bulkley) MD thesis on hernias in the groin. She then took up a career in the Army from 1813 to 16 before developing a career in the British Colonies.

From 1817 to 1827, he/she spent a decade in Cape Town, South Africa, where he/she performed the first documented Caesarean Section in the English speaking world. He/she enjoyed a close friendship developed with the Governor General of the Cape Province, Lord Charles Somerset. Barry introduced improved sanitary standards and had a reputation for being a good clinician exhibiting excellent rapport with patients. He/she continued his/her career as Colonial Medical Officer, with postings in Mauritius, Jamaica, St Helena, and Trinidad, served in the Crimean war in 1855, and eventually rose to become Inspector General in Canada 1857–1859. When in the Crimea, Barry had a run-in with Florence Nightingale who described him as arrogant and obnoxious. His/her gender, or rather her female anatomy, was only discovered by the maid servant, Sophia Blake, after his death. She clearly possessed a frame that enabled her to appear male in male clothing.

Another option was for a woman was to practice unlicensed. Unable to attend university until much later in the century, many women, such as the Swedish Hanna Svensdotter (1798–1864), practiced as "cunning folk" or "wise folk" as their forbearers had done.

9.2.1.1 Lovisa Åhrberg (1801–1881) (Fig. 9.1)

Lovisa Åhrberg (1801–1881) is reputed to be the first female Swedish doctor, practicing from 1840, but was only informally educated in medicine, learning likes a tradesperson through observation and hands-on experience. She established an independent practice in Stockholm gaining a good reputation earned through her patient outcomes. Yet Åhrberg was normally not referred to as "doctor" but rather was called "the wound healer doctoress" and "maiden Åhrberg." Once she was accused of quackery and brought before the authorities, but under examination she was found to have adequate knowledge of the conditions she was treating. Her defense also relied on her practice as a surgeon, and so, as she prescribed only herbal remedies internally, she was not found guilty of trespassing in the practice of physicians! Indeed such was her reputation that in 1852, she was awarded the King's medal for her services to the poor [6, 7].

9.2.2 USA

9.2.2.1 Harriet Hunt (1805–1875)

Sisters, Harriot and Sarah Hunt, began practice in Boston in 1835 having completed their medical apprenticeships.[1] Harriot was inspired by Sarah's illness (consumption) and by the lack of efficacy of a Boston doctor's treatment.[2] So she went to unlicensed quacks, Richard and Elizabeth Mott, who had set up their practice in 1832, having immigrated from England. The local qualified physicians had only very limited treatment options, so often recommended chemicals, laxatives, and bloodletting. Harriot was in practice for over 20 years and became a strong advocate for women's emancipation. She applied for Harvard Medical School when the supportive Oliver Wendell Holmes was Dean. Although he considered accepting her, he was criticized by the all-male student body so her application was rejected in 1847. She was eventually awarded an MD by the female Medical School of Pennsylvania in 1853. However, it was not until almost a century later, in 1945, that Harvard actually admitted its first female class, initially only for a 10-year trial [8].

Hunt endured much criticism for undertaking a role that upset the traditional view of a woman's role at that time. In 1858, the New York Times described her as "one of the dozen women in the United States who pine because Nature did not make them men." Hunt countered that women were eminently suited to the medical role stating, "What could be more delicately feminine, more truly womanly, than to take the hand of a sister, afflicted in body and mind, and to show her the cause of her diseases?" Hunt was also a strong advocate that women wanted to be treated by female doctors, particularly as in the nineteenth century many women felt it indelicate to present to a doctor, and were reluctant to seek help for their difficulties [8]. Martha Swain defined the rights of women not as "their right to legislate or rule the nation, but their right to fully understand the physical laws which govern their own organisation." [letter to Boston Medical and Surgical Journal 1849;41:202].

Before 1847 only members of the Boston Medical Society were able to register as physicians or surgeons and the society did not admit women. Female physicians such as Harriot Hunt had to put female physician after her name. When the Massachusetts Medical Society reorganized in the late 1840s, the Boston Medical Association was replaced by the Suffolk District Medical Society with three categories: Members of Massachusetts' Medical Society, Physicians, and Physicians Female.

Progress would continue slowly but steadily throughout the second half of the nineteenth century. In 1850, the Boston City Directory listed only six female doctors, 2% of medical listings. This number would increase to 210 (18%) by 1890. Harvard continued to refuse female entrants to medicine, rejecting Lucy Sewall and Anita Tyng in 1866, and then also Susan Dimock and Sophia Jex-Blake in 1867.

[1] http://www.womenhistoryblog.com/2013/04/harriot-kezia-hunt.html

[2] Hunt HK. Glances and Glimpses, John P Jewett and Co, Boston 1856.

9.2.2.2 Elizabeth Blackwell (1821–1910) (Fig. 9.3)

Elizabeth Blackwell was born in Bristol, England, but her family moved to the USA in 1831. She eventually obtained her MD from the University of Geneva, New York State, in 1849. She then travelled to Britain and Europe (Paris) to obtain clinical experience and became the first woman to be registered in the UK. She had two eminent champions for her cause in Britain, Sir James Paget [Paget's disease] in London, and James Young Simpson in Edinburgh, of chloroform fame.

In his graduation address to the 1849 medical class, Charles Lee, Dean of Geneva Medical College, referred to the extraordinary event of the day and declared his wholehearted admiration for the first female M.D. However, when he had the graduation address printed he added a footnote stating that, though he supported medical education for qualified women, the *"inconveniences attending the admission of females to all the lectures in a medical school, are so great, that he will feel compelled on all future occasions to oppose such a practice...."*

Her younger sister, Emily Blackwell (1826–1910) (Fig. 9.3), duly had her application rejected to study at Geneva Medical College but was accepted by Rush Medical College in Chicago. Emily studied there for only one semester, because the State Medical Society censured the College for taking in a female medical student.

She was, however, accepted by Cleveland Medical College, Ohio, where she graduated MD in 1854.

Although now seen as a champion for the cause and a pioneer, Elizabeth Blackwell found being the first female doctor in the USA and the UK with a medical degree a lonely and difficult situation.

> *A blank wall of social and professional antagonism faces the woman physician that forms a situation of singular and painful loneliness, leaving her without support, respect or professional counsel.*

9.2.2.3 The Boston Female Medical College (1848–1873)

A medical school in the USA required a faculty of four, a classroom, a dissecting room, and a few educational supplies. The first medical school for women in the world was the Boston Female Medical College (1848–1873), founded by Samuel Gregory. It had 12 women enrolled for midwifery training in November 1848. Yet Gregory while wanting to give women the opportunity to study medicine did not see them as equals. He published his public lectures *"Man-Midwifery Exposed and Corrected together with Remarks of the use and abuse of ether in Labour"* which sold 18,000 copies (Boston 1848). In his writings about the school, he reassured readers that the women would limit themselves to the treatment of children and their own sex *"in the delicate disorders and conditions peculiar to them..... that nice sense of delicacy which the ornament of the female character, the soul of virtue, and the safeguard of morals"* would be maintained.

Dr. Marie Zakrzewska (1829–1902) (Fig. 9.3)

Forty scholarships were awarded to women of Massachusetts in 1855. In 1858, the city of Boston purchased the former Boston Lying-in Hospital (Closed in 1856 because of its reputation over infections) and then sold it to the Female Medical College. Dr. Marie Zakrzewska (1829–1902), a 27-year-old protégé of Elizabeth Blackwell, was appointed Professor of Obstetrics and Diseases of Women and Children and also resident physician at the hospital. Gregory objected to some improvements recommended by Zakrzewska (microscopes etc.) and denounced them as "a new fangled European notion." One of the instructors even said when agreeing to pass a borderline candidate "nobody in Boston would employ a woman doctor in serious cases anyhow." Indeed Gregory in 1860 proposed that the school should consider naming the degree as "doctress," but this was strongly opposed by women including graduates of the College. He still introduced the qualification of "doctress of medicine" in 1864 but was forced to withdraw it in 1868 when the school was struggling to attract students. His style of leadership and management was such that he wanted to run things himself and was unable to delegate. He neither trusted his female managers, nor did he heed their advice.

The college had 98 graduates from 1854, 24 of whom practiced in Boston for some period of time, around 5–13 per year. Their graduates included notable high achievers such as Mary Putnam Jacobi, Mercy Bisbee Jackson (aged 57, died 1877), Mary Harris Thompson (1863), and Rebecca Lee who was the first black woman to receive a medical degree in 1864. However, the medical education provided was mediocre and not the first-rate education that would have resulted in a self-confident and well-respected product. Zakrzewska commented:

The public treated the school's graduates more like well-trained nurses than physicians who assume an authority which creates confidence.

In 1845, most medical schools had no clinical instruction or, if clinical instruction, no hospital instruction. In 1862, Gregory sold the hospital facility associated with the school. However, this was counter to the trend as by 1865 two-thirds of medical schools in the USA provided hospital facilities for education. By 1868, Gregory's school was one of only five medical schools in the country without its own hospital facility.

Zakrzewska resigned in 1862, in protest at the Trustee's reversal of their decision to reappoint Gregory as Secretary and Administrative officer.

Not one of my expectations for a thorough medial education for women has been realized… If it were the intention of the trustees to supply the country with underbred, ill-educated women under the name of physicians… I think the New England Female Medical College is on the right track.

When Gregory died in 1872, the school was to be merged, and one possible merger was with Harvard. This plan was thwarted by the Boston Fire which affected the livelihoods of some of the trustees, so the school went to Boston University, despite objections given that Boston University's medical curriculum was then based on the unorthodox homeopathy [6, 7].

9.2.2.4 Pennsylvania Woman's Medical College

The second women's medical school was the Pennsylvania Woman's Medical College was founded in 1850 (Fig. 9.2). Ann Preston (1813–1872) graduated MD from Pennsylvania Woman's Medical College in 1852 and became the first female Dean of any medical school in the USA in 1866. Unlike the Boston Female Medical College the Pennsylvania College has withstood the tests of time. The School first took male students in 1970, merged with the Hahnemann medical college in 1993 before their merged school became part of Drexel University Medical College in 2003.

Examples of State and County Medical Society opposition to women in medicine was rife. In 1847, the Pennsylvania Medical Society did not bar women from its ranks but, nonetheless, adopted a resolution that there was nothing to commit the society *"to acknowledge the right of women's medical colleges and association of female physicians to representation in this society."* However, the fledgling Women's Medical College of Pennsylvania did survive.

In 1859, the Philadelphia County Medical Society passed *"resolutions of excommunication against every physician who should teach in the women's medical college, every woman who graduated from it and everybody else who would consult with such teachers."* On the other side of the Atlantic, the British Medical Association was no different.

In 1857, Elizabeth and her sister, Emily Blackwell (1826–1910), (Fig. 9.3) and Marie Zakrzewska (intern) founded the New York Infirmary for Indigent Women and Children. Emily took on the management and fund-raising, which enabled the facility to grow from a rented 16-roomed house to a full-fledged hospital. By 1874 it was treating 7000 patients a year. In 1869, Emily Blackwell was Professor of Obstetrics and became Dean of the New York Women's Medical College which trained 364 women by 1899.

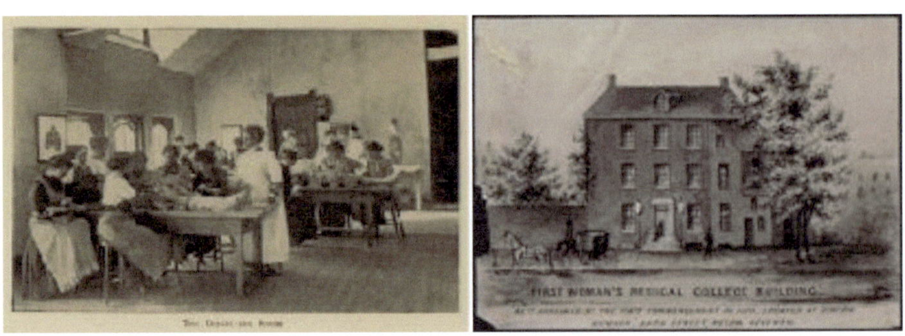

Fig. 9.2 The Dissecting room (L) and the original Pennsylvania Women's Medical College (R). https://upload.wikimedia.org/wikipedia/commons/3/3a/First_Female_Medical_College_of_Pennsylvania_Building.JPG

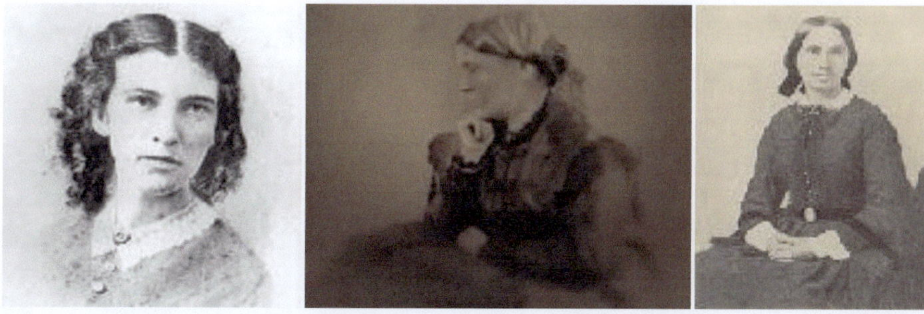

Fig. 9.3 Elizabeth Blackwell (left) Emily Blackwell (middle). Marie Zakrzewska (right), Public domain. https://en.wikipedia.org/wiki/Elizabeth_Blackwell#/media/File:Copy_of_a_portrait_of_Elizabeth_Blackwell_seated_in_profile,_ca._1850-1860._(16223865345).jpg

Marie Zakrzewska (1829–1902)

Marie Zakrzewska (1829–1902) (Fig. 9.3) was born in Berlin and trained as a midwife at the Charité Hospital. She became the chief of midwifery but emigrated to the USA in 1852 where she met Elizabeth Blackwell. Blackwell persuaded her to enter medical school in Cleveland, Ohio, from which she graduated in 1856. She gained clinical experience with the Blackwells at the New York Infirmary for Indigent women and children in 1857 but moved to Boston to teach at the Boston Female Medical College in 1859 until resigning in 1862 as detailed above. In 1862, she founded the New England Women and Children's Hospital in Boston.

Mary Edwards Walker (1832–1919) (Fig. 9.4)

She gained her medical degree from Syracuse Medical University in New York in 1855. Hers was an "eclectic" training avoiding chemical substances in favor of vegetable substitutes, acceptant of both allopathic and homeopathic medical models. She married one of her classmates, and they opened a joint practice. The marriage failed, and they divorced, with her adulterous husband being banned by the Supreme Court of ever marrying during her lifetime. When the American Civil War (1861–1865) broke out, she sought to join the Unionists, but it was not until 1863 that secured a position as a contract Assistant Surgeon. She was renowned for her work tending the injured even across military lines and was eventually captured as a "spy" by the Confederates but after 4 months returned in a prisoner exchange. The New York Times reported, "she can amputate with the skill of a surgeon and administer medicine just as well." However, she believed that too many amputations were being performed. These had a high mortality during the civil war, with perhaps 60% of people dying following a below-knee amputation and 80% if above-knee. The death rate from sepsis was halved if done within the first 24 h rather than after 48 h, but the surgeons amputating were performing the procedures with unwashed hands and dirty, blood-stained aprons. Lister's publications on asepsis would not be

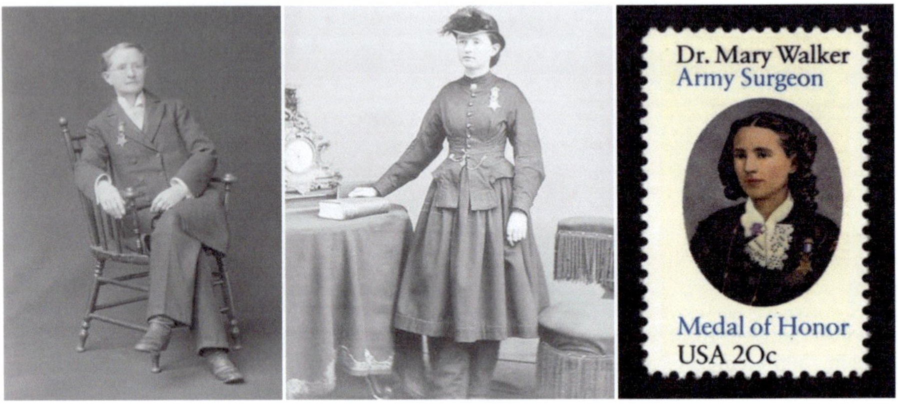

Fig. 9.4 Mary Edwards Walker later in life in her chosen military uniform and on 1982 stamp. (https://upload.wikimedia.org/wikipedia/commons/d/db/Dr._Mary_Walker.jpg)

published until after the war, although there were already proponents of cleanliness and antisepsis. Mary Walker was one of those who advocated clean water and dressing, a nutritious diet, and avoiding amputation for minor wounds. After examining their wounds, she would counsel soldiers they had the right to refuse an amputation if she believed it was not necessary.

> *Dr. Walker met with considerable abuse over her persistent demands to be made a surgeon but also earned considerable respect for her many good works. Meanwhile, she abandoned bloomers and adopted a modified version of male attire, with a calf length skirt worn over trousers, keeping her hair relatively long and curled so that anyone could know she was a woman.* (https://www.ausa.org/dr-mary-e-walker)

After the war she was decorated with the Congressional Medal of Honour. The Medal was retracted in 1917, on the grounds that she (and 900 male recipients) had not won it in active service in battle. The honour was reinstated by President Jimmy Carter in 1977. Since 2016, the American College of Surgeons has offered a "Mary Edwards Walker Inspiring Women in Surgery award" in her honour. The American Army also offers a Mary Edwards Walker Award in memory of this woman who was the first female to be employed by the American military and the only female recipient of the Congressional Medal of Honour. She was active in suffrage movement, and the year after her death in 1920, American women were given the right to vote.

9.2.2.5 Abuse and Rejection and Overcoming Prejudice

Dr. Amanda Sanford, who had studied at the Woman's Medical College of Pennsylvania, as well as New England Hospital, was able to complete her medical school program in 1 year, graduating MD with honours. She had to suffer being hooted at, and showered with, abusive notes at her graduation.

The struggle for women doctors to be accepted by the male medical profession continued throughout the nineteenth century and beyond. Not only was it difficult to obtain training and enter the profession, but then the early women faced exclusion from the professions' societies. Dr. Sara Brown submitted a research paper to the Boston Medical and Surgical Journal in 1874. It was rejected because she was female and had to be published in the Archives of Ophthalmology and Otology.

The discrimination and prejudice that existed is well described in the words of Dr. Edward Clarke who succeeded Bigelow as Professor of Materia Medica at Harvard (1855). Although he acknowledged that women were knocking on the door of the profession and deserved *"the same right to every function and opportunity which our planet offers, that man has." "Let the experiment … be fairly made… in 50 years we shall get the answer."* But *"God forbid that I should ever see men and women aiding each other to display with the scalpel the secrets of the reproductive system; or charmingly discuss together the labyrinthine ways of syphilis."*

Clarke somehow believed that the education of girls was at odds with the development of their reproductive system and postpubertal functions. *"They cannot be educated as males. The results would be: monstrous brains and puny bodies; abnormally active cerebration and abnormally weak digestion; flowing thought and constipated bowels."*

In an 1869 address to Harvard (which fell on deaf ears) and then a later 1872 lecture to the New England Women's Club of Boston (overnight fame), he discussed the relationship between the education and physiology of women, finding that women are limited by their biology. *His Sex in Education; or, a Fair Chance for the Girls* (1873) went through 17 editions over the next 13 years.

Mary Putnam Jacobi and the Harvard Boylston Prize

The storm of controversy that was aroused by women entering medicine demanded scientific study. Mary Putnam Jacobi won the Harvard Medical School Boylston Prize for her essay on *"Do women require mental and bodily rest during menstruation and to what extent?"*. In 1881, a study of 430 women doctors who had graduated since 1870 found only 13 were in poor health, while only 34/307 were periodically incapacitated by menstruation.

Massachusetts's Medical Society Admits Women (1884)

Boston's Massachusetts's Medical Society vigorously discussed female membership, but their Council resisted admitting women until 1884. Their first female member was Dr. Emma Louisa McCall (1847–1937), an 1873 graduate of the University of Michigan, which had admitted their first five women students in 1869. She practiced at the New England Hospital for Women and Children from 1875 to 1902 and thereafter continued practice as a consulting obstetrician until 1928.

Table 9.1 Women Medical Students in American Medical Schools 1893–4 [9]

Medical Schools	Females	% Total
Boston[a]	52	23.7
Chicago	0	0
Los Angeles	6	15.4
Minneapolis	12	4.7
New York	0	0
Philadelphia	0	0
San Francisco	40	11.9

Mary Roth Walsh p 183
[a]3 of 4 Medical Schools in Boston were open to women, only Harvard was not Michigan 19%

Women Doctors Registered in 1900

Despite the prejudice and opposition, by 1900, there were 7000 women registered as doctors in the USA (Table 9.1). Although this represented only 5–6% of the total number of doctors and these women still faced many prejudices, particularly a lack of equal opportunity in their careers that needed to be addressed, this was the end of the beginning. The twentieth century would see further advances for the cause of women and their careers in medicine, in all specialties, in research, and in academia.

9.2.2.6 Harvard Accepts Female Medical Students (1945)

However, it took Harvard until 1945 to accept female medical students. During the late 1800s a number of substantial endowments were offered to them on the provision that they would accept women. These they rejected, and in 1899 one of $500,000 was then offered to Johns Hopkins' University which went co-educational in 1893 [10–11].

9.2.3 Women Doctors in Europe

9.2.3.1 Dorothea Erxleben (1715–1762)

The first woman in the Modern Era to obtain the MD [University of Halle] was Dorothea Erxleben (1715–1762) in Germany in 1754 (Fig. 9.5). Her father was Christian Polycarp Leporin, a physician in Prussia. In 1742, she published a tract arguing that women should be allowed to attend University and was granted special dispensation by Frederick the Great. Her tract addressed male and female readers and was critical of women not wanting to educate themselves, recognizing nonetheless the burden of their housework and caring for children.

At the start of the nineteenth century, although women practiced medicine as midwives, nurses, or quacks, they did so informally. What options were then open to a woman who dared to dream of being a doctor and wanted to bring that dream to reality? No universities in Europe would accept women to study medicine until the second half of the nineteenth century.

However, by the late 1860s and early 1870s, there were at least seven universities that offered degrees in Europe; - Zurich, Paris, Berlin, Leipzig, Berne, Montpellier, and Brussels. However, their degrees did not allow medical practice without sitting a local examination that entitled those passing to become licensed to practice.

9.2.3.2 Sweden

The first Swedish-born woman to obtain a University degree was Charlotte Yhlen (1839–1920) (Fig. 9.5), who graduated from the Women's Medical College of Pennsylvania in 1873. Only in 1870, did Swedish universities begin to admit women, with Karolina Widerström (1856–1949) becoming the first medical graduate in 1884 (Fig. 9.5).

There were many challenges women faced to obtain a university education. The first was finding a university that would allow them to matriculate. Then they had to find and pay faculty members who were willing to teach them as often their classes had to be separate from those for the male students. Then for clinical experience, they had to find a hospital with sufficient patients and doctors willing to train them. Lack of clinical experience prompted women's hospitals to be founded in the major training cities. Finally, a female student had to apply for permission to sit their examinations. Women were obstructed at each of these stages by men determined to ensure that medicine remained closed to women and that a woman's place was effectively in the home. Some feared competition; others were just prejudiced. However, the cause for women to enter university and study medicine also had some enlightened male champions and increasing public support toward the end of the 1800s.

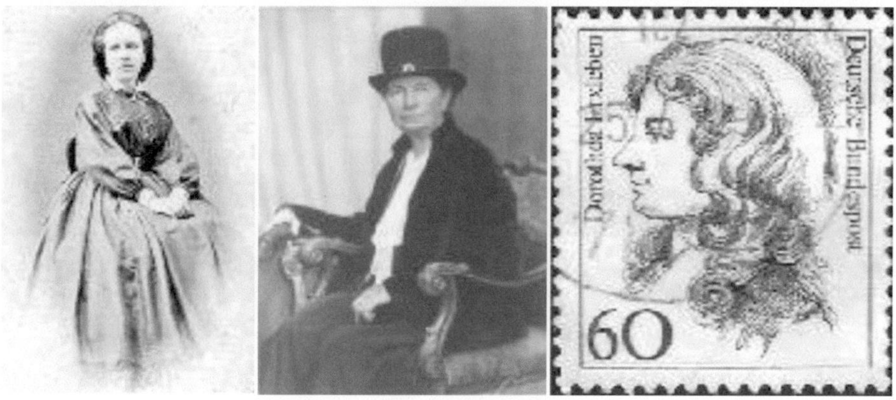

Fig. 9.5 Left to Right: Charlotte Yhlen, Karolina Widerström, Dorothea Erxleben (German commemorative Stamp). Wikipedia Public domain. (https://en.wikipedia.org/wiki/Charlotte_Yhlen#/media/File:Charlotte_Yhlen.jpg)

9.2.3.3 Russia

In 1864, the University of Zurich began accepting female medical students, with their first female graduates qualifying MD in 1867.

Nadezhda Suslova (1843–1918)

The first woman medical doctor in Russia, and to graduate MD from Zurich, was Nadezhda Suslova (1843–1918) (Fig. 9.6), who published a collection of short stories espousing a feminist, nihilist philosophy in 1861. She was permitted to attend the Imperial Military Medical Academy in St Petersburg in 1862 along with Mariia Obrucheva (Bokov).

However, in Russia, women were banned from universities in 1865. Suslova moved to Zurich and graduated MD in 1867. Her thesis was on the muscular reflexes of frogs, with the research conducted at Graz University in Austria. To register to practice medicine in Russia, she had to pass a further examination which she did in 1868, and then practiced in gynecology and pediatrics in St Petersburg.

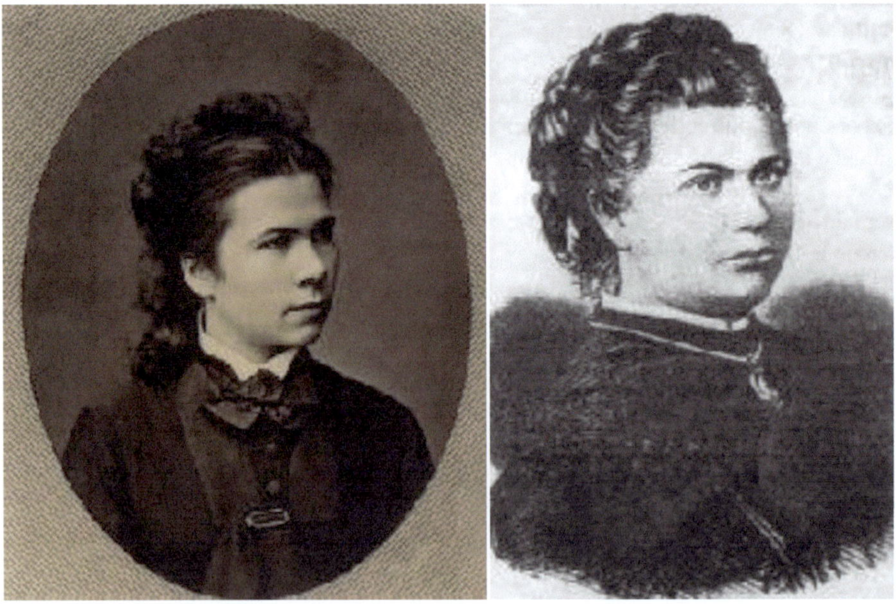

Fig. 9.6 Left: Nadhezhda Suslova (1843–1918) Figure Right: Kashevarova-Rudneva Varvara Alexandrovna (1842–1899). Wikipedia public domain. https://en.wikipedia.org/wiki/Varvara_Rudneva#/media/File:Kashevarova-rudneva.jpg

Kashevarova-Rudneva Varvara Alexandrovna (1842–1899)

Kashevarova-Rudneva (Fig. 9.6) trained at the midwifery institute, St Petersburg, in 1862. In 1863, she became the first woman to enroll in the St Petersburg Medical and Surgical Academy, graduating in 1868 with her diploma of doctor in the Specialty of Obstetrics and Gynaecology. She successfully defended her MD thesis on "*Materials for pathological anatomy of the uterine vagina*" in 1876, the first Russian woman to do so in the country. She became the first Russian woman to be accepted into the Society of Russian doctors in St Petersburg. She published a number of gynecological papers over the next 20 years.

9.2.3.4 Switzerland

After the Russian, Nadezhda Suslova (1843–1918), the next three women doctors to graduate MD from Zurich were Frances Morgan (1843–1927) from Wales also in 1870, later to graduate with a Licentiate from RCSI allowing her to register to practice in the UK. She was followed by an American, Susan Dimock (1847–1875) in 1871, who had been rejected by Harvard, and, in 1873, by the first Swiss graduate, Marie Heim Vögtlin (1845–1916).

9.2.3.5 France

Madeline Brès (1839–1925)

In Paris in 1866, the Dean of the Faculty of Medicine, Charles Adolphe Wurtz (1817–1884), supported the cause of a woman, Madeleine Brès (1839–1925), who wanted to undertake medical studies. He recommended she sit her Baccalaureate in preparation. Meanwhile, Wurz sent Doctor Alexis Dureau (1831–1904) to Zurich to learn of their methodology of admitting female medical students. There was considerable opposition to female admission from some of the faculty, notably the famous, Jean-Martin Charcot (1825–1893) who argued that *"the nature of a woman"* would be inhibitory.

However, Wurz permitted three foreign women to be admitted to the medical school to study for the MD: The first was Mary Putnam Jacobi MD (1842–1906), an American graduate of the Women's Medical College in Philadelphia in 1864, but born in London. The second was Catherine Gontcharoff, a Russian, and the third, Elizabeth Garrett LSA, was English and would be the first female to graduate from Paris with the MD in 1870.

Madeleine Brès (1839–1925) (Fig. 9.7), having gained her baccalaureate, was able to undertake her medical training from 1869 to 1875. She gained experience as an intern at L'hôpital de la Pitié de Paris in 1870 but also during the two sieges of Paris during the 1870–1871 Franco-Prussian war. Her medical work was well respected, and prominent physicians including Wurz wrote of her,

> *We are pleased to declare that Mrs. Brès, through her impeccable behavior, her hard work and her zeal in the hospital, gained the respect of all the students she had to interact with, and justified the opening of our courses to other female students.*

However, in 1871, she had been initially denied the right to sit her internal and external medical examinations for fear of setting a precedent though she was to finally graduate MD *summa cum laude* in 1875. It still took until 1881 for other female students to be allowed to sit external examinations and still later, in 1885, to sit internal examinations.

Caroline Schultz (1867–1926)

Caroline Schultz (1867–1926) (Fig. 9.7) was Polish and following her Baccalaureate (1884) defended her MD Thesis in 1888 on "*The Woman Physician in the Nineteenth Century.*" Her successful defense was made under the questioning of Jean Marie Charcot who remained opposed to women in medicine. Schultze's thesis inspired many women to consider careers, previously regarded as "men only."

9.2.3.6 Great Britain

The First British Trained Doctor: Elizabeth Garrett Anderson (1836–1917)

In 1860, Elizabeth Garrett nursed at the Middlesex hospital. In 1861, her application to study medicine, supported financially by her wealthy father, was rejected by the medical schools of Edinburgh, Glasgow, Oxford, and Cambridge. In 1862, she was denied admission to London by one vote and Edinburgh by two, while the University of St Andrews returned her matriculation fee after one term of tuition. However,

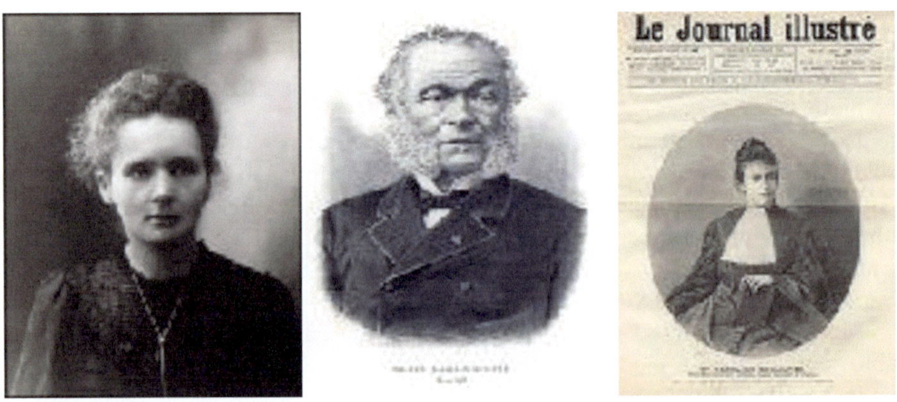

Fig. 9.7 Madeleine Brès, Charles Adolphe Wurtz, Caroline Schultze. Wikipedia Public domain. https://en.wikipedia.org/wiki/Madeleine_Brès#/media/File:Madeleine_Brès_(1842-1921).jpg

with the support of her father, she began medical training under willing teachers despite not being allowed to matriculate. London University would not open its doors to women until 1877.

The 1815 Act which permitted the Society of the Apothecaries to examine doctors and so provide a recognizable qualification (LSA) for registration stated they could examine any who had fulfilled the required apprenticeship to a qualified doctor for a period of 5 years and received instruction from recognized university tutors in the syllabus. So despite considerable opposition from many in the profession, including the Lancet, the LSA could not prevent Elizabeth Garrett from sitting the exam which she passed. She was then able to register with the General Medical Council (GMC) as a doctor, the second woman to do so after Elizabeth Blackwell.

However, the Society of Apothecaries then changed its constitution and so was able to prevent another woman, Frances Hogan (1843–1927), from sitting their examination in 1867. She went to Zurich and gained her MD in March 1870, the first British woman to do so. Seven years later she would obtain her Licentiate to practice from the King and Queen's College of Physicians in Ireland.

Garrett opened her own practice at 20 Upper Berkeley Street, London. At first, patients were scarce but the practice gradually grew. In 1865, there was an outbreak of cholera in Britain, affecting both rich and poor, and in their panic, some people forgot any prejudices they had in relation to a female physician. In 1866, Garrett opened St Mary's Dispensary for Women and Children, at 69 Seymour Place, and in the first year, had 3000 new patients, who made 9300 outpatient visits to the dispensary. It later became the New Hospital for Women and Children and later named the Elizabeth Garrett Anderson Hospital. From 1868, Garrett studied for her MD in Paris becoming the first woman to graduate MD from Paris in 1870. She even had to defend her thesis on migraine in front of Jean-Marie Charcot who was staunchley opposed to women becoming doctors! She married in 1871, had three children, two of whom survived to adult life. She was the first woman elected to the British Medical Association in 1873 and later became Dean of the London Hospital for Women and Children in 1883. In 1908 she became the Mayor of Aldeburgh and was active in the suffragette movement.

Sophia Jex Blake (1840–1912) and the Edinburgh Seven

Jex Blake's (Fig. 9.8) application to Harvard Medical School was rejected in 1867. However, the sympathetic and supportive Dean, Oliver Wendell Holmes arranged for her to have some clinical teaching at the Massachusetts' General. She then returned to Bristol, England, for further teaching, but her father fell ill and so her studies in medicine were interrupted.

In Edinburgh, Professor James Balfour was a sympathetic Dean of the Faculty. Champions of the women's cause in Edinburgh included Sir James Simpson (1811–1870) who advocated for. However, the Senate was unwilling to rule and make concessions for just one woman. Sophia Jex Blake thus sought out other interested women, recruiting Isabel Thorne, Edith Pechey, Helen Evans, and Matilda

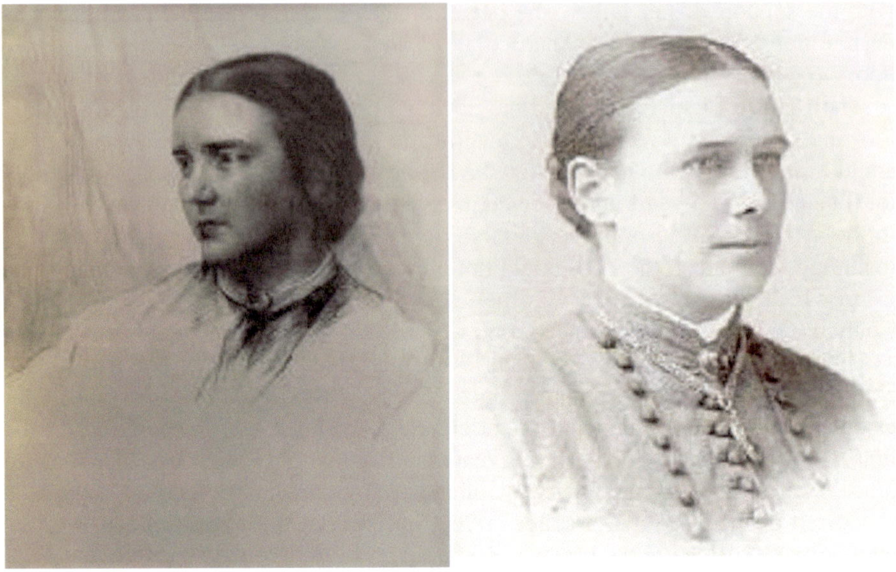

Fig. 9.8 Sophia Jex-Blake (1840–1912) (Left). Edith Pechey (1845–1908) (Right), Wikipedia, public domain. https://en.wikipedia.org/wiki/Sophia_Jex-Blake#/media/File:Sophia_Jex-Blake_Aged_25.jpg

Chaplin. They applied to matriculate accepting they would be taught in separate classes from the men and would pay the appropriate tuition fees. The admission of Sophia and the other female medical students was vehemently opposed by Professor Christison (1797–1882), the Professor of Medicine and Therapeutics since 1822, who was religious, an elder of the Church of Scotland, and a member of five influential University committees including the Senate. The five female students enrolled in October 1869. Some of their opponents were biding their time, expecting the women to fail. However, all five passed, four with honours. Edith Pechey topped the class but was denied the scholarship that went with the honour because she was a woman. The University's reputation then came under fire in the Press.

In 1870, Mary Anderson and Emily Bovell joined them; the seven women became known as the "Edinburgh Seven." Some male medical students made life difficult for the women, and matters came to a head when there was a riot at an anatomy exam held at Surgeons' Hall (Fig. 9.9). The women were pelted with mud and other objects, and during the exam, a sheep was introduced to the examination hall causing further chaos. The University was further criticized by the Times, the Scotsman, the Spectator, the British Medical Journal (BMJ), and the Lancet. It was only on International Women's Day on March 8, 2018, that the Royal College of Surgeons of Edinburgh erected a plaque in honor of the seven women, who were Britain's first female University Medical Students. However, such was the injustices they faced, they were never allowed to sit their final examinations in Edinburgh, but rather had to find alternative places to finish their training and undergo examinations in order to register with the GMC as medical practitioners.

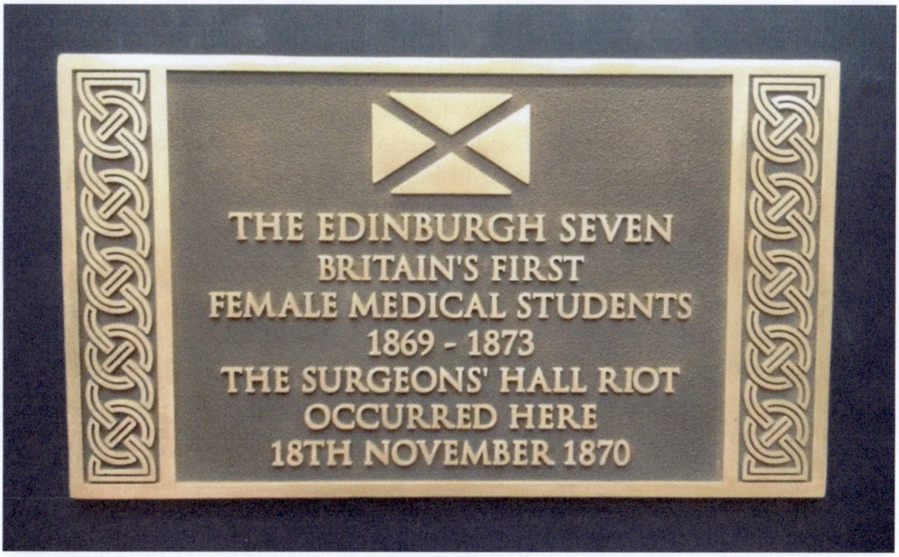
THE EDINBURGH SEVEN
BRITAIN'S FIRST
FEMALE MEDICAL STUDENTS
1869 - 1873
THE SURGEONS' HALL RIOT
OCCURRED HERE
18TH NOVEMBER 1870

Fig. 9.9 Edinburgh, Britain first med students, Wikipedia, Public domain. https://en.wikipedia.org/wiki/Edinburgh_Seven#/media/File:Edinburgh_Seven_Plaque.jpg

9.2.3.7 The London Hospital for Women

In 1874, the London Hospital for Women was founded but this was small and only treated women, insufficient to cover the entire medical curriculum and all specialties. Fourteen students enrolled, 12 of whom had been in Edinburgh, and a further 6 joined during the first term. Francis Anstie (1833–1874), a physician, helped found the hospital with 13 donations of 100 pounds sterling, but he died at the age of 40, and William Norton became Dean. Initially, the Royal Free Hospital refused to take female medical students in 1876 but relented in 1877. It had two physicians and two surgeons on staff. The two physicians agreed to teach the women as did one of the two surgeons, though the unwilling surgeon later began teaching as well. Although the women could then undertake their clinical training, such was the prejudice against them, they still struggled to be admitted for examination despite there being 19 medical examining bodies in the UK between 1874 and 1876.

John Simon, Medical Officer of the Privy Council in Britain, asked the registration (not examination) body, the GMC, for its views, and received this reply:

> *that the study and practice of medicine and surgery, instead of affording a field of exertion well fitted for women, do, on the contrary, present special difficulties which cannot be simply disregarded; but the Council are not prepared to say that women ought to be excluded from the profession.*

King and Queen's College of Physicians in Ireland (1876)

However, in 1876, the King and Queen's College of Physicians in Ireland passed a rule allowing the admission of women for the licentiate examination, which, if passed, would allow registration with the GMC. Eliza Louisa Walker Dunbar became their first woman graduate, with Edith Pechey and Sophia Jex-Blake following in the same year, having previously obtained MD's in Bern, Switzerland.

9.2.3.8 London University

London University also had to undergo considerable debate and considerable delay before finally admitting women in 1878. The London School of Medicine for Women (LSMW) and the Royal Free Hospital were accredited as training institutions the same year.

Sir William Jenner (1815–1898), later President of the Royal College of Physicians (1881–1888), opposed their admission, while Sir James Paget (1814–1899) was in favor. Paget, President of the London Medical and Chirurgical Society, won the day as the convocation vote to admit women to all faculties of the University was finally carried in January 1878 by 241 votes to 132. Jenner, leading the anti-women matriculation case, stated during the fierce debate that he:

> *had but one dear daughter, and he would rather follow her to the grave than allow her to go through such a course of study.*

Edith Shove (1848–1929) and Mary Scharlieb (1845–1930)

Edith Shove (1848–1929) and Mary Scharlieb (1845–1930) (Fig. 9.10) were the first two female graduates from London University in 1882. Mary Scharlieb, accompanying her husband, had undertaken some of her study as one of the first four female medical students in Madras, India, as well as the LSMW. She was to graduate from London with honours in all subjects as well as the Gold Medal and Scholarship in Obstetrics. She returned to India in 1883 and became a lecturer in midwifery and gynecology at the Madras Medical College. She returned to London in 1887, as a surgeon at the LSMW, along with Elizabeth Garrett Anderson. She undertook a Master of Surgery in 1897. She was also appointed forensic pathologist at the Royal Free Hospital and later Chief Gynaecologist from 1902 to 1909. She was made a Dame in 1917.

The early history of the LSMW, later called the Elizabeth Garrett Anderson Hospital, was successful in terms of graduation/qualification outcomes. Thirty-two students entered from 1877 to 1879 and a further 36 in the next 3 years. In 1877, five of six intending to qualify did so. In 1878, Julia Cock completed and she later became Dean. Also, Matilda Chaplin originally in the Edinburgh cohort, qualified KQCPI and MD Paris 1879 but died in 1883. Katherine McDonough was later struck off for advertising in Australia. The others qualified. In 1879, there were two

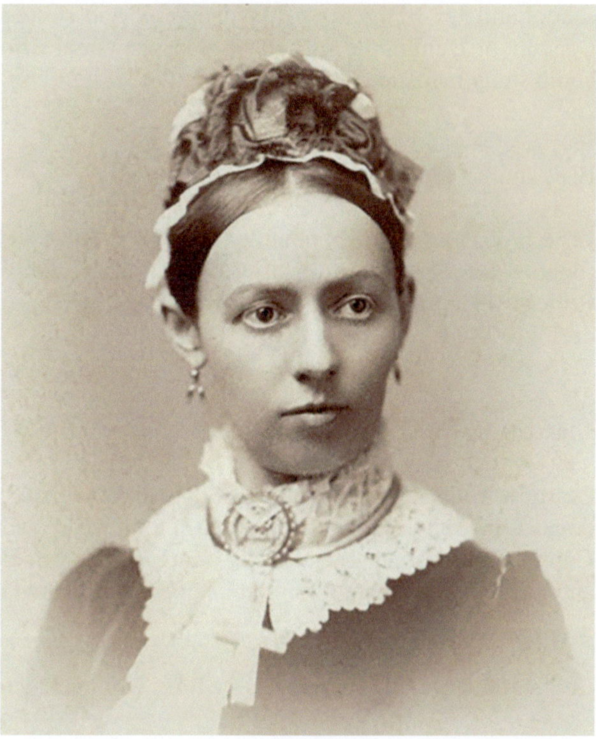

Fig. 9.10 Mary Scharlieb (1845–1930). https://en.wikipedia.org/wiki/Mary_Scharlieb#/media/File:Mary_Scharlieb_c1875.jpg

who left before qualifying, one of whom was Mary Scharlieb who went to Madras but later did complete with honours (see above), and the other was Janet Harriet Walker. In the 1880–1882 cohort of 36, 18 qualified, while 13 of them had never had an intention of doing so.

9.2.3.9 Scotland

In 1886, the Royal Colleges of Physicians and Surgeons of Edinburgh admitted women to the licentiate examination for their Joint Qualification.

The Edinburgh School of Medicine for Women

The Edinburgh School of Medicine for Women was founded by Sophia Jex-Blake in 1886 and ran for 12 years until 1898. Women were still forbidden to attend clinical teaching in the Royal Infirmary though separate clinical teaching was provided for them in Leith Hospital from 1887. The Edinburgh School was to host 80 students, 33 of whom graduated in medicine. Jex-Blake had an uncompromising approach towards discipline, and this led to problems. When two sisters won a court case challenging their expulsion from the school, bad publicity meant that both the school and Jex-Blake herself lost support, and some students moved to Glasgow, London, or Dublin, the only other places in Great Britain or Ireland where women could study medicine at that time.

Elsie Inglis (1864–1917)

Elsie Inglis (1864–1917) qualified with an Edinburgh Licentiate in 1892, and then founded the Scottish Women's Hospital. She established an alternative Medical College for Women and was a suffragist and became a military surgeon in Serbia during WWI.

Glasgow University: First Scottish Graduates in 1894

Glasgow University was the first Scottish University to have women graduate as doctors in 1894. There were four in that year, Marion Gilchrist, Alice (Lily) Cumming, Elizabeth Lyness, and Margaret Dewar. Edinburgh's early opposition and misbehavior meant it missed its opportunity and Glasgow became the first.

Edinburgh University Graduates Its First Women Doctors (1896)

In 1892, women were formally admitted to Edinburgh University for the first time following the Universities of Scotland Act (1889). By 1914, a thousand women had degrees from Edinburgh University. In 1894, the University announced that it would admit women for graduation in the Faculty of Medicine, but for many years, they continued to be taught separately. In 1896, the first two women graduated. Jessie MacGregor (1863–1906), who had studied at Sophia Jex Blake's Edinburgh School of Medicine for Women, gained a first class honours in every subject in the curriculum and gained the Arthur Scholarship. The other graduate was Alexandra Mary (Mona) Campbell Geddes. Subsequently there were 51 medical graduations between 1896 and 1900.[3] Jessie MacGregor added the MD in 1899, achieving a gold medal for her thesis on the comparative anatomy of the auditory nerve. She set up in practice with Elsie Inglis, and in 1901, they established a maternity hospital for working-class women on the Royal Mile. She moved to Denver, Colorado, in 1905 but died of meningitis the following year.

It was only in 1916, with the First World War bringing a much higher percentage of female students and a growing demand for their medical skills, that the Edinburgh University Faculty of Medicine finally admitted women on an entirely equal footing to men.

---

[3] http://collections.ed.ac.uk/alumni/search/*:*/Collection:%22female+medical+graduates+1896-1900%7C%7C%7CFemale+Medical+Graduates+1896-1900%22

The Extramural School of Medicine of the Royal Colleges (1895–1948)

The Extramural School of Medicine of the Royal Colleges (1895–1948) was a body consisting of lecturers recognized by the Royal College of Physicians of Edinburgh and the Royal College of Surgeons of Edinburgh, with its remit to assist in the provision of extra academical instruction in all branches of medicine and surgery. It was open to male and female students—who for varied reasons, including being women or from marginal groups, did not attend university—to train and qualify in medical and surgical practice. This was normally achieved by following a course of study leading to the Triple Qualification as an alternative to a University degree that would satisfy registration requirements [11].

By the year 1900, there were 258 registered doctors in England, 95 in France and 7000 in the United States of America (Table 9.2).

9.2.3.10 Latin America

Marie Josefina Mathilde Durocher, Medical Graduate in 1834

Marie Josefina Mathilde Durocher (1809–1893) was a Brazilian and the first female doctor in Latin America. Durocher was the daughter of French immigrants. She was born in Paris and moved to Brazil with her parents at the age of 8. Widowed young with two children, she was the first to be granted a medical degree from the newly founded Medical School of Rio de Janeiro in 1834. This was 15 years before Elizabeth Blackwell became the first female medical graduate of the English speaking world. Durocher was active in her profession for 60 years. She aroused attention with her habit of dressing in men's clothes, as she considered them more practical in her profession than the contemporary women's clothes. Midwife of the grandchildren of Emperor Pedro II of Brazil, Durocher became the first female member of the Academia Nacional de Medicina in 1871.

9.2.3.11 Japan

Ogino Ginko (1851–1913)

Ogino Ginko (1851–1913) was the first female doctor in Japan. She had an arranged marriage aged 16 but contracted gonorrhea from her husband whom she then divorced in 1870. She described feeling ashamed of being treated for 2 years by only male doctors, thus making the case for the need for women to become doctors

Table 9.2 Registered female doctors in 1900

Country	Registered female Drs	Population
France	95	38 m
England	258	38 m
USA	7000	76 m

to help other women, and so she decided to study medicine herself. She moved to Tokyo in 1873 to complete her basic education, which she achieved with honours, before entering the Tokyo Women's Normal School (now Ochanomizu University), where all the other students were male. She graduated in 1882, but was not allowed to sit her examinations until 1885, in which she achieved full marks. She specialized in Obstetrics and Gynaecology and founded the Ogino Hospital in Yushima. She married Yukiyoshi Shikata, a protestant clergyman, in 1890, and moved to Hokkaido in 1894, where she ran a medical practice.

Dr. Yoshioka Yayoi (1879–1951)

The Tokyo Women's Medical School, now called Tokyo Women's Medical University, was the first female Medical School in Japan, founded in 1900 by Dr. Yoshioka Yayoi (1879–1951). However, the graduates of the school were not permitted to practice medicine until 1912, as they were not able to sit the examination.

Yayoi was awarded the Order of the Precious Crown in 1955, and the Order of the Sacred Treasure posthumously in 1959. The Japan Medical Women's Association has named its two awards after Drs Yoshioka Yayoi and Ogino Ginko (Fig. 9.11).

Keiko Okami (1859–1941)

Keiko Okami (1859–1941) graduated from the Pennsylvania Women's Medical College in the USA in 1889. She returned home and opened a clinic in Akasaka, Tameike. She also worked at the Jikei Hospital (now Tokyo Jikei University School of Medicine). In 1897, she opened an Akasaka Hospital Branch Hospital to provide a respite service for sick women which also provided a nurse dispatch system (Fig. 9.12).

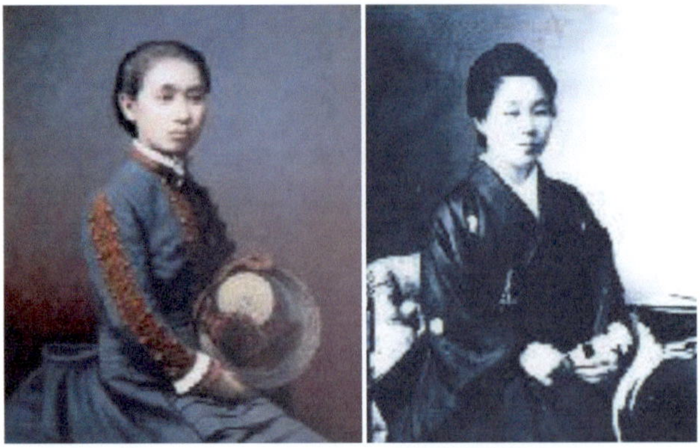

Fig. 9.11 Left: Ogino Ginko (1851–1913). Right: Yoshioka Yayoi (1879–1951), Wikipedia, public domain. https://en.wikipedia.org/wiki/Yoshioka_Yayoi#/media/File:YoshiokaYayoi1901.jpg

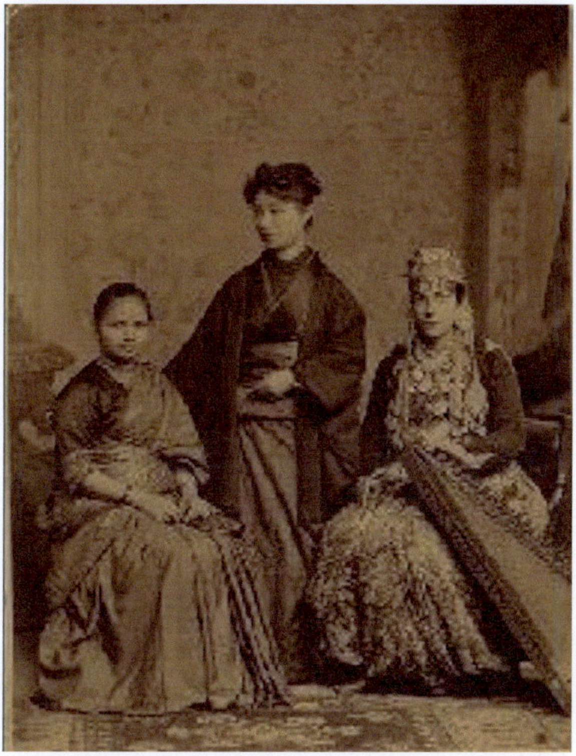

Fig. 9.12 From left: Anandibai Joshi, Keiko Okami, and Sabat Islambouli, students of the Woman's Medical College of Pennsylvania. Photo dated: October 10, 1885 (Public domain via Wikimedia Commons). https://en.m.wikipedia.org/wiki/File:Anandibai_Joshee,_Kei_Okami,_and_Tabat_M._Islambooly.jpg

9.2.3.12 China

Hu King Eng (1865—1929)

Hu King Eng (1865–1929) was born to a Christian Chinese family in Fuzhou. She went to America to study at Ohio Wesleyan Female College (1884–1888) and then the Woman's Medical College of Philadelphia, graduating in 1894. She returned to Fuzhou in 1895, working in the Foochow Hospital for Women and Children. When the supervising doctor returned to the USA, she was put in charge. In 1899, she became resident physician at Woolston Memorial Hospital where from 1899 to 1901, she trained two medical students, one of whom was her younger sister, Hü Seuk Eng. As Hu's reputation in the community increased, the hospital case load grew from 1837 in 1899 to 24,091 in 1910. Tragically the hospital was burned down by bandits in 1927, and Hu relocated to Singapore where she died of a stroke in 1929.

Dr. Mary Fulton (1854–1927), an American Presbyterian missionary, founded the Hackett Medical College for Women, the first in China, in 1902. It offered a 4-year curriculum. It was registered under control of the Chinese government in 1932, and affiliated with Guangzhou Hospital and Lingnan University to form the

Sun Yat-Sen College in 1936. The hospital had to relocate several times when the Japanese invaded.

Kin Yamei (1864–1934)

Kin Yamei's father, Rev. Kying Ling-yiu (Fig. 9.13), was a Christian convert, but her parents died in a cholera epidemic when she was aged 2. The orphan was adopted by American missionaries. She attended the Women's Medical College of the New York Infirmary founded by the Blackwells, graduating top of the class in 1885. She was the first Chinese woman to receive a medical degree in the USA in 1888. She published a book on medical photomicrography while in medical school. From 1890 to 1894 she ran a hospital in Kobe, Japan. She was superintendent at a women's hospital and nursing training program at Tianjin and also founded the Northern Medical School for Women at Zhili in 1907. She spent World War I in the USA where she wrote and promoted the use of soya beans but also is credited with introducing Tofu to the USA.

9.2.3.13 India

Early in the nineteenth century, medical training was only available to men. A Native Medical Institution in Calcutta provided medical training from 1822 to 1835. The Calcutta Medical College was established in 1835 to provide a 4–6 "native doctor" program leading to a certificate to practice surgery and medicine. In Bombay, surgeon John McLennan began a school to train Indian doctors, but the school only lasted 6 years. The Governor, Sir Robert Grant, became distressed at the lack of proper medical care and the resulting mortality. In 1835, after the formation of the medical and physical society of Bombay, their members also advocated for a

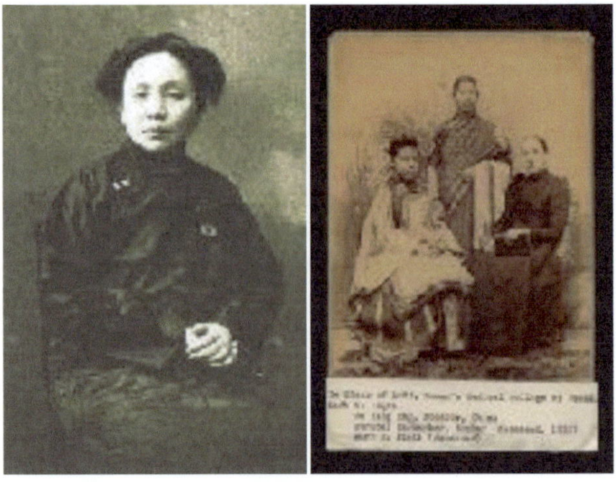

Fig. 9.13 Kin Yamei in 1905. Hu King Eng (Left) 1892, Wikipedia, public domain. https://en.wikipedia.org/wiki/Hü_King_Eng#/media/File:Gurabai_Karmarkar,_Hu_King_Eng,_and_Mary_H._Platt,_members_of_the_Class_of_1892_at_the_Woman's_Medical_College_of_Pennsylvania.jpg

Medical College which would train Indians. The Grant Medical College opened in 1845, again only taking male students. In Madras, medical education began in 1835. In Goa, the Portuguese initiated Medical and Pharmacy Licentiates. University-affiliated medical education (initially men only) was introduced in the 1850s after the opening of the first three Indian universities in Madras, Bombay, and Calcutta. Culturally Hindu and Muslim women were forbidden to consult male doctors on matters relating pregnancy, childbirth, and the female reproductive system. This meant that women often neglected their health or went to other health providers. When female medical missionaries started working in India coming from Great Britain, the USA, and Australia, this provided them with a Western Medicine option for care. However, this was only late in the nineteenth century or early twentieth century.

The Indian Mutiny of 1857 led to the dissolution of the East India Company, and the British Government was established in India. This led to the initiation of the Indian Medical Service (1869), the Central and Provincial Medical Services, and the Subordinate Medical Services. The vast majority of practitioners were trained in the Ayurvedic or other indigenous systems of medicine. In 1877, of some 8000 registered (male) practitioners, only 450 were trained in Western medicine [12].

Madras Medical College

Medical Education for women in India began in Madras (Chennai) Medical College. Surgeon General Edward Green Balfour (1813–1889) championed their admission. Four women were admitted in 1875 including Mary Scharlieb (née Bird, 1845–1930) who had migrated to India with her barrister husband, having begun her medical training at the London Medical Women's Hospital. On graduation, the Madras Medical College offered women a Licentiate in Medicine and Surgery (LMS) qualification which allowed registration for medical practice in India, but not elsewhere. The longer 4.5 year program leading to a MBCM was only open to men.

Mary Scharlieb would later complete her MB ChB in London top of her class, one of the first two female graduates from London in 1882. With her scholarship prize, she undertook 4 months further training in operative midwifery under Gustav August Braun at Vienna's Allgemeines Krankenhaus (General Hospital). Thanks to the personal interest of Lady Grant Duff, the wife of the Governor of Madras, the Royal Victoria hospital was established for Caste (Hindu) and Gosha (Mohammedan) women under the superintendence of Mary Scharlieb. The Scharlieb's left for the UK in 1887. The hospital was further developed and relocated to Triplicane, a suburb of Madras on the coast, in 1890. The management of the hospital was taken over by the government of Madras in 1921 and renamed the Kasturba Gandhi Hospital for women and children in 1948.

Annie Jaganadhan qualified from Madras with the LMS in 1883. She studied further at Sophie Jex-Blake's Edinburgh School of Medicine for Women in 1888. She returned to India to work at Cama Hospital, Bombay in 1892 but died of tuberculosis in 1894 [12, 13, 14].

Kadambini Ganguly (1861–1923)

In Calcutta, Kandamini Basu (1861–1923) (Fig. 9.14), and Chandramukhi Basu became the first female graduates of the University in 1882. In 1883, Kandamini applied to Calcutta Medical College and was admitted, thanks to the Lieutenant Governor giving consent overruling the Medical Council. Soon after she married Dwarakanath Ganguly, who was a 39-year-old widower who mentored and supported her career aspirations in medicine. She graduated GBMC (graduate of Bengal Medical College) in 1886, having passed all the written examinations but failed one essential part of the practicals. She was appointed Doctor at the Lady Dufferin Women's Hospital in 1888. Conservative Hindus subjected her to discrimination and abuse and even launched a slander campaign against her. One journalist called her a "whore," but Kambini took successful legal action against him. She also suffered from racial discrimination:

> *The Indian medical women will miss all the advantages of such professional duties by their exclusion from medical charge of important hospitals, or by being placed in an inferior position there, for in the inferior class of hospitals few cases of importance will ever go for treatment, an in the large and important hospitals the major operations and other important duties will always be performed by the senior person in charge.*

In order to promote the position of and respect for women in society, Kandamini Ganguly went on to become Secretary of the Bengal Ladies' Association and organized the Women's Conference in Calcutta in 1906 [13, 14].

Haimabati Sen (1866–1933)

The Calcutta Medical College ran a 3-year course for any woman over the age of 16, offering a Vernacular Licentiate in Medicine and Surgery. They would then work as hospital assistants. In 1888, the Campbell School admitted 15 women including Hindus, Brahmos, native Christians, and Eurasians. The first Muslim

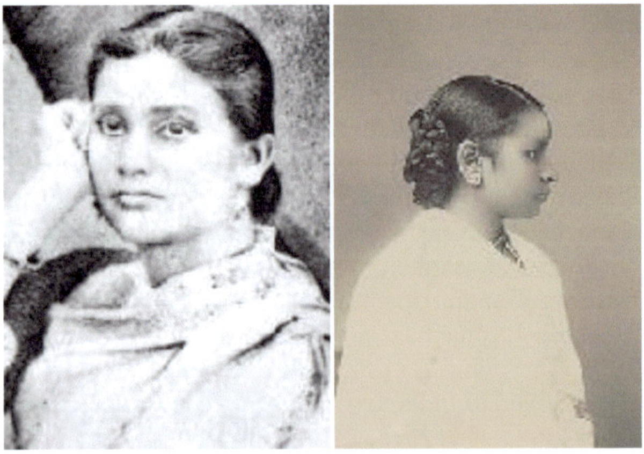

Fig. 9.14 Left: Kandamini Ganguly (1861–1923). Right: Anandibai Joshee (1865–1887), Wikipedia, Public Domain. https://en.wikipedia.org/wiki/Kadambini_Ganguly#/media/File:Kadambini_Ganguly.jpg

was admitted in 1891. Between 1888 and 1905, over 50 Bengali women graduated, one of whom was Haimabati Sen who was admitted in 1891. She practiced medicine in Chinsurah from 1894 to 1933. Her early life (maiden name H. Mitra) included being married at 10, widowed a year later, with her parents and mother-in-law also passing away. Ill-treated by her brother in law she left to become a teacher at a girls' school. She moved to Calcutta and remarried a Brahmo, Kunjabehari Sen. In her second year, she obtained the highest marks in Anatomy, Physiology, and Materia Medica but had to decline the Gold Medal in favor of a Silver because the male students opposed her accepting it. She obtained a low-paid job at Dufferin Hospital as an assistant to the Assistant Surgeon, Dr. Badrikanath Mukherjee who sexually harassed her. Her complaint to the Civil Surgeon resulted in her being rebuked for arrogance. Her memoir describes the violence against women in India at that time and her balancing the roles of professional and family life. She had eight pregnancies and five children. Her husband was sometimes abusive. She died of breast cancer in 1933.

Anandibai Joshee (1865–1887) (Fig. 9.14)

She was married to Gopalrao Joshee at 10 and became a mother at the age of 12 but lost her infant son. She was not in good health but continued to study and so was sent to the USA with the support of her husband; also Pandita Ramabai, a Masharashtian champion of feminism and an American benefactor, Ms. Carpenter. In 1883, she attended the Women's Medical College of Philadelphia from which she graduated in 1886, the first Indian woman to obtain a Western Medical degree. She was appointed as a lady doctor in Kolhapur in the Bombay Presidency but succumbed to tuberculosis prior to commencing at the age of 21.

Another overseas Indian graduate was *Rakhmabai* (1864–1955) who graduated MD from London in 1894, having trained at the London Medical School for Women and the Royal Free Hospital. She became the Principal Medical Officer at Surat Women's Hospital, Gujarat, for many decades, dying at the age of 90.

Hospitals providing care for women began to be created through an initiative of the wife of the then Viceroy of India, Lady Dufferin. The Dufferin hospitals were established from 1885, also a fund that also supported Indian women with scholarships to study medicine [12, 13].

Lady Hardinge Medical College, New Delhi

In 1914, the Times of India reported (18/3/14) that in the Medical Colleges of Calcutta, Bombay, Lahore, and Madras, there were 89 female medical students. However, few of these were Hindus or Mussulmans, being rather Parsis, native Christians, or expatriate Europeans. The Association of Medical Women of India, formed in 1907, had been advocating that there should be a medical college for women run by women. Lady Hardinge (Fig. 9.15) was the wife of the Viceroy of

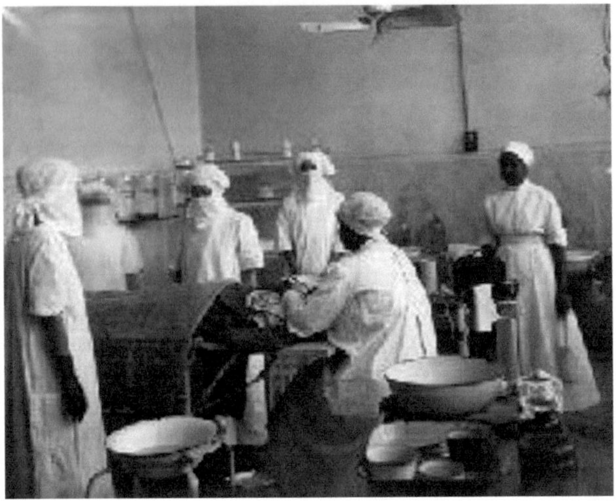

Fig. 9.15 Lady Hardinge Medical College and Hospital, Delhi: an operation taking place. Photograph, 1921. Wellcome Collection. In copyright. Source: Wellcome Collection. https://wellcomecollection.org/works/z3ba6mj2

India who strongly supported the proposal but died after the Foundation stone was laid in New Delhi. This led to the College being named after her; the Lady Hardinge Medical College was opened in 1916.

9.2.3.14 Early Twentieth-Century Pioneers in India

Ida Scudder (1870–1960)

Ida Scudder (1870–1960), the daughter of a medical missionary to India, established what would become the now famous Christian Medical College of Vellore. She was a graduate of Cornell University, USA, and began practice in Vellore in 1900, establishing nursing training in 1909 and a Missionary Medical School offering LMP diplomas in 1918. The famous missionary surgeon, Paul Brand (1913–2003), worked at CMC Vellore where he established many of the principles for treating leprosy patients, whose injuries were related to a loss of sensation. CMC Vellore trained many world-leading Indian doctors throughout the twentieth Century and beyond.

Hilda Lazarus (1890–1978)

Hilda Lazarus (1890–1978) was the first Indian Christian to qualify as a doctor with a MBCM from Madras Medical College (MMC). She joined as an Obstetrician and Gynaecologist working in the Lady Hardinge Medical College and Hospital, New Delhi, becoming its first Indian Principal. She was the first Indian woman doctor in government service and then worked at the Dufferin Hospital, Calcutta, before retiring in 1947. She then directed CMC&H at Vellore from 1948 to 1954 [14].

9.3 Daring to Dream of Equal Opportunity: Twentieth Century

By 1900, women could enter university and study medicine in many countries of the world. However, their qualification and registration as a doctor did not mean they would be appointed to hospital positions which were usually given to men. This restricted their ability to gain sufficient experience to specialize and to advance their careers. They were often dependent on hospitals run by women, or on a few hospitals that began to offer limited opportunities for female doctors to gain postgraduate experience.

This chapter covers the pioneers who achieved Fellowship of a Surgical College, the struggle faced by women doctors to enter the military and serve in theaters of war, and those who succeeded in advancing their academic careers and being appointed as Professors or Chairs of Departments.

9.3.1 Specialist College Fellowship

9.3.1.1 Royal College of Surgeons of Ireland

The first female to be elected to Fellowship of a College was *Emily Winifred Dickson (1866–1944)*. In 1887, she had been refused entry to Trinity College Dublin on the grounds that she was a woman, so she undertook medical training at the Royal College of Surgeons of Ireland, obtaining her licentiate in 1891 and her MB in 1893 with honors. She was elected a Fellow the same year and became an examiner in gynecology and midwifery.

9.3.1.2 Royal College of Physicians and Surgeons of Glasgow

Anne Louise McIlroy (1874–1968) (Fig. 9.16) was born in Ireland and became the first Fellow of the Royal College of Physicians and Surgeons of Glasgow. She applied for admission in 1910, but this was refused, but after a change of policy, the Council accepted her application in 1911. She served in the Scottish Women's Hospitals in France and Serbia during WWI (see below). She was also the first female Medical Professor appointed in the UK, as London University's Professor of O&G at the London Medical Women's College in 1921. She was a founding fellow of the Royal College of Obstetricians and Gynaecologists (RCOG) in 1929, and the first woman to serve on its Council. She was appointed OBE and DBE for her services to Obstetrics.

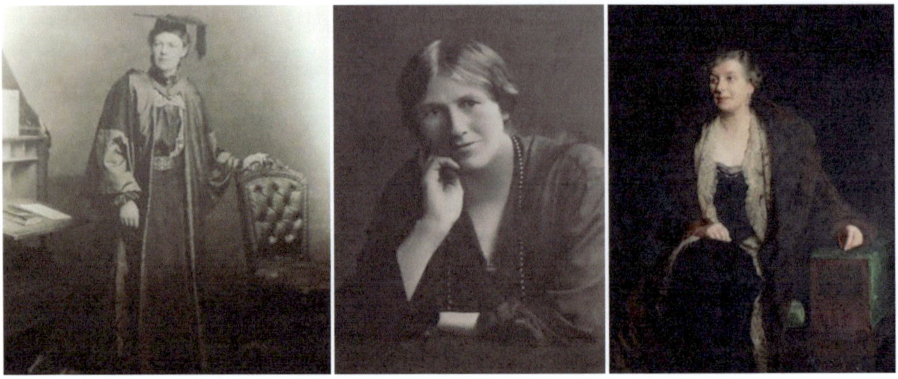

Fig. 9.16 Left: Emily Winifred Dickson. Middle: Eleanor Davies-Colley. Right: Anne Louise McIlroy, Wikipedia, Public domain. https://en.wikipedia.org/wiki/Emily_Winifred_Dickson#/media/File:Emily_Winifred_Dickson.jpg, https://wellcomecollection.org/works/q67k7fk2, https://en.wikipedia.org/wiki/Louise_McIlroy#/media/File:Scottish_Women's_Hospital_-_Dr._Louise_McIlroy.png

9.3.1.3 Royal College of Surgeons of England

Eleanor Davies-Colley (1874–1934) (Fig. 9.16) was the first woman to sit the Fellowship examination of the RCS in 1911. She had trained at the London School of Medicine for Women where she did her residency under Maud Chadburn and became a Senior Obstetrician at the Elizabeth Garrett Anderson Hospital and one of the Founding members of the Medical Women's Foundation. A lecture theatre in the Royal College of Surgeons in London is dedicated to her and women surgeons. She was also appointed as a surgeon to the Marie Curie Cancer Hospital. By 1919, there were only four women Fellows of the Royal College of Surgeons of England; by 1990, this number had risen to 320 and by 2009, to 1184.

9.3.1.4 Royal College of Surgeons of Edinburgh

In early 1920, the RCSEd Council concluded that the 1919 Sex Disqualification (Removal) Act applied to both public and private bodies alike. Thus women should be admitted to the Fellowship of the College on exactly the same basis as men and that, furthermore, they should enjoy exactly the same rights and privileges. The first woman to sit the Fellowship Exam was *Alice Mabel Headwards Hunter (d 1973)*. She then married and never practiced as a surgeon though was admitted to the Fellowship in October of that year along with *Miss Gertrude Herzfeld (1891–1991)*. Herzfeld, the first female practicing surgeon in Scotland, took an active interest in College life until she died in 1981 at the age of 90. She was the first female house surgeon at the Royal Hospital for Sick Children in Edinburgh, and specialized in paediatric surgery.

9.3.1.5 American College of Surgeons

The American College of Surgeons was founded in 1913. Out of a convocation of 1057 Fellows, there were five females selected in 1913, all of whom lived in Boston and had privileges at the New England Hospital for Women and Children. Four were US graduates from the Woman's Medical Colleges in New York (Alice Bryant [1862–1942], 1890), Pennsylvania (Emma Culbertson[d1920],1881) Tufts College Medical School (Florence Duckering [1869–1951],1901) (Fig. 9.17), and Northwestern University (Jane Kelly Sabine [1863–1950] (Fig. 9.17). The fifth, Mary Almira Smith [1850–1923], had graduated MD from Zurich in 1880 and, following her return to America, was Head Surgeon at the New England Hospital for Women and Children until 1918. Alice Bryant specialized in otolaryngology.

9.3.1.6 RACS in Australia and New Zealand

The Royal Australasian College of Surgeons (RACS) was formed in 1927. Lilian Violet Cooper (1861–1947), a General Surgeon, was a Foundation Fellow in June of that year. She had studied medicine at the LSMW and taken the Triple Licentiate from the Colleges of Physicians and Surgeons in Edinburgh and Glasgow in 1890. She then practiced in Brisbane and was the first woman doctor to be appointed at the Brisbane Hospital for Sick Children. She also graduated MD from the University of Durham in 1912. She worked in the Scottish Women's Hospital with Drs Agnes Bennett and Mary De Garis on the Eastern Front in Macedonia from 1916 to 1917. She returned to Brisbane after the war and retired from practice in 1941. She was a foundation member of the Queensland Medical Women's Society in 1929. Her house was donated by her lifelong friend, Miss Josephine Bedford, to the Anglican church for the Mount Olivet Hospital of the Sisters of Charity.

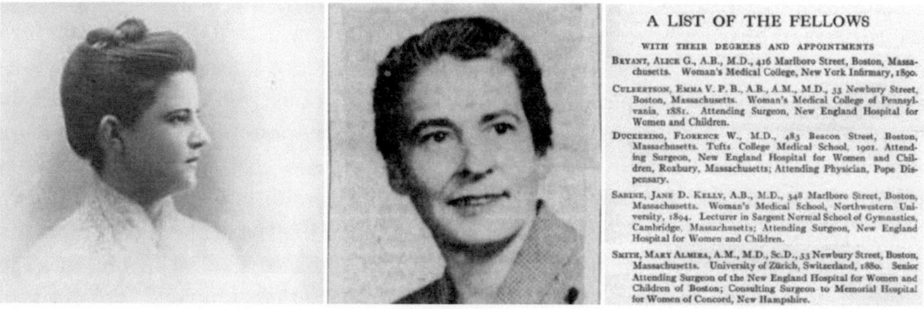

A LIST OF THE FELLOWS

WITH THEIR DEGREES AND APPOINTMENTS

BRYANT, ALICE G., A.B., M.D., 416 Marlboro Street, Boston, Massachusetts. Woman's Medical College, New York Infirmary, 1890.

CULBERTSON, EMMA V. P. B., A.B., A.M., M.D., 33 Newbury Street, Boston, Massachusetts. Woman's Medical College of Pennsylvania, 1881. Attending Surgeon, New England Hospital for Women and Children.

DUCKERING, FLORENCE W., M.D., 483 Beacon Street, Boston, Massachusetts. Tufts College Medical School, 1901. Attending Surgeon, New England Hospital for Women and Children, Roxbury, Massachusetts; Attending Physician, Pope Dispensary.

SABINE, JANE D. KELLY, A.B., M.D., 348 Marlboro Street, Boston, Massachusetts. Woman's Medical School, Northwestern University, 1894. Lecturer in Sargent Normal School of Gymnastics, Cambridge, Massachusetts; Attending Surgeon, New England Hospital for Women and Children.

SMITH, MARY ALMIRA, A.M., M.D., Sc.D., 33 Newbury Street, Boston, Massachusetts. University of Zürich, Switzerland, 1880. Senior Attending Surgeon of the New England Hospital for Women and Children of Boston; Consulting Surgeon to Memorial Hospital for Women of Concord, New Hampshire.

Fig. 9.17 Left: Jane D Kelly Sabin: Centre: Florence Duckering [Duckering image at https://sheboyganpress.newspapers.com/article/the-sheboygan-press/14874521/]. Right: Figure from 1913 ACS Yearbook. https://www.facs.org/for-medical-professionals/news-publications/news-and-articles/bulletin/2019/09/the-first-women-elected-to-college-fellowship/

Constance Elizabeth Darcy (1879–1950) was a gynaecologist and the second female to be elected a RACS Foundation Fellow in 1927. She had graduated from Sydney in 1904, worked at the Royal Hospital for Women in Paddington (Sydney), an opened a private practice in Macquarie St. She devoted her professional life to reducing maternal mortality. From 1919 to 1949 she was a member of the University of Sydney Senate and an honorary gynaecologist to St Vincent's Hospital, 1923–1945 and lecturer in clinical obstetrics 1923–1939. She was appointed a Dame of the British Empire in 1935, and honored by the Pope in 1940 with the *Cross Pro Ecclesia et Pontifice*. She was Deputy Chancellor of the University of Sydney 1943–46.

9.3.2 Women Doctors at War

9.3.2.1 Princess Vera Ignatievna Gedroits (1870–1932)

Princess Gedroits was born in Kyiv, Ukraine, and studied medicine initially at St Petersburg until she was involved in revolutionary politics and expelled from the University. She married her close friend Nikolai Belozerov and moved to Switzerland to complete her studies in the University of Lausanne (1898). She worked in Cesar Roux's clinic, learning particularly about hernia repairs. She returned to Kyiv in 1900, where she worked at a cement factory performing over 250 surgical procedures. When the Russo-Japanese war broke out in 1904, she joined as a surgeon to the Russian Red Cross, performing many life-saving procedures. She advocated early laparotomy (within 3 hrs) for penetrating abdominal injuries, something opposed by British and French doctors at the time:

> *Among those who went to the Front in the service of the Red Cross as surgeons [was] the Princess Gedroits, chief surgeon of the hospital train furnished by the associated nobility of 40 Russian "governments," who was always at the front, operating in a specially constructed car, till the enemy's fire threatened the train.*

Gedroits was awarded the Gold Medal of diligence from the Order of Saint Anna, the Ribbon of St George with the silver medal for bravery, Russian Red Cross' third highest distinction and the silver neck medal of the order of Saint Vladimir. She was appointed as the first female physician of the Royal household at Tsarskoye Selo Court hospital for "a salary of 2100 Rubles and a State apartment." She became the first woman to earn a MD from the University of Moscow in 1912, for her work on hernia repair. Early in World War 1, she trained nurses including Countess Dmitrieva Maria Nirod, who became her lifelong partner. In 1917, she was physician to the sixth Siberian Rifle Regiment with the equivalent rank of Lt Col in the Russian Army. She became the first woman to be a Professor at the University of Kyiv in 1923, becoming head of the surgery department in 1929. She published 58 papers and kept sound records of her cases. In 1904, she had 1255 patients with 138 bullet wounds to the head and 61 to the abdomen. She published a paper on 183 laparotomies for abdominal war wounds in 1914. In 1916, she saved the life of the then Chief of Staff of the Russian Imperial Army and a Japanese Prince (Japan and

Russia were allies in WWI). She also published poetry under the pseudonym Sergei Gedroits. She was well ahead of her time in her surgical treatment; however, publishing in Russian limited her academic exposure to the rest of Europe.

9.3.2.2 World War I (1914–1918)

In August 1914, World War I began when Germany invaded Belgium prompting Britain and its Allies to declare war on Germany. Although there would be shortages of doctors, the British War Office clearly stated they did not want to recruit women doctors. However, women were determined to play their part and formed their own volunteer hospital units, served with the Red Cross or St John Ambulance, until later in the war when the Royal Army Medical Corps recognized that they needed women doctor volunteers and began to contract them, although they did not gazette their appointments, nor officially commission them despite offering them a rank. However, the Australian expeditionary force did not agree to recruit women doctors at all, and so the Australians, at least 25 of the 129 womenregistered to practice in Australia, served with the British (RAMC), or Volunteer Hospitals such as the Scottish Women's Hospital (SWH) on the Eastern Front.

The Women's Hospital Corps

Flora Murray (1869–1963) was educated at Durham University (MB Bsc 1903; MD 1905) and the London School of Medicine for Women. She was a medical officer at the Belgrave Hospital for Children in London and then an anaesthetist at the Chelsea Hospital for Women [15].

Louisa Garrett Anderson (1873–1943) was the eldest of Elizabeth Garrett Anderson's three children and educated at St Leonards School in St Andrews. She graduated from the London School of Medicine for Women (MB ChB 1898; MD 1900). She was not able to secure a hospital position and so, following postgraduate studies in Johns Hopkins and observerships in Paris and Chicago, took a position at the New Hospital for Women in London, founded by her mother where she became senior surgeon. She was an active and radical suffragette and in 1912, briefly imprisoned, but later found herself treating the war wounds of the policeman who arrested her in France!

Flora Murray and Louisa Garrett Anderson founded the Women's Hospital Corps (WHC). Initially, between September 1914 and January 1915, with the support of the French Red Cross, they ran a volunteer hospital at Claridge's Hotel on the Champs Elysees in Paris, treating British and French soldiers who had been transferred some 60 miles from the front. They overcame initial skepticism that women doctors could treat war injuries and gained a reputation for a well-run, caring, and efficient hospital. When senior officers of the British Army inspected the Women's Hospital they would ask, "But why are you a French Hospital? You ought to be working with us." The women replied, *"The War Office would never look at women doctors*." A second WHC unit was established in November 1914, at a chateau in Wimereux near Boulogne and operated until there was a relative lull in the fighting due to the cold winter weather. The RAMC then asked the WMC to run a military hospital at Endell St, Bloomsbury, London, and which remained in operation tending the sick and wounded until October 1919.

Flora Murray was given the rank of Lt Col during the war and appointed CBE together with Louisa Garret Anderson, her partner, in 1917. She died of cancer in 1923.

Australian Women Doctors

At the outbreak of war, there were 129 women doctors registered as medical practitioners in Australia. There are 26 serving women Australian doctors who contributed to the war effort in Europe and Egypt according to Sheard and Lee's book covering women doctors of the Great War [Women to the Front, Ebury Australia, 2019]. Many of these women were able to serve in RAMC hospitals, despite being denied the right to serve with the Australian Army Medical Corps (AAMC). These included Eleanor Bourne (1878–1957), Sydney 1903 graduate, and Phoebe Chapple (1879–1967), an Adelaide graduate in 1904, who worked at the Cambridge Military Hospital in Aldershot. Rachel Champion (1890–1965), a graduate of the University of Melbourne, served in Endell St, Military hospital in 1916–1917. Emma Buckley (Turkington) (1879–1953) was a 1911 Sydney graduate who worked in London during WWI at the Lister Institute, King George Military Hospital, and briefly at Endell St. Elizabeth Hamilton-Browne (1882–1985), a 1910 Sydney graduate, served at Endell St from March 1916–March 1918, and then at the No 19 General Hospital in Egypt. Vera Scantlebury (Brown) (1889–1946), a Melbourne 1914 graduate, worked in Endell St from May 1917 until January 1919. Tasmanian, Dr. Eveline Benjamin (Cohen) (1879–1922), one of the first Tasmanian-born women to graduate in Medicine, served in 1915–1916 at British military hospitals in England, Salonika, and Malta.

Scottish Women's Hospitals

Elsie Inglis (1864–1917) from Edinburgh and *Louisa McIntyre* (1874–1968) from Glasgow founded the Scottish Women's Hospitals (SWH) with funds from the National Suffragette Union, the American Red Cross and other Donors. During World War I, there 14 units of the SWH, involving over 1000 women in 6 countries, serving on both the Western and Eastern fronts.

Inglis set up the first hospital at Royaumont in France before moving to Serbia in April 1915. As the Germans and Austro-Hungarian Empire advanced, the Inglis-led Serbian SWH unit had to retreat through Albania. They treated the wounded of both sides and were eventually captured but repatriated through Vienna in February 1916. The Serbians requested the SWH to return so after a period of fund-raising Inglis, as CMO with 75 women and 16 vehicles, set off from Liverpool through

Archangel to join the Serbians fighting in Romania from August 1916. The Serbians were again in retreat as the Germans and Bulgarians advanced. One Serbian doctor described how the Inglis and the SWH handled themselves:

> *Elsie Inglis maintained a unique discipline…during the terrible retreat when her hospitals were ceaselessly bombed…she worked without a day's rest, not shrinking from the most arduous or loathsome tasks. We shall never forget these days when we saw the Scottish women collecting our wounded from the firing line in their own ambulances.*

Inglis' unit eventually had to retreat into Russia in 1917, but when the Russian revolution occurred in October of that year, they were ordered home. By then she was unwell, probably dying of gastric cancer, and passed away the day after returning home. She was honoured with a state funeral at St Giles' Cathedral in Edinburgh. She was also awarded the Serbian Order of the White Cross, their highest honor. Edinburgh's Elsie Inglis Memorial Maternity Hospital was established in her honour in 1925 and treated patients until 1988.

Louise McIlroy was posted to a SWH unit in Troyes in France and later served in Salonika and Serbia. She was awarded a Croix de Guerre by France in 1916 and the OBE in 1920.

Australian women doctors who served with SWH include Lilian Cooper (1861–1947) had graduated from LSMW in 1890, also had a MD from Durham University (1912), and served in SWH in Macedonia in 1916–1917. Agnes Bennett (1872–1960) was a graduate of Sydney in 1894, who had first worked with the NZAMC in Egypt in 1915–1916, before serving in the SWH in Macedonia in 1916–1917. Laura Fowler (Hope) (1868–1952) was the first MB BS graduate from the University of Adelaide in 1891 and served with SWH in Serbia from October 1915 until captured in February 1916. Mary De Garis (1881–1963), a University of Melbourne graduate in 1905 served in 1916 at Manor Hospital, London, and then with SWH in Macedonia, in 1917 and 1918.

Millicent Fawcett Hospitals for Russia

Millicent Fawcett was a political activist for the Suffragette movement and other causes who supported hospital units in Russia during World War I.

Mabel Eliza May (1874–1971) graduated from Manchester in 1911, and served as a house surgeon at Ashton Infirmary and then during World War I in Mrs. Stoddart's unit in Serbia (1915) and later with a Millicent Fawcett Unit in Russia (1916–1917).

Helena Adelaide Hall (1867–1926) served with Mrs. Stoddart's unit in Serbia and then in Russia until the revolution in 1917 and subsequently worked in Egypt.

Laura Foster (1858–1917) was a graduate of the University of Berne in 1894 and served with a Belgian Field Hospital from September 1914 until early 1915 and then in St Petersburg and the Caucasus with the Russian Red Cross (1915–1917) and in Galicia. She died of typhoid in Zaleschiki, Galicia, in January 1917.

9.3.2.3 World War II

Major Barbara Stimson (1898–1986) was an orthopaedic surgeon who graduated in medicine from the third-class that admitted women at the Columbia Medical School (1923) and was the second female surgical resident to complete training at the Columbia Presbyterian Medical Centre. She was admitted (elected) to the ACS in 1934 as the only female fellow of the New York group. She wrote a textbook *A Manual of Fractures and Dislocations* published in 1939. The American Board of Surgery (ABS) was formed in 1936, to introduce more rigor to the training program requiring 4 years of post-internship training in surgery and then passing the ABS examinations. In 1940, when she decided to sit for examination to become Board Certified woman, there were already 850 certified men. During WWII, it would not be until December 1941, that the USA entered the war, but the British Medical Service was asking for American doctors to volunteer to work in civilian hospitals. Barbara Stinson, together with her lifelong friend, Dr. Achsa Bean MD, volunteered and served at the Royal Free Hospital in London. The US military still did not commission women to service. Dr. Bean was commissioned a RAMC captain, while Stimson was given the rank of RAMC major, and deployed, at her request, to military hospitals in North Africa and Italy as senior surgeon on the orthopaedic team. She was awarded two Distinguished Service medals and appointed a Member of the British Empire (MBE). When stationed in Rome, she developed expertise in knee injuries and had to treat the bucket handle tear of Major Randolph Churchill, the son of the wartime British Prime Minister. After the war she returned to practice in New York. She became the first woman president of the Dutchess County Medical Association in 1960, the first female member of the New York Surgical Society, and the American Association for the surgery of trauma. She retired in 1963, and wrote a memoir, *Major Barbara's memories of WWII* which was published posthumously by her sister in 1987.

9.3.3 Career Advancement in the Twentieth Century

9.3.3.1 Canada

Dr. Jennie Smillie Robertson (1878–1981) was the first recorded female surgeon in Canada, graduating in 1909 from the University of Toronto. She undertook her residency at the Philadelphia Women's Medical College. She helped establish the Women's College Hospital where she was the Chair of Gynaecology from 1912 to 1942. She married Alex Robertson at the age of 70, because, despite meeting him in 1898, she believed she couldn't have both a career in medicine and be married.

Dr. Jessie Gray (1910–1978) was the first registered female general surgeon in Canada having graduated from the University of Toronto as the gold medal recipient. She was the first female surgical graduate of the Gallie Program at the University of Toronto. In 1941, she was named Canada's "First Lady of Surgery," and she served, starting in 1946, as the chief of surgery at the Women's College Hospital. In 1954, she was honoured with the Elizabeth Blackwell Medal.

9.3.3.2 USA

Patricia Numan (b1941), later President of the ACS (2011–2012), founded the ACS' Association of Women Surgeons (AWS) in 1981 which, as it grew, incorporated in 1986. The AWS established the Olga Johansson lecture at the ACS in 2007, in honor of *Olga Johansson (1934–2006*), the first female head of an academic surgical department in the USA, being appointed at Cook County Hospital in 1977. Olga, a kidney transplant surgeon, was later chair of Ohio State University Department of Surgery (1987–1993). She then joined the staff of the American College of Surgeons, as Director of the then Education and Surgical Services Department, the first woman to hold a senior position at the College.

9.3.3.3 Scotland

Margaret Fairlie (1891–1963) was the first female Professor of Obstetrics and Gynaecology, appointed to Dundee University in 1940. She grew up in Angus, Scotland, and graduated from St Andrews Dundee University. She trained in O&G in St Mary's Hospital, Manchester. She was appointed head of O&G at Dundee Royal Infirmary in 1936, and this led to a protracted impasse in her appointment as the Professor at St Andrews University until 1940, partly due to the principal's reluctance to appoint a woman as a Professor. When she retired in 1956, she was still the only female Professor in Scotland.

Agnes Marshall Cowan (1880–1940) (Fig. 9.18) was the first Scottish Professor in O&G but one based overseas, appointed by RCOG in 1934. She graduated from the University of Edinburgh in 1906 and obtained a position at Leith hospital, which was the first to accept female doctors. In 1911, she left Scotland for Manchuria where, until 1915, she worked at Mukden Medical College (now Sheng Jing Hospital), originally founded by Scottish Presbyterian missionary, Dr. Dugald Christie. She returned to Scotland to work with Queen Mary's Army Auxiliary Corps, attached to the RAMC, in Gretna where there was an explosives factory. After the war she returned to Manchuria (now Shenyang, China). MMC had strong links to the University of Edinburgh, so became the first College outside the UK to have its medical degree recognized in Scotland. RCOG elected her a Fellow, and awarded her a Professorship in 1934. The Japanese invaded Manchuria in 1931, but Cowan stayed until 1939, only returning before the outbreak of WWII. By then her health was poor and she died in Cambridge in 1940.

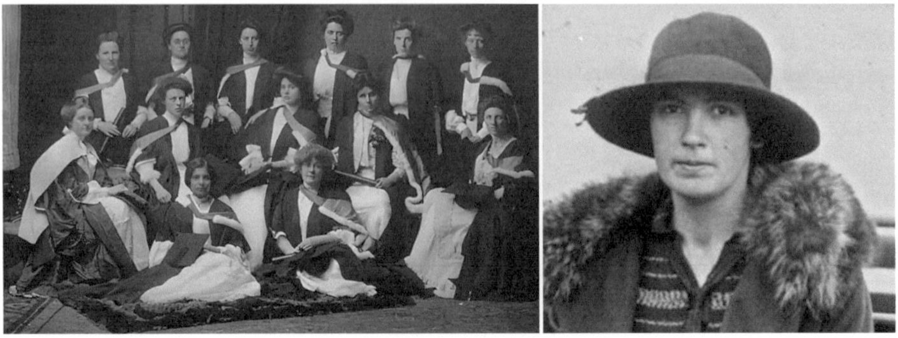

Fig. 9.18 Left: Edinburgh University Female Medical Graduates 1906. Right: Agnes Marshall Cowan (1880–1940), aged 31. Archives @ University of Edinburgh. November 12, 2013. Accessed March 22, 2024. https://upload.wikimedia.org/wikipedia/commons/2/2e/The_female_graduates_in_Medicine_at_Edinburgh_University_in_July_1906.png

9.3.3.4 England

Averil Mansfield (b1937), a graduate of Liverpool University, was the first female Professor of Surgery in the UK. She was appointed a consultant vascular surgeon in Liverpool in 1972, and moved to St Mary's Hospital, London, where she worked from 1982 to 2002, becoming Professor of vascular surgery in 1993 (Fig. 9.19). In 1991, she founded the Women in Surgical Training (WIST) Committee at the RCS. She was also President of the BMA (2009–2010). She was appointed Dame of the British Empire in 2023. In 1987, she married John (Jack) Bradley, a surgeon, who died in 2013.

Anne Christine Bayley - Professor of Surgery in Zambia (1984–1988)
Anne Christine Bayley (1934–2025) was a graduate of Girton College, Cambridge, and the Middlesex Hospital Medical School, qualifying as a doctor in 1958. As a junior doctor, she rotated through various hospitals in England but also worked at St Francis' Hospital, Katete, Zambia in 1961–1962, then returned to England to train for the FRCS which she gained in 1968. She was appointed as Lecturer in Surgery, first at the Korle Bu hospital, Accra, Ghana, from 1968 to 1970, and then in the University of Zambia (UNZA) and the University Teaching Hospital in Lusaka in 1971. Her career progressed until she was appointed Professor of Surgery from 1984, overseeing the development of a MMed program to train Zambian surgeons. During Anne's tenure, the first seven candidates were enrolled and graduated. She served on the Council of the Association of Surgeons of East Africa (ASEA), was its first female President in 1983–1984. Her specialty was surgical oncology, but later, as HIV was spreading rapidly South and across sub-Saharan Africa, she focused on surgical aspects of this condition including atypical aggressive Kaposi's sarcoma. She was appointed OBE and awarded an honorary fellowship of the Royal College of Surgeons of Edinburgh in 1986. In 1990, somewhat burned out by the rapid spread of the HIV pandemic in sub-Saharan Africa, Bayley left Zambia to undertake

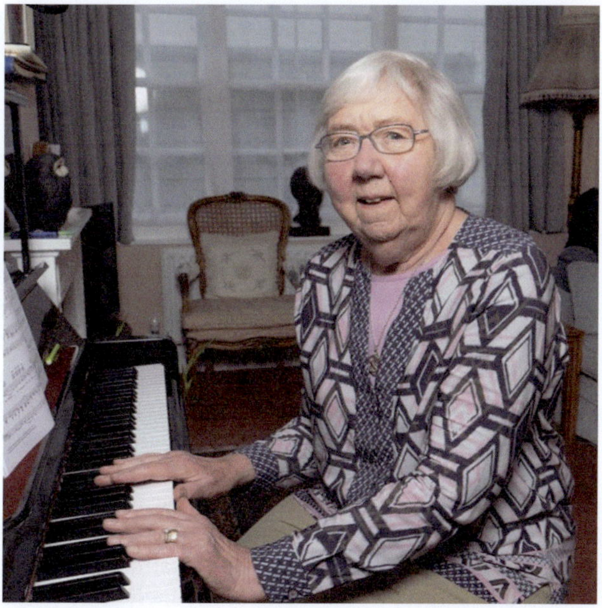

Fig. 9.19 Professor Averil Mansfield (b1937)

theological training in England. In 1992, the General Synod of the Church of England finally agreed, after 19 years of debate and division, to ordain female priests. The first 32 women were ordained in March 1994, the year Anne was also ordained into the Anglican priesthood.

9.3.3.5 Other Female Doctor Pioneers of Twentieth Century

Dorothy Lavinia Brown (1914–2004), born in Philadelphia, Pennsylvania, was raised in an orphanage until the age of 12 and was the first African American from the Southeastern United States to become a surgeon. Following a BA, she studied medicine at Meharry Medical College from 1944 and was an intern in Harlem, New York City, graduating in 1948. She was the Chief Surgeon at the Riverside hospital in Nashville, Tennessee, from 1957 to 1983 and was also elected to Tennessee State Legislature for 2 years in 1966. In 1959, she was the first black female American to be elected a Fellow of ACS. She never married but adopted two children.

Dr. Brown received many honors including the naming of the Dorothy L. Brown Women's Residence at Meharry College in 1970; a humanitarian award from the Carnegie Foundation in 1993; and the prestigious Horatio Alger Award in 1994. She was proud to be a role model, *"not because I have done so much, but to say to young people that it can be done."*

Alexa Irene Canady (b 1950), a 1975 graduate cum *laude* of the University of Michigan, was the first African-American woman to become a neurosurgeon in the USA in 1984. She became Chief of neurosurgery at Children's Hospital of Michigan 1987–2001.

9.4 Daring to Dream of Equal Opportunity: The Twenty-First Century

In 2017, for the first time, there were more women than men enrolled in medical schools in the USA. In Europe, the UK, and Australia, this had been the case for some decades though the female gender representation in surgery were much lower. Of all Fellows of Surgical Colleges, the numbers of women as a proportion of the total are little more than 10–15%. In 2014, 11% of Fellows of the RCS in England were female; the proportion was similar in Australia. However, the proportion of women choosing a career in surgery and being successfully selected currently hovers around the 30% mark, though this still suggests that young women are not as attracted to surgery as men. Hopefully increasing number of women in surgery will convince more girls, female medical students, and junior doctors that the surgical specialties offer a valid and rewarding career choice. More women surgeons will lead to increasing opportunities for aspiring female surgeons to have role models who are women. The women who enter the profession have a right to equity, to be respected, to earn the same financial rewards, and to enjoy a profession without experiencing discrimination, bullying, or sexual harassment, such as their pioneers had to endure in the 19th and 20th centuries. All surgeons, whether male or female, have a responsibility to promote gender equity [16, 17].

9.4.1 Addressing Discrimination, Bullying, and Sexual Harassment

The surgical workplace has been experienced as an overtly "male culture," toxic, and humiliating environment for surgical education, training, and practice. Discrimination, bullying, and sexual harassment have often been accompanied by a failure by hospitals to address these issues adequately, particularly dealing with perpetrators (who are often surgical consultants and leaders) when they occur. Women doctors and trainees frequently do not report harassment for fear of it influencing their career advancement, despite the distress it causes. Discrimination (on the basis of race or gender), bullying, and other forms of harassment are even more common, more likely to be experienced by women than men, and cause considerable distress, impairing performance in the surgical workplace. The approach to complaints or addressing culture in health and other professions has often been to deny, deflect, or disagree, sweeping the broader problem under the carpet in an effort to avoid effectively tackling such difficult issues. Yet up to 50% of women have reported experiencing and/or witnessing these behaviors in the workplace. The first formal apology to those who had experienced discrimination, bullying, or sexual harassment in surgery was made by the President of the Royal Australasian College of Surgeons (RACS) in 2015. An Operate with Respect campaign was launched in Australia and New Zealand during 2016. This led to a wider recognition and acceptance by other Colleges of Surgeons around the world, with the Royal Colleges of Ireland, Edinburgh, England and Malaysia conducting reviews and launching their own initiatives to address the cultural issues and harassing behaviors. For example, RCSEd then launched a Bullying and Undermining campaign "Lets Remove It" in 2017, while RCSI published a progress report on "Promoting gender equity in Surgery." The New Yorker launched a cover campaign showing female surgeons beneath an operating light [16, 17] (Fig. 9.20).

Many have reported that there are significant longer-term effects of experiencing discrimination, bullying, and sexual harassment in medicine. These include lack of self-esteem, depression, anxiety, use of prescription medications, alcohol abuse, suicide ideation, impaired workplace performance, and leaving their chosen profession altogether. These are in addition to their impact on team performance and patient outcomes.

9.4.1.1 #MeToo (2017)

The year 2017 also saw the launch of the Twitter (now X) hashtag, #MeToo, to raise awareness of sexual harassment in all occupations. There have been significant reviews and inquiries of the problem in many previously much respected professions including legal, police, healthcare in general, military and politics. Additionally in 2017, Harvey Weinstein was arrested (and later convicted), raising the issue of not only his behaviour and abuse of power, but also exposing sexual and other forms of harassment in the Movie industry [17, 18].

As this book of Surgical History is being written in 2023–2025, it is acknowledged that the problems of discrimination, bullying, and sexual harassment are not over. Processes and policies have been improved, complaints are taken more seriously, and the evidence suggests that at least 80% of complaints are likely to be substantiated. However, too many victims still suffer, and their complaints are often inadequately addressed with limited feedback.

A 2023 review of the British Surgical Workforce published in the British Journal of Surgery reported that:

> *Among women, 63.3 per cent reported being the target of sexual harassment versus 23.7 per cent of men (89.5 per cent witnessing versus 81.0 per cent of men). Additionally, 29.9 per cent of women had been sexually assaulted versus 6.9 per cent of men (35.9 per cent witnessing versus 17.1 per cent of men), with 10.9 per cent of women experiencing forced physical contact for career opportunities (a form of sexual assault) versus 0.7 per cent of men* [19].

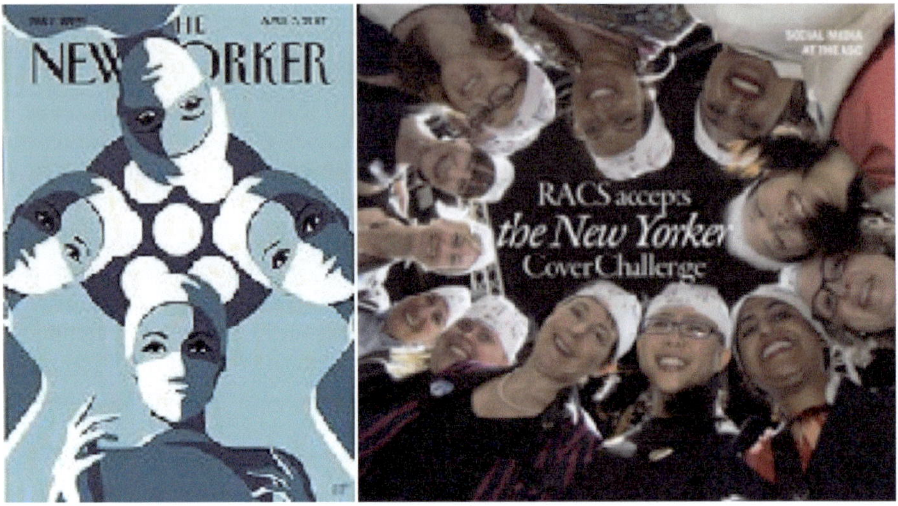

Fig. 9.20 The New Yorker Cover Challenge 2017 (left) and the RACS response (right), typical of the response of many hospitals and Professional Surgical Associations across the world

The review also found that complaints are still inadequately investigated and resolved, with only 15% satisfactorily resolved for the complainant by a health service though this rose to 31% for a College.

In the mid 2020's, these figures remain unacceptable. There are still too many individuals who abuse their power, who discriminate against other races and cultures, sexually harass, and/or intimidate women in the workplace. There are also too many silent bystanders who observe the unacceptable behaviors but do not address them. It should be acknowledged that not all complaints are about men; some are also about how women behave [20].

But the right to equity, the right for everyone to be treated with respect, is no longer disputed despite the need to recognize that in the third decade of the twenty-first century, there is still much to be done to ensure everyone feels safe to be a doctor, surgical trainee, or surgeon at work.

9.4.1.2 Career Advancement and Surgical Leadership

Career advancement and opportunity also remains a gender equity issue for women. In 2018, the New England Journal of Medicine published a perspective on ending sexual harassment in Academic Medicine stating:

> *Although 2017 marked the first time more women than men enrolled in U.S. medical schools (after the proportion had hovered near 50% for more than a decade), women are still vastly outnumbered in academic leadership positions. According to the Association of American Medical Colleges, only 38% of faculty members, 15% of department chairs, and 16% of deans are women. Within certain specialties, the numbers are even worse—in 2014, women chaired only 11% of neurology departments, 10% of emergency departments, and less than*

1% of surgery departments. Women are also paid less, are less likely to be promoted, and receive less recognition from academic societies. Unfortunately, these concerns are not without basis [21].

Nonetheless women surgeons are being elected increasingly to the surgical leadership roles they did not have in the twentieth century. In terms of Surgical College leadership, New Zealander, Anne Kolbe, a paediatric surgeon, was the first female President of a "Western" Surgical College in 2003–2005 [Royal Australasian College of Surgeons]. In Obstetrics and Gynaecology, she was preceded by Heather M Munro AO, who was President of the Royal Australasian College of Obstetrics and Gynaecology (RACOG) in 1994–1996. RACOG was renamed the Royal Australian and New Zealand College of Obstetrics and Gynaecology (RANZCOG) in 1998, and Prof Christine Tippet was RANZCOG's first female President in 2006-8. Kathryn D Anderson, a paediatric surgeon, was the first President of the American College of Surgeons in 2005–2006, followed by Patricia J Numan in 2011–2012, a breast and endocrine surgeon, and then Barbara L Bass in 2017–2018. Clare Marks (1954–2022), an orthopaedic surgeon, was the first President of the Royal College of Surgeons in England between 2014 and 2017. Anne C Bayley, a surgical oncologist from England (see above), was the first female President of the Association of Surgeons of East Africa (ASEA) (1983–1984) which, in 1999, became the College of Surgeons of East, Central, and Southern Africa (COSECSA). Dr. Fualal Jane Odubu from Uganda became the first female President of COSECSA in 2022. The formation of the Women in Surgery in Africa (WISA) in 2015, has resulted in the number of female trainees increasing in a region where currently only 9% of surgeons are women. In 2022 Emeritus Professor Dato' Yip Cheng Har, a Malaysian breast surgeon, was elected the first female President of the International Surgical Society, the oldest International Surgical Association in the world having been constituted in 1902. She was also the first female President of the College of Surgeons of Malaysia between 2010 and 2013.

9.4.1.3 Representation at Surgical Conferences and Interview Panels

Surgical conferences are now reporting the rates of women chairing sessions, being keynote speakers and other presenters, ensuring there is sufficient measurement to drive greater equity. Surgical departments and their Hospital or University employers also consider the gender balance of their interview panels to ensure equal opportunity among applicants.

9.4.1.4 Gender Pay Gap

The gender pay gap is also a critical topic and still exists in many countries as shown in a review of the topic in the American Journal of Surgery in 2022. To promote equity, the authors recommended open reporting on regional pay scales, acknowledgment of gender and racial pay inequalities by departmental and institutional leadership, and more training on contract negotiation during training. The pay gaps occur in countries with widely varying health systems [22]. There is also a considerable gender pay gap in Japan (Tomizawa) [23].

References

1. Callo P, Proto MC, Patruno C, Del Sorbo A, Bifulco M. The first cosmetic treatise of history. A female point of view. Int J Cosmetic Sci 2008;30:79–86.
2. Ferraris ZA, Ferraris VA. The women of Salerno: contribution to the origins of surgery from medieval Italy. Ann Thorac Surg. 1997 Dec;64(6):1855–7. https://doi.org/10.1016/s0003-4975(97)01079-5. PMID: 9436596.
3. Wyaman AL. The Surgeoness: The female practitioner of Surgery 1400-1800. Medical History 1984;28:22–41.
4. Kubba AK. The life, work and gender of Dr James Barry MD (1795-1865). Proc R Coll Physicians Edinb 2001;31:352–6.
5. Rehman A, Rahman NG, Harris SM, Cheema FH. Mary Edwards Walker: the soul ahead of her time. JAMA Surg. 2015;150(2):173–4. https://doi.org/10.1001/jamasurg.2014.877.
6. Klifto KM, Quan A, Lee DA. Mary Edwards Walker (1832–1919): approach to limb salvage therapy. Wound Repair Regen. 2019;27(3):285–7. https://doi.org/10.1111/wrr.12695. Epub 2019 Jan 25
7. Tan SY, Sung H. Mary Edwards Walker (1832–1919): surgeon, feminist and war heroine. Singapore Med J. 2008;49(3):186–7.
8. Hunt HK. Glances and glimpses. Boston: John P Jewett and Co; 1856. http://www.womenhistoryblog.com/2013/04/harriot-kezia-hunt.html.
9. Walsh MR. Wanted Doctors. No women need apply. Sexual barriers in the medical profession (1835–1975). Yale University Press; 1979.
10. Bhadra M. Indian women in medicine: an enquiry since 1880. Indian Anthropol. 2011;41(1):17–43. http://www.jstor.org/stable/41921931.
11. http://collections.ed.ac.uk/alumni/search/*:*/Collection:%22female+medical+graduates+1896-1900%7C%7C%7CFemale+Medical+Graduates+1896-1900%22.
12. Mukherjee S. Women and medicine in colonial India: A CASE study of three women doctors. Proc Indian Hist Congr. 2005;66:1183–93. http://www.jstor.org/stable/44145930.
13. Raman R, Raman A. Women Doctors and women's hospitals in Madras with notes on the related influencing developments in India in the late 19th and early 20th centuries. Curr Sci. 2019;117(7):1232.
14. Anshu, Supe A. Evolution of medical education in India: the impact of colonialism. J Postgrad Med. 2016;62(4):255–9. https://doi.org/10.4103/0022-3859.191011. PMID: 27763484; PMCID: PMC5105212.
15. Murray F. Women as army surgeons. being the history of the Women's Hospital Corps in Paris, Wimereux and Endell St, September 1914 to October 1919. London: Hodder and Stoughton; 1920.
16. Crebbin W, Campbell G, Hillis DA, Watters DA. Prevalence of bullying, discrimination and sexual harassment in surgery in Australasia. ANZ J Surg. 2015;85(12):905–9. https://doi.org/10.1111/ans.13363. Epub 2015 Oct 29
17. McNally S. Sexual harassment and bullying in UK surgery: no room for complacency. BMJ. 2016;354:i4682. https://doi.org/10.1136/bmj.i4682.
18. Coopes A. Operate with respect: how Australia is confronting sexual harassment of trainees. BMJ. 2016;354:i4210. https://doi.org/10.1136/bmj.i4210.
19. Dzau VJ, Johnson PA. Ending sexual harassment in academic medicine. N Engl J Med. 2018;379(17):1589–91. https://doi.org/10.1056/NEJMp1809846. Epub 2018 Sep 12

20. Begeny CT, Arshad H, Cuming T, Dhariwal DK, Fisher RA, Franklin MD, Jackson PM, McLachlan GM, Searle RH, Newlands C. Sexual harassment, sexual assault and rape by colleagues in the surgical workforce, and how women and men are living different realities: observational study using NHS population-derived weights. Br J Surg. 2023;110(11):1518–26. https://doi.org/10.1093/bjs/znad242. Erratum in: Br J Surg. 2023 Nov 07;: PMID: 37697690; PMCID: PMC10564399.
21. Slama EM, Arjani S, Sulciner ML, Riner AN, Yu YR, Maxwell J. The gender gap in surgeon salaries – striving to achieve pay equity. Am J Surg. 2023;225(2):436–8. https://doi.org/10.1016/j.amjsurg.2022.09.037. Epub 2022 Sep 23
22. Halim UA, Qureshi A, Dayaji S, Ahmad S, Qureshi MK, Hadi S, Younis F. Orthopaedics and the gender pay gap: A systematic review. Surgeon. 2023;21(5):301–7. https://doi.org/10.1016/j.surge.2023.02.003. Epub 2023 Mar 12
23. Tomizawa Y. Commentary: role modeling for female surgeons in Japan. Tohoku J Exp Med. 2019;248:151–8.

Chapter 10
Surgical Specialization in Reconstructive Surgery, Orthopaedics, Ophthalmology, Neurosurgery, Cardiothoracic Surgery, Vascular Surgery and Transplantation

10.1 Skin and Skin Grafts

Skin can be considered the largest organ in the body. It plays a major role in mechanically protecting inner tissues against external injuries, also providing a defense against infection and desiccation. It is essential for physiological homeostasis including thermoregulation and fluid and electrolyte balance. It is the part of the body people see, and therefore its appearance, shape, and contour are fundamental to cosmesis.

Today, one of the basic techniques of surgery is the ability to perform a skin graft to cover large epithelial defects that would otherwise heal with unacceptable scarring. There are essentially three types of skin graft, an autograft (skin from the same person to a different site, also called an isograft), an allograft or homograft (from same species but another person), and a xenograft (from another species). Each type skin graft can be partial (split) thickness or full thickness, with partial-thickness skin grafts being more likely to "take" and thus more suitable for wider defects, while full-thickness skin grafts will heal with a better cosmetic appearance but are limited to smaller wounds [1, 2].

Skin grafts were described in ancient Hindu times, more than 3000 years ago. According to *Sushruta Samhita*, the graft was described as a free graft of skin and subcutaneous fat from the gluteal region. Skin grafting was also documented by the ancient Egyptians in the "Ebert Papyrus" around 1600 BCE [2].

Some of the inspiration to, and underlying principles for, performing skin grafts came from attempts to treat tissue defects associated with wounds and, in particular, severed noses as a result of war, punishment, or sword fighting. Rhinoplasty and facial defect reconstruction are covered in an accompanying section.

S. Abbas, D. Watters, *The Road to Modern Surgery*,
https://doi.org/10.1007/978-981-96-4337-0_10

Today, at least in countries where medicine is highly specialized, skin grafts are performed largely by plastic and reconstructive surgeons. However they were a fundamental procedure for all general surgeons throughout the twentieth century and would still be regarded as such in many low- and middle-income countries. Where a skin graft no longer represents the best procedure to cover a limited-sized defect and achieve best function, appearance, and cosmesis, reconstructive surgeons may choose to perform rotation flaps and, from late in the twentieth century, free flaps using microsurgical techniques combined with a detailed knowledge of flap anatomy and blood supply. The challenge to survival presented by major full-thickness burns has also led from the 1990s to the development of skin cultures based on skin cells from the patient's own skin, often supported by xenografts or artificial skin cover to provide temporary wound cover while the cultures were being grown.

10.1.1 Burns

Currently burns are one of the most devastating of all injuries, representing a major cause of global death and disability. The management of a burn wound and its outcome is dependent on whether it is a partial-thickness burn or a full-thickness burn, and in the case of the former how deep is its extent. Another determining factor is the body surface area that is burned. Without modern burn management and skin coverage, anyone burned in excess of 20–30% of their body surface area would be likely to succumb either early to burn shock or later to infection.

Burns and their treatments are as old as human history, certainly since our ancestors discovered fire. Archaeologists have found cave paintings of Neanderthal man treating burn wounds with plant-based extracts. Throughout history, topical applications have often represented the only available treatment.

10.1.2 Management of Burns in Ancient Times

One of the earliest records described in an Egyptian Smith Papyrus (1600 BCE) utilized resin and honey salve, combined with religious intonations to the Goddess Isis. For good measure, the salve was sometimes followed by a dressing soaked with the milk of the mother of a male infant [2, 3].

In 600 BCE, the Chinese described the use of tea leaf abstracts and tinctures for burns. Hippocrates (circa 400 BCE) described the use of dressings impregnated with pig fat, alternated with vinegar soaks, and then supplemented with tanning solutions made from oak bark [3].

In the first century CE, Celsus described the use of wine and myrrh as a lotion for burns; these conveyed some antiseptic properties. Muhammad ibn Zakariya al-Razi (Rhazes), an Arabian physician in the ninth to tenth centuries CE, recommended cold water for the relief of pain from burns.

The problem with waiting for spontaneous healing in full-thickness burns is that, if death from infection is avoided, larger burn wounds will heal with ugly, hypertrophic scars, and burns sited over a joint heal with contracture that impedes joint function. After a period of years, neglected and chronic burns scars are also prone to undergo malignant transformation or Marjolin's ulcer, named after Jean Nicolas Marjolin (1780–1850), a French surgeon in Paris.

In Roman times, Celsus and Galen described using skin grafts for treating facial defects. Celsus also described it to reconstruct the foreskin of circumscribed Jewish men. Galen's *De Medicina*, also depicted skin flaps to repair facial defects of the ears, noses, and lips.

10.1.3 Burns Management in Sixteenth-Century Europe

The ancient salves of the Egyptians, Indians, and Chinese appear to have been forgotten in Roman times. Galenic doctrine recommended boiling oils to clean or disinfect (detoxify) burn wounds. This was an agonizing treatment which continued to be employed throughout the Middle Ages and beyond, even until the time of the French Barber surgeon Ambroise Paré (1510–1590) in the sixteenth century. In the battle of Pas de Suze, Paré ran out of oil and had to improvise by concocting a balm made of egg yolk, turpentine, and rose oil; he noticed that this treatment made the burned or wounded patient far more comfortable than those previously treated with boiling oil. The turpentine carried antiseptic properties, and the balm was efficacious. On the basis of his first-hand battle wound experience, Paré then broke with Galenic doctrine and later (1545) published his observations in his first book, *the method of curing wounds caused by arquebus and firearms*. Paré also introduced burn wound excision, but although he wrote about skin grafts, he was skeptical about their benefits [2, 3].

10.1.4 Skin Grafting in the Seventeenth to Eighteenth Centuries

Wilhelm Fabricius Hildanus (1560–1634) was the first to write a book *De Combustionibus,* devoted to the management of burn injuries in 1607. He was either ignorant of, or did not acknowledge, Paré's methods, described some 70 years earlier. However, a lack of scientific understanding of burn pathophysiology meant that successful treatment remained limited to small surface areas and partial-thickness burns. Progress with skin grafts was also protracted given the use of inappropriately thick grafts and a lack of understanding of wound healing.

Two centuries after Ambroise Paré, Italian physician Giuseppe Baronio (1759–1811) successfully and reproducibly performed a series of (free) skin grafts on sheep. Baronio reported three different experiments. The first harvested skin from the back of a ram and grafted it to a new site on the back of the ram. The graft was secured with adhesive dressings without sutures. In the second experiment, a similar procedure was tried but with an 18 min delay between graft harvesting and placement. In the third experiment, there was 60 min delay. The first graft was successful, the second developed superficial necrosis, while the third graft failed completely. The surviving grafts were cut into 10–12 days after transplantation and were found to be adequately vascularized. Sadly, his achievement was not appreciated at the time and Baronio died single, young, and in obscurity [4–6].

10.1.5 Full-Thickness Grafting

10.1.5.1 Christian Heinrich Bünger (1823)

The next advance was made by a German anatomist and surgeon, Christian Heinrich Bünger (1782–1842), reconstructing a nasal defect using free skin graft inspired by the old Indian method. In1823, he reconstructed the nose of a 33-year-old woman, who had suffered skin loss and disfigurement from skin necrosis. Bünger transferred a full-thickness skin graft from the buttock. His graft was thin with all the subcutaneous tissue excised. This operation was considered by many as the first verified (free) skin graft performed in Europe. Having said that, his peers were not convinced that his results were reproducible.

10.1.5.2 Jaques-Louis Reverdin (1869)

In 1869 a Swiss surgeon, Jaques-Louis Reverdin (1842–1929) reported a successful skin graft using the tip of the scalpel to harvest small epidermal pieces from the arm and laid in the wound. He called his procedure "epidermal grafting," but it is now better known as a "pinch graft." Initially he applied a 1 mm piece of very thin skin on a granulating wound, where he noticed it produced an epithelial island. Although the results were not aesthetically pleasing, it paved the way for partial skin graft in burn victims [7, 8].

10.1.5.3 George Pollock (1870)

In 1870, George Pollock (1817–1897) performed the first successful pinch skin grafts on an 8-year-old girl suffering a large burn to her right thigh. Pollock used two small pieces of skin from the lower abdomen and transplanted it to the lower part of the defect; 3 weeks and 6 weeks later, he performed a second and third series of autografts. He also attempted homografting in combination with pinch autografts, but although the autografts took, the homografts failed.

Pollock presented his work titled "Cases of Skin Grafting and Skin Transplantation" before the Clinical Society of London in 1870. He described 16 cases of thin skin grafts applied to open wounds, of which 8 were successful. Pollock gave due credit to Reverdin in his presentation, but was the first to document a case series of successful skin grafts for burn wounds in the modern era [8].

10.1.5.4 George Lawson: Full-Thickness Correction of Ectropion

At the same time, George Lawson (1831–1903), another British surgeon corrected a complete ectropion of the upper eyelid using a 32 mm full-thickness graft from the forearm, in which all the subcutaneous tissue had all been excised from the dermis. He presented his findings to the Clinical Society of London, but somehow his pioneering of this procedure was overlooked in history as it is Wolfe, following publication of his cases in the BMJ that is given major credit for the full-thickness graft and to which his name is attached [2, 3].

10.1.5.5 John Reisberg Wolfe (1874)

John Reisberg Wolfe (1823–1904) was a Polish born, ophthalmologist who graduated from Glasgow University in 1856. He introduced the modern, full-thickness, free skin graft. In 1874, Wolfe wrote comparing his graft to the pedicle flap:

> *This pedicle (flap) has, in my opinion, been a source of great embarrassment to surgeons, and tended rather to retard the progress of plastic surgery. I have long held it demonstrated, that in most cases the pedicle is not essential, if indeed it (does) contribute anything, to the vitality of (the) flap.*

Wolfe later used even larger grafts (2.5 cm × 5 cm) from the forearm to reconstruct lower eyelid ectropion.

10.1.6 Split-Thickness Skin Graft

The evolution of split-thickness graft occurred parallel to the full-thickness graft. Reverdin's pinch grafts were historic in the origins of skin graft of all thicknesses. Although originally called epidermal grafts, Reverdin admitted that they contained a small portion of dermis. The split-thickness skin grafts were further developed by Ollier (1872) and Thiersch (1886) [9–12].

10.1.6.1 Léopold Ollier (1872)

In 1872, a French surgeon, Louis Xavier Édouard Léopold Ollier of Lyon (1830–1900) published a series of thin skin grafts ranging from 4 to 8 cm^2 in size, significantly larger than previously used by Reverdin or Pollock. Due to the technologic limitations of instruments at the time, the harvesting of such split-thickness grafts required considerable technical expertise. The partial-thickness skin grafts were harvested using scalpels adapted for surgical procedures, such as the Catlin knife, a double-bladed instrument 17 × 1.5 cm wide, but lacking any mechanism to control the depth of excision. In addition to this, the blade was relatively blunt, and one can understand that its effective use was very challenging.

10.1.6.2 Carl Thiersch (1886)

A German surgeon, Carl Thiersch (1822–1895) in Leipzig, also developed partial-thickness grafts with minimal dermal inclusion at a similar time to Ollier [13].

> *The only alternative, therefore, is elimination of the superficial portion of the granulation (layer) and implantation of the skin (graft) directly upon the tense underlying tissue. This substratum is exposed by sharp, horizontal incision, hemorrhage is permitted to run its course completely, and then skin graft is placed upon this greyish wound surface, whose vessels and tissues are in excellent condition for immediate inflammatory adhesion.* (Carl Thiersch)

10.1.7 Skin Graft Knives

10.1.7.1 Thiersch

The Thiersch knife (named posthumously after Thiersch) was developed in 1920. Its rectangular, single-bladed with a handle design is the basis of nearly all subsequent skin grafting knives where the skin graft is taken by hand.

10.1.7.2 Humby

Today, skin grafts when taken by hand utilize the Humby (1930) or the Watson knives that allow a setting for different depths of cut. Braithwaite in 1955 modified the Humby knife to include a fully supported replaceable blade (Fig. 10.1).

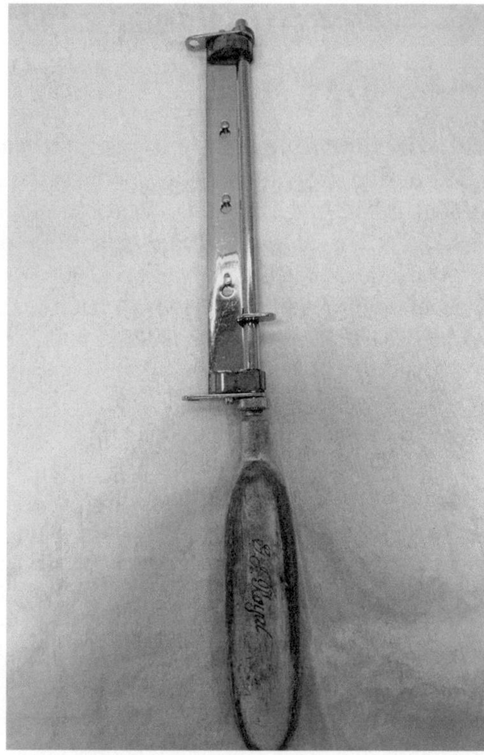

Fig. 10.1 Humby knife. (Photo by the Author SA)

10.1.7.3 Watson

Then came the Watson knife, introduced by John Watson (1914–2009). Watson had served as a pilot in the British Royal Air Force during World War II, then trained under Sir Archibald McIndoe (1900–1960), and had operated on many former air-crew who had sustained war injuries. Inspired by a potato peeler and wanting to create a user-friendly instrument, he produced a knife that is easier to work with and is still widely used today.

Split-thickness skin grafts became popular in the 1930s after Blair and James Brown (1899–1971) further defined the differences between full-thickness, intermediate-thickness, and epidermal skin grafts. They demonstrated that donor sites healed by epithelization from the basal layer and epithelial outgrowth from hair follicles and that donor sites could, in time, be reused [13–15].

10.1.8 Progress in Managing Major Burn Wounds

10.1.8.1 Rule of Nines

Late in the nineteenth century, it was appreciated that survival from major burns was based on the proportion of the body surface burned and the depth of the burn. Various complicated formulae were developed to estimate the body surface area (BSA), but the easiest to utilize is the Rule of Nines published by Scottish plastic surgeon, Alexander Burns Wallace (1906–1974) in 1951. This reduced BSA from a calculation to a simple matter of addition and was based on an earlier proposal made by American surgeons, Pulaski and Tennison in 1947 [18].

10.1.8.2 Resuscitation

Concurrent developments focused on resuscitation during the early phase of burn injuries. Initially burns are associated with significant fluid extravasation so that when involving a large surface area, there is a significant risk of hypovolemic shock. In 1921, Frank Underhill treated the burn victims of a fire at the Rialto theatre (New Haven) and noticed the fluid in the burn blisters resembled normal plasma. He then realized that the victims had lost large volumes of fluids, were thus hypovolemic, and needed aggressive resuscitation with intravenous fluids including plasma or colloids. Twenty years later Frances D. Moore and Oliver Cope (Massachusetts) treated 40 victims of a fire at Boston's Coconut Grove Nightclub and recommended that the volume of fluid replacement required to prevent shock in early phases should be determined by the surface area of the burn. Moore developed a formula based on replacement fluid and body surface area burned, which went through a number of modifications based on age and type of fluid required. Today, the Parkland formula or a modification thereof, based on crystalloid rather than colloid resuscitation fluids, is widely used, as recommended by Baxter and Shires in 1968 [15–17].

10.1.8.3 Early Excision of Full-Thickness Burns

Then, Forrest Young at Rochester University recognized that the rapid colonization of burn wounds by bacteria, after a few days, inevitably resulted in septic shock. This led him to advocate for early excision of full-thickness burns and early application of skin grafts. This doctrine of "early surgical intervention "was introduced to reduce mortality by removing the source of sepsis. However, it was slow to be accepted by the surgical profession, with the majority of cases still being delayed for about 10 days before surgery.

In the 1970s, **Zora Janžekovič** (1918–2015), a Slovenian surgeon, abandoned the accepted, delayed practice and boldly performed early excision down to the healthy bleeding tissue in the base of the burn and then applied a split-thickness skin graft within the first 5 days of the burn. She reported that patients with up to a 20% of the total body surface area could be healed within 10 days, which was unheard-of at the time even in major burns centers.

Janžekovič would become the first woman to receive the Evans Medal from the American Burn Association and also received the Zora Janžekovič (Golden Razor) Award from the European Club for Paediatric Burns. Surgeons from all over the world travelled to learn her technique and took the practice back to their local hospitals [15, 17, 18].

10.1.8.4 Early Excision and Immediate Grafting

John Francis Burke (1922–2011) from Harvard University showed that the combination of early excision for smaller burns and full excision for larger burns followed by immediate skin graft markedly reduced mortality and enabled successful treatment of children even with large burns up to 80% total body surface area [19].

Dermatomes and Skin Graft Meshers

In 1938 **Earl Calvin Padgett** (1893–1946), an American physician from Kansas City in collaboration with his colleague George J. Hood from the Department of Engineering designed a simple to use dermatome that allowed calibrated collection of skin grafts. In 1948, Harry Brown (American surgeon) modified the dermatome to become electric [17–19].

Cicero Parker Meek (1914–1979) from South Carolina introduced a novel micrografting technique in 1958 that enabled a graft to be utilized over a wound by up to ninefold greater in size. Meek built on the principle of Reverdin's pinch grafts by recognizing that epithelialization occurred from the graft edge.

So the surgeon would cut each square inch of harvested graft in a 16 by 16 grid pattern using the Meek–Wall microdermatome.

In 1964, James Tanner (1921–1996) and his chief resident Jacques Vandeput (Grady Memorial Hospital in Atlanta, Georgia) invented a device called the Tanner–Vandeput mesh-dermatome that could expand STSG by a ratio of 1:3. Today skin graft meshers can allow expansion of donor grafts up to a ratio of 1:9 or more [20–22] (Fig. 10.2).

Skin Banks

During the Second World War, research into skin banks found a method of preserving skin in glycerol-based cryo-preservative at 79° Fahrenheit. This allowed hospitals to store skin and have a sufficient reserve for mass wartime injuries.

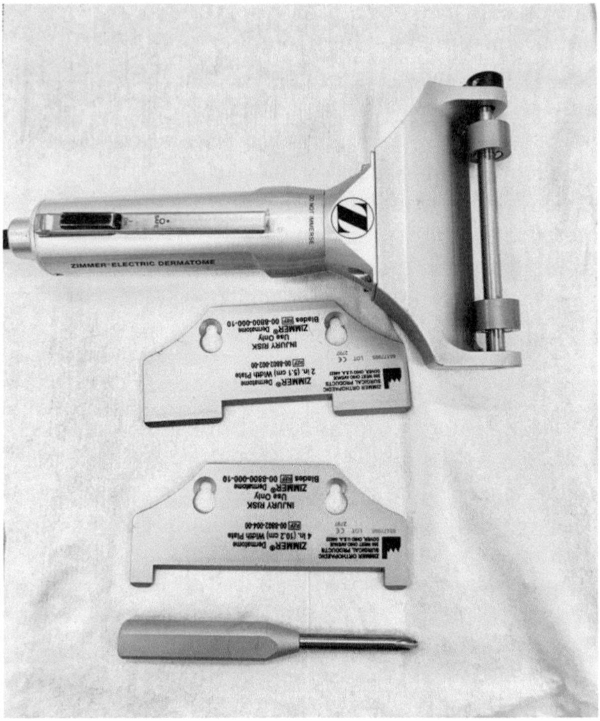

Fig. 10.2 Modern dermatome. (Photo by the Author SA)

Homografts and Their Rejection

During the battle of Britain 1940, a plane crashed near the home of Immunologist Peter Medawar (1915–1987). The surgeon treating the badly injured pilot consulted with Medawar; they thought skin graft would save him, but unfortunately the pilot did not survive. But that incident triggered Medawar's curiosity about immunology of the skin grafting. He then collaborated with plastic surgeon Thomas Gibson to perform autografts and homografts for burn victims. They noticed that the homografts seemed to incorporate initially but later get rejected after 2 weeks, while the autografts survived. Also repeat homografts would get rejected even quicker. This convinced Medawar that the rejection was immune-mediated. Medawar took the experiment further in cooperation with others, in particular with an Australian virologist, Frank Burnet (1899–1985), who introduced the concept of immune tolerance. Their work is now regarded as the foundation of modern transplant immunology, and Medawar and Burnet were awarded Nobel Prize in Medicine (1960) for their discovery of immune tolerance. They were also both knighted for their contributions to medicine.

10.1.8.5 Skin Substitutes

More recent skin substitutes have been investigated such as the Integra. Integra® consists of a layer of cross-linked bovine collagen and shark chondroitin (glycosaminoglycan) with a silicon top layer. The collagen-chondroitin matrix facilitates the regeneration of the dermal layer, while the silicone acts as a temporary protective layer. After the excision of a full-thickness burn, Integra® allows the wound bed to regenerate a layer equivalent to the dermis. After approximately 3 weeks, the silicon layer is removed and replaced with a standard partial-thickness graft [23, 24].

Skin Cultures

Howard Green (1925–2015) and his PhD student, James Rheinwald, were the first to successfully culture human keratinocytes in 1975. Their discovery was accidental as they were trying to grow a teratoma cell line. In 1983, Green was successful in providing large volumes of cultured epithelial autograft (CEA) to save the lives of two young boys with greater than 95% burns.

The 1980s and 1990s then saw the wider use of cell-based therapies utilizing cultured keratinocytes or CEAs. The finding that wounds closed within 10 days has the best cosmetic outcomes, which presents some challenges for skin cultures which may take days to yield sufficient cells. This led to therapies using cell suspensions, some of which had added fibrin glue to promote cellular adhesion to the burn wound base.

10.1.8.6 Fiona Wood and Spray on Skin Cells

During the 1990s, the British-Australian plastic surgeon, Fiona Wood (b 1958), found that CEAs could be successfully applied to the wound at 10 days rather than waiting the 2–3 weeks for adequate culture growth. Edwin Deitch reported that a burn wound closed at 21 days had a 70% risk of hypertrophic scar formation compared with 4% if closed within 10 days. Wood's team then worked on keratinocyte culture suspensions and reduced the time to application to 5 days by culturing in suspension, harvesting at the pre-confluent stage and then aerosolization of the culture, allowing it to be applied by spray. The resultant spray on skin was commercialized and used in Wood's own unit. A lack of randomized trials, comparing with controls treated by the then gold standard of a meshed split-thickness skin graft (STSG), resulted in skepticism from Wood's global peers and insufficient evidence for TGA approval. However, in 2002 when 28 severely burned patients from the Bali bombing were transferred to Wood's Australian unit in Perth, spray-on-skin was liberally used and 25 of the patients survived. This made the world take notice of the technique and the product. Wood's team then developed an aerosolized epidermal suspension, ReCell®, that could be sprayed on. Subsequent trials conducted in other units have shown its non-inferiority to STSG, but also patients experienced much less pain and quicker healing compared with those with painful STSG donor sites. Today ReCell® is used in many burns units across Australia and New Zealand and has received TGA approval [24, 25].

In conclusion, the history of skin grafting and soft tissue reconstruction is millennia old with documentation of its having been practiced in India and Egypt thousands of years ago. The autograft remains the most likely graft to take though porcine and artificial skin can provide temporary cover prior to autografting. For major burns we can now apply individual cell suspensions to wounds, and we recognize that the earlier the wound surface is covered, the less likelihood there is of infection, and the greater the chance of survival and the better the cosmetic outcome. The future of skin grafting may soon include 3D printing, possibly with nanotechnology, and/or enriching with specific cellular growth factors. These will represent new chapters in the management of burns and the restoration of skin coverage. Developments after 1846 were facilitated by being able to provide anaesthesia to patients and provide painless procedures noting that local anaesthesia using cocaine was not introduced to surgery until 1884 [26].

10.2 Flaps for Reconstructive Surgery

10.2.1 Sushruta's Development of the Pedicle Skin Flap in India

The first operative description of tissue transplantation was performed by Sushruta (approximately 600 BCE), the father of Indian surgery. The instruments and surgical techniques in are described in the Sanskrit hymns (the Vedas). Sushruta was the pioneer of the modern pedicle skin flap in his techniques of rotating and advancing flaps of skin and subcutaneous tissues from the face, also called the "Indian cheek flap," and mainly used for nasal reconstruction. Sushruta also documented more than 15 methods to repair mutilated ears and lips. Today, the Indian cheek flap would be considered an advancement of a sliding flap. Many of these techniques were later rediscovered and adopted by the Greeks, Arabs, and Romans. Reconstructive techniques were also described by the Egyptians.

Facial mutilation used to be a common type of punishment in antiquity, usually delivered through amputation of ears or noses. It was also believed to deter potential criminals. The nose was synonymous with respect. One of the oldest descriptions of such nasal mutilation comes from an ancient Indian epic (1500 BCE), the Ramayana, in which Lady Surpunakha (Meenakshi), angry at Prince Rama, attacks his wife, Sita, amputating her nose. These mutilations also inspired surgeons to start thinking about reconstruction [27].

10.2.2 Reimplantation of a Severed Nose

Leonardo Fioravanti (1517–1588), a charismatic Italian surgeon, was renowned for his vocal rejection of Galenic doctrine and is reputed to have performed the first splenectomy in Italy. He was also the first European to document the successful reattachment of a severed body part, in this case a nose of a 29-year-old who had fought with a soldier [27, 28].

> *A Spaniard) upon a time walked in the field, and fell at words with a soldier, and began to draw (his sword); the soldier seeing that, struck him with the left hand, and cut off his nose, and there it fell down in the sand. I then happened to stand by, and took it up, and pissed thereon to wash away the sand, and dressed it with our balsama artificiato, and bound it up, and so left it to remain 8 or 10 days, thinking that it would have come to matter; nevertheless when I did unbind it I found it fast conglutinated, and then I dressed it only once more, and he was perfectly whole.*

The above practice of tissue restitution laid the foundation for the development of modern reimplantation and reconstruction. Numerous similar descriptions of nasal reconstruction subsequently appeared throughout the literature as criminal punishment with nasal disfigurement was a common practice in those days.

10.2.2.1 Branca de Branca Method of Nasal Reconstruction

Tagliacozzi (1545–1599) was a surgeon and anatomist in Bologna. His principle work was *De Curtorum Chirurgia per Insitionem* (1597) (*On the Surgery of Mutilation by Grafting*). He described the Italian method of nasal reconstruction that had been practiced by the Branca and Vianeo families of Sicily since the previous century.

As a pioneer of reconstructive surgery, one of the popular quotes from his book has become a plastic surgeon's mantra:

> *We restore, rebuild, and make whole those parts which nature hath given, but which fortune has taken away. Not so much that it may delight the eye, but that it might buoy up the spirit, and help the mind of the afflicted.*

The Branca de Branca method used a flap from the cheek, but Antonio de Branca, his son, also developed a pedicle flap from the arm. The Italian rhinoplasty was based on the Indian accounts of Sushruta, which had been translated into Arabic and later brought to Italy. Following Tagliacozzi's death, the practice was forgotten for two centuries until rediscovered by Joseph Carpue in England and Karl Ferdinand von Gräfe in Germany [28–30].

10.2.2.2 Joseph Carpue Rhinoplasty (1814): Modified Indian Method

In 1814, Joseph Carpue (1746–1840) revived a version of the ancient Indian method, preferring it to the modified Italian method (median forehead flap), previously described by Tagliacozzi. In doing so he achieved the first modern-day successful rhinoplasty in Europe. However, in India the skill to perform a rhinoplasty had already been handed down through two millennia and was still current practice. Carpue's rhinoplasty was based upon illustrated reports by two British surgeons observing the procedure in India in 1793 and published in the Gentleman's Magazine of London.

10.2.2.3 Karl Ferdinand von Gräfe (1818) Textbook on Rhinoplasty

Karl Ferdinand von Gräfe (1767–1840), Professor of Surgery and head of the Ophthalmological Institute in Berlin, also revived the Tagliacozzi's Italian method of rhinoplasty based on the ancient Indian techniques. He published a text on rhinoplasty in 1818 and introduced other surgical reconstructive procedures including for cleft lip and palate. He was also superintendent of the Prussian military hospitals in the sixth coalition against Napoleon (March 1813–May 1814) prior to Napoleon's first defeat and capture, leading to imprisonment on the island of Elba.

10.2.2.4 Johann Friedrich Dieffenbach (1823–1847)

Johann Friedrich Dieffenbach (1792–1847), based in Berlin, is credited with the introduction of leeches in plastic surgery, a therapy then forgotten for some 150 years. He was appointed under Gräfe in Berlin in 1823 and focused his work on plastic and reconstructive surgery. He published three volumes and an atlas on rhinoplasty and succeeded Gräfe to the Berlin chair. In addition to the above contributions, he also studied tenotomy in club foot and experimented with blood transfusion. He died in 1847, at work, and while about to start operating [30, 31, 34].

Remarkably, all of the advances described above were conducted without general or local anaesthesia. General anaesthesia was only introduced in 1846 and local anaesthesia for ophthalmological procedures using cocaine in 1884.

10.2.3 The Early Development of Plastic Surgery as a Surgical Specialty

During latter part of the nineteenth century, the major advances in plastic surgery were made through the introduction of pinch grafts, full-thickness (Wolfe) grafts, and split-thickness skin grafts. Their historical development is intertwined with other advances in reconstruction but has been dealt with in a separate section earlier in this chapter.

10.2.3.1 Victor von Brun in Tübingen (1843–1881)

Victor von Brun (1812–1883), MD graduate of Tübingen, who had undertaken further study in clinics at Halle and Berlin, before qualifying as a physician at Braunschweig in Germany, was Professor of Surgery in Tübingen from 1843 until 1881. He was to be succeeded by his son, Paul. His view on surgery was, according to Hauben:

> *Prüft alles und das Beste behaltet* [Test everything and keep the best of it for yourself]

Although better known for his contributions to laryngeal surgery, he also developed original techniques in reconstructive surgery (see below). He invented a laryngeal mirror and was the first surgeon to remove a laryngeal polyp via an endolaryngeal approach. He devised a circular incision for an amputation that created an anterior flap to cover the stump. From 1868 to 1873, he wrote a *Handbuch der Chirurgischen Praxis* which summarized 100 years of surgical experience and also an approach to war injuries which included antisepsis and cotton-wool bandages.

In reconstruction following excision of a cheek tumor, his meloplasties employed either a wedge excision with two lateral flaps for closure to form a T or an H plasty. He also devised a mandible advancement procedure for a boy with osteomyelitis and a septic ulcer with fixed mandible. He also made original contributions to flaps for lip reconstruction (cheiloplasty) which were used by Gillies (see below) and throughout the twentieth century. His operation for unilateral and bilateral cleft lip used similar principles to the current Millard technique [34, 35].

10.2.3.2 Hippolyte Morestin in Paris (1914)

Hippolyte Morestin (1869–1919) was Professor of Anatomy in Paris and a surgeon whose work during World War I resulted in his treating injuries of the face and jaw. In 1914, he inspired Harold Gillies to take an interest in reconstructing the face while Gillies was a surgeon at the British General Hospital in Rouen. Gillies watched Morestin remove a tumor of the jaw and the grafting of skin to the resulting defect. At the end of the war, Morestin was to die of influenza during the pandemic of 1919.

10.2.3.3 Harold Gillies WWI to WW2 in London

Harold Delf Gillies (1882–1960) was born in Dunedin, NZ. He studied medicine at Cambridge University and St Bartholomew's Hospital and gained his FRCS in 1910. He specialized as an ENT surgeon, and his reconstructive work was to become legendary during World War I (1914–1918). A specialist unit was established under his command where some 11,000 cases were treated. He championed multidisciplinary teams, and his operations on the mouth and jaw always included a dentist. As his operations took place on the face he persuaded his anesthetists to intubate the trachea to give him greater access to his surgical field. He published his first book, *Plastic surgery of the face,* in 1920. Later in the 1930s, two other New Zealand surgeons, Archibald McIndoe and Rainsford Mowlem, trained under him. During World War II (1939–1945), three plastic surgery units were established under Gillies, McIndoe and Mowlem. In 1946, after the war, Gillies was elected the Foundation President of the British Association of Plastic Surgery, and later, honorary President of the International Society of Plastic Surgeons. Gillies was also an accomplished artist and, in his youth, had represented England at golf [29, 32, 33, 34].

10.2.3.4 John Staige Davis in Virginia (1920s)

John Staige Davis (1875–1946), the son of an anatomist and Confederate civil war surgeon, was the first American surgeon to specialize in plastic surgery. He wrote the first North American textbook on the subject in 1918, describing reconstructive procedures from head to toe. During the 1920s he developed a plastic surgical training program in Virginia [30, 31, 36, 37].

10.3 Cleft Lip and Palate Repair

The first documented repair of a cleft lip was in 390 BCE in China. The patient was Wey Young-Chi, an 18-year-old, and the operation was performed in Nanking. Wey Young-Chi was recruited into the Imperial Army and went on to become a general.

The condition was largely unknown in Greek and Roman times because the children who were born with such defects were euthanased or discarded and left to die. In Sparta they were abandoned on Mt. Targete, while in Rome they were drowned in the Tiber river or thrown off a cliff. There is an Egyptian mummy with a cleft and Greek statue of a clown has also been found with full representation of the cleft and its secondary defects. Thus, in the ancient world, where clefts and other congenital defects were seen as a sign of possession, evil, or an error of the mother while pregnant, survivors to adult life were rare.

Jean Yperman (1295–1351) described the congenital nature of the disease and outlined the different defects and how they might be treated. His method involved scarifying the margins with a scalpel then suturing them. A needle was inserted through the two sides of the lip and held in place by fixing its shaft with a figure-of-8 thread over the lip. Fabricius ab Aquapendente (1537–1619) suggested that there was an embryological failure of development as the upper lip only fuses late. Frederick Blandin (1838–1896) suggested it was a failure of the premaxilla and maxilla to unite, while Meckel proposed five separate processes toward closure, three for the upper, and two for the lower lip. William His of Leipzig (1831–1904) noted five processes around the stomodeum, with any two failures of fusion resulting in some form of cleft.

In 1460, Heinrich von Pfolsprundt described a technique in which he sutured all the layers introducing the concept of ensuring a good muscle repair. In 1497, Hieronymus Brunschwig, a military surgeon from Alsace, scarified the edges with scissors and then applied a pinching clamp to hold the edges together before suturing with waxed stiches. The sutures and clamp were then left in place until there was secure union of the wound [38–40].

Pierre Franco (1505–1578), a pupil of Paré, wrote, in1856, a short treatise *Petit Traité* that covered hernias, lithotomy, and cataracts. However, in his 1861 major work, *Traité des Hernies*, he devoted two chapters to clefts classifying them as a congenital malformation, with various types. He called bilateral cleft lip as a *dent de lièvre* (hare tooth), due to the marked protrusion of the premaxillary bone and teeth.

His technique of repair was two-staged, mobilizing the cheeks and not hesitating to resect the premaxilla. Paré in *Les Oeuvres* provided one of the earliest illustrations showing the suturing method for cleft lip repair.

For the next three centuries, surgeons continued to scarify the margins of the cleft and then use various techniques and sutures to hold the edges together, albeit with an ugly, vertical scar and shortened lip. It wasn't until 1844 that Germanicus Mirault (1796–1879) made a horizontal medial incision and introduced a triangular flap from the lateral side to provide extra tissue to lengthen the lip as well as creating a nostril floor. In 1848, Werner Hagedorn (1831–1894) of Magdeburg, a pupil of von Langenbeck in Berlin, introduced a quadrangular flap into the vertical repair, which, for bilateral clefts, exerted pressure on the protruding premaxilla. Hagedorn was the first surgeon to close a bilateral cleft lip in one stage, also operating on two babies within 1 week of their birth. He was also a strong advocate for antisepsis and its introduction in Germany. In the twentieth Century, Hagedorn's technique was modified by Le Mesurier in 1849, Tennison in 1952, and Peter Randall in 1959 [41].

There was ongoing debate from the sixteenth to nineteenth centuries as to what age to repair the lip. Most advised operating by 4–5 months of age. Nonetheless, for those with limited access to surgical care, surgical techniques need to adapt to older children up to adult life, as with the first cleft lip repair in China on an 18-year-old. Today, the ideal timing is 10 weeks for the lip and 10 months for the palate.

Excision of the protruding premaxilla to achieve bilateral lip repair is accompanied by mid-face retrusion. In 1872, Jacob August Estlander (1831–1881), a Finish surgeon, left the premaxilla intact with a wedge resection of the vomer which would allow the premaxilla to be pushed back. However, this did not achieve the desired outcome. In 1935, another Finnish surgeon, Faltin, recommended the procedure be abandoned but only published in Swedish which led to a 50-year delay in the adoption of preoperative orthodontic treatment to replace preoperative vomerine resection [40–43].

10.3.1 Cleft Palate

Whereas repair of a cleft lip is about cosmetic appearance, repair of the palate is about speech, dentition, and normal facial growth. All of the functions/senses of the face other than vision can be affected if the palate is not adequately repaired—smell, taste, speech, and hearing.

The principles of repair require closure of the defect, tension-free suturing, reorientation of the abnormal soft palate to reconstruct levator veli palatini, lengthening and retro-positioning of the soft palate, minimizing denuded areas of bone and oral or nasal mucosa, and a layered closure of the hard and soft palate.

The palate is key to normal speech production. The focus of soft palate repair is lengthening the palate, closing the defect, and reconstructing the levator sling. The first documented soft palate closure was in 1764. A French dentist, Le Monnier, cauterized the edges of the soft (not hard) palate and sutured them closed.

The first successful repairs of a cleft palate, as opposed to the lip, were performed by Karl Ferdinand von Gräfe (1787–1840) in 1816 and Roux in 1819. However, the repairs involved large sutures holding the palate together under some tension and rendered the palate rather immobile, thus impairing normal speech [44, 45].

In Berlin, Johann Friedrich Dieffenbach (1792–1847) performed a hard palate closure by elevating the hard palate mucosa (1828), while his successor, Bernhard von Langenbeck (1810–1887), performed a bipedicle mucoperiosteal elevation (1859). In 1931, Victor Veau (1871–1949), at the Enfants-Malades Hospital in Paris, described how the soft palate musculature runs parallel to the cleft, whereas in a normal person, it should be transverse. He introduced a unipedicle mucoperiosteal flap (1931), before Wardill and Kilner lengthened the soft palated through a V-Y pushback technique (1940). These involved an incision in the nasal mucosa with release incisions anteriorly and laterally to create triangular flaps that could be closed in V-Y fashion. Bardach introduced a two-flap palatoplasty to limit bone exposure (1967), while Krien, in 1969, suggested an intravelar veloplasty to reconstruct the velopharyngeal muscle sling. Furlow's double opposing Z-plasty (1986) achieved closure of the hard palate without the need for release incisions, lengthening of the soft palate, reconstruction of the velopharyngeal sling, reducing palatal scarring, increasing palatal mobility, and limiting any impact on maxillary growth [45–48].

Today, different high-income countries have different schedules for cleft lip and palate closure. In America the tendency is to close the lip early (less than 10 weeks) and perform a single-stage palate repair at 10–18 months. In low-middle-income countries, a single-stage palate repair is also appropriate, given a second-stage repair may not be feasible due to challenges with surgical access. At Great Ormond Street in London and in Oslo, the hard palate is reconstructed at about 3 months using a vomer flap, followed by the soft palate as a second stage at 18 months using a similar technique to Langenbeck. As cleft lip and palate closure require specialist reconstructive skills, various options to deliver services in low-middle-income countries have had to be developed including Smile Train, a charity, and visiting specialist supporting teams such as those delivered by Interplast, supporting local surgical services [48, 49].

10.4 A History of the Management of Fractures and Orthopaedic Eponyms

Fractures are as old as mankind, and bonesetters were specialists in their management in the ancient world. Today's bonesetters are orthopaedic surgeons, who are trained doctors unlike the bonesetters of the ancient world who reduced, splinted, dressed, and applied traction to fractures. Around 1500, the Aztecs even described an early form of intramedullary nail using a wooden peg for fracture nonunion.

A simple definition of a fracture that has important implications for clinical practice is "a soft tissue injury in which a bone is also broken." In terms of clinical outcome and return of function, the management of the soft tissues is as important as that of the bone. Fractures may also be classified as closed and open fractures. Open fractures in the past were often subjected to immediate amputation close to the field of battle. Even today, if not well managed, they are prone to complications of infection, including acute and chronic osteomyelitis which may impact upon union, health, and function.

Open fractures were diagnosed and treated in Ancient Egypt and other ancient civilizations. The fractures were manually reduced, with splints applied to attempt to hold the reduction (probably not with a lot of success). Wounds were dressed with honey, grease, and lint from vegetable fibers. However, this treatment had a poor prognosis, confirmed by the bodies excavated from graves of those who died with their open fracture [50–52].

Today's classification of open (compound) fractures was introduced by a Filipino surgeon, Rámon Gustilo (1930–2024; see below), based on the size of the wound, soft tissue injury, and any vascular involvement [53]. The term "complicated" when applied to a fracture implies an associated injury from (or adjacent to) the fracture to nerves or vessels or some other major structure.

Fractures may also be classified by their pathological appearance on imaging. These include simple, comminuted (many parts), transverse, oblique, spiral, or greenstick. If accompanied by a dislocation, the term fracture dislocation is used. Fractures into joints are more prone to joint stiffness and impairment of function if not accurately reduced and internally fixed.

Fractures heal by periosteal reaction through forming callus with later remodeling. They may unite in good alignment or may suffer malunion through angulation or shortening, particularly when involving long bones. When a fracture is internally fixed in tight alignment, there may be no callus and only endosteal healing. Nonunion may result from tissue interposition between the fracture ends, from avascular necrosis of the bone, or from chronic infection or instability.

Fracture healing may result in no long-term deformity when the bone involved remains in good alignment (e.g., the fractured metatarsal without dislocation, fractured neck of humerus, or fractured sternum). However, many fractures need to be reduced, brought into alignment with bone length restored. Reduction can be achieved by manipulation under anaesthesia (MUA) or by traction applied through the skin or the skeleton. For lower limb fractures, traction can be applied through the skin or by a pin passed through the proximal tibia (for femoral shaft fractures), calcaneum (for tibial fractures). George Perkins (1892–1980), Professor of orthopedic surgery at St Thomas' Hospital in London, combined skeletal traction through a tibial pin, with cutting the base of the bed in half to allow the bottom board (supporting the legs) to be removed to encourage flexion and extension of the knee and promote healing through maintenance of the quadriceps muscle and avoid knee stiffness. This is still a valid method of treating mid-femoral shaft fractures today, where internal fixation cannot be done without a high risk of infection. Halo traction for cervical spine fracture/dislocations uses pins screwed into outer table of the skull and a circular (halo) device for traction to reduce pedicular fracture dislocations of the neck. A particular type of skin traction for femoral shaft fractures in children aged under 2–3 years is a Gallow's (Bryant's) traction which suspends the legs through skin traction and uses the weight of the body to maintain reduction and length. Suspension was also used in ancient Egypt and by the Greeks at the time of Galen. Dr. John Dunlop's (1877–1964) traction was introduced for displaced supracondylar fractures of the humerus in children and proved an effective treatment at times when operative reduction and internal fixation was less commonly used [52].

A reduced fracture then needs to be kept in alignment during the healing process until it is both united (4 weeks) and stable (6–8 weeks). These timelines are for adults. A child's femoral shaft fracture in Gallows traction may unite in 2–4 weeks depending on its age.

Fixation can be achieved by external or internal fixation. External fixation can often be achieved for undisplaced fractures by plaster of Paris (POP) or any of its modern, lighter substitutes. As the tightness of POP and its ability to hold a fracture in position reduce with the reduction of swelling in the first 2 weeks after a fracture, it is important to check position of the bones (usually by imaging) around 10–14 days to avoid malalignment and malunion despite a satisfactory initial reduction or position. When there is an open fracture and both bone and open wound need to be treated, external fixation may be more appropriate. Internal fixation is indicated for femoral and forearm long bones in particular, which may be achieved by either intramedullary nail (best to lock them so rotatory malunion does not occur) or with plates and screws. Other reasons for fixation may be to limit pain and improve ventilation as for patients with rib fractures [51, 52].

Fractures involving joints are often best treated by internal fixation when available, particularly fractures of the ankle where there may be displacement of fracture medial, lateral, or posterior malleoli. A shoulder dislocation with significant glenoid labrum fracture (Bankart lesion) will result in recurrent dislocations if the labrum is not restored.

Physeal injuries in children and adolescents are a special type. The current Salter-Harris classification indicates their severity and likelihood of impairing growth.

The current classification of physeal (growth plate) injuries was introduced by Robert B Salter (1924–2010) and W Robert Harris (1922–2005) in 1963. There are five grades from I to V indicating increasing severity, while the mnemonic *Salter* helps to remember them: I (Slip), II (above the physis, away from the joint), III (lower: below the physis in the epiphysis, IV (through everything: the metaphysis, physis, and epiphysis), and V (rammed or crushed: a crushed physis) [54].

This chapter now briefly describes some of the common fracture eponyms, their significance, and those who described them. Inevitably the eponyms are named after those who described them in the eighteenth to twentieth centuries, although some of these fractures were recognized and treated in the millennia before the modern-day descriptions.

10.4.1 Sir Percival Pott

Sir Percival Pott (1714–1788) was an English Barber surgeon, admitted to the Company of Barbers in 1736. He trained under Edward Nouse at St Bartholomew's hospital in London and was also appointed there as assistant surgeon in 1745 and then full-time in 1749. Pott had a riding accident in 1756, sustaining an open (compound) fracture of his ankle. The first doctors who attended to him advised amputation which he refused; he was stretchered home at his instruction, his mentor Nouse summoned, who recommended reduction and wound management. The leg healed and Pott's case resulted in alternatives to amputation being subsequently considered!

Percival Pott was famous for many conditions he described including cancer of the scrotum in chimney sweeps (1775), an early example of cancer due to occupational exposure. He described treatments for cataract, nasal polyps, as well as describing, of importance to orthopedics, Pott's disease of the spine (1779) due to tuberculous chronic osteomyelitis [51, 55].

10.4.1.1 Fractures of the Wrist and Hand

If one enters the Royal College of Surgeons of Ireland (RCSI) in Dublin, there are two rooms as in the vestibule, one on the right and one on the left. They are named after the two common fractures of the wrist, Colles and Smith. Both eponyms were coined from Irish Surgeons.

Abraham Colles (1774–1843) was Professor of anatomy, surgery, and physiology at RCSI (from 1805) and also President of the College in 1802 and 1830. Although his father died when he was sick, the family owned a Kilkenny black marble quarry that his mother continued to run and provided the income to ensure Colles received an education. He studied medicine at Trinity College Dublin and gained the RCSI licentiate in 1795, before moving to Edinburgh for an MD (1795). He spent time with Astley Cooper in London undertaking inguinal dissections. In 1799 he was appointed to Dr. Steevens' hospital, where he was to work for the next 42 years, in addition to the rotunda and lying-in hospitals. His paper on *Fracture of the Carpal Extremity of the Radius* was published in 1814, and his wrist fracture with dinner fork deformity and ulnar deviation was thereafter known as a Colles fracture. His name is also associated with a fascial layer of the abdomen and a ligament. He wrote a two volume *Lectures on the theory and practice of surgery.* He died from gout. His son, William, was elected Chair of Anatomy at RCSI in 1863 [50, 55, 56].

Robert William Smith (1807–1873) studied medicine in Dublin at RCSI, Trinity College, and the Richmond Hospital. He was awarded the RCSI Licentiate in 1832 and the MD from Trinity College in 1842. He became the inaugural Professor of Surgery at Trinity College in 1847. He co-founded the Dublin pathological society with Abraham Colles, Sir Dominic Corrigan, and William Stokes in 1838. In 1847, he wrote a *Treatise on Fractures in the vicinity of joints and on certain forms of accidental and congenital dislocations* in which he described a Smiths fracture which involves and anterior dislocation of the carpus on the radius. He also published a correction on Colles' description:

> *The situation of the fracture is not so high as Mr. Colles states it to be; I have never seen it more than an inch above the carpal end of the bone; in the majority of cases it is not so much.*

He also described neurofibromatosis 33 years before von Recklinghausen. He died while Vice President of RCSI. A third, Irish-named fracture is the Bennett fracture. Edward Hallaran Bennett (1837–1937) was Professor of Surgery at Trinity College Dublin and described the thumb base fracture *that* "passed obliquely across the base of the bone, detaching the greater part of the articular surface, and the separated segment was very large and deformity that resulted there-from seem more a dorsal subluxation of the first metacarpal."

John Reah Barton (1794–1871) was a graduate of the University of Pennsylvania in 1818, and he returned to the Pennsylvania Hospital as surgeon 1823. He described a wrist fracture with a carpal dislocation (Barton fracture) in 1838. He was, training in the days before anesthesia, a quick surgeon and once was said to perform an osteotomy of the hip in 7 min. He was also renowned for the figure-of-8 bandage for the jaw (Barton bandage) and obstetric forceps (Barton forceps).

10.4.1.2 Fractures of the Forearm

Two Italian surgeons are famous for describing the classic fracture dislocations of the forearm. These fractures are important in that they are best treated by internal fixation and that each can be missed by not imaging the joint above and below the obvious fracture [54, 57, 58].

Giovanni Battista Monteggia (1762–1815) trained in Milan and gained his MD from the University of Pavia in 1789. In 1795, he was appointed Professor of Anatomy and Surgery in Pavia. He contracted syphilis from a laceration obtained performing an autopsy. He was also the second person to describe the Monteggia fracture, which involves the proximal third of the ulna and a dislocation of the head of the radius.

His publications include Fasciculi Pathologici (1789), a translation of a Compendium of venereal illnesses by German, Johann Friedrich Fritz (1792), and his own practical annotations on venereal diseases (1794). In 1808, he was examiner for aspiring surgeons to the army. His career took many routes, and he was responsible for small pox vaccination in Maggiore, lectured in surgery and wrote on a wide variety of surgical and medical conditions. During his life he collected a rich library [56].

The Galeazzi fracture was first described by Sir Astley Cooper in 1842.

Professor Ricardo Galeazzi (1866–1952) studied in Turin, graduated in 1890, and was Director of Orthopaedic Surgery in Milan and described the fracture in 1934. He was also renowned for his work on congenital hip dislocation (CDH) [cf the Galeazzi test], scoliosis, skeletal tuberculosis, and juvenile osteochondritis. He was the Editor in Chief of the *Archivio di Ortopedia*, the oldest journal devoted to orthopaedic surgery. He published his experience of 18 Galeazzi fractures.

10.4.2 Volmann's Ischemic Contracture

Richard von Volkmann (1830–1889) graduated from Berlin in 1854. He was Professor and head of surgery in Halle from 1867. He performed the first excision of carcinoma of the rectum in 1878. His description of Volkmann's ischemic fracture resulting from a supracondylar fracture compromising the brachial artery in the cubital fossa was in 1881. He invented a surgical retractor and was a strong advocate for aseptic surgery. In addition to his surgical works, he also published poetry and fiction under the pseudonym of Richard Leander.

10.4.2.1 Fractures of the Foot and Ankle

Jacques Lisfranc de St Martin (1787–1847) was a preeminent French surgeon in Paris in the early nineteenth century prior to the introduction of general anesthesia. He was an assistant to Guillaume Dupuytren prior to assuming the Directorship at the Parisien Hôpital de la Pitié in 1826. In 1815, he described his eponymous Lisfranc injury in French cavalrymen, an injury which involves a dislocation of one or more metatarsal bones in the foot. Lisfranc contributed to the development of rectal surgery, lithotomy, as well as publishing significant works on gynecological surgery with *Maladies de l'utérus, d'après les leçons cliniques*, and the treatment of aneurysms *Des diverses méthodes et des différens procédés pour l'oblitération des artères dans le traitement des anévrysmes.*

The ankle is a complex hinge joint with stabilizing medial (deltoid) and lateral ligaments attached to the medial and lateral malleoli and tarsal bones. The tibia and fibular are held together by an interosseus membrane which if damaged leads to tibiofibular syndesmosis. The tibia also has a posterior protuberance, sometimes called the posterior malleolus.

The initial classification of ankle fractures was the work of a Belgian surgeon, Robert Danis (1880–1962) with a later modification in 1972, by Swiss orthopedic surgeon, Bernhard Georg Weber (1929–2002). The Danis-Weber classification divides ankle fractures into Types A, B, and C. Type A involves a fracture of the fibula distal to the syndesmosis. It is usually a stable fracture, with an intact deltoid (medial) ligament, though there may be an avulsion fracture of the tip of the medial malleolus. Type B is a fracture of the distal fibula the level of the syndesmosis extending superiorly and laterally. The medial malleolus may be fractured or the deltoid ligament torn with variable stability of the ankle joint. Type C is a fracture of the fibula above the ankle joint proximal to the syndesmosis, disrupting the syndesmosis with a fracture of the medial malleolus or disruption of the deltoid ligament. The fracture is unstable and requires operative reduction and internal fixation.

Robert Danis published two early books on osteosynthesis: *Technique de l'Ostéosynthèse* (1932) and *Theorie et pratique de l'osteosynthese* (1949). He was at least 20 years ahead of his time (see below) and was to be one of those who inspired Müller to devote his career to internal fixation and osteosynthesis [52, 53, 56].

10.4.2.2 Open (Compound) Fractures

Josep Trueta i Raspall (1897–1977) had to flee to England after the Spanish Civil War as he was a Catan Nationalist. Prior to this and during the war, he had been the chief of trauma services in Barcelona's main hospital. He wrote a book on the *Treatment of war wounds and fractures with special reference to the closed method as used in the war in Spain.* This was first published in Catalan and then in English in 1939. During World War II, he was posted in the RAMC, where his plaster cast method of treating open wounds and fractures saved many lives and limbs. He joined Florey and Chain's team in Oxford, holding the first animal to be given penicillin. From 1949 to 1966, he was the third Nuffield Professor of Orthopaedic Surgery in Oxford, Directing the Nuffield Orthopaedic Centre. Every year, Trueta medals and plaques are awarded to professionals and institutions that excel in the Catalan medical field. The Josep Trueta University Hospital in Girona is named after him.

Rámon Gustilo (b 1930) is a Philippine orthopaedic surgeon who graduated from the University of Philippines in 1957 and from the University of Minnesotal orthopaedic training program in 1964. Gustilo and Anderson described their initial classification of open long bone fractures in 1976, based on the size of the wound and degree of soft tissue injury. Their classification was revised to include in grade III, further subclassifications of A, B, and C depending on the degree of periosteal stripping (B) and vascular involvement (C). The classification system is easy to use and is associated with prognosis, but studies have shown there is significant interobserver variation, so that treatment decisions, for example, to perform an amputation, should not be made based on the classification system alone. The Gustilo-Anderson represents the input also of John Anderson [57–59].

10.4.2.3 Shoulder Dislocation

Arthur Sidney Blundell Bankart (1879–1951) was the son of a surgeon, James Bankart, and qualified from Guy's Hospital in 1906. He was awarded his English Fellowship (FRCS) in 1909. His early orthopedic training was at the Royal National Orthopaedic Hospital in London but was also appointed at three other hospitals, practicing neurosurgery and paediatric surgery as well as orthopaedics. He worked under Robert Jones at the Shepherd's Bush Military hospital during WWI. He performed most of the spinal operative procedures at Maida Vale until 1933. After the War he was appointed as an orthopaedic surgeon at the Middlesex Hospital. He worked at Mt. Vernon Hospital during WWII and died in 1951 after a full day of operating aged 72. His name provides the eponym for the fracture of the glenoid labrum in shoulder dislocation—the Bankart lesion—and for an operation to reconstruct the unstable shoulder prone to recurrent dislocation (1923 and 1938).

10.4.2.4 Spinal Fractures

Certain spinal fractures have been given eponymous names either after the person who first described them or in relation to the mechanism of injury.

The Jefferson fracture was described by Sir Geoffrey Jefferson (1886–1961), who reported four cases of boney fracture of the anterior and posterior arches of C1 (the Atlas) in 1920. A Jefferson fracture is caused by a load on the back of the head, incurred from diving into shallow water, and impact against the roof of a vehicle and falls. Having served in at Anglo-Russian hospital in Petrograd and RAMC in France during WWI, he became a neurosurgeon. After the war, he worked in Manchester where he also performed the first successful embolectomy in England in 1925. He became Britain's first Professor of Neurosurgery at the University of Manchester and Manchester Royal Infirmary in 1934. He was awarded the Lister medal in 1948. His Lister oration to the Royal College of Surgeons of England in 1949 was titled *the Mind of the Mechanical Man* in which he described the Manchester Mark 1, one of the first electronic computers. His lecture even touched on the possibility of artificial intelligence.

In 1948, George Quentin Chance (b 1904) was an Irish radiologist working in Manchester who described three cases of the flexion fracture of the spine (first lumbar vertebra). The addition of shoulder harness to motor vehicle seat belts as opposed to lap belts has made this fracture less common that it was in the 1950s.

The Hangman's fracture affects the axis (C2) cervical vertebra, with hyperextension and distraction causing bilateral pedicular fractures. When the mechanism of injury is not hanging (e.g., unrestrained front seat driver), the hyperextending distracting force tends to widen the space between the bone and though unstable may spare the spinal cord [58, 59].

10.4.2.5 Trendelenburg Gait and Trendelenburg's Sign

Friedrich Trendelenburg (1844–1924), though born in Berlin, studied in Glasgow and Edinburgh before completing his studies under Bernhard von Langenbeck in Berlin. He was awarded his doctorate in 1866. He practiced in Rostock and Bonn before becoming head of surgery at the University of Leipzig from 1895. He was a founder of the German Surgical Society in 1872. He died of a cancer of the mandible. His student, Martin Kirschner (1879–1942) performed the first successful pulmonary embolectomy in 1924, which was called the Trendelenburg operation as Trendelenburg had spent much time studying pulmonary embolism. He gave his name to the gait, exhibited by weakness of the abductor muscles of the hip, usually associated with osteoarthritis. The sign or gait is positive when the person stands on one leg when walking and the contralateral hip drops rather than slightly rising. Another "Trendelenburg operation" involves high ligation of the greater saphenous vein for varicose veins. His position involves a head down, feet up position of a bed or an operating table.

10.4.2.6 Perthes Disease

Austrian **Karel Maydl** (1853–1903) was the first to describe avascular necrosis of the femoral epiphysis in children. However, it was **Georg Clemens Perthes** (1869–1927), a pupil of Trendelenburg, who has had his name attached to Perthes' disease, and this because he took the first radiograph of a patient with this condition in 1898. He called the condition *arthritis deformans juvenilis*. The report and radiology of his case was not published until 1910. Perthes became head of surgery in Tübingen in 1910. After WWI he became Professor of Surgery in Bonn. The term, Legg-Calvé-Perthes disease may be more accurate because in 1910, **Arthur Legg** (1874–1939), an American, published a series of five cases, while **James Calvé** (1875–1954) in France reported a series of ten cases [60].

10.4.2.7 Garden's Classification of Subcapital Fractures of the Hip

Scottish orthopedic surgeon, **Robert Symon Garden** (1910–1982), classified subcapital fractures of the neck of the femur according to their risk of avascular necrosis due to the blood supply to the head of the femur running up the neck, in the event that, in the elderly, the ligamentum teres supply is likely to have dried up. His classification involves four grades, the first two of which can be treated by screw fixation, whereas grades 3 (partially displaced with varus with all three trabeculae disturbed) and 4 (completely displaced head, no contact with fracture fragments) require hemi or total hip arthroplasty. Garden commanded the No 3 orthopedic hospital during WWII in Egypt and North Africa and practiced in Preston after the war.

10.4.2.8 Facial Fractures

René Le Fort (1869–1951), the son of a physician and nephew of a surgeon, was born and trained in Lille, France. He served in the first Balkan War (1912) and WWI. After the war, he became Professor of orthopaedics and paediatric surgery. In 1901, his treatise *Étude expérimentale sur les fractures de la mâchoire supérieure* dealt with fractures of the maxilla. He used clubs and bars, or kicked and threw against tables and walls, 35 cadaver heads to study the patterns of fractures. He was then able to classify facial fractures into three types. Although the original classification has been modified in by Robert Marciani in 1993, the classification is widely used. Essentially, Le Fort I is a floating palate due to a horizontal force, Le Fort II is a floating maxilla due to a pyramidal fracture, and in Le Fort III, the whole face is floating due to a transverse force [51, 54, 55].

10.4.2.9 The Association for Osteosynthesis (AO)

By the 1940s and 1950s, a system of conservative management of fractures had been established by Lorenz Böhler (1885–1973) in Vienna, George Perkins (1892–1980) in London, and many others. Bohler's 1929 textbook, *Die Technik der Knochenbruchbehandlung* (*Treatment of Fractures*) was a best seller, and translated into eight languages. Perkins wrote an influential book on *Fractures and Dislocations* (1958) after his retirement. Although methods involving reduction and holding fractured bones in position by splints, plaster of Paris (POP), or traction was often effective, they relied upon weeks of fracture union (e.g., 6 weeks for a fractured femur), limited or no mobility during this period, usually accompanied by deconditioning and muscle wasting. Both Bohler and Perkins advocated exercising as many muscle groups as possible to promote blood supply to the fracture site, maintenance of muscle mass, and general health.

However, the management of fractures in the second half of the twentieth century was about to radically change.

Gerhard Küntscher (1900–1972) was a German surgeon who first implanted an intramedullary nail into a fractured femur at the University of Kiel hospital in November 1939. He presented his first series of cases to a meeting in Berlin the following year and was met with stiff disapproval. However, the German military approved his technique in 1942. Küntscher was posted to Lapland where he taught the technique to Finnish surgeons. Because of the war his operation was not known during the war years outside of Germany. However, he was later reposted to the Luftwaffe in Berlin to treat Luftwaffe Prisoners of War, many of whom had fractured their femurs on landing as paratroopers. When these Allied POWs returned to their countries, they carried the news of his intramedullary nailing and its success and that they were up walking within days. Küntscher's nail was clover-leafed in cross section. It worked well for fractures of the mid-shaft, but it did not control rotation and Küntscher introduced a locked (detensor) nail in 1968, with a proximal and distal screw [51, 52].

Professor Flavio Pires de Camargo (1916–1999), in Sao Paulo, Brazil, designed an early distal self-locking device to improve axial and rotatory instability. His 1952 thesis included 240 patients treated between 1946 and 1951 using his adaptation of the Küntscher IM nail. It is an example of how many surgeons around the world began to adapt Küntscher's technique, improve nail design, and have their patients mobilized early and thus less prone to the complications of lying in bed.

Maurice Edmond Müller (1918–2009), a Swiss-trained doctor and soon to be orthopaedic surgeon, studied medicine in Neuchatel, Bern, and Lausanne (1944) before graduating with a MD from Zurich (1946). During WWII, in 1944, he had met a patient who had had a femoral shaft fracture treated by Gerhard Küntscher with an intramedullary nail. In 1950, aged 32, he visited the then 70-year-old Robert Danis in Brussels, Belgium (see above), who had been internally fixing selected fractures for 25 years. His 1949 book, *Theorie et pratique de l'osteosynthese*, inspired him to study internal fixation and become an orthopaedic surgeon. Following his specialty qualification in orthopaedics in 1957, he co-founded, the *Arbeitsgemeinschaft für Osteosynthesefragen* (*Association of the study of internal fixation*) in 1958. The first AO course was run in Davos in 1960. Müller was Professor of Orthopaedics at the University of Bern from 1963 to 1980.

The AO society became a foundation in 1984 and is now a nonprofit organization dedicated to improving the care of patients with musculoskeletal injuries through education and research. He had to develop new tools and techniques which were marketed by two Swiss Companies (Mathys and Stratec) and later by Synthes USA, though the three companies have since combined. Over the next 40 years, royalties from sales of AO instrumentation grew progressively. Eventually the AO instrumentation side of the business was sold to separate surgeons profiting from the instruments, plates, and screws that they used on their patients. An annual (fixed) royalty fee is paid to the AO foundation to enable it to continue its mission of providing education and research for musculoskeletal injuries.

Müller also founded another company (Protek AG) to market his 1960s hip prosthesis, and, from 1974, the profits went to the Maurice E Müller foundation to provide education and research in orthopaedics. Protek AG was sold to Sulzer Medica in 1990 and later became part of Zimmer [50–53].

10.5 Joint Replacement

Osteoarthritis is one of the commonest conditions affecting aging populations. It involves the destruction of articular cartilage in the joint resulting in bone on bone, with inflammation, osteophyte formation, and deformity. Patients experience pain on movement but eventually pain at rest. Although the condition is most common in those over 60 years of age, it is accelerated by previous injury to ligaments, or damage to articular cartilage from trauma, inflammation (e.g., rheumatoid arthritis), or infection. Joint replacement, particularly in large weight-bearing joints of the lower limbs comprise some of the commonest procedures performed in high-income countries of the world.

In the eighteenth century the spread of modern firearms and the wars that afflicted Europe from Ireland to the Black Sea led to unprecedented number of young people crippled by injuries requiring amputation and/or disarticulation. These were the only available surgical options. Some surgeons were horrified by the fact that those operations were performed without antisepsis or anesthaesia and started promoting limb-saving approach, such as a Prussian surgeon, Johann Ulrich Bilguer (1720–1796).

The first resection arthroplasty of the hip was performed by Anthony White in 1821, for a 9-year-old girl with tuberculosis. In New York in 1854, Lewis Sayre (1820–1900), Professor of orthopaedic surgery, performed the first excision arthroplasty for ankylosis in America. Subsequently, he operated up to 59 patients, though only 39 survived. Although in the USA this technique was well received, the European surgeons, like Volkmann and Calot adopted a conservative approach [61].

Henry Park (1744–1831) in Liverpool, UK, told his mentor, Percival Pott (1744–1778), that the only treatment was extirpation of the joint by excision of the head of the femur and hoping for callus formation to effect healing. Vitezslav Chlumsky (1867–1943) experimented with interposition materials in Breslau (Poland), including muscle, silver plates, rubber struts, zinc, glass, decalcified bones, and wax.

The first total hip replacement occurred in Germany by Themistocles Glück (1853–1942). Glück was a Romanian-born German orthopaedic surgeon who is credited with developing the first successful artificial hip joint. In 1891, he designed a ball and socket joint made from ivory and fixed it to the bone with nickel-plated screws. Glück presented his results at the tenth International Medical Conference in 1891. Glück showed the use of ivory to replace femoral heads of patients whose hip joints had been destroyed by tuberculosis [62].

He later improved the fixation of the joint by using plaster of Paris and powdered pumice with resin. Glück was born in 1853 in Iasi, which was then part of the Principality of Moldavia (modern-day Romania). His father was a physician who served as the personal physician to King Charles I of Romania. Glück studied medicine in Vienna and Berlin and eventually settled in Berlin, where he became a Professor of orthopaedic surgery at the Charité Hospital. During his time as a military surgeon, Glück experimented with using screws and steel plates to fix bone fractures, developing an early form of open reduction and internal fixation (ORIF) surgery. This technique involved making an incision in the skin and using screws and plates to hold the broken bones in place while they healed [61, 62].

William Steven Baer (1872–1931) was an American surgeon renowned for his work in reconstructive surgery. In 1918, Baer used pig bladder as an interposition material in a patient who had suffered a facial injury. This was a pioneering use of biological materials in plastic surgery. Informed consent was less likely to be obtained in the early twentieth century as it is today, so many surgeons had a great deal of freedom in adopting novel surgical approaches and/or materials.

A major breakthrough occurred in 1923. Marius Smith-Petersen (1886–1953) from Boston described the mould interposition arthroplasty with glass. Petersen noticed that glass was well tolerated by the body, so when a patient had a piece of glass in his back, Petersen noticed a fibrous membrane. Therefore, he concluded that glass molded onto the femoral head could stimulate the formation of that fibrous membrane and relieve pain, improving range of motion and patient mobility. Despite glass being a biocompatible material, it failed to withstand the shear forces going through the hip joint and shattered. Vitallium, suggested by his dentist, helped him implant almost 500 hip molds with good clinical results.

The first attempt at replacing the joint surfaces was made by a French surgeon named Pierre Delbet (1861–1925). He used rubber prostheses to replace the femoral head in 1919 [62, 63].

In the 1930s and 1940s, scientists and surgeons began experimenting with using plastic and other synthetic materials for joint replacements. These early plastic joint replacements were also not very successful and had a high failure rate. Dr. Austin T. Moore (1899–1963) from North Carolina and Dr. William H. Thompson from New York separately designed cobalt-chrome hip replacements in the 1940s and 1950s, which were among the first to succeed. These prostheses were made of a metal stem that was inserted into the femur and a metal ball that replaced the head of the femur, which articulated with a plastic socket in the hip bone.

While these designs were revolutionary at the time, they did not always have the same longevity and success. The Austin Moore and Thompson prostheses were known to cause wear and tear on the plastic socket, leading to loosening of the implant and potential failure [62–64].

Gathorne Robert Girdlestone (1881–1950) in Oxford popularized the girdlestone arthroplasty of the hip in the 1940s—an excision of the femoral head for tuberculosis or infection of the hip, though this operation had been described over a century before. The first to use a metal-on-metal prosthesis on a regular basis was the English orthopedic surgeon George Kenneth McKee (1906–1991). In 1953, he began by using the modified Thompson stem (a cemented hemiarthroplasty used for neck of femur fracture treatment) with a new one-piece cobalt-chrome socket as the new acetabulum. This arthroplasty involves using a metal ball and socket to replace the damaged hip joint. The metal surfaces of the implant are designed to glide against each other, creating a smooth and durable joint though they were subject to wear and to releasing metal into the tissues [62–64].

British orthopedic surgeon, Sir John Charnley (1911–1982) (Fig. 10.3) of Manchester Royal Infirmary, was working in his garage to design a hip replacement which was destined to be so successful that the results and longevity are still considered a gold standard. He was a very hands-on person: both an orthopaedic surgeon and an engineer. After working in an orthopaedic unit for several years, he would come home and work in his garage workshop on various implant designs. He used Plexiglas or acrylic cement for his projects.

John Charnley developed the concept of low-friction arthroplasty with regard to three distinct ideas: the idea of low-friction torque arthroplasty, the use of acrylic cement to fix components to bone, and the introduction of high-density polyethylene as a bearing material. Charnley created a prosthesis inspired by dental prostheses by fashioning an implant with acrylic bone cement. This cemented hip replacement proved very successful due to the cement's two main features: its strength and ability to be used as grout to fit the implant. These three ideas came together to create a new way of thinking about arthroplasty that has since been adopted by the surgical community. Charnley's low-friction arthroplasty had a 80% survivorship at 25 years follow-up. Until Charnley, hip components were fashioned with the same size and shape as the patient's femoral head and acetabulum. He noticed that this setup was prone to failure, so he created a system with a steel ball on a PTFE/Teflon acetabular cup. The ball had a size of 22 mm. This meant that the surface bearings were close to native joint friction torque, and by decreasing the size of the femoral head from 40 mm to 22 mm, he ensured a greater range of motion up to 90 degree [65].

Charnley's materials and design resulted in the take-off of hip arthroplasty in 1966, when it was presented at the tenth International Surgical meeting. Swiss orthopedic surgeon, Maurice Edmond Müller (1918–2009), increased the size of the femoral head up to 32 mm, thus increasing the range of motion up to 106°. Müller was Professor of orthopaedic surgery in Bern from 1963 to 1980.

Teflon had a high failure rate, so Charnley used a different bearing material in the form of ultrahigh-molecular-weight polyethylene (UHMWPE). In the 1950s, he introduced (polymethyl methacrylate) bone cement. In 1960, his article "Anchorage of the femoral head prosthesis to the shaft of the femur" explained the basic principles, which included reaming the medulla of the femur before cementing and fixing the stem within the femur. The problem with this is that it is a surgeon's choice. The mix is made in the operating room, which means there is a chance it could be wrong. In 1984, Askew showed that pressurisation of cement increased its penetration into bone, but this resulted in increased tensile and sheer forces at the bone-cement interface. These cementing techniques are also applicable when one is cementing the acetabular cup. In the 1950s and 1960s, advances in metallurgy and plastics technology led to the development of more durable and long-lasting joint replacements. Additionally, the development of new surgical techniques, such as cementing and press-fit fixation, allowed for more secure and stable fixation of the joint replacements [65].

After Sir John Charnley introduced his innovative hip replacement design in the 1960s, other orthopaedic surgeons began experimenting with different materials and approaches to joint replacement surgery. In the 1960s, Peter Ring (1922–2018), an orthopaedic surgeon at Redhill hospital, developed a cementless metal-on-metal (MoM) arthroplasty. In the 1960s and 1970s, the use of cobalt-chromium and stainless steel alloys or ceramic as well as new surgical techniques such as the cementless fixation improved durability and longevity of the joint replacements.

In the twenty-first century, advances in materials science, computer-assisted design and manufacturing, and robotic-assisted surgery have led to the development of more advanced joint replacements with improved durability and longevity. Additionally, the development of customized, patient-specific joint replacements has improved the outcomes and recovery for some patients.

Prosthesis development has continued to progress since 1990, with the introduction of high cross-linked polyethylene (UHXLPE). This was followed in 1995, with BIOLOX® forte and, in 2003, BIOLOX® delta. The "forte" implant is a pure alumina ceramic mixed with magnesium oxide. The "delta" implant had zirconia fortified with alumina ceramic with strontium and yttrium. In 1999, Trabecular Metal® implants were introduced for revision arthroplasty with a tantalum structure. Another innovation is vitamin E-enriched poly introduced in 2010, which is useful for young and active patients [66–68].

The hip replacement today is a highly successful operation. The ball and socket nature of the joint means that replacement is generally successful with over 95% of patients being relieved of their pain with much improved mobility. However, there has been a major class action with a Johnson & Johnson hip arthoplasty.

In the late 2000s, the Australian National Joint Replacement Registry identified that Johnson & Johnson's Pinnacle hip replacement was defective with a high rate of removal. This was confirmed by the UK National Joint Registry in 2010. The joints were not being manufactured to advertised specifications, so cobalt and chromium ions were leaking from the implants, poisoning patients, and necessitating their removal in at least 12% of cases. More than 5500 Depuy J&J joints were inserted in Australia but also more than 100,000 worldwide. This led to a class action which was finally settled in 2019, for over US$1bn, involving over 6000 cases. Metal-on-metal implants are particularly prone to these complications and have been largely discontinued for hip arthroplasty. A similar problem occurred with a metal-on-metal version of Smith-Kleine's Birmingham hip also.

Metal allergy is another rare complication of metal and metal alloy implants. Allergic reactions may cause significant morbidity for the affected individual—including aseptic loosening, pseudotumour formation, and frank device failure. The ability to predict this complication is limited with those who already have metal allergies or who may react to a patch test the most at risk [66, 69, 70].

10.5.1 Knee Arthroplasty

The pain, disability, and deformity associated with knee osteoarthritis intrigued surgeons and frustrated their patients for millennia before the introduction of a successful total knee arthroplasty in 1968 and a unicompartmental arthroplasty during the

1980s. The knee is a hinge joint for which the stability depends upon four major ligaments (anterior and posterior cruciates, medial and lateral collaterals) and the strength of the surrounding muscles, particularly the quadriceps femoris. In addition the bone of the tibial and femoral condyles is not only covered with articular cartilage, but the tibial condyles are also further cushioned by the medial and lateral menisci.

Early efforts to ameliorate the symptoms arising from a damaged knee involved interpositions between the femur and tibial condyles using biological materials such pig bladder or fascia lata from the ninth century and later synthetic material such as nylon. These efforts were not successful. In 1890, Themistocles Glück (1853–1942) (Fig. 10.3), at the Charité Hospital in Berlin, inserted an ivory prosthetic hinged

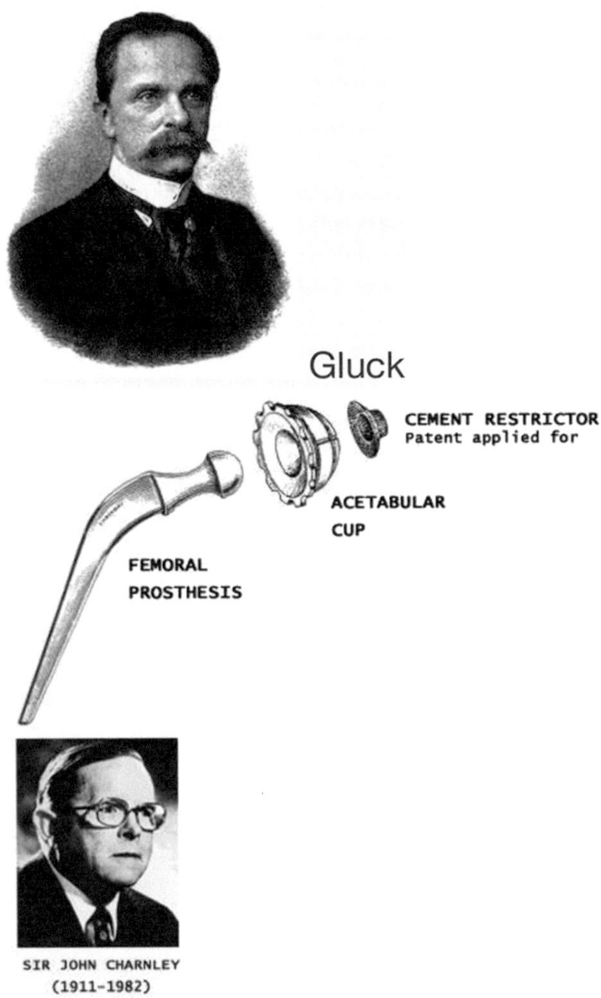

Fig. 10.3 Public domain, no restrictions. (https://madeupinbritain.uk/Hip_Replacement)

joint held into a 17-year-old girl. Postoperatively, the joint was held in place by plaster. He did 14 arthroplasties in that year, but many of them were for tuberculous destruction of the joint, and so although initially the patients recovered, the joints later had to be removed because of further chronic infection. He then made tuberculosis and other chronic infections a contraindication to joint replacement. Glück was a remarkable pioneer in orthopaedics performing hip, knee, shoulder, and wrist arthroplasties using ivory. He made many other significant contributions to orthopaedics. One of his knee joint replacements was able to be left in situ [71].

The total condylar knee prosthesis was developed in 1970, to align function and anatomy but with a simpler joint. This involved a Chrome Cobalt femoral shield plus two polyethylene tibial and patellar components. The cruciate ligaments were excised. There were then various modifications and improvement including an uncemented horseshoe tibial component that allowed sparing of the cruciates (Kodama and Yamamoto). This was followed by Townley's polycentric geometry and others contributing a mobile meniscus bearing resurfacing prosthesis. These developments were fundamental to the eventual low contact stress prostheses of today.

Constrained hinged prostheses were also introduced, but these showed a high degree of wear and tear or dislocation due to the rotational forces that occur during flexion and extension. They are today only used where there is significant ligamental instability. There is also an unhinged variety, the constrained condylar knee, which is sometimes used for revisions. The femoral rollback is the posterior movement of the femur as the knee progressively flexes. In the normal knee, this is controlled by the cruciates, so to achieve a good outcome with TKA, there is a need to both have good quadriceps function and ensure a good range of flexion by preventing posterior impingement during deep flexion. Thus, there are now various designs based on maintaining cruciate ligament (CR) and/or posterior stabilized (PS) components.

10.5.2 Unilateral (unicompartmental) Knee Arthroplasty (UKA)

In 1957, McKeever used the metal, vitallium, and reported the hemiarthroplasty was particularly effective in patients with rheumatoid arthritis. However, Campbell was probably the first to use a tibial plateau plate of vitallium in 1940. DL MacIntosh, in 1958, then began to perform hemiarthroplasties for persons with painful and significant varus (bow) or valgus (knock) knees. He inserted a tibial acrylic plateau to correct the deformity but switched to vitallium in 1964. MacIntosh and McKeever presented their combined 6-year results in Switzerland in 1967, and because one of the problems was migration of the plate, McKeever added a keel (like that of a boat) to prevent this complication.

The Gunston and polycentric prostheses were introduced for unilateral arthroplasty in the 1970s. This was the first time that both femoral and tibial surfaces were implanted. However, the device had a 10% removal rate at 2 years. The 1970s and 1980s were a period of introduction of new devices (St Georg sled, Brigham and Marmor) and awaiting longer-term results. Orthopaedic knee surgeons were also learning more regarding appropriate case selection. Variable results were reported from 32% to 90% 4-year successful outcomes for unilateral knee replacement. Patients with unstable joints and the presence of rheumatoid arthritis were unsuitable for a UKA.

Today, there are suitable UKA devices such as the Unispacer and ComfortMIS for appropriately selected patients. However, during the 1980s–2000s, the results of TKA improved dramatically. There were European champions of UKA who continued to report successful results throughout the 1990s and early 2000s.

The use of computer-assisted technology in joint replacement surgery has become increasingly common over the past few decades, and it is true that one of the earliest examples of this was a knee replacement surgery performed in 1997.

The procedure involved using a computer to generate a 3D image of the patient's knee joint, which was then used to guide the placement of the implant during surgery. This approach is sometimes referred to as computer-assisted surgery (CAS) or computer-assisted navigation (CAN) and is designed to help improve the accuracy and precision of joint replacement procedures [71, 72].

Since that initial knee replacement in 1997, computer-assisted technology has continued to evolve and has been used in a wide range of joint replacement surgeries, including hip replacements and shoulder replacements. Today, many orthopedic surgeons use computer-assisted technology to help plan and execute joint replacement procedures, with the aim of achieving better outcomes for their patients.

The Mako device adds a robotic arm in combination with 3D CT imaging. This minimizes bone resection and allows more accurate orientation of the various prosthetic components with allowance for the soft tissue dynamics. Greater individualization is bringing TKA on a journey toward a point where a prosthesis is becoming more personalized with greater conformity in function to the patient's original knee. The complexity of the knee joint and biomechanical challenges means that good outcomes are still not guaranteed though around 80–90% of persons will achieve their desired result as measured by 10-year follow-up. Prosthetic infection, which often results in removal and revision of the prosthesis should occur at a rate of less than 1%. Dislocation or instability should also be rare [72, 73].

10.6 Cataract Surgery

A cataract is a medical condition where the eye's normally clear lens becomes opaque and affects vision, leading to symptoms like blurriness, altered colors, halos around light, and, eventually, complete blindness. The purpose of the lens is to refract light entering the eye through the pupil and onto the retina, and impulses are sent through the optic nerve to the occipital cortex of the brain.

There are several factors and causes that can lead to opacification of the lens and cataract formation, but the most common one is the age-related senile cataract. Cataracts make a significant contribution to vision impairment worldwide. As populations age, their incidence is rising. In 2010, it was estimated that more than 20 million were affected, with that number projected to increase in the future. In high-income countries, cataract surgery is the commonest operative procedure performed. The unmet need for surgical procedures in low- and middle-income countries includes a large number of patients with cataracts who must live with impaired vision without surgery. To see the joy that lights up on the faces of those who, on removal of their eye pad, can see clearly again is one of the most satisfying experiences for any healthcare practitioner.

In the past, people believed that cataracts were due to a liquid material flowing through the lens, which is why the term "*cataracta*" comes from the Latin word for "waterfall," although it may also be because dense cataracts can look like a waterfall to imaginative viewers. There is good evidence that the Indian, Suśruta, who lived as early as 600 BCE, conducted cataract surgery and subsequently documented it [74]. In one form or another, cataract surgery has been practiced throughout the ages.

The practice of couching, one of the earliest surgical methods described to treat cataracts, dates back to the fifth century BCE. The term "couching" is derived from the French word "*coucher*," which means "to put to bed." This technique involves using a sharp needle to puncture the eye near the limbus, allowing the surgeon to manually move the mature cataract from the visual axis, usually pushing it into the vitreous chamber [75].

As per current understanding, cataract surgery is still the only known way to treat a visually significant cataract, which is defined as a visual acuity of 20/40 or poorer. This definition has evolved over time. In the early stages of cataract surgery, a visually significant cataract would have been considered as an advanced or mature cataract, resulting in such severe vision impairment that the patient was almost blind [76].

The ophthalmic historian, Julius Hirschberg (1843–1925) wrote: *"At the present time it is impossible to answer this important historical question as to which nation (or even which man) first performed a cataract operation, the historical evidence suggests that cataract surgery possibly originated in one location and then spread to other parts of the world, or being independently developed in multiple locations at different times"* [77, 78].

During the ancient Egyptian period, the Ebers papyrus, the Edwin-Smith papyrus, and other medical papyri included various medical recipes for treating eye conditions, but there is no reference to cataract surgery in these documents [79].

The Babylonian code of Hammurabi (1792–1750 BCE) specified the rewards for making an incision which heals a man's eye, and the severe penalty of inflicting blindness with surgery gone wrong. This may be referring to cataract surgery.

> *If a physician [asû]...opened a man's temple with a bronze scalpel and healed the man's eye, he shall charge 10 shekels of silver (as his fee)... If an asû-physician has...opened a man's temple with a bronze scalpel and blinded the man's eye, they shall cut off his hand... If he opened his (the commoner's slave's) temple with a bronze scalpel and blinded his eye, he shall weigh out silver equal to half his value.* [80]

Al-Hasan Ibn al-Haytham, also known as Alhazen in the Western world, was a pioneering scientist of the Islamic Golden Age, born around 965 CE in Basra, present-day Iraq. He made groundbreaking contributions to various fields, including optics, mathematics, astronomy, and physics. His most influential work, the "*Kitab al-Manazir*" (Book of Optics), laid the foundation for modern optics by correctly explaining the theory of vision and the nature of light and color. Ibn al-Haytham was a strong advocate for the scientific method, emphasizing the importance of experiments and mathematical reasoning to validate hypotheses. His innovative approach earned him the title of the "father of modern optics" and influenced many later scientists, including Isaac Newton and Johannes Kepler. Beyond his scientific achievements, he also wrote extensively on philosophy, theology, and medicine (Figs. 10.4 and 10.5).

In the *Paradise of Wisdom* (Firdaws al-Hikma), written by the Muslim physician Ali ibn Sahl al-Tabari in the ninth century, both Suśruta and Vāgbhaṭa (Indian physicians) are cited. The book referred to cataract as "*mâ*" but did not discuss its surgical treatment. Al-Razi's (Rhazes) *Kitāb al-ḥāwī*, also known as the *Comprehensive Book* and later as *The Continens*, is an extensive encyclopedia. The majority of Arabic authors who wrote about cataract surgery, including Hunain Ibn Ishaq (809–877 CE) and Ali ibn Isa el-Kahhal (c. 940–1010 CE) from Baghdad, and Ammar ibn Ali al-Mawsili from Cairo (fl. c. 1000 CE), frequently referenced Greek authors but did not explicitly mention Indian authors. However, there are certain aspects of the descriptions of cataract surgery in Arabic literature that imply a plausible connection with Indian literature, as elaborated below [80, 81].

There is some evidence to suggest that a thorn or needle-like object may have been used for cataract couching in ancient times. While there is no direct reference to this technique in historical texts, there are some clues that point toward its possible use. For instance, ancient Greek and Latin texts mention a "stilus" or "style," which was a sharp instrument used to puncture the eye and extract the cataract. Similarly, ancient Egyptian hieroglyphics depict a procedure where a sharp object is used to pierce the eye and remove the cataract. These descriptions may be referring to the use of a thorn or other pointed object, rather than a specifically designed surgical instrument. Furthermore, there are reports of traditional healers in rural areas of some developing countries using thorns or other sharp objects to perform

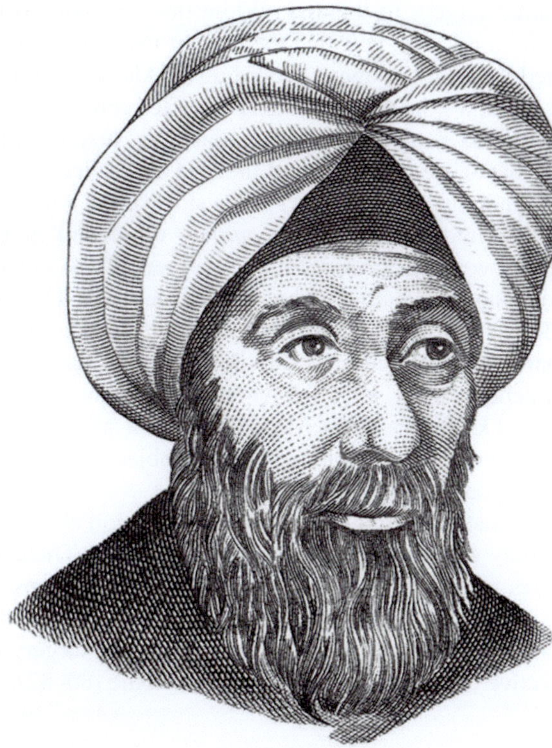

Fig. 10.4 Ibn al-Haytham. (Illustrated by Michel Bakni, Wikimedia Commons. https://upload.wikimedia.org/wikipedia/commons/a/a3/Ibn_Al-Haytham_portrait.jpg)

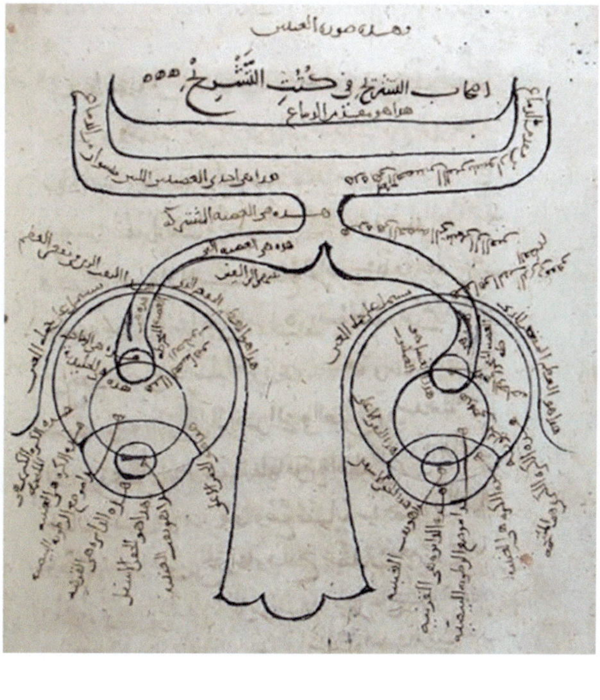

Fig. 10.5 A sketch showing the structure of the human eye, as described by Ibn al-Haytham in the eleventh century CE, is detailed in a copy of the *Kitab al-Manazir.* (Wikimedia commons, public domain. https://www.laternamagica.co/cine-ibn-al-haytham/)

cataract surgery to this day. While this technique is considered unsafe and unhygienic, it does suggest that the idea of using a thorn for cataract couching has persisted through the ages. According to Alexandrian traditions, there is a story that describes a goat as performing cataract couching by accidentally running into a thorn. This story is not substantiated by historical texts but is often cited as an example of the persistence of the idea that a sharp object can be used to move cataracts and improve vision [81]. The story of the goat couching a cataract in its eye by running into a thorn was a widely circulated narrative among Graeco-Roman authors who mentioned cataract surgery. This suggests that the story was well-known and had gained popularity in their day. The fact that multiple authors from different regions and time periods included the story also suggests that it had become a part of a larger cultural tradition and may have served as a teaching tool. In the thirteenth century, Khalifah Al-Halabi, a medieval oculist from Aleppo, compared a surgical knife to a thorn. This comparison suggests that there may have been a historical precedent for the use of sharp objects for ancient surgical practices, such as cataract couching.

Cataract couching, as stated in the section above, does not remove the cataract, but only dislodges it from the line of vision. There was a need for surgical techniques to evolve, first removing the lens (extracapsular extraction) and providing refraction through spectacles. Today, following removal, an intraocular lens is placed allowing much better vision. Cataract surgery is regarded as one of the most effective treatments in the field of medicine [80–82].

10.6.1 Extracapsular Cataract Extraction (ECCE)

The first modern cataract extraction is credited to Jacques Daviel (1696–1762) in 1747, in Paris. His technique involved a large corneal incision, puncturing the capsule of the lens and extracting the nucleus in fragments. This was progress, but the early operations were prone to complications of poor wound healing and retained lens fragments. The posterior capsule was also prone to opacify, particularly if there was infection. ECCE was the treatment of choice for the next 200 years but then was progressively replaced by intracapsular methods of extraction. By the 1970s improved methods of performing ECCE with manual small incisions (MSICS) resulted in a return to ECCE with an overall success rate of 90–95 per cent. ECCE is still the preferred method in many parts of the world [84].

10.6.2 Intracapsular Cataract Extraction (ICCE)

In 1753, Samuel Sharp (1709–1778) was a British surgeon working at Guy's Hospital in London, who performed an intracapsular extraction. He was a Barber-Surgeon having spent a 7 year apprenticeship with William Cheselden (1724–1731).

He wrote a text on operative techniques in Surgery. The ICCE he performed involved removing the entire lens through a large limbal incision. Sharp used his thumb to expel the cataract, and fracturing the zonular fibers that suspend the lens to the eye was essential to the procedure. The technique used to fracture the zonules has evolved from the use of forceps to hold the lens while manually disrupting them to the introduction of chemical dissolution with the enzyme alpha chymotrypsin by Joaquin Barraquer of Barcelona (1927–1916) in 1957. Another technique involved cryoextraction with a frozen probe was used to evacuate the cataract/lens from the eye. ICCE was also prone to complications, as the lens separates the anterior from the posterior chambers of the eye. Retinal detachment, macular degeneration, and corneal decompensation are more likely when there is no barrier to vitreous prolapsing forwards. The larger incision took longer to heal and made the eye prone to astigmatism (imperfection of the curvature of the eye affecting near and far vision). ICCE remained the main procedure performed for cataract in the USA until the 1970s.

Modern cataract surgery involves and ECCE with phacoemulsification. Improved instrumentation resulted in the extracapsular approach becoming safer and better than the intracapsular. The introduction in the 1970s of ophthalmic viscosurgical devices (OVD) means that the space within the anterior chamber prior to cataract extraction can be retained while not interfering with the steps of the procedure. In 1967, Charles Kelman (1930–2004) introduced phacoemulsification which utilizes an ultrasound probe through a 3–4 mm incision to emulsify and aspirate the lens. This technique is widely used in the developed world as the 3–4 mm incision ensures a much more stable anterior chamber.

Kelman had been experimenting with how to better dissolve the lens prior to extraction allowing a smaller incision to remove the lens. He had tried 40 prototypes, and all were failures. He was on the verge of giving up. The idea to use ultrasound came in the dentist's chair. His Lancet obituary gave a brief account in Kelman's own words:

"But when he went to his dentist, Larry Kuhn, an early adopter of the ultrasonic probe to remove tartar, he "felt an exquisite vibration and heard a high-pitched sound". He jumped out of his chair, asked what device Kuhn was using, hugged Kuhn and his assistant, and ran back to his lab to pick up a cataract that had just been removed. Returning to the dentist's office, he picked up the probe and used it to make grooves in the cataract. "I knew that it wouldn't be quite that easy, that the instrument would have to be modified perhaps a hundred times, but I also knew that I had found, finally, in the eleventh hour, the road that would lead to a small incision cataract surgery" [83].

In 2008, femtosecond laser technology was first used to assist even smaller incisions in cataract surgery in Budapest, Hungary.

All of the techniques described above resulted in an aphakic (without a lens) patient whose vision depended upon powerful, hyperopic spectacles to refract light onto the retina.

10.6.3 Intraocular Lens (IOL)

The intraocular lens was introduced by Sir Harold Ridley in 1949. Ridley realized that the anterior chamber of the eye would tolerate plastic implants as there were many WWII pilots who had fragments of plastic in their anterior chambers. His first lens, made of polymethyl methacrylate (PMMA), was prone to cause infections such as uveitis, glaucoma, and dislocation of the implanted lens. However, when the early IOC's were inserted, the predominant method of cataract removal was ICCE.

Modern IOL's were first introduced by Stephen Shearing (1934–2011), a Las Vegas ophthalmologist, who developed a compressible lens that could sit where the original one did, behind the iris. It was understood that the best place for the lens to sit was within the capsular gag. In the 1980s foldable lenses made with acrylic or silicone were introduced which enabled even smaller incisions. As the lenses improved, the complications reduced, and patients were able to have cataract surgery that resulted in their having no need for spectacles. In 1992, astigmatism correction became possible [83, 84].

IOLs can now be fashioned to be multifocal (1990s) and support near and far vision simultaneously. There are also accommodating IOLs (since 2000) that respond to whether the person needs near or far vision. The mathematical calculations to design the right lens for the right patient to maximize the likelihood of good vision without spectacles are becoming increasingly sophisticated. Cataract surgery has come a long way in the days since couching. The challenge for the future is to meet the needs of the vision impaired, as cataract is the world's commonest, but not the only cause, for blindness.

10.7 A History of Neurosurgery

The Edwin Smith Papyrus, dated around 1600 BCE but probably a copy of an even older text around 3000–2500 BC, is so-called because Edwin Smith purchased the papyrus in Egypt in 1862. The Ancient Egyptian text is currently housed in the New York Academy of Medicine, on permanent loan from the New York Historical Society. It describes history taking, examination, diagnosis, and recommendations for treatment of 48 injuries, involving different body parts including the head, face, neck, and trunk, with six that involve the spine—five cervical and one lumbar. For example, the decision-making advice in the papyrus only advised treatment for some boney or soft tissue injuries of the spine but did not advise treatment if there was clinical evidence of spinal cord involvement. Case 8 provides a head injury scenario and what to do with and without a scalp wound, whether there is a fracture, and also how not to proceed in the case of a base of skull fracture recognized by blood being discharged from the nose or ear. Case 12 scenario is a nasal fracture, an injury which can be treated by reduction. The papyrus confirms the considerable clinical skills of ancient Egyptian doctors, skills that were probably lost (or not written down) for over a millennium until the time of Hippocrates (see below) [85–87].

10.7.1 Trepanation

However, in ancient times, medical and surgical skills were certainly passed on from surgeon to apprentice in many ancient societies as is evidenced from the skill to perform a successful trepanation. In Anatolia (Asia Minor and part of Turkey today), 35 skulls with trepanations have been found, 19 of which show signs of healing and survival after the procedure. These skulls date back thousands of years though the indications for surgery are largely unknown and some may have been for religious, superstitious, misguided, or mystical reasons such as letting the demons escape. Similar skulls have been excavated in South America, sub-Saharan Africa, and Melanesia. A report of 66 Peruvian skulls from around 1000 AD showed not only an 85% survival with minimal rate of infection, but increased survival rates over time. In Papua New Guinea's Bismarck archipelago, even in the nineteenth century, the proceduralist was often on the site of a tribal fight performing the surgery for head injuries including open depressed fractures, although trepanation was also being carried out for other conditions such as convulsions, mental illness, or perceived demon possession [87–89].

10.7.2 Hippocrates and Neurosurgery (Fourth Century BCE)

Hippocrates (460–377 BC) based his practice of medicine on scientific principles and observation. He established a medical school on the Island of Cos and wrote ten volumes of medical texts. He rejected the influence of religious and magical beliefs in favor of science. For example, he wrote the first book on epilepsy called "*The Sacred Disease*" noting "*It is thus with regard to the disease called Sacred: it appears to me to be nowise more divine nor more sacred than other diseases, but has a natural cause like other affections*" [85, 87].

Hippocrates also wrote extensively on different types of head injuries describing six types including fractures, depressed fractures, and closed head injuries without a fracture including injuries in other parts of the brain remote from the site of injury (contra-coup). He also established clinical and decision-making principles for the assessment and treatment of spinal injuries and conditions, adopting a conservative, no treatment approach for spinal cord damage, reaffirming the advice of the ancient Egyptians.

10.7.3 Herophilus and Erasistratus: Neuroanatomical Descriptions from Alexandria (Third Century BCE)

Herophilus Chalcedon (335–280 BC) and Erasistratus (310–250 BC) were two Greek physicians who founded a school of anatomy in Alexandria, benefitting enormously from the right to undertake human dissections in the kingdom of Ptolemy, under the reign of the Ptolemic Pharaohs for a period of about 40 years. Erasistratus recognized that nerves originated from the brain, the first description of cranial nerves, including the hypoglossal nerve. They identified the difference between motor and sensory nerves and recognized seven pairs of cranial nerves, as well as other neuroanatomical structures such as the meninges, ventricles, and dural sinuses. The fourth ventricle was regarded as the seat of the soul [87, 88].

10.7.3.1 Meges of Sidon and Trepanation (First Century BCE)

Meges of Sidon, Phonecia, was a prominent surgeon of the first century BCE. His surgical innovations that include instruments to extract bladder stones, cutting setons for anal fistula, but also, relevant to this chapter, the trephining of head injuries, are cited by Aulus Cornelius Celsus, (25–50 AD), who was an encyclopedist not a surgeon. Celsus' *De Medicina* has eight volumes, the first of which is devoted to the history of medicine and the last on orthopaedics. Although none of Meges' works remain, he was also cited by Galen [89, 90].

10.7.3.2 Soranus of Ephesus: Convulsions, Hydrocephalus, and Neonatal Neurology (Second Century CE)

Soranus of Ephesus (98–138 AD) studied neurologic issues in newborns and pregnancy, wrote about pre-eclampsia, eclampsia, fits and epilepsy, hydrocephalus, and migraine.

10.7.3.3 Aretaeus of Cappadocia and Trigeminal Neuralgia (Second Century CE)

Aretaeus of Cappadocia (second century CE) described trigeminal neuralgia. He wrote about the whole range of medical conditions but was also the first to give an account of diabetes and coeliac disease [87, 88].

10.7.3.4 Herophilus, Marinus, and Galen Identifying Cranial Nerves

During the ancient Greek and Roman era, human dissections did take place in Alexandria around the third century BCE, enabling that generation of doctors to be better informed about human anatomy. Following the first descriptions of cranial nerves by Herophilus Chalcedon (335–280 BC) and Erasistratus (circa 310–250 BC) in Alexandria, the first classification of cranial nerves was introduced by Galen's mentor, Marinus, who had identified seven pairs of cranial nerves. Galen (129–200 AD) also advanced the understanding of the pathology of spinal injuries through his experiments on animals, including identifying the Brown-Sequard phenomenon which occurs when the spinal cord is hemisected. However, he also did not recommend treating spinal injuries where they involved the spinal cord. Among many other advances, Galen also introduced the terms of kyphosis, scoliosis, and lordosis [88, 89].

10.7.3.5 Paulus of Aegina (Seventh Century CE): Laminectomy

Paulus of Aegina (625–690 AD), during the Byzantine period, was trained in the Greek tradition but also influenced by the Islamic medical teachings. He became a leading physician of his day, or at least the one whose writings survived the passage of time. His works, including his magnum opus *Epitomae Medicae Libri Septem* was translated into Arabic in the ninth Century by Hunayn ibn Ishaq. These seven books were not translated into European languages until the sixteenth century and not into English until 1843. In the sections on spinal injuries, he advocates operating to remove loose fragments that are crushing the "spinal marrow"—the first ever description of laminectomy! This was a strategy that was subsequently undertaken by some leading Arab and Middle-Eastern surgeons such as Albucasis (936–1013 AD) and Avicenna (980–1037 AD) who had the benefit of his texts translated into their language. Avicenna follows the recommendation for some form of decompression made by Paulus and advises *to* "remove the compressing bone that causes the neurological deficit…. If the crushed bone is removed even in part then the remaining bone chips must also be taken away." There is no evidence that European surgeons attempted to perform laminectomy for many centuries despite this advice by Avicenna.

10.7.3.6 Salerno in Twelfth Century CE: Trepanation

In Salerno, Rogerius Salernitanus Frugardi (1140–1195) published *Practica Chirurgiae* in 1180. This brief, practical manual of surgery was based on anatomical studies, describing different injuries and surgical techniques including trephination. In 1345, Guido da Vigevano published *Anathomia designate per figures* with 24 plates, 6 of which were about the anatomy of the central nervous system, depicting the head, brain, meninges, and spinal cord.

10.7.3.7 Arab and Ottoman Contributions to Neurosurgery Eleventh to Fifteenth Centuries

Ibn-al Quff (1233–1286) was a Christian surgeon born in what today would be Jordan but who trained and worked in Damascus (Syria). He was also a military surgeon stationed with the army in Jordan where he gained considerable clinical experience. His book *Basics in the Art of Surgery* is by far the largest Arab surgical text to survive the medieval era. He introduced the most novel use of a bridlelike instrument for anterior cervical fracture through the oral route. By introducing the device in the mouth, he described a pushing maneuver to the cervical vertebrae from the ventral site and a simultaneous pulling maneuver by cupping on the neck from the dorsal site.

During the Ottoman era, Şerafeddin Sabuncuoğlu (1385–1468) practiced in Amasya during the reign of Mehmet the Conqueror (1432–1481). His textbook *Imperial Surgery* is written in Turkish and is remarkable for its color illustrations. On neurosurgical topics it covers low back pain, spinal injuries, epilepsy, facial paralysis, hydrocephalus, and head injuries.

Ibrahim bin Abdullah in the early sixteenth century wrote in *Ala'im-i Cerrahin* the first account of cranioplasty in the Arab world suggesting a cranial defect could be replaced by a bone graft from a slaughtered capricorn (a horned goat). He also cited Hippocrates and Galen with regard postoperative progress: "if the person develops a fever after three days, you have to know this is not a good sign." Ibrahim bin Abdullah also wrote about neurosurgical anatomy, trauma and other surgical topics [90–92].

The Italian wars occurred during a 60-year period between 1494 and 1559. There were also Ottoman-Venetian wars recurring from the end of the fourteenth century until the early eighteenth century.

10.7.3.8 Berengario: The First Printed Textbook on Head Injuries (1518)

Jacopo Berengario (1460–1530), was a polymath, anatomist, and surgeon (and son of a barber surgeon) who had received his medical degree from the University of Bologna in 1489. He was appointed a lecturer in Bologna and, in 1518, was to publish the first printed book devoted to head injuries *De Fractura Calvae sive Cranei* [92].

Giovanni Andrea Dalla Croce (1514–1575), a physician and son of a barber surgeon, was a military surgeon at the time of the Venetian naval victory at the battle of Lepanto in 1571. The University of Padua was the center for medical training in the Venetian State. The training involved a 3-year study of the works of Galen and Mondino de Luzzi and an examination in Latin. Giovanni was awarded a license to practice as a public doctor by the Venetian College of Surgeons in 1532. He was appointed Professor of anatomy and from 1537, practiced in Feltre, before returning to Venice in 1546. There he became chief practitioner to the Naval fleet and wrote an illustrated text *The universal and perfect surgery of all the parts necessary for the optimal surgeon* that includes woodcuts of trephination and the instruments of the day. It is a text of seven books which cover tumours; head, neck, and trunk traumas; ulcers; fractures; and dislocations, the instruments used and a variety of other topics (e.g., phlebotomies, leeches, childbirth, bladder stones, cataracts), antidotes, and treatments. Fifty-two pages of the second book describe head injuries and their treatment. There is advice on how to manage wounds as well as how to remove arrows and bullets from different body parts. "It is the aim of the surgeon to cut, separate and unite anatomical parts, therefore it's part of the surgical art to know each element of the anatomical art" [92, 93].

10.7.3.9 Further Progress on the Anatomy of the Cranial Nerves VII–XI

A German anatomist, Thomas von Sömmering (1755–1830), gave the abducens nerve its name in 1788. He also separated the facial nerve (VII) from the vestibulocochlear (VIII) and the glossopharyngeal (IX) from the vagus (X) and accessory (XI). What is remarkable is that despite being a 23-year-old medical student at the time, his classification of 12 pairs of cranial nerves were submitted as part of his doctoral dissertation on the base of the brain and the nerves that emerge from it. On his travels, he studied also under John Hunter in London and Munro Secundus in Edinburgh. He became Professor of Anatomy in Kassel, Mainz, but had to move to Frankfurt (1795), then later to Munich (1804), after the French annexed Mainz as part of Napoleon Bonnaparte's French Republic. He was a strong advocate for the newly introduced smallpox vaccination. He also was the first to identify the macula in the eye [91, 93].

Carl Hueter (1838–1882), a German Surgeon based in Marburg, was the first to document the epineural suture repair of a peripheral nerve and to document recovery in 1873. He was a general and orthopeedic surgeon who also named the condition of hallux valgus. In 1880, Francis Parker in South Carolina, also repaired a severed posterior interosseus nerve with restoration of function [95].

Francesco Durante (1844–1934), an Italian surgeon and Professor of Surgery in Rome, removed the first meningioma (left frontal causing anosmia, memory loss, and exophthalmos) by means of a craniotomy in 1884. The tumor weighed 70 g and was the size of an apple. The patient survived and had surgery for recurrence in

1897, but was still alive in 1905. Durante was also the author of a major textbook in surgery that had three volumes and underwent three editions from 1895 to 1913 and was used by students and surgeons for decades [94, 96, 97].

Feder Krause (1857–1937) was one of the fathers of German and world neurosurgery. He had worked initially in Halle (1883–1890), as assistant to Richard von Volkmann (1830–1889). His career progression took him to Frankfurt am Main (1890–1892), Hamburg (1892–1900), and then, as head of Department and Associate Professor, at the Augusta Hospital, Berlin (1900–1931). He performed the first recorded lumbar discectomy in 1908. He also ligated the feeding vessel of an arteriovenous malformation the same year. However, Krause had already performed pioneering surgery for trigeminal neuralgia (1894) and tinnitus (1898) and, in 1904, had taken a frontal, transcranial approach to remove a meningioma from the sella tuberculum. In 1909, he removed a pituitary adenoma accessing the pituitary above the sellar ridge.

10.7.4 The First 50 Pituitary Operations

The early history of pituitary surgery was the subject of a treatise by Giovanni Verga (1879–1923) in which he reviewed the first 50 cases operated including 10 performed by Victor Horsley (1857–1916). The Viennese surgeons, Anton von Eiselsberg (1860–1939) and Oskar Hirsch (1877–1965), were surgeons who led the development of pituitary surgery in Europe. The operative mortality was 36% [101], and the pathology was available for 42 cases—28 adenomas and 15 craniopharyngiomas. He described palliative (n = 6), frontal or temporal transcranial (n = 13), endonasal-transeptal (n = 12), and transsphenoidal-transethmoidal approaches (n = 19) [96, 97].

10.7.5 Hydrocephalus

German surgeons such as Ernst von Bergmann (1836–1907) promoted the need to base early treatments for hydrocephalus on an understanding of anatomy and accurate diagnosis. This required collaboration between surgeons, neurologists, and psychiatrists. Late in the nineteenth century, early German pioneers were based at the University of Halle, with surgeons such as Fedor Krause (1857–1937) and Gustav von Bramann (1854–1913), as well as psychiatrist, Gabriel Anton (1858–1933). Bramann and Anton established a transcallosal method of internal drainage (Balkenstich) for hydrocephalus, avoiding the need for and risks of repeated external tapping. In 1917, Viktor Schmieden (1874–1945) introduced a drainage approach through the atlanto-occipital membrane, resulting in continuous drainage of CSF to the neck musculature. In 1938, Arne Torkildsen (1899–1968), published a ventriculocisternostomy shunt which was more successful and replaced the Balkenstich method.

Imaging is essential to the practice of neurosurgery. Feder Krause used X-rays to guide neurosurgical procedures early in the twentieth century. Egas Moniz (1874–1955), a Portuguese neurologist, was the developer of cerebral angiography. His contributions are covered in the chapter on radiology (Chap. 7). The use of ultrasound, computed tomography, and magnetic resonance imaging (MRI) is also covered in Chap. 7 [96–98].

10.7.6 The Introduction of Neurosurgery Services and Departments Around the World

Neurosurgery began to develop as a specialty in the 1920s in North America and Europe. Those establishing departments in the USA tended to do so with the support of Harvey Cushing. In the UK, Sir Victor Horsley had pioneered neurosurgery in London but died of typhoid during World War I. The British Society of Neurosurgeons was established in 1926. Cushing and Bovie introduced monopolar electrocautery in 1928, but otherwise early efforts at hemostasis involved small pieces of muscle or sliver clips. With electrocautery larger tumors could be excised with a diathermy loop.

10.7.6.1 10.7.6.1 Hugh Cairns

Hugh Cairns (1896–1952), was born in South Australia, studied medicine in Adelaide, but after war was awarded a Rhodes scholarship to Oxford where he rowed in the 1920 Oxford Cambridge boat race. He trained with Harvey Cushing in Boston before returning to become Britain's first full-time neurosurgeon, establishing the Neurosurgery Unit at the London Hospital before becoming the first Nuffield Professor of Surgery in Oxford and setting up its first neurosurgery department in 1938. Howard Florey, also an Adelaide University graduate, and also a Rhodes scholar, was appointed Professor of Pathology in 1935. During WWII, Cairns was appointed to St Hugh's, a military hospital for head injuries, with Sir Charles Symonds, a neurologist. Together with younger neurologists, Derek Denny-Brown (later Professor at Harvard) and William Ritchie Russell (later Professor of neurology at Oxford), they established a service for soldiers with post-traumatic amnesia (PTA) and epilepsy and requiring rehabilitation after head injury. Their team also included Ludwig Guttmann, a Jewish doctor who had escaped from Nazi Germany, who led the work on the role of surgery and physiotherapy for patients with peripheral nerve injuries and who went on to establish the spinal injuries unit at Stoke Mandeville Hospital in 1943. In 1943, Cairns and Florey were sent to North Africa to trial penicillin. Although penicillin does not readily cross the blood-brain barrier, they found that topical penicillin directly applied after cranial debridement reduced the infection rate from 4.4% to 0.9%. They also introduced intrathecal injections reducing the mortality rate from brain abscess from 27% to 3% in 1945. He also introduced the mandatory wearing of helmets for military motorcyclists after showing that they reduced the rate of skull fractures by 75%, hospital admission by 50% and PTA by a third. Cairns was someone who knew how to assemble the right multidisciplinary teams and coordinate their skills to collectively achieve great things. In 1935, he also treated TE Lawrence (of Arabia) following his motorbike accident, though this was unsuccessful [99, 100].

Adams Andrew McConnell (1884–1972) was the first neurosurgeon in Ireland, and for many years the only neurosurgeon in Ireland. He had observed the work of Harvey Cushing and Walter Dandy in the USA and of Hugh Cairns and Geoffrey Jefferson in England. He is known for introducing the technique of air ventriculography to Europe, which he had learned from Walter Dandy. In addition to his roles in the British Society of Neurosurgeons (President 1936–1938), he was also President of the Royal College of Surgeons in Ireland [101].

10.7.6.2 Norman Dott (Edinburgh)

Norman Dott (1897–1973) practiced in Edinburgh from 1928 to 1965. He gained his FRCSEd in 1923, then went to study neurosurgery under Harvey Cushing in Boston. He was appointed Professor of neurosurgery at Edinburgh University in 1947 and established a neurosurgical department at the Western General Hospital in Edinburgh where he operated on the author's (DW) grandfather, removing (successfully) a pituitary adenoma.

10.7.6.3 Fritz König (Würzburg)

In Germany, the first independent neurosurgical unit was established in Würzburg in 1934, under the leadership Fritz König (1866–1952) and Wilhelm Tönnis (1898–1978). Tönnis underwent training in Stockholm with Herbert Olivecrona who had trained with Walter E Dandy. Thanks to the clinical skills and imaging from pneumoencephalography, air or contrast ventriculography, and angiography, 96% of intracranial lesions were able to be correctly localized prior to surgery. Electroencephalography was still in its early development having been discovered by Hans Berger in 1924. Of 52 brain operations over 7 months, the surgical mortality was a remarkably low 10% for that era. Tönnis returned to Würzburg in 1932 and persuaded König to allow him to do the brain surgery (König was by then 66!). In the first year, 60 patients came from all over Germany, 10 of whom were operated with only one mortality. In 1933, the value of intracranial surgery was established when the nine survivors paraded at a psychiatry conference in Würzburg carrying their tumours! The argument against specialization raged for some time with prominent German detractors in the German Surgical Society (Ferdinand Sauerbruch) arguing that all surgeons should be general and that neurosurgery specialization should be resisted, as with thoracic surgery. However, König argued that Cushing could not have achieved what he did if he had had to head a general surgery department as well as being Chief of neurosurgery, and so in Würzburg he handed over all neurosurgery to Tönnis. Tönnis founded the first neurosurgical journal with an international editorial board in 1936. There was a joint British-German neurosurgical meeting in Berlin and Breslau in 1937. In Breslau, Otfrid Foerster (1873–1941) presented his lifelong experience of brain tumours. Foerster had also been one of Lenin's (1870–1924) physicians in the last two years of his life. Tönnis moved to Berlin in 1938, and this and the war brought further development of neurosurgery in Würzburg to a halt. During the war, Tönnis focused on neurosurgical injuries and in 1948 accepted the Chair in Köln (Cologne) where he built up a new department until retiring in 1968. He was also Dean of Medicine, and later, Vice-Chancellor of the University of Köln [97, 98].

10.7.6.4 Cemil Topuzlu (Turkey)

In Turkey, Dr. Cemil Topuzlu (1868–1958) was the founder of modern surgery in Turkey. Dr. Abdulkadir Cahit Tuner became the first neurosurgeon with a degree in Turkey in 1923. The first neurosurgery department was established in Istanbul in 1923, but the first training program did not begin until the late 1940s. The Turkish neurosurgical society was founded in 1968. Over 1200 neurosurgeons were registered in Turkey by the year 2013.

10.7.6.5 Neurosurgery in Asia

In China, Song-Tao Guan and Yi-Chen Zhao pioneered neurosurgery at the Peking University Medical College Hospital during the 1930s. There they did over 1200 neurosurgical procedures [102].

In 1949, the first neurosurgical department was established in India at Christian Medical College, Vellore, under Jacob Chandy [103].

In Malaysia, neurosurgical services were developed in 1963, and the first local comprehensive neurosurgical training program was established in 2001 [104].

10.7.6.6 The First Female Neurosurgeons

Sofia Ionescu (1920–2008), a Romanian surgeon, first operated on the brain in 1944 and practiced for 47 years, performing all the neurosurgical procedures of her day. She was inspired to study medicine and become a neurosurgeon because a school friend had died of a brain abscess complicating neurosurgery. She entered medical school in Bucharest in 1939, but, as an intern, during the Allied bombing of Bucharest in 1943–1944, she performed surgical procedures, particularly amputations, but also operated on the brain of an injured boy. She was finally registered as a doctor in 1945. After the war she trained as a neurosurgeon and was a member of the Hospital 9 neurosurgical team, later called, "the golden team."

Diana Beck (1900–1956) was the first female British neurosurgeon and, perhaps, the first trained female neurosurgeon in Europe. She studied under Hugh Cairns in Oxford where she also researched intracranial hypertension and graft materials for cranioplasty. She was appointed consultant neurosurgeon at the Royal Free Hospital in 1943 and as head of neurosurgery at the Middlesex in 1947. She published research on intracerebral hemorrhage and even operated on AA Milne, author of Winnie the Pooh, following his stroke. She died of a pulmonary embolism following surgery to resect a thymoma for myasthenia gravis. She was awarded a British Heritage Blue Plaque in 2024 to commemorate her achievements.

Sofia Ionescu worked in the field of neurosurgery for 47 years, performing all the known neurosurgical procedures of the time. She made herself known through her incredible surgical skill and her enormous work power. Due to her incredible modesty and workload, she never participated at international congresses or manifestations. Her nomination as first woman in neurosurgery took place in Marrakech, Morocco, during the 2005 WFNS Congress. Some claim that Diana Beck was the first woman neurosurgeon in the world. The first documented surgical intervention performed by Diana Beck dates to 1952. Sofia Ionescu operated for the first time on a human brain as early as 1944. Furthermore, Diana Beck's actions surfaced in the year 1947, long after the war had ended, when Sofia Ionescu had become a neurosurgeon [106, 107].

10.7.7 Neurosurgery After World War II

Neurosurgery further advanced as a specialty after the War, both as a result of advances in its field but also with the introduction of intensive care units, mechanical ventilation, intracranial pressure monitoring, and imaging including CT, MRI, and less invasive cerebral angiography.

The clinical assessment of head injuries and conscious levels has been considerably improved by Graham Teasdale and Bryan Jennett's introduction of the Glasgow Coma Scale in 1974. This 15-point scale, based on best eye opening and verbal and motor responses, has been introduced all around the world in the last 50 years. The Glasgow team also developed a Glasgow Outcome Score and a Glasgow Assessment Schedule to aid in assessing the longer-term outcome of head injuries and their treatment.

10.7.7.1 The Glasgow Coma Scale (1974)

The clinical assessment of head injuries and conscious levels has been considerably improved by Graham Teasdale and Bryan Jennett's introduction of the Glasgow Coma Scale in 1974. This 15-point scale, based on best eye opening and verbal and motor responses, has been introduced all around the world in the last 50 years. The Glasgow team also developed a Glasgow Outcome Score and a Glasgow Assessment Schedule to aid in assessing the longer term outcome of head injuries and their treatment.

10.7.7.2 Hydrocephalus Shunts

During the first half of the twentieth century, treatments for hydrocephalus were largely experimental involving external drainage, internal drainage, or endoscopic choroid plexectomy all of which carried a high morbidity or were ineffective. In the 1950s, the introduction of valve-regulated shunts made with nonreactive synthetic materials (such as silicone) resulted in safe and effective treatment. Today the majority of shunts are ventriculoperitoneal or ventriculoatrial, though more recently the procedure of endoscopic third ventriculostomy has also been reintroduced for obstructive hydrocephalus [107, 108].

The introduction of neurovascular microsurgery, stereotactic and endovascular procedures, all supported by advances in imaging, offer minimally invasive and less morbid options for treatment. The twenty-first century should see effective treatments for many, previously untreatable neurological conditions, with maximal maintenance and/or restoration of function [100, 107].

10.8 Open-Heart Surgery

The history of open-heart surgery can be traced back to the early twentieth century, when scientists and doctors first began exploring the possibility of operating on the heart.

It was during the late nineteenth and early twentieth centuries when surgery was still a relatively new and risky field, and there were many unknowns and uncertainties surrounding the surgical treatment of heart disease. Many doctors and society at large viewed heart surgery as a last resort or even as an outright violation of the body.

It wasn't until the mid-twentieth century that advances in anaesthesia, surgical techniques, and technology made heart surgery safer and more reliable. Today, heart surgery is a common and accepted treatment for many types of heart disease, and it has saved countless lives [109].

10.8.1 Early Attempts at Cardiac Surgery

10.8.1.1 Henry Dalton: Repair of Pericardial Wound (1891)

Henry C. Dalton, a surgeon in St. Louis, Missouri, is credited with performing the first successful repair of a pericardial wound in a human being in 1891. Dalton's pioneering work helped to establish the feasibility of pericardial repair.

Professor Theodor Billroth in Vienna during the late nineteenth century, like many of his contemporaries, was skeptical of the idea of performing surgery on the heart. In particular, Billroth was wary of attempts to suture wounds of the heart, which he saw as an extremely risky and dangerous procedure. According to some reports, he expressed his disapproval of such attempts at a meeting of the Vienna Medical Society in 1881, stating that:

> *"no surgeon who wished to preserve the respect of his colleagues would ever attempt to suture a wound of the heart."*

10.8.2 Ludwig Rehn Repair of Stab Right Ventricle (1896)

Another early attemps at heart surgery was performed by Dr. Ludwig Rehn (1849–1930) in Frankfurt, Germany, in 1896. He successfully repaired a stab wound to the right ventricle of a patient's heart, but the procedure was met with skepticism and criticism from many of his colleagues despite a favorable patient outcome. In the years that followed, few other doctors attempted similar procedures, and those that did were often criticized.

However, Rehn was not deterred and later compiled a summary of 124 cases of cardiac wound repair that had been performed in Europe during the 1890s and early

1900's. Rehn's work, which was published in 1906, represented a major milestone in the development of cardiac surgery and helped to establish the feasibility and safety of surgical interventions on the heart.

10.8.3 The First Ligation of a Patent Ductus Arteriosus (1938)

Robert Edward Gross (1905–1988), an American surgeon, performed the first successful ligation of a persistent patent ductus arteriosus (PDA) in 1938. This was a landmark achievement for cardiac surgery, as it was the first extracardiac procedure performed on the heart. Prior to this, most cardiac procedures involved opening the chest and operating directly on the heart itself. Gross's work laid the foundation for the development of a wide range of extracardiac procedures including coarctation of the aorta (see below) [109, 110].

In the early 1900s, scientists such as Dr. Alexis Carrel, a French surgeon and biologist, developed techniques for suturing blood vessels and joined the first successful organ transplant [109].

In the 1920s and 1930s, advances in thoracic surgery, such as the development of the thoracoscope, allowed doctors to visualise the inside of the chest without making a large incision.

10.8.4 Clarence Crafoord Repair of Aortic Coarctation (1944)

In 1944, Swedish surgeon Clarence Crafoord (1899–1984) performed the first successful surgical repair of an aortic coarctation [110].

10.8.5 First Blalock-Taussig Procedure (1944)

The Blalock-Taussig procedure is a surgical technique used to treat the congenital heart defect known as Tetralogy of Fallot, which causes cyanosis (bluish discoloration of the skin and mucous membranes) due to decreased oxygen levels in the arterial blood.

The procedure was developed in the early 1940s by American surgeon Alfred Blalock (1899–1964) and paediatric cardiologist, Helen Taussig (1898–1986). It involves creating a connection between the subclavian artery and the pulmonary artery, which allows blood to bypass the blocked or narrowed pulmonary valve and enter the lungs to pick up oxygen.

The Blalock-Taussig procedure was a major advance in the treatment of congenital heart disease, as it allowed many children with Tetralogy of Fallot to survive and grow large enough for more definitive surgery. Prior to the development of this procedure, there were few effective treatments for this condition, and many affected children died in infancy or childhood.

Today, the Blalock-Taussig procedure, or a modification of the original, is still employed for some cases of pulmonary valve stenosis or pulmonary atresia without significant left to right shunt, prior to complete repair of the Tetralogy of Fallot. It remains an important historical milestone in the field of paediatric cardiology and has saved the lives of countless children [111].

10.8.6 Ball and Cage Device for Aortic Regurgitation (1950s)

The ball-and-cage device was an extracardiac surgical procedure developed by American surgeon Charles Hufnagel (1916–1989) in the 1950s. It was used to treat severe aortic regurgitation, a condition in which the aortic valve does not close properly, causing blood to flow back into the heart instead of out to the body, so causing cardiac failure [112].

The ball-and-cage device consisted of a stainless steel ball that was inserted into the aorta and held in place by a cage-like structure made of stainless steel wires. The ball prevented blood from flowing back into the heart through the aortic valve, while the cage allowed blood to flow out of the heart and into the aorta [113].

The ball-and-cage device was an effective treatment for severe aortic regurgitation, and it allowed many patients to avoid more invasive procedures until the advent of aortic valve replacement [114].

10.8.7 Mitral Valve Surgery

10.8.7.1 Mitral Commissurotomy

Mitral commissurotomy is a surgical technique used to treat mitral stenosis, a condition in which the mitral valve in the heart is narrowed, causing blood flow from the left atrium to the left ventricle to be restricted. Pulmonary oedema develops presenting with difficulty breathing, tiredness, and exercise intolerance.

The first direct surgical repair of mitral stenosis was performed in 1923 by American surgeon Dr. Elliot Cutler (1888–1947). Cutler developed a technique for dividing the fused commissures (valve leaflets) of the mitral valve, which allowed the valve to open more fully and improve blood flow. The procedure was initially performed through a left thoracotomy (an incision on the left side of the chest) and later through a median sternotomy (an incision down the center of the chest through the sternum or breast bone). Mitral commissurotomy became a widely used surgical technique for treating mitral stenosis, and it remained the primary treatment option for many years [115].

However, as techniques for mitral valve replacement and repair have improved, mitral commissurotomy has become less common. Today, it is usually reserved for patients who are not good candidates for other types of surgical intervention. Nonetheless, the development of mitral commissurotomy was a major milestone in the history of cardiac surgery, as it represented the first successful surgical repair of a common, chronic structural abnormality of the heart [115].

10.8.7.2 Henry Souttar: Mitral Stenosis and Insufficiency (1925)

Henry Souttar (1875–1964) was a Scottish surgeon who is credited with performing one of the first successful surgical repairs of mitral stenosis and mitral insufficiency.

In 1925, Souttar, at the London Hospital, performed surgery on a patient with severe mitral stenosis and mitral insufficiency, which involved repairing the damaged mitral valve by suturing the valve leaflets together. The patient's symptoms improved significantly following the surgery, and the repair was successful in the long term.

Souttar's successful surgery was a significant breakthrough, as it demonstrated that it was possible to repair damaged heart valves using surgical techniques. However, this was followed by widespread criticism and Souttar's colleagues stopped him from performing the procedure on other patients, leading to the procedure being abandoned until the 1940s [115].

In the years following World War II, both Charles P. Bailey in Philadelphia and Dwight E. Harken in Boston independently developed and refined the technique of closed mitral commissurotomy, a surgical procedure used to treat mitral stenosis. Closed mitral commissurotomy involves making a small incision in the left atrium of the heart and using a special instrument called a dilator to widen the narrowed mitral valve. The procedure can often be performed without the need for cardiopulmonary bypass, which made it a less invasive and risky option for patients with mitral stenosis. Bailey and Harken both achieved significant successes with the procedure, with reported mortality rates of less than 5% in their early series of cases.

F. John Lewis and his colleagues at the University of Minnesota performed the first successful repair of an atrial septal defect (ASD) using hypothermia in 1952. This technique paved the way for the development of open-heart surgery and other complex cardiac surgeries [115].

10.8.8 Cardiopulmonary Bypass and Open-Heart Surgery (1953)

The invention of the cardiopulmonary bypass (CPB) machine is credited to several individuals who contributed to its development over several decades. In the early twentieth century, researchers began to explore the possibility of using a mechanical device to replace the heart and lungs by temporarily oxygenating and pumping the blood during surgery, but the technology was not yet advanced enough to make this a reality.

One of the key breakthroughs came in the 1930s, when John Gibbon Jr. (1903–1973), a young surgeon at Jefferson Medical College in Philadelphia, began experimenting with a primitive heart-lung machine using an oxygenator and roller pumps. He was initially inspired to do this in 1931, when a patient died of a pulmonary embolus and he was not able to save her. In 1937, he reported his experiments on cats that showed he was able to keep them alive for 4 h on cardiopulmonary bypass. Then the war intervened and he was posted to the Far East. It wasn't until the 1950s that Gibbon and his team were able to successfully perform the first open-heart surgery using the CPB machine in 1953. The patient, an 18-year-old girl with a congenital heart defect, survived the procedure and lived for several more years [116–118].

This marked the beginning of a new era in the treatment of heart disease and open heart surgery [116].

John Kirklin (1917–2004), a cardiac surgeon at the Mayo Clinic, performed the first series of open-heart surgeries using a heart-lung machine in 1955. During surgery, the heart-lung machine is used to perform the roles of both the heart and lungs, enabling the surgeon to operate on a heart that is not beating. This technique paved the way for more complex cardiac surgeries, including valve replacements and coronary artery bypass grafting [117].

The first series of open-heart surgeries using the heart-lung machine was small, with only eight patients, and the mortality rate was high by current standards, at 50%. However, this early work laid the foundation for the development of safer and more effective open-heart surgical procedures, as well as better selected patients, and has led to saving many lives over the past several decades. Richard DeWall made a simpler, disposable bubble oxygenator at the University of Minnesota. It was clinically effective and increased surgical facility greatly. With effective bypass, cardiac surgeons were able to operate on a variety of cardiac conditions under direct vision. Leaders in this work were Michael E. DeBakey (1908–2008) and Denton A. Cooley (1920–2016) in Houston [118].

10.8.9 Coronary Artery Bypass Grafting

In the 1960s and 1970s, advances in surgical techniques and equipment, such as the introduction of the coronary artery bypass grafting (CABG) and heart valve replacement, further expanded the range of conditions that could be treated with open-heart surgery.

The decline in the prevalence of rheumatic heart disease in high-income countries and the successful treatment of congenital heart disease led to a decreased demand for valvular heart surgery in the industrialized world, though this is not true in low-middle-income countries. Instead, the focus shifted to coronary artery disease, which became more prevalent in the post-World War II years, leading to a new set of challenges for cardiac surgeons. Alexis Carrel had originally proposed the idea of surgically relieving coronary obstruction in 1913. He suggested that the occlusion of a coronary artery could be treated by anastomosing the coronary artery to another vessel to bypass the obstruction. However, it was not until the mid-twentieth century that this idea was able to be put into practice with the development of techniques for coronary artery bypass surgery and the availability of cardiopulmonary by-pass. The idea was initially doubted and resisted until the 1960s.

10.8.10 Robert Hans Goetz (1960)—the first successful coronary artery bypass graft (CABG)

In 1960, Dr. Robert Hans Goetz (1910–2000) performed the first successful coronary artery bypass graft (CABG) surgery in New York, in which he grafted the right internal mammary artery to the right coronary artery to bypass a blockage. The patient, who had had angina, lived for 1 year. This was a pioneering procedure that would eventually become a standard treatment for coronary artery disease [119].

However, at the time, many of Goetz's colleagues in the medical and surgical communities were highly critical of his having performed the procedure. They saw CABG surgery as experimental and untested, and they were concerned about the risks and potential complications of the surgery. Some doctors believed that the procedure was unnecessary and that coronary artery disease could be managed effectively with medication and lifestyle changes.

Despite this criticism, Goetz continued to refine and develop his technique, and over time, the procedure became widely accepted and has become standard practice.

10.8.11 Edward Garrett: CABG with Saphenous Vein Graft (1964)

In 1964, Dr. H. Edward Garrett (1926–1996) and his colleagues performed the first successful coronary artery bypass graft (CABG) surgery using the saphenous vein as a graft material. This was a significant breakthrough in the field of cardiac surgery; as the saphenous vein was found to be a reliable and durable graft material for bypassing blocked coronary arteries. Angiographic follow up revealed that the graft was still patent after 7 years.

10.8.12 *Vasilii I. Kolesov CABG with Internal Mammary Bypass Graft (1964)*

Vasilii I. Kolesov (1904–1992) was a Soviet cardiac surgeon in St Petersburg who was also a pioneer in the field of coronary artery bypass graft (CABG) surgery. Also in 1964, Kolesov performed his first successful coronary bypass surgery using a saphenous vein graft, which bypassed a blocked coronary artery in a patient's heart. He continued to refine and develop his technique over the years, and his work was also instrumental in establishing CABG surgery as a safe and effective treatment for coronary artery disease. Kolesov's work was particularly notable because he was working in the Soviet Union, where resources and access to advanced medical technology were more limited [119].

Today, open-heart surgery is a well-established and widely accepted method and is, in fact, the commonest cardiac procedure performed in many cardiac centers where the prevalence of atherosclerotic disease is high. The expected mortality of planned CABG surgery is now as low as 1–2%, with clinical quality registries measuring outcomes such as return to theatre for bleeding, new onset acute kidney impairment, deep sternal wound infection, and mortality. Risk adjusted cardiac surgery outcomes in the UK are even reported publicly whilst other national registries report their results by unit. Recently, minimally invasive techniques including the use of robots in open-heart surgery have been introduced, with the promise (yet to be realised) of more precision, and better outcomes. As coronary angioplasty and stenting have emerged, an increasing proportion or coronary disease is being treated by interventional cardiologists without the need for surgery. Even some valve replacements can now be performed intraluminally such as transcatheter aortic valve implantation (TAVI), which was first performed in 2002, by Dr Alain Cribier (1945-2024) in Rouen, France.

10.8.13 *The First Heart Transplant (1967) by Christian Barnard in South Africa*

On December 3, 1967, Dr. Christiaan Barnard (1922–2001) and his surgical team at Groote Schuur Hospital in Cape Town, South Africa, performed the world's first human-to-human heart transplant. The recipient of the transplant was Louis Washkansky, a 53-year-old man who was suffering from end-stage heart disease (Fig. 10.6).

The surgery was a groundbreaking achievement that captured the attention of the world, and Barnard became an instant celebrity. However, the success of the surgery was also accompanied by controversy and ethical questions about the use of human organs for transplantation. The idea cannot be totally credited to Barnard himself, as other surgeons such as James Hardy and Vladimir Demikhov, Richard Lower, and Norman Shumway had already described the technical aspects of the operation [120].

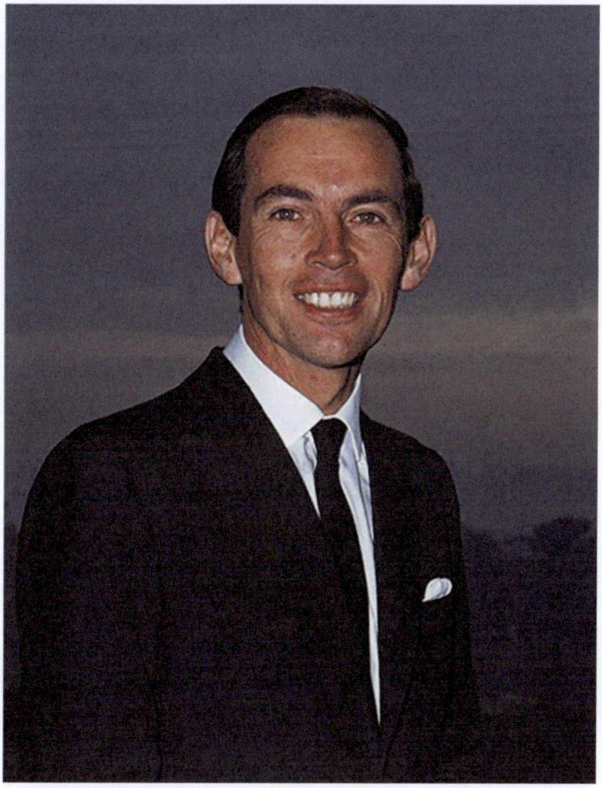

Fig. 10.6 Portrait of Christiaan Barnard in 1967. (https://upload.wikimedia.org/wikipedia/commons/5/54/Christiaan_Barnard_1968.jpg)

Adrian Kantrowitz (1918–2008), a surgeon at Maimonides Hospital in Brooklyn, was another pioneer in the field of paediatric cardiac surgery and transplantation. Prior to the first human-to-human heart transplant performed by Dr. Christiaan Barnard in 1967, Kantrowitz had been experimenting with heart transplantation using anencephalic babies as donors. To develop and refine his technique, Kantrowitz conducted a series of experiments using more than 400 puppies as subjects. He was able to successfully transplant hearts from one puppy to another, and he used this knowledge to refine his technique for human heart transplantation.

Despite ethical concerns, the development of heart transplantation represented a significant advance in the field of cardiac surgery, and it has since become an established treatment for end-stage heart disease. Today, thousands of heart transplants are performed each year around the world, each successful one a life-saving procedure. The introduction of cyclosporine as an immune suppressive drug in the 1970, improved the long-term survival by reducing immune rejection.

One of the major challenges in heart transplantation, as well as other organ transplantations, is the shortage of donor organs relative to the number of patients who need them. This has been an ongoing issue for many years, and despite efforts to increase organ donation rates and improving the allocation of organs, the gap between the number of patients waiting for organs and the number of available organs remains significant. As a result of the shortage of donor organs, many patients who are candidates for transplantation must wait months or even years for a suitable donor organ to become available. During this time, their condition may deteriorate, and some patients may die before a suitable donor organ is found. This has led to the development of alternative treatments for end-stage heart failure, such as ventricular assist devices and artificial hearts, which can help to extend the lives of patients who are awaiting transplantation [120, 121].

10.8.13.1 Metal Heart Valve

The history of metal heart valves can be traced back to the mid-twentieth century, when scientists and engineers first began exploring the possibility of using metal to replace diseased heart valves.

In the 1950s and 1960s, Dr. Charles Hufnagel (1916–1989) and Dr. Albert Starr (1926–2024), both American surgeons, developed the first successful metal heart valves. The Hufnagel valve, also known as the "all-metal" valve, was made entirely of metal and was the first heart valve to be mass-produced. The Starr-Edwards valve, also known as the "ball-and-cage" valve, consisted of a metal ball that was held in place by a metal cage.

These early metal heart valves were made of stainless steel and were designed to be durable and long-lasting. However, they had some limitations, such as the potential for blood clots to form on the valve and the need for lifelong anticoagulation therapy.

In the 1970s, the development of new materials, such as pyrolitic carbon and titanium, led to the production of more advanced metal heart valves that were more biocompatible and less prone to clotting.

Today, metal heart valves are widely used in surgical procedures to replace diseased or damaged heart valves. They are made of a variety of materials such as stainless steel, titanium, and cobalt-chromium alloy. Heart valve replacements can be mechanical, which are actuated by a mechanical means, or bioprosthetic, which are made from animal tissue.

Advancements in design and materials continue to improve the durability and longevity of these devices, and new technologies such as transcatheter valve implantation have offered effective, but less invasive options [114, 115, 122–124].

10.8.13.2 Tissue Heart Valve

The history of tissue or pig heart valves can be traced back to the early twentieth century, when scientists and surgeons first began experimenting with using animal tissue to replace diseased heart valves.

In the 1920s and 1930s, Dr. Charles Hufnagel and Dr. Albert Starr, both American surgeons, also performed the first successful heart valve transplants using animal tissue. They used tissue from cows and pigs to replace the diseased heart valves of their patients.

However, these early tissue valves had some limitations, such as a relatively short lifespan and the potential for infection and calcification.

In the 1960s and 1970s, advances in technology and materials, such as the development of cryopreservation and the use of glutaraldehyde as a tissue fixative, led to the production of more advanced tissue valves that were more durable and less prone to infection and calcification.

Today, tissue valves are widely used in surgical procedures to replace diseased or damaged heart valves. They are made from a variety of animal tissues, such as porcine (pig) and bovine (cow) pericardium, and they are freeze-dried, sterilized, and treated with various chemicals to improve their durability and biocompatibility.

Tissue valves have a more natural feel and motion than mechanical valves, and they don't require lifelong anticoagulation therapy like mechanical valves. However, tissue valves have a finite lifespan and may need to be replaced over time [112, 125–127].

10.8.14 Anticoagulation

10.8.14.1 Heparin

Heparin is a very important anticoagulant medication that is used to prevent blood clots during procedures such as cardiopulmonary bypass surgery, as well as in the prevention and treatment of deep vein thrombosis, pulmonary embolism, and other conditions prone to thrombosis and/or embolism. Heparin is used during cardiopulmonary bypass surgery to prevent the formation of clots in the extracorporeal circuit, which could potentially cause serious complications if such clots embolised back to the patient's circulation.

Heparin was the first anticoagulant to be discovered and isolated for medical use and is one of the oldest drugs still in widespread clinical use. It was first discovered in 1916 by a group of scientists at the Johns Hopkins University School of Medicine. They extracted it from a type of dog liver and found that it had significant anticoagulant properties. Since then, it has been studied and refined in order to improve its effectiveness and safety.

Jay McLean (1890–1957)was a second-year medical student at Johns Hopkins Medical School in Baltimore, Maryland, in 1916. He was working on Cephalin in the lab of physiologist, William Henry Howell (1860–1945). Cephalin was thought to be a procoagulant substance that neutralized antithrombin and thereby allowed the activation of prothrombin, leading to clotting which could help to reduce bleeding. Howell then continued the work with T Emmett Holt, publishing a paper in which he gave heparin its name in 1918. In 1929, Charles Best, with Arthur Charles, tried to improve heparin by reducing or eliminating the bad effects and show it could stop thrombus formation. In 1933, Arthur Charles and colleague, David Scott, published a series of three papers describing how it prevented blooding clotting in injured dogs.

Although Best and many others contributed to its development into a clinically usable product. In 1963, a plaque was revealed at Johns Hopkins University in honor of Jay McLean MD (1890–1957), *"in recognition of his major contribution to the discovery of heparin in 1916 as a second-year medical student"* in collaboration with Professor William H. Howell.

Heparin as anticoagulant is essential medicine to prevent blood clotting while using the cardiopulmonary bypass machine [121]. It's action is reversed by protamine sulphate. Low molecular weight heparin (enoxaparin sodium) was introduced in 1993, and is widely used today for thromboprophylaxis of venous thromboembolism (VTE).

10.8.14.2 History of Anticoagulation with Warfarin

Warfarin is an anticoagulant medication that works by inhibiting the action of vitamin K, which is necessary for the production of several clotting factors in the blood. The history of anticoagulation with warfarin can be traced back to the early twentieth century. Warfarin was first discovered in the early 1920s, when cattle in the northern USA were observed to be bleeding uncontrollably after eating spoiled hay. Many farmers fed moldy hay to their cattle even though the recommendation was not to do so. Ten years later, sweet clover disease was still prevalent. Desperate, Ed Carlson, a Wisconsin farmer, drove a dead cow 200 miles to an agricultural experimental station. There, Karl Link presented him with a milk can of unclotted blood. Link and colleagues eventually identified the compound causing the bleeding as a derivative of 4-hydroxycoumarin, a compound found in spoiled sweet clover hay. The synthetic derivative, warfarin, was first used as a rat poison before being approved for human use as an anticoagulant in the 1950s.

In 1951, a member of the US Army tried to end their life by consuming warfarin but was able to recuperate after being administered vitamin K in a medical facility. Studies then began on the use of warfarin as a therapeutic anticoagulant. The main advantages of warfarin were high water solubility and oral bioavailability; its effect could still be reversed by vitamin K. Therefore, warfarin transitioned into clinical use to treat deep vein thrombosis (DVT) and pulmonary embolism (PE) under the trade name Coumadin, being approved by the FDA in 1954.

Warfarin quickly became the most widely used oral anticoagulant worldwide, as it was safe, effective, and cheap. It is also used to prevent and treat thromboembolic disease such as atrial fibrillation in patients who have prosthetic heart valves, as well as deep vein thrombosis.

However, warfarin has a narrow therapeutic window, which means that the dosage must be carefully monitored to ensure that the patient's blood is not too prone to clot nor too prone to bleed. Warfarin therapy requires regular blood testing and dose adjustments to maintain the optimal level of anticoagulation [128, 129].

In the twenty-first century, new oral anticoagulants (NOAC) such as rivaroxaban, apixaban, and dabigatran were developed. These are more predictable in their effects, and they do not require routine monitoring of blood levels, though they also carry a bleeding risk.

10.9 Abdominal Aortic Aneurysm

The history of modern repair of abdominal aortic aneurysms (AAA) can be traced back to the early twentieth century, when doctors and surgeons first began exploring ways to treat this condition.

An abdominal aortic aneurysm is a weak spot in the wall of the aorta, which causes the vessel to first dilate and then, over the passage of time, rupture. Treatment for a AAA was mainly surgical, but the surgical options were limited when reuptured, and the mortality rate is high, often as high as 50%.

The ancient Egyptians have described aneurysms in the Ebers Papyrus:

> *Treat it with a knife and burn it with a fire so that it bleeds not too much.* [This is unlikely to have been successful]

Antyllus was a Greek physician and surgeon who lived during the second century AD. He′s credited with performing one of the earliest known surgical procedures for the repair of an aneurysm, likely in relation to extremities—in his writings, he describes aneurysms on physical examination as "localized pulsatile swellings." The "Antyllus method" consisted of proximal and distal ligation and removal of the thrombus. This remained the standard treatment of peripheral false aneurysms for over 1000 years to follow with little further progress. However, the writings of Celsus (30 BCE to 50 CE) also wisely warned against unwittingly incising an aneurysm (which is pulsatile), and not mistaking it for an abscess.

Andreas Vesalius (1514–1564) was a friend and colleague of Paré and apparently was the first to describe thoracic and abdominal aortic aneurysms.

Paré (1510–1590) suggested the application of a proximal ligation to aneurysms. He also described a ruptured aneurysm of the thoracic aorta, writing *"The aneurysms which happen in the internal parts are incurable."*

John Hunter (1728–1793) was a Scottish surgeon who was known for his pioneering work in surgery and anatomy. One of the most well-known surgeries he conducted involved tying off the popliteal artery for an aneurysm behind the knee [130, 131].

John Hunter's older brother, William (1718–1783), was also a physician and anatomist who made important contributions to the study of aneurysms. William Hunter is also famous for his research on the human uterus.

Astley Cooper (1768–1841), a pupil of John Hunter, undertook pioneering work on aneurysms, including a successful ligation of the abdominal aorta in a patient with an aortic aneurysm. In 1817, Cooper was called to care for a 38-year-old patient with an external iliac artery aneurysm that had ruptured. He performed a transperitoneal exploration and ligation of the common iliac artery, which was the only practical option given the patient's condition. The patient survived for 48 h after the operation before succumbing to his illness. The post-mortem specimen remains on display in the Gordon Museum of Pathology at King's College London [130, 131].

Fast forward to the end of the nineteenth century, Rudolph Matas (1860–1957) tried to use electrothrombosis in 1900, for the treatment of a large abdominal aneurysm. Earlier, he had explained how peripheral aneurysms can be treated using endoaneurysmorrhaphy. In 1923, he used these techniques to successfully treat an infrarenal AAA. The patient survived for 18 months, which is the first recoded modern repair of AAA [132].

Alexis Carrel (1873–1944) was a French surgeon and biologist who made significant contributions to the fields of vascular surgery, transplantation, and microbiology. He was awarded the Nobel Prize in Physiology or Medicine in 1912, for his work on vascular suturing and the transplantation of blood vessels and organs and thus regarded by many as a father of modern vascular surgery [133].

10.9.1 Albert Einstein's AAA

In 1949, Albert Einstein (1879–1955) was suffering from intense abdominal pain. He consulted the famous Rudolf Nissen (1896-1981), in the days before modern CT scans. Nissen suggested exploration by laparotomy and found an AAA. He used cellophane to wrap around the aneurysm. Einstein survived for more than 5 years after this operation but ultimately succumbed to a ruptured aneurysm April 18, 1955. When it ruptured he declined to have surgery as he was 76 and frail.

10.9.2 The First Successful AAA Repair (1951)

A breakthrough took place on the 29th of March 1951. Charles Dubost (1914–1991), a French surgeon, performed the first successful aneurysm resection and interposition graft using a cadaveric aortic allograft. This procedure was a big step forward in treating aortic aneurysms. It made it possible to develop other surgical techniques and materials [133, 134].

During the 1950s and 1960s, the preferred method for treating AAA was through open surgical repair by laparotomy. This was a major advancement in the treatment of AAA, but the procedure was still considered high-risk, and the mortality rate was still high.

A paper titled "Successful Resection of an Aneurysm of the Abdominal Aorta: A Case Report" described using a Dacron graft to repair an abdominal aortic aneurysm. This paper was another major milestone in the development of modern vascular surgery. It established the potential to use a synthetic graft as a standard of care for aneurysm repair. Michael Debakey, Denton Cooley, and E. Stanley Crawford were all pioneers in the field of vascular surgery, particularly the surgical treatment of abdominal and thoracic aortic aneurysms [135].

10.9.3 *Michael DeBakey (1908–2008)*

Michael DeBakey (1908–2008) (Fig. 10.7) was one of the most influential surgeons of the twentieth century. He was born in Louisiana on September 7, 1908. His parents, Shiker and Raheeja Dabaghi (the name was anglicized to DeBakey before Michael's birth), were immigrants from Marjeyoun, Lebanon. His parents were fluent in French, which is the likely reason they settled in Louisiana. He studied medicine at Tulane University. He was trained with Rudolph Matas. He was also sent to Strasbourg and Heidelberg universities to complete his training. In 1948, DeBakey became a member of the teaching staff at Baylor University College of Medicine, specializing in general and cardiovascular surgery [135].

In the 1950s, his pursuit of the ideal material to make grafts led him to a department store that had run out of nylon, so he bought a piece of polyethylene terephthalate (Dacron). Using his wife's sewing machine, he produced the first arterial Dacron grafts to repair AAA. He later collaborated with researchers from Philadelphia College of Textiles and science associates from the university to create a knitting machine for the graft [133–135].

Debakey holds the credit for performing the first modern carotid endarterectomy in 1953, using a Dacron or vein to patch the artery and prevent narrowing. He revolutionized cardiovascular surgery and aneurysm repair, contributing to coronary artery surgery, cardiopulmonary bypass, artificial heart, and left ventricular support devices.

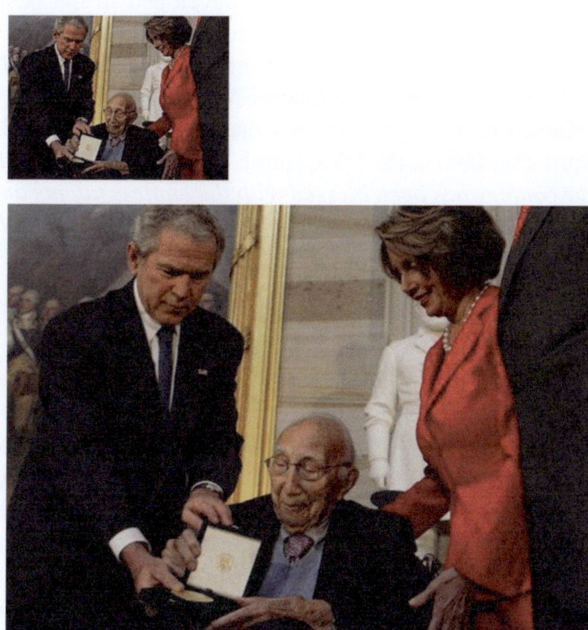

Fig. 10.7 President George W. Bush presents the Congressional Gold Medal to famed heart surgeon Dr. Michael Ellis DeBakey. (https://commons.wikimedia.org/w/index.php?search=Michael+debakey+and+president+bush&title=Special:MediaSearch&go=Go&type=image)White House photo by Chris Greenberg

Debakey and Cooley's (1920–2016) work in Houston, Texas, in developing techniques for complex aneurysm repair and spinal cord protection during thoracic aortic surgery paved the way for modern aortic surgery. Their success in the resection of a fusiform thoracic aneurysm on January 5, 1953, marked a significant milestone in the field. They continued to build on this success, reporting a series of 245 successful aneurysm repairs by July 1955.

It must be acknowledged that there was a dispute about who did the first carotid endarterectomy due to the decades-long rivalry between the two towering figures of vascular surgery, Debakey and Denton Cooley, because Debakey didn't report his case until the 1970s. The rivalry ended after Debakey was honored with the Congressional Gold Medal [136, 137].

He operated on so many prominent people, including Russian President, Boris Yeltsin. His surgical career spans almost seven decades and he operated on 60,000 people. He pioneered modern thoracic aortic aneurysm treatment with his colleague Cooley. He received innumerable awards and honors.

Debakey received the Presidential Medal of Freedom in 1969.

President Ronald Reagan awarded him the National Medal of Science in 1987. In addition to these honors, DeBakey received numerous other awards and recognitions throughout his career, including the Lasker-DeBakey Clinical Medical Research Award, the French Legion of Honour, and induction into the National Inventors Hall of Fame. Also the congressional gold medal in 2008.

In 1980, DeBakey was a consultant in the care of the exiled Shah of Iran, Mohammad Reza Pahlavi, who had advanced lymphoma. On March 28, 1980, in Cairo, the Shah had his spleen removed by DeBakey for the condition of hypersplenism. Several complications developed in the postoperative period, probably caused by a pancreatic leak that led to a subphrenic abscess and respiratory complications. The Shah succumbed from his malignancy on July 27, 1980 [138, 139].

In Fig 10.7, President George W. Bush presents the Congressional Gold Medal to famed heart surgeon Dr. Michael Ellis DeBakey during a ceremony Wednesday, April 23, 2008, at the US Capitol. Said the President, *"For nearly a hundred years, our country has been blessed with the endless talents and dedication of Dr. Michael DeBakey. And he has dedicated his career to a truly noble ambition – bettering the life of his fellow man."*

10.9.4 Endovascular Aneurysm Repair (EVAR)

In the 1990s, another revolution was in the making. It was the endovascular aneurysm repair (EVAR), which was developed as a endovascular alternative to open surgery. EVAR involves using a stent-graft, a metal mesh tube that's inserted into the aneurysm through a small incision in the femoral artery, which serves as a scaffold to repair the aneurysm from within. Today, EVAR is considered the standard of care for the treatment of AAA, with a lower mortality rate and faster recovery compared to open surgery. Advancements in technology, such as the development of custom-made stent-grafts, have further improved the safety and outcomes of the procedure.

Juan Parodi (b1942) was an Argentinean vascular surgeon who's credited with developing the first catheter-based arterial approach to AAA intervention, known as endovascular aneurysm repair (EVAR). He first performed the procedure in 1990 on a patient in Buenos Aires, Argentina, and it was the first successful EVAR operation.

The field of AAA repair continues to evolve with the integration of new technologies and research, which aim to improve the safety and outcomes of these procedures. Parodi received numerous awards and honors for his contributions to the field of vascular surgery, and he's widely recognized as a pioneer in the development of endovascular techniques for the treatment of arterial diseases.

There was a twist to the story of EVAR. It turns out that Nicholas Volodos (1934–2016) and his colleagues in the late 1980s in Ukraine performed the first reported cases of endovascular aneurysm repair (EVAR). Volodos developed and used both bare and covered stents in his procedures, and he reported his findings in a 1988 article published in the Soviet Journal of Surgery.

However, due to the political climate at the time, news of Volodos' procedures did not spread widely in the global medical community, so it was not until years later that most surgeons in the West learned of his pioneering work and the primacy of his procedure [139].

Frank J. Criado was also an early champion of EVAR and a friend of Juan Parodi, and he played an important role in advancing the technique and raising awareness of its potential benefits. Thanks to the work of Dr. Parodi, Dr. Criado, Dr. Volodos, and many others, endovascular techniques for the treatment of arterial diseases have continued to evolve and improve, and they have become an important part of the modern vascular surgeon's toolbox. There's no doubt that EVAR has significantly and enduringly transformed the field of AAA surgery.

The development and acceptance of endovascular aneurysm repair (EVAR) wasn't an easy journey. Despite the early successes of pioneers like Juan Parodi and Nicholas Volodos, the technique faced resistance from many members of the vascular surgery establishment who were skeptical of the long-term efficacy and safety of EVAR.

However, as more and more evidence of the benefits of EVAR emerged, some influential figures within the field began to take notice. John Bergan, MD, and Ramon Berguer, MD, were two such individuals, and their advocacy played a crucial role in bringing EVAR to wider attention.

After seeing Juan Parodi present his work at a meeting in Miami in 1991, John Bergan called Ramon Berguer, who was the editor of The Annals of Vascular Surgery, and urged him to publish an article on the technique. Ramon Berguer recognized the potential of EVAR and quickly accepted the article for publication, and it appeared in the November 1991 issue of the journal [163, 164].

10.10 Organ Transplantation

The history of organ (as opposed to skin) transplantation begins in the early twentieth Century. Transplants or grafts may be from another species (xenograft), another human (homo or allograft), or from oneself (autografts). Autotransplants are relevant for skin, fascial, and nerve grafts but not for organs.

The techniques for successful vascular repair and anastomosis were not well established at the end of the nineteenth century. The first documented successful repair of a gunshot laceration of the femoral artery was only performed in 1897 in Chicago, by J B Murphy (1857–1916). Murphy was a graduate of Rush Medical College in Chicago and spent his career there other than 2 years working in Vienna under Billroth. He also gave his name to Murphy's sign for acute appendicitis, and developed the Murphy button for intestinal anastomosis [140].

10.10.1 Xenografts

The first attempts used xenografts. In 1902, Emerich Ullmann (186–1937) in Vienna transplanted a dog's kidney into the animal's neck and showed that it functioned. The renal vessels were joined to the carotid artery and jugular veins by means of magnesium tubes, with the urine draining via the ureter in the neck. The graft lasted 5 days. Ullmann also showed that grafting from one dog to another or from a dog to a goat resulted in early failure [141].

In 1905, a surgeon named George Landerer attempted to transplant a rabbit kidney into a child, but the transplant was unsuccessful, and the child died a few days later. In 1906, other surgeons attempted to transplant organs from pigs and goats into humans, but these attempts also failed within days due to graft thrombosis and other complications.

In 1906, Mathieu Jaboulay (1860–1913), Professor of Surgery in Lyon, France, attempted to transplant a pig's kidney into the elbow of a patient in renal failure human but the graft failed and had to be removed. He performed a similar operation with a goat's kidney without success. Neither kidney secreted urine.

In 1910, Ernst Unger (1875–1938) in Berlin performed a xenotransplant using the kidney of a monkey and transplanting it into the groin of a 21-year-old woman with progressive kidney failure. She died after 32 h and the autopsy showed patchy necrosis of the graft [141].

10.10.1.1 Alexis Carrel

Alexis Carrel (1873–1944) was a graduate of the University of Lyon and had studied under Jaboulay. His publication on techniques of vascular anastomosis and transplantation of viscera in 1902, marked a significant step forward in understanding the operative techniques required for organ transplantation. The Carrel patch fashioned a button of aorta sutured into the feeding vessel (e.g., the carotid in many of his experiments) thus allowing smaller vessels whose orifices were in the button to be perfused and supply the end organ [141, 142].

Carrel moved to Chicago in 1904, and, from 1908, worked with Charles Guthrie (1880–1963). Carrel and Guthrie's kidney experiments on a dogs showed that the dog would survive with its own kidney transplanted to its neck, even if the other kidney was removed. However, if another dog's kidney was transplanted, the kidney would fail within a few days. Carrel mastered the techniques of transplantations but was not able to understand the biology of rejection [141].

In addition to kidneys, they also transplanted a donor heart into the neck of a dog, anastomosing the coronary arteries to the carotid (using the button technique) and venous return by inserting the pulmonary artery into the jugular vein of the host. The heart supported the dog for 2 h.

Carrel was awarded the 1912 Nobel Prize for work on vascular anastomosis. This spurred the possibility of organ transplantation. Although some have suggested Guthrie should have shared the 1912 Nobel Prize with Carrel, they did not work together until 1908, and Carrell had already published his paper on the triangulation method of vascular (end to end) anastomosis in 1902) [142].

10.10.2 Kidney Transplantation

In 1933, Ukrainian surgeon Yuri Vornyi (1895–1961) did the first allograft transplant for six transplants for patients with acute renal failure due to mercury poisoning. They had ingested the mercury to commit suicide. The transplants failed because of a misunderstanding about the harmful effects of warm ischaemia in the cadavers that provided the donor kidneys. For example, the first kidney was retrieved 6 h after the donor died. Also, there was ABO incompatibility between some of his donor kidneys and the recipients [143–145].

10.10.2.1 Dialysis

Peritoneal dialysis was first introduced in the 1920s and 1930s but the results were poor. In 1959, a single dialysis catheter was introduced with better constituted commercially prepared solutions. In 1968, a permanent indwelling catheter was developed which allowed for continuous ambulatory peritoneal dialysis.

The first efficient artificial kidney or dialysis machine was developed by Willem Kolff (1911-2009) in Holland during the German occupation of World War II. He used cellophane tubing wound around a drum rotating in dialysis solution. Arterial blood was heparinized to prevent it clotting and returned to a vein [146].

The modern development of organ transplantation was inspired by the story of Charles Woods. Charles Woods was a United States Army Air Forces pilot who suffered extensive burn injuries after his plane, loaded with aviation fuel, exploded on takeoff during World War II. He was treated by Dr. Bradford Cannon, a plastic surgeon who was part of the team that pioneered skin grafting techniques during the war.

In Woods' case, Dr. Cannon used a technique called "pinch grafting" to transplant skin from other parts of his body to cover the burns on his face and hands. Charles Woods also received a skin transplant from a recently deceased soldier about 6 weeks after his accident. This was a relatively new and experimental procedure at the time, known as homograft or allograft skin transplantation [140].

Joseph Murray (1919–2012) was a member of Charles Woods medical team at Valley Forge General Hospital during World War II. Murray was a surgical resident at the time, and was drafted into the US Army Medical Corps in 1943. He was assigned to Valley Forge General Hospital, where he worked alongside other medical professionals to treat wounded soldiers and develop new surgical techniques. During his time at Valley Forge, Murray became interested in the field of transplantation and began conducting research on the subject. After the war, he continued his research at Harvard Medical School and eventually became a pioneer in the field of organ transplantation. In 1954, [140] Murray performed the first successful kidney transplant between identical twins, one of whom had developed chronic nephritis at the age of 22. The donor kidney functioned immediately in the twin recipient. There were no signs of rejection, the transplant was a success, the patient married his nurse, had two children and lived for a further 8 years before dying of cardiac failure [140, 147].

Murray's work on transplantation earned him numerous accolades and awards, including the Nobel Prize in Physiology or Medicine in 1990. The prize was awarded to him jointly with Edward Donnall Thomas (1920–2012), who pioneered bone marrow transplantation and stem cell research. The first successful bone marrow transplants (allografts) were achieved in the 1970s in Seattle.

10.10.2.2 Preventing Rejection

Early research on kidney transplantation was focused on understanding the immune system and developing techniques to prevent rejection of the transplanted organ. In the 1950, several researchers, including Murray, developed methods to match donors and recipients based on blood type, which helped to reduce the risk of rejection.

The first transplant to a non-genetically identical human was in Louisiana, at Charity Hospital in 1959, by a team of physicians led by Dr. John A. Mann. The patient was a 23-year-old man who had been suffering from chronic kidney disease. The donor was his 22-year-old brother. At the time there were no immune suppressive medications. Before kidney transplantation the recipient had sublethal total body irradiation (TBI). This experiment was based on success with bone marrow transplantation after total body irradiation. TBI was used to suppress the recipient's immune system and prevent rejection of the transplanted kidney. However, the exact role of TBI in kidney transplantation was not well understood at the time. TBI works by damaging the recipient's immune system, particularly the lymphocytes, which are responsible for rejecting foreign tissue. This allows the transplanted kidney to be accepted by the recipient's body without triggering an immune response. The surgery was successful, and the patient's new kidney functioned normally and he lived for another 25 years [141, 147].

Sir Peter Medawar (1915–1987) (Fig. 10.8), was a British immunologist who made significant contributions to the understanding of the immune system's role in the rejection of transplanted tissues and organs. Medawar's work on skin grafts during and after World War II demonstrated that the immune system could recognize and attack foreign tissues, leading to the rejection of transplanted organs. Medawar' research also helped to establish the concept of histocompatibility, or the degree to which the tissues of one individual can be tolerated by another, as a critical factor in the success of transplantation. This work laid the foundation for the development of immunosuppressive drugs and other strategies aimed at preventing or minimizing the rejection of transplanted organs by the recipient's immune system. Medawar was awarded the Nobel Prize in Physiology or Medicine in 1960, together with an

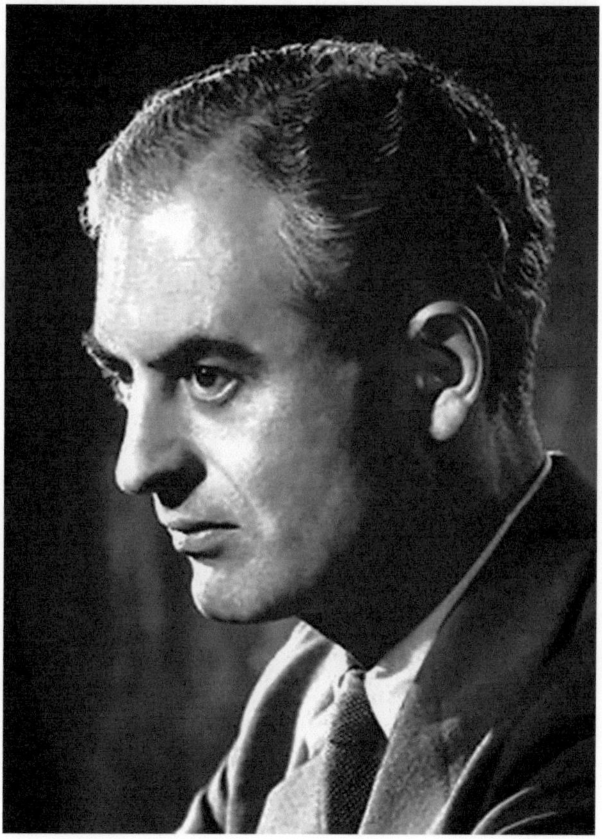

Fig. 10.8 Sir Peter Medawar, Nobel laureate in 1960 for the discovery of immune tolerance. (Wikipedia, public domain. https://upload.wikimedia.org/wikipedia/commons/c/ca/Peter_Brian_Medawar.jpg)

Australian immunologist, Sir Frank McFarlane Burnet (1899–1985) "for the discovery of acquired immune tolerance" [148].

The next breakthrough was immune suppression medications. In the early days of kidney transplantation, it was believed that the best chance of success was with transplants from genetically identical or related donors. However, as the demand for kidney transplants grew and the availability of suitable donors remained limited, researchers began to explore other options.

10.10.2.3 Early Immunosuppression

In the early 1960s, Dr. Roy Calne and his team at Peter Bent Brigham Hospital in Boston, Massachusetts, conducted a series of experiments on dogs to test the effectiveness of a medication called 6-mercaptopurine in preventing rejection after kidney transplantation. Their findings, which were published in 1962, showed that 6-mercaptopurine (6MP) was effective in prolonging survival after renal transplant in dogs. This was a significant breakthrough, as it provided a therapeutic way of preventing rejection and improve the success rate of kidney transplantation. However, 6MP is toxic and would not prove safe in humans [147].

Roy Calne (1930–2024) worked in Boston in 1960–1961 before he returned to London (1961) and then Cambridge (1965). While in Boston, he developed a combination of immunosuppressive medications that became known as the "Boston Cocktail." This cocktail, which included medications like azathioprine (a derivative of 6MP) and prednisone, was widely used in the 1960s and 1970s as, despite its toxicity, it helped to increase the success rate of kidney transplantation [147].

In Cambridge, Roy Calne worked on cyclosporin, a drug which had originally been developed as an anti-fungal. After animal experiments in which it was successful in countering rejection, it was introduced for human transplantation in 1978.

In the early 1960s, due to a shortage of human donor kidneys, some researchers began to investigate the possibility of using kidneys from nonhuman sources, such as chimpanzees.

Between November 5, 1963, and February 4, 1964, a team of researchers led by Dr. Keith Reemtsma (1925–2000) at Tulane University performed six renal chimpanzee (blood group O) xenotransplants on humans. While the surgeries were initially successful, all six patients eventually experienced organ rejection and the transplanted kidneys failed. Some patients lived for 9 months and this was considered as relative success. Xenotransplants are still being explored as an option today through genetic modification of the relevant animal [149].

10.10.2.4 Brain Death

Until the 1960, organs for transplants were retrieved from persons who had died because their heart had stopped beating and they had no circulation. In the late 1950s, Guy Alexandre (1934–2024) of Brussels, Belgium, encountered several patients who had suffered catastrophic brain injuries and were being kept alive on life support machines. Although these patients had no detectable brain activity and were clinically dead, they were still being maintained on life support due to the lack of a clear definition of death. Alexandre recognized the need for a new definition of death that took into account the irreversible loss of brain function. He coined the term "*coma dépassé*," which translates to "*beyond coma*," to describe this state of irreversible brain damage [150].

Dr. Alexandre's work in the 1960s helped to pave the way for the development of the concept of brain death, which is now widely recognized as the standard for determining death in many countries around the world. Today, the determination of brain death is an important consideration in the process of securing organ donation and facilitating transplantation, as it allows for the recovery of viable organs for transplant from donors who have irreversible brain damage but still have functioning organs albeit on artificial ventilation [150].

In 1963, the first successful organ transplant from a brain-dead donor was performed. The donor was a young man who had suffered a traumatic brain injury and had been declared brain-dead by Dr. Alexandre. Dr. Alexandre requested permission to perform a kidney transplant using the patient's organs, and this request was approved by the departmental chair, Jean Morelle. The transplant was successful, and the recipient, who had end-stage renal disease, went on to live for several years with the transplanted kidney. Alexandre and Morelle performed several more kidney transplants before presenting a case series in London in 1966. The Harvard Ad Hoc Committee largely adopted Alexandre's definition of brain death in 1968.

Alexandre showed that organs could be safely and effectively transplanted from brain-dead donors and that these organs had not suffered warm ischaemia because they were removed from persons with intact circulations [150].

Stewart Welch (1909–1980) performed the first experimental liver transplant on a dog in 1955. In this procedure, the donor liver was placed heterotopically (i.e., in a different location from the native liver) in the abdomen without removing the native liver. The experiment was successful in that the transplanted liver maintained its function, and the dog survived for several days. This experiment laid the groundwork for subsequent research and further development of liver transplantation in humans [151].

Thomas Starzl (Fig. 10.9) performed the first liver transplant in a human in 1963 in Denzer. His team also performed the first successful liver transplant in 1967. Their contributions and those of Roy Calne's team, in Cambridge, England, who performed the first liver transplant in Europe in 1968 are further discussed in the chapter on liver surgery [Chap. 8, p.].

Many units worked to refine surgical techniques, organ preservation, and make immunosuppression more effective and less toxic throughout the 1970s. Early survival rates remained below 25% [152].

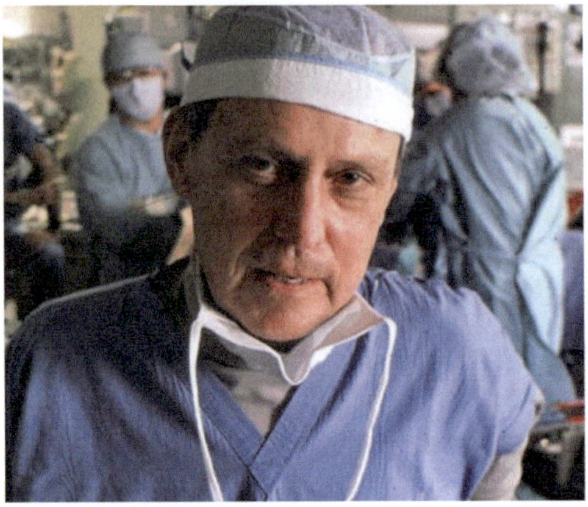

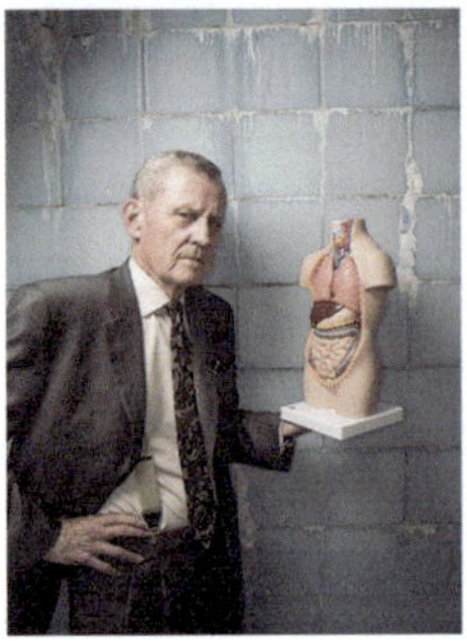

Fig. 10.9 Thomas Starzl. (Wikkimedia, Public domain, https://upload.wikimedia.org/wikipedia/commons/0/04/Thomas_starzl_transplant_surgeon_by_bill_cramer.jpg)

10.10.2.5 Further Advances in Immunosuppression

The next milestone was the development of immune suppressing agent cyclosporine. Cyclosporine was discovered in the 1970s by a team of researchers led by Dr. Jean-Francois Borel at Sandoz Pharmaceuticals (now part of Novartis) in Switzerland. The drug was initially identified as a potential antifungal agent during a screening process of soil samples, but it was found to be ineffective against fungi. However, further tests showed that the drug had potent immunosuppressive properties, and Roy Calne requested a sample to study its effectiveness in preventing rejection.

Dr. Borel and his team conducted a series of experiments in animals to test the safety and efficacy of cyclosporine in preventing rejection of transplanted organs. Their initial experiments showed promising results, and in 1978, cyclosporine was first used in a human liver transplant performed by Dr. Thomas Starzl. The use of cyclosporine helped to significantly reduce the risk of rejection and improve long-term outcomes for transplant patients. In the 1960s survival rate of transplanted kidneys longer than a year was about 50–60%. Once cyclosporine was introduced 90–95% of transplanted kidneys survived [147, 148].

Today, cyclosporine is one of the most commonly used immunosuppressive drugs in transplantation and has been instrumental in the success of organ transplantation as a lifesaving treatment for patients with end-stage organ failure.

In the 1980s, the discovery of the T-cell receptor and the role of the T-cell in transplant rejection led to the development of new immunosuppressive drugs, such as rapamycin (also known as sirolimus) and tacrolimus which target the T-cell, and have become the backbone of transplant immunosuppression.

In the twenty-first century, the development of new immunosuppressive drugs, such as belatacept and alemtuzumab, has been carried out. These drugs target different pathways in the immune system, and have been found to be more effective in preventing transplant rejection with fewer side effects, for transplantation of solid organs like kidney, liver, and pancreas.

It's worth noting that the field of immunosuppression is a rapidly evolving field with new drugs and therapies being continually developed and tested. The immunosuppressive therapy regimen is typically managed by a multidisciplinary team including transplant surgeons, transplant physicians, and nephrologists. The goal is to find the most effective and safe immunosuppressive regimen that balances the risk of rejection with the risk of side effects in order to improve the best long-term outcomes for transplant patients.

Lung Transplantation

James Hardy (1918–2003) at the University of Mississippi, was performing experimental lung transplants on dogs in the 1950s and early 1960s. In 1963, he transplanted a lung for a 58-year-old patient with bronchial carcinoma. After a period of initially breathing better, the patient died after 18 days, succumbing to kidney failure. The immune suppressive regimen at the time was radiation, azathioprine, and prednisolone. In 1964, Hardy also transplanted a chimpanzee heart into a dying patient performing the first xenograft heart transplant. Although the heart beat for an hour, the patient never regained consciousness. The first successful human lung transplant was finally performed by Joel D Cooper and his team at Toronto General Hospital in 1983, more than 20 years after Dr. Hardy's work with dogs [153].

Heart Transplantation

In the mid-1960s, it appears that there was a global race to perform the first heart transplant. Given that there were little alternatives for patients whose life was severely compromised by heart failure not amenable to revascularization or valve repair, there were patients willing to undergo what was at best an experimental procedure that offered some hope as well as contributing to scientific advancement.

Christiaan Barnard (1922–2001) at Groote Schuur Hospital, Cape Town, South Africa, performed the world's first successful human-to-human heart transplant on December third 1967. His team used the heart of 25-year-old, Denise Darvall, who had suffered irreversible brain damage following a car accident. After declaring her brain dead using criteria that he had helped to establish, Barnard and his surgical team removed her heart and transplanted it into 54-year-old Louis Washkansky, who had end-stage heart disease.

Before the surgery, Darvall was placed on a ventilator to maintain her breathing and circulation. After she was declared brain dead, Barnard and his team waited for approximately 6 min until the electrocardiogram indicated the absence of cardiac output before removing her heart for transplantation. This was done to ensure that her heart was in the best possible condition for transplantation. Washkansky lived 18 days but died of pneumonia [154].

Three days later, at Maimonides Hospital in Brooklyn, New York, Adrian Kantrowitz (1918–2008) led a team that undertook a paediatric heart transplant, although the new heart stopped beating after 7 h and the child died [155].

On January 6, 1968, a team led by Norman Shumway (1923–2006) and Randall Griepp (1940–2022) performed the second adult transplant at Stanford Hospital, USA. During the surgery, Shumway's chief resident assisting him asked whether the procedure was legal, to which Shumway simply responded, "I guess we'll see." At the time, there were no clear guidelines or regulations in place regarding the definition of death or the use of brain death criteria for organ donation. It wasn't until the 1980s that brain death criteria became widely accepted as the standard for declaring a patient dead for the purpose of organ donation [156].

Donald Ross (1922–2014), a classmate of Christian Barnard's in Cape Town, but who worked in London at the National Heart hospital, led the first British heart transplant in May 1968. The patient was a 45-year-old male who lived 46 days before dying of "overwhelming infection." Ross' team stopped after three transplants until the problems of rejection were able to be overcome [155].

In 1969, Denton Cooley (1920–2016), in Houston, Texas, inserted the first artificial heart into a human. The patient Haskell Karp lived 65 h. In 1970, he inserted another artificial heart for a patient for whom no heart donor was available [156].

Despite some success with the first heart transplants, there were also concerns raised about the ethical implications of the procedure. One of the main concerns was whether the removal of the heart from a brain dead patient constituted killing the donor.

The first heart lung transplant was performed by Norman Shumway and Bruce Reitz in 1981 [156, 157].

The first totally artificial heart was developed by Vladimir Demikhov; he was also the first to perform coronary arteries bypass. The artificial heart was tow pumps driven by a motor; he was also the first to perform successful heart-lung transplant on a dog which reportedly survived for 30 days, and he preserved the organs with closed circuit circulation [158].

Robert Jarvik (b 1946) invented the Jarvik-7, a completely artificial heart, after his own father died of heart disease. In Salt Lake City, at the University of Utah, Jarvik and his team developed the device, which was designed to be a bridge to transplant for patients with end-stage heart disease who were awaiting a donor heart. The first successful implantation of the Jarvik-7 in a human was performed in

1982 by William DeVries (b 1940) and his team at the University of Utah. The patient, Barney Clark, was a retired dentist who had severe heart disease and was not a candidate for a heart transplant. Clark survived for 112 days after the implantation but ultimately died due to complications related to the device.

The Jarvik-7 was not without its limitations and drawbacks. The device was large and heavy, weighing in at 350 pounds, and required the patient to be attached to an air compressor. Additionally, patients who received the Jarvik-7 were required to remain in the hospital for the duration of their use of the device.

Despite these limitations, the Jarvik-7 paved the way for the development of other artificial heart devices. It was implanted in more than 150 patients during the 1980s and 1990s, and while it is no longer in use today, its legacy lives on in the ongoing development of new technologies and treatments for heart disease [159].

Pancreas Transplant

In 1966, Richard Lillehei (1927–1981) at the University of Minnesota, performed the first unsuccessful and first successful combined pancreas-kidney transplant for patients with diabetic end-stage kidney disease. The successful operation involved the whole pancreas, accompanying duodenum and one kidney. Their transplant was the result of years of experimentation in dogs. Although the early results of pancreatic transplants were poor, by 2000, graft survival was around 78% at 1 year. These figures were consistent whether the pancreas was transplanted alone, or whether transplanted after the kidney or simultaneously though the simultaneous transplant survival was slightly better at 84% for the pancreas [160].

Intestinal Transplant

An intestinal transplant spares the individual who has lost all or most of their small intestine from a life supported by parenteral nutrition. The first reported intestinal transplant was by Richard Lillehei (1927–1981) at the University of Minnesota in 1967. Starzl performed a multivisceral transplant in 1983, and in 1990, David Grant performed a combined liver and intestinal transplant in Canada [161, 162].

10.10.2.6 Ethics of Organ Donation

Government involvement in the USA started with the National Uniform Anatomical Gift Act (NUAGA) which was first drafted in 1968 and has since been revised and adopted by all 50 US states. The act allowed individuals to make a legally binding gift of their organs and/or tissues for transplantation upon their death. The act also established the use of the uniform donor card, which serves as a legal document indicating an individual's decision to donate their organs and/or tissues after death. In 1968, a committee at Harvard Medical School, led by anesthetist, Dr. Henry

Beecher (1904–1976), established criteria for determining brain death based on Guy Alexandre's earlier work in France. The report defined brain death as "irreversible coma" and established the criteria for determining when brain death had occurred. The report aimed to clarify the definition of death and to provide a legal and ethical basis for organ donation.

The United Network for Organ Sharing (UNOS) was established in 1984 as a private, nonprofit organization that manages the nation's organ transplant system under contract with the federal government. However, its precursor, the South-Eastern Organ Procurement Foundation (SEOPF), established a computer database in 1977 that was the first of its kind and aimed to increase the efficiency of organ matching. This database was a significant step forward in the organ donation and transplantation process, allowing organs to be matched with compatible patients at any member institution more efficiently.

Although in the twenty-first century, many countries in the world have established similar laws regulations to control organ donation, there are countries where the only donors permitted are live donors. There remains concern that, in some countries, live donors may be exploited and their organs sold, or forcibly removed, because they are criminals. However, organ transplant offers new life to the recipient who might otherwise die and when carried out ethically, with full informed consent in the case of a live donor, carries a low risk to the donor. It is incumbent on regulators to ensure that organ donation is carried out ethically and in keeping with the law and that neither donors nor recipients are exploited [156, 157].

References

Skin and Skin Grafts

1. Ozhathil DK, Tay MW, Wolf SE, Branski LK. A narrative review of the history of skin grafting in burn care. Medicina (Kaunas). 2021;57(4):380. https://doi.org/10.3390/medicina57040380. PMID: 33920783; PMCID: PMC8071142
2. Kohlhauser M, Luze H, Nischwitz SP, Kamolz LP. Historical evolution of skin grafting-a journey through time. Medicina (Kaunas). 2021;57(4):348. https://doi.org/10.3390/medicina57040348. PMID: 33916337; PMCID: PMC8066645
3. Shen JT, Weinstein M, Beekley AC, Yeo CJ, Cowan SW. Ambroise Paré (1510 to 1590): a surgeon centuries ahead of his time. Department of Surgery Gibbon Society Historical Profiles; 2014. Paper 41. https://jdc.jefferson.edu/gibbonsocietyprofiles/41
4. https://livesonline.rcseng.ac.uk/client/en_GB/lives/search/detailnonmodal/ent:$002f$002fSD_ASSET$002f0$002fSD_ASSET:375043/one?qu=%22rcs%3A+E002860%22&rt=false%7C%7C%7CIDENTIFIER%7C%7C%7CResource+Identifier
5. Joseph K, Trehan A, Cherian M, Kelley E, Watters DA. Assessment of acute burn management in 32 low- and middle-income countries. World J Surg. 2016;40(4):791–800. https://doi.org/10.1007/s00268-015-3355-3. PMID: 26661635
6. Majno G. The healing hand: man and wound in the ancient world. Cambridge: Harvard University Press; 1975.

7. Ehrenfried A. Reverdin and other methods of skin-grafting: historical. Boston Med Surg J. 1909;161:911–7. https://doi.org/10.1056/NEJM190912231612601.
8. Barrow RE, Herndon DN. Total burn care. Amsterdam, The Netherlands: Elsevier BV; 2007. History of treatments of burns. p. 1–8.
9. Ang GC. History of skin transplantation. Clin Dermatol. 2005;23:320–4. https://doi.org/10.1016/j.clindermatol.2004.07.013.
10. Almast S. History and evolution of the Indian method of rhinoplasty. In: Sanvenero-Rosselli G, editor. Transactions of the fourth international congress of plastic and reconstruction surgery. Rome, Italy: Exerpta Medica Foundation; 1969. p. 49.
11. Thornton JF. Skin grafts and skin substitutes. Sel Read Plast Surg. 2004;10:1–23.
12. Davis JS. Address of the president: the story of plastic surgery. Ann Surg. 1941;113:641–56.
13. Schwokowski CF. Erinnerungen an Carl Thiersch—Zum 100. Todestag [In memory of Carl Thiersch—on the 100th anniversary of his death]. Zentralbl Chir. 1996;121(5):426–9. German. PMID: 8677706
14. Koch SL. The transplantation of skin and subcutaneous tissue to the hand. Surg Gynecol Obstet. 1941;72:157–77.
15. Janžekovič Z. Once upon a time … how west discovered east. J Plast Reconstr Aesthetic Surg. 2008;61:240–4. https://doi.org/10.1016/j.bjps.2008.01.001.
16. Trop M. Zora Janzekovic (September 30, 1918-March 17, 2015). Burns. 2015;41(6):1374. https://doi.org/10.1016/j.burns.2015.05.012. PMID: 26523298
17. Baxter CR, Shires T. Physiological response to crystalloid resuscitation of severe burns. Ann N Y Acad Sci. 1968;150:874–94.
18. Wallace AB. The exposure treatment of burns. Lancet. 1951;257:501–4.
19. Lee KC, Joory K, Moiemen NS. History of burns: the past, present and the future. Burns Trauma. 2014;2(4):169–80. https://doi.org/10.4103/2321-3868.143620. PMID: 27574647; PMCID: PMC4978094
20. Burke JF, Bondoc CC, Quinby WC. Primary burn excision and immediate grafting. J Trauma Injury Infect Crit Care. 1974;14:389–95. https://doi.org/10.1097/00005373-197405000-00005.
21. Rogers BO. Historical development of free skin grafting. Surg Clin N Am. 1959;39:289–311. https://doi.org/10.1016/S0039-6109(16)35732-2.
22. Kamolz L, Schintler M, Parvizi D, Selig H, Lumenta D. The real expansion rate of meshers and micrografts: things we should keep in mind. Ann Burn Fire Disasters. 2013;26:26–9.
23. Dragstedt LR, Wilson H. A modified sieve graft; A full thickness skin graft for covering large defects. Surg Gynecol Obstct. 1937;65:104–6. Anger B. Sur l'heteroplastie. CR Acad. Sci. 1874;79:1210–12
24. Ameer F, Singh AK, Kumar S. Evolution of instruments for harvest of the skin grafts. Indian J Plast Surg. 2013;46(1):28–35. https://doi.org/10.4103/0970-0358.113704. PMID: 23960303; PMCID: PMC3745118
25. Freshwater MF. Joseph Constantine Carpue and the bicentennial of the birth of modern plastic surgery. Aesthet Surg J. 2015;35(6):748–58. https://doi.org/10.1093/asj/sju157. Epub 2015 Mar 19. PMID: 25795909; PMCID: PMC4520582
26. Ruetsch YA, Böni T, Borgeat A. From cocaine to ropivacaine: the history of local anesthetic drugs. Curr Top Med Chem. 2001;1(3):175–82. https://doi.org/10.2174/1568026013395335. PMID: 11895133

Flaps for Reconstructive Surgery

27. Gräfe KF Rhinoplastik (1818)—Rhinoplasty.
28. Rogers BO. Hippolyte Morestin (1869–1919). Part I: a brief biography. Aesth Plast Surg. 1982;6(3):141–7. https://doi.org/10.1007/BF01570633. PMID 6758545. S2CID 9881793.

29. Rex Wright-St Clair. 'Gillies, Harold Delf', Dictionary of New Zealand Biography, first published in 1996. Te Ara - the Encyclopedia of New Zealand. https://teara.govt.nz/en/biographies/3g9/gillies-harold-delf. Accessed 27 December 2023.
30. Sargent LA, Morgan RF, Davis WB. John Staige Davis: pioneer American plastic surgeon. Clin Plast Surg. 1983;10(4):653–6. PMID: 6360481
31. NB: his father was John Staige Davis (1824–1885) also a Professor at the University of Virginia, an anatomist and a confederate surgeon during the American Civil War.
32. Freshwater MF. A critical comparison of Davis' principles of plastic surgery with Gillies' plastic surgery of the face. J Plast Reconstr Aesthet Surg. 2011;64(1):17–26. https://doi.org/10.1016/j.bjps.2010.03.009. Epub 2010 Mar 30. PMID: 20356811
33. https://www.whonamedit.com/doctor.cfm/1421.html
34. Dieffenbach JF. Chirurgische Erfahrungen, besonders über die Wiederherstellung zerstörter Theile des menschlichen Körpers nach neuen Methoden. (Surgical observations on the Restoration of the Nose).
35. 3 volumes [in 4] and atlas. Berlin, T. C. F. Enselin, 1829–1834. English translation of the section on rhinoplasty, with additional cases and notes by the translator, John Stevenson Buchnan; London, 1833.
36. Ozhathil DK, Tay MW, Wolf SE, Branski LK. A narrative review of the history of skin grafting in burn care.
37. Hauben DJ. Victor von Bruns (1812–1883) and his contributions to plastic and reconstructive surgery. Plast Reconstr Surg. 1985;75:120–7.

Cleft Lip and Palate Repair

38. Bhattacharya S, Khanna V, Kohli R. Cleft lip: the historical perspective. Indian J Plast Surg. 2009;42(Suppl(Suppl)):S4–8. https://doi.org/10.4103/0970-0358.57180. PMID: 19884680; PMCID: PMC2825059
39. Naidu P, Yao CA, Chong DK, Magee WP 3rd. Cleft palate repair: a history of techniques and variations. Plast Reconstr Surg Glob Open. 2022;10(3):e4019. https://doi.org/10.1097/GOX.0000000000004019. PMID: 35492233; PMCID: PMC9038491
40. Markatos K, Karamanou M, Korres D, Tsourouflis G, Damaskos C, Garmpis N, Androutsos G. Pierre Franco (1505–1578): an innovative surgeon of the 16th century in the treatment of hernia and lithotomy. Surg Innov. 2019;26(1):129–33. https://doi.org/10.1177/1553350618812280. Epub 2018 Nov 25. PMID: 30472922
41. Dupoirieux L, Penneau M. La contribution de Germanicus Mirault à la chirurgie maxillo-faciale en général et à celle du Bec-de-lièvre (1) en particulier [The contribution of Germanicus Mirault to maxillofacial surgery in general and to surgery of the cleft lip in particular]. Rev Stomatol Chir Maxillofac. 1996;97(4):195–201. French PMID: 8927924
42. Randall P. Triangular flap operation for unilateral clefts of the lip. Plast Reconstr Surg. 1959;23:331.
43. Faltin R. History of plastic surgery in Finland. Finsk Lak Sallsk Handl. 1937;80:97.
44. Manchester WM. The repair of bilateralcleft lip and palate. Br J Surg. 1965;52:878–82.
45. Millard RC. Cleft craft, vol. 1.3. Boston: Little Brown; 1976.
46. Victor Veau 1871–1949. https://livesonline.rcseng.ac.uk/client/en_GB/lives/search/detailnonmodal/ent:$002f$002fSD_ASSET$002f0$002fSD_ASSET:377034/one?qu=%22rcs%3A+E004851%22&rt=false%7C%7C%7CIDENTIFIER%7C%7C%7CResource+Identifier
47. Nandoskar P, Coghlan P, Moore MH, Ximenes J, Moore EM, Karnon J, Watters DA. The economic value of the delivery of primary cleft surgery in Timor Leste 2000–2017. World J Surg. 2020;44(6):1699–705. https://doi.org/10.1007/s00268-020-05388-3. PMID: 32030441

48. Michael AI, Okoli C, Olusanya AA, Akintayo AJ, Onah II, Yiltok S, Oluwatosin OM. Multicenter pattern of cleft surgeries and factors associated with late primary cleft surgery in Nigeria. Plast Reconstr Surg Glob Open. 2024;12(5):e5795. https://doi.org/10.1097/GOX.0000000000005795. PMID: 38746947; PMCID: PMC11093566
49. Roldán JC, Pape HD, Koch H, Koller M. Ten-year cleft surgery in Nepal: achievements and lessons learned for better cleft care abroad. Plast Reconstr Surg Glob Open. 2016;4(5):e711. https://doi.org/10.1097/GOX.0000000000000702. PMID: 27579235; PMCID: PMC4995715

A History of the Management of Fractures and Orthopedic Eponyms

50. Knothe U, Knothe-Tate ML, Perren SM. 300 years of intramedullary fixation—from Aztec practice to standard treatment modality. Eur J Trauma. 2000:217–25.
51. 300 Years of Intramedullary Fixation—from Aztec Practice to Standard Treatment Modality Ulf Knothe, Melissa L. Knothe Tate, Stephan M.
52. Dodge HS. Displaced supracondylar fractures of the Humerus in children-treatment by Dunlop's traction. J Bone Joint Surg Am. 1972;54(7):1408–18.
53. Gustilo RB, Simpson L, Nixon R, et al. Analysis of 511 open fractures. Clin Orthop Relat Res. 1969;66:148–54.
54. Salter RB, Harris WR. Injuries involving the physeal plate. J Bone Joint Surg Am. 1963;45(3):587–622.
55. Kevau I, Watters DA. Conservative management of femoral shaft fractures. P N G Med J. 1996;39(2):143–51. PMID: 9599987
56. Rehim SA, Maynard MA, Sebastin SJ, Chung KC. Monteggia fracture dislocations: a historical review. J Hand Surg Am. 2014;39(7):1384–94. https://doi.org/10.1016/j.jhsa.2014.02.024. Epub 2014 May 3. PMID: 24792923; PMCID: PMC4266382
57. Kim PH, Leopold SS. In brief: Gustilo-Anderson classification. [corrected]. Clin Orthop Relat Res. 2012;470(11):3270–4. https://doi.org/10.1007/s11999-012-2376-6. Epub 2012 May 9. Erratum in: Clin Orthop Relat Res. 2012;470(12):3624. Erratum in: Clin Orthop Relat Res. 2019;477(10):2388. doi: 10.1097/CORR.0000000000000950. PMID: 22569719; PMCID: PMC3462875
58. Yim GH, Hardwicke JT. The evolution and interpretation of the Gustilo and Anderson classification. J Bone Joint Surg Am. 2018;100(24):e152. https://doi.org/10.2106/JBJS.18.00342. PMID: 30562299
59. Gustilo RB, Mendoza RM, Williams DN. Problems in the management of type III (severe) open fractures: a new classification of type III open fractures. J Trauma. 1984;24:742–6.
60. Brand RA. Biographical sketch: Georg Clemens Perthes, MD (1869–1927). Clin Orthop Relat Res. 2012;470(9):2347–8. https://doi.org/10.1007/s11999-012-2432-2. Erratum in: Clin Orthop Relat Res. 2013;471(1):345. PMID: 22723245; PMCID: PMC3481115

Joint Replacement

61. Gomez P, Morcuende JA. Early attempts at hip arthroplasty-1700s to 1950s. Iowa Orthop J. 2005;25:25–9.
62. Brand RA, Mont MA, Manring MM. Biographical sketch: Themistocles Gluck (1853–1942). Clin Orthop Relat Res. 2011;469(6):1525–7. https://doi.org/10.1007/s11999-011-1836-8. PMID: 21403990; PMCID: PMC3094624

63. Learmonth ID, Young C, Rorabeck C. The operation of the century: total hip replacement. Lancet. 2007;370:1508–19.
64. Fenton P, Rampurada A, Qureshi F. Bone cement, its history, its properties and developments in its use; 2009.
65. Charnley J. Anchorage of the femoral head prosthesis to the shaft of the femur. J Bone Joint Surg Br. 1960;42B:28–30.
66. Niculescu M, Solomon BL, Viscopoleanu G, Antoniac IV. Chapter 29: Evolution of cementation techniques and bone cements in hip arthroplasty. In: Antoniac IV, editor. Handbook of bioceramics and biocomposites. 1st ed. Germany: Springer; 2016.
67. Ring PA. Total replacement of the hip. Clin Orthop Relat Res. 1970;72:161–8.
68. Brown SR, Davies WA, DeHeer DH, Swanson AB. Long-term survival of Mckee-Farrar total hip prosthesis. Clin Orthop Relat Res. 2002;402:157–63.
69. Reininga IH, Zijlstra W, Wagenmakers R, et al. Minimally invasive and computer-navigated total hip arthroplasty: a qualitative and systematic review of the literature. BMC Musculoskelet Disord. 2010;11:92.
70. Cech O, Dzupa V. The European school of total hip arthroplasty and 35 years of total hip arthroplasty in The Czech Republic. Acta Chir Orthop Traumatol Cechoslov. 2005;72(1):57–76.
71. Dall'Oca C, Ricci M, Vecchini E, Giannini N, Lamberti D, Tromponi C, Magnan B. Evolution of TKA design. Acta Biomed. 2017;88(2S):17–31. https://doi.org/10.23750/abm.v88i2-S.6508. PMID: 28657559; PMCID: PMC6178992
72. Macintosh DL. Hemiarthroplasty of the knee using space occupying prosthesis for painful varus and valgus deformities. J Bone Joint Surg. 1958;40:1431.
73. Bruni D, Iacono F, Akkawi I, Gagliardi M, Zaffagnini S, Marcacci M. Unicompartmental knee replacement: a historical overview. Joints. 2013;1(2):45–7. PMID: 25606516; PMCID: PMC4295698

Cataract Surgery

74. Davis G. The evolution of cataract surgery. Mo Med. 2016;113(1):58–62. PMID: 27039493; PMCID: PMC6139750
75. Priority Eye Diseases. World Health Organization; 2018., www.who.int/blindness/causes/priority/en/index1.html
76. Cataracts: Overview. InformedHealth.org. 10-Oct-2019. [Online]. Available: https://www.ncbi.nlm.nih.gov/books/NBK390302/.
77. Pascolini D, Mariotti SP. Global estimates of visual impairment: 2010. Br J Ophthalmol. 2012;96(5):614–8.
78. Hirschberg J, Blodi FC (trans.). The history of ophthalmology. Vol. 1. Antiquity. Bonn: Wayenborgh Verlag; 1982, pp. 34–349.
79. Blomstedt P. Cataract surgery in ancient Egypt. J Cataract Refract Surg. 2014;40:485–9.
80. Geller MJ. Ancient Babylonian medicine: theory and practice. Oxford: Wiley-Blackwell; 2010. p. 58–184.
81. Meyerhof M. Alî at-Tabarî's "Paradise of Wisdom", one of the oldest Arabic Compendiums of Medicine. ISIS. 1931;16:6–54.
82. Leffler CT, Schwartz SG, Peterson E, et al. Cataract couching and the goat's eye. Acta Ophthalmol. 2018;96:755–6.
83. Oransky I. Charles Kelman. Lancet. 2004;364(9429):134. https://doi.org/10.1016/S0140-6736(04)16646-4. PMID: 15281216
84. Hubbell AA. Samuel Sharp, the first surgeon to make the corneal incision in cataract extraction with a single knife: a biographical and historical sketch.

A History of Neurosurgery

85. Chang A, Lad EM, Lad SP. Hippocrates' influence on the origins of neurosurgery. Neurosurg Focus. 2007;23(1):E9. https://doi.org/10.3171/foc.2007.23.1.9.
86. Stefanou MI. The footprints of neuroscience in Alexandria during the 3rd-century BC: Herophilus and Erasistratus. J Med Biogr. 2020;28(4):186–94. https://doi.org/10.1177/0967772018789349. Epub 2018 Aug 31
87. Pearce JM. The neuroanatomy of herophilus. Eur Neurol. 2013;69(5):292–5. https://doi.org/10.1159/000346232. Epub 2013 Feb 23
88. Solaroglu I, Acar F, Bavbek M, Ture U, Beskonakli E. The history of neurosurgery in Anatolia and Turkey: the Turkish Neurosurgical Society. World Neurosurg. 2013;79(1):16–24. https://doi.org/10.1016/j.wneu.2012.11.042. Epub 2012 Nov 19. PMID: 23174152
89. Watters DA. Skull trepanation in the Bismarck archipelago. PNG Med J. 2007;50(1–2):20–4.
90. Andrushko VA, Verano JW. Prehistoric trepanation in the Cuzco region of Peru: a view into an ancient Andean practice. Am J Phys Anthropol. 2008;137(1):4–13. https://doi.org/10.1002/ajpa.20836.
91. Jang K, Rosenfeld JV, Di Ieva A. Paulus of Aegina and the historical origins of spine surgery. World Neurosurg. 2020;133:291–301. https://doi.org/10.1016/j.wneu.2019.10.026. Epub 2019 Oct 15. PMID: 31627004
92. Aciduman A, Belen D, Simsek S. Management of spinal disorders and trauma in Avicenna's canon of medicine. Neurosurgery. 2006;59:397–403.
93. Aciduman A, Belen D. An early description of using oral route for the management of cervical vertebra fracture by Ibn al-Quff in the thirteenth century. World Neurosurg. 2018;120:476–84. https://doi.org/10.1016/j.wneu.2018.09.005. Epub 2018 Sep 8
94. Mattei TA. "Reinventing the wheel": reflections on a recurrent phenomenon in the history of neurosurgery. J Neurosurg. 2018;129(6):1641–8. https://doi.org/10.3171/2018.4.JNS18652.
95. Hubbard ZS, Cunningham CM, Saway BF, Weber AC, Sowlat MM, Henderson FC, Patel S, Varma A. An early case of successful peripheral nerve repair in 1880
96. Parker FL. J Neurosurg. 2024:1–5. https://doi.org/10.3171/2024.2.JNS232614. Epub ahead of print. PMID: 38728759
97. Tomasello F, Germanò A. Francesco Durante: the history of intracranial meningiomas and beyond. Neurosurgery. 2006;59(2):389–96; discussion 389–96. https://doi.org/10.1227/01.NEU.0000223444.18909.9A.
98. Pascual JM, Mongardi L, Prieto R, Castro-Dufourny I, Rosdolsky M, Strauss S, Carrasco R, Winter E, Mazzarello P. Giovanni Verga (1879–1923), author of a pioneering treatise on pituitary surgery: the foundations of this new field in Europe in the early 1900s. Neurosurg Rev. 2017;40(4):559–75. https://doi.org/10.1007/s10143-017-0864-6. Epub 2017 May 27
99. Atwood JE, et al. Sir High Cairns: a pioneering collaborator. Acta Neurochir. 2019;161:1491–5. https://doi.org/10.1007/s00701-019-03934-0.
100. Stone JL, Patel V, Bailes JE. Sir Hugh Cairns and World War II British advances in head injury management, diffuse brain injury, and concussion: an Oxford tale. J Neurosurg. 2016;125(5):1301–14. https://doi.org/10.3171/2015.8.JNS142613. Epub 2016 Feb 19. PMID: 26894455
101. Duddy JC, Kennerk B. Adams Andrew McConnell (1884-1972): Pioneer of Irish neurosurgery. Br J Neurosurg. 2015;29(1):4–8. https://doi.org/10.3109/02688697.2014.994472.
102. Ching L, Ng A, Rosenfeld JV, Di Ieva A. World Neurosurg. 2019;128:299–307. https://doi.org/10.1016/j.wneu.2019.05.036. Epub 2019 May 15
103. Rajshekhar V. History of neurosurgery at Christian Medical College, Vellore: a pioneer's tale. Neurol India. 2016;64(2):297–310. https://doi.org/10.4103/0028-3886.177625.
104. Raffiq A, Abdullah JM, Haspani S, Adnan JS. History of neurosurgery in Malaysia. Malays J Med Sci. 2015;22(Spec Issue):5–8.
105. The legacy of Renaissance surgeon Giovanni Andrea Dalla Croce on the history of military surgery and neurosurgery.

106. Di Ieva A, Rosenfeld JV. Cranial nerve nomenclature: historical vignette. Neurosurg Focus. 2022;53(3):E3. https://doi.org/10.3171/2022.6.FOCUS22243.
107. Priola SM, Raffa G, Abbritti RV, et al. The pioneering contribution of Italian surgeons to skull base surgery. World Neurosurg. 2014;82:523–8.
108. Hiçdönmez T, Ozek MM. Hydrocephalus in Sabuncuoğlu's textbook of surgery: Cerrahiyyet' ul Haniyye. Childs Nerv Syst. 2006;22(6):545–6. https://doi.org/10.1007/s00381-006-0099-2.

Open-Heart Surgery

109. Weisse AB. Medical odysseys–the different and unexpected pathways to twentieth-century medical discoveries. New Brunswick, NJ: Rutgers University Press; 1991. p. 229. 112. Landmark article Feb 25, 1939: Surgical ligation of a patent ductus arteriosus. Report of first successful case. By Robert E. Gross and John P. Hubbard. JAMA 1984;251(9):1201–2
110. Crafoord C, Nylin G. Congenital coarctation of the aorta and its surgical treatment. J Thorac Surg. 1945;14:347–61.
111. Landmark article May 19, 1945Blalock A, Taussig HB. The surgical treatment of malformations of the heart in which there is pulmonary stenosis or pulmonary atresia. JAMA. 1984;251(16):2123–38.
112. Hufnagel CA, Harvey WP. The surgical correction of aortic regurgitation preliminary report. Bull Georgetown Univ Med Cent. 1953;6(3):60–1.
113. Weisse AB. The surgical treatment of mitral stenosis: the first heart operation. Am J Cardiol. 2009;103(1):143–7.
114. Starr A, Edwards ML. Mitral replacement: clinical experience with a ball-valve prosthesis. Ann Surg. 1961;154:726–40.
115. Lewis FJ, Taufic M. Closure of atrial septal defects with the aid of hypothermia. Surgery. 1953;33(1):52–9.
116. Gibbon JH Jr. The development of the heart-lung apparatus. Am J Surg. 1978;135(5):608–19.
117. Kirklin JW, Dushane JW, et al. Intracardiac surgery with the aid of a mechanical pump-oxygenator system (gibbon type): report of eight cases. Proc Staff Meet Mayo Clin. 1955;30(10):201–6.
118. Dewall RA, Gott VL, Lillehei CW, et al. A simple, expendable, artificial oxygenator for open heart surgery. Surg Clin North Am. 1956:1025–34.
119. Konstantinov IE, Robert H. Goetz: the surgeon who performed the first successful clinical coronary artery bypass operation. Ann Thorac Surg. 2000;69(6):1966–72.
120. Griepp RB, Ergin MA. History of experimental heart transplantation. Heart Transpl. 1984;III:145–51.
121. Lim G. Discovery and purification of heparin. Nat Rev Cardiol. 2017; https://doi.org/10.1038/nrcardio.2017.171.
122. Starr A. The thoracic surgical industrial complex. Ann Thorac Surg. 1986;42:124–33.
123. Edwards M, Edwards M. Miles Lowell Edwards. In: Miles Lowell Edwards... his ancestors and descendants. Santa Ana, CA: Pioneer Press; 1972. p. 11–26.
124. Kay EB. Early years in artificial valve development. Ann Thorac Surg. 1989;48:S24–5.
125. Björk VO. The development of artificial heart valves: introduction and historical perspective. In: Morse D, Steiner RM, Fernandez J, editors. Guide to prosthetic cardiac valves. New York, NY: Springer; 1985.
126. Manji RA, Ekser B, Menkis AH, Cooper DK. Bioprosthetic heart valves of the future. Xenotransplantation. 2014;21:1–10.
127. Kumar T, Singh A, Thakre S, Acharya S, Shukla S, Kumar S. Scientific evolution of artificial heart valves: a narrative review. Cureus. 2023;15(7)

128. Wardrop D, Keeling D. The story of the discovery of heparin and warfarin. Br J Haematol. 2008;141(6):757–63.
129. Barritt DW, Jordan SC. Anticoagulant drugs in the treatment of pulmonary embolism; a controlled trial. Lancet. 1960;1:1309–12.

Abdominal Aortic Aneurysm

130. Slaney G. A history of aneurysm surgery. In: The cause and management of aneurysms. London: WB Saunders; 1990. p. 1–18.
131. Barker WF. Clio: the arteries. Austin, TX: RG Landers; 1992. p. 2–502.
132. Cooley DA, DeBakey ME. Ruptured aneurysms in the abdominal aorta — excision and homograft replacement. Postgrad Med. 1954;16:334–42.
133. Thompson JE. Early history of aortic surgery. J Vasc Surg. 1998;28:746–52. https://doi.org/10.1016/S0741-5214(98)70107-7.
134. Dubost C, Allary M, Oeconomos N. Resection of an aneurysm of the abdominal aorta. AMA Arch Surg. 1952;64:405–8. https://doi.org/10.1001/archsurg.1952.01260010419018.
135. De Bakey ME, Cooley DA, Crawford ES. Clinical application of a new flexible knitted Dacron arterial substitute. Am Surg. 1958;24:862–9.
136. Miller C. A time for all things: the life of Michael E. DeBakey. Oxford University Press; 2019. p. 523–30.
137. Gotto AM. Profiles in cardiology; Michael DeBakey. Clin Cardiol. 1991;14(12):1007–10.
138. Criado FJ. EVAR at 20: the unfolding of a revolutionary new technique that changed everything. J Endovasc Ther. 2010;17:789–96.
139. England A, McWilliams R. Endovascular aortic aneurysm repair (EVAR). Ulster Med J. 2013;82:3–10.

Organ Transplantation

140. Murray J. The man who lost his face; how a severely burned World War II pilot with a will to live helped launch the age of organ transplants. Newsweek; 2005.
141. Matevossian E, Kern H, Hüser N, Doll D, Snopok Y, Nährig J, Altomonte J, Sinicina I, Friess H, Thorban S. Surgeon Yurii Voronoy (1895-1961) - a pioneer in the history of clinical transplantation: in memoriam at the 75th anniversary of the first human kidney transplantation. Transpl Int. 2009;22(12):1132–9. https://doi.org/10.1111/j.1432-2277.2009.00986.x. PMID: 19874569
142. Carrel A. Lyon Med. 1902;98:859–64.
143. Twin's life may hang on fingerprint today. Boston Herald, December 22, 1954.
144. Murray JE, Merrill JP, Dammin GJ, Dealy JB Jr, Alexandre GW, Harrison JH. Kidney transplantation in modified recipients. Ann Surg. 1962;156(3):337–55. https://doi.org/10.1097/00000658-196209000-00002.
145. Voronoy Y. Sobre el bloqueo del aparato reticulo-endothelial del hombre en algunas formas de intoxicacion por el sublimado y sobre la transplantacion del rinon cadaverico como metodo de tratamiento de la anuria consecutive a aquella intoxicacion. El Siglo Med. 1936;97:296.
146. Wieringa FP, Søndergaard H, Ash S. Father of Artificial Organs - The story of medical pioneer Willem J. Kolff (1911–2009). Artif Organs. 2021;45(10):1136–40. https://doi.org/10.1111/aor.13990. Epub ahead of print. PMID: 33948975; PMCID: PMC851839
147. Calne RY, Alexandre GP, Murray JE. A study of the effects of drugs in prolonging survival of homologous renal transplants in dogs. Ann N Y Acad Sci. 1962;99(3):743–60.

148. Simpson E. Medawar's legacy to cellular immunology and clinical transplantation: a commentary on Billingham, Brent and Medawar (1956) 'Quantitative studies on tissue transplantation immunity. III. Actively acquired tolerance'. Philos Trans R Soc Lond B Biol Sc. 2015;370(1666):20140382. https://doi.org/10.1098/rstb.2014.0382. PMID: 25750245; PMCID: PMC4360130
149. Reemtsma K. Xenotransplantation: a historical perspective. ILAR J. 1995;37(1):9–12. https://doi.org/10.1093/ilar.37.1.9.
150. Mollaret P, Goulon M. Coma dépassé (preliminary memoir). Rev Neurol (Paris). 1959;101(1):3–15.
151. Welch C. A note on transplantation of the whole liver in dogs. Transplant Cull. 1955;2:54–5.
152. Starzl TE, Demetris AJ. Liver transplantation: a 31-year perspective. Part I Curr Probl Surg. 1990;27(2):49–240. https://doi.org/10.1016/0011-3840(90)90021-v.
153. Lung Transplant Foundation. History of Lung Transplantation. http://lungtransplantfoundation.org/facts-history/
154. Barnard CN. The operation. A human cardiac transplant: an interim report of a successful operation performed at Groote Schuur Hospital, Cape Town. S Afr Med J. 1967;41(48):1271–4.
155. Kantrowitz A, Haller JD, Joos H, Cerruti MM, Carstensen HE. Transplantation of the heart in an infant and an adult. Am J Cardiol. 1968;22(6):782–90. PMID: 4880223
156. White T. Magical moment: the enormity of the first U.S. adult heart transplant. Stanford, CA: Stanford University Medicine; 2018.
157. Organ Procurement and Transplantation Network. Transplants in the U.S. by State, U.S. Transplants Performed: January 1, 1988–March 31, 2021. April 26, 2021.
158. Konstantinov IE. At the cutting edge of the impossible: a tribute to Vladimir P. Demikhov. Tex Heart Inst J. 2009;36(5):453–8.
159. Khan S, Jehangir W. Evolution of artificial hearts: an overview and history. Cardiol Res. 2014;5(5):121–5. https://doi.org/10.14740/cr354w. Epub 2014 Oct 6. PMID: 28348709; PMCID: PMC5358116
160. Toledo-Pereyra LH, Sutherland DE. Richard Carlton Lillehei: transplant and shock surgical pioneer. J Invest Surg. 2011;24(2):49–52. https://doi.org/10.3109/08941939.2011.558433. PMID: 21345003
161. Gondolesi GE. History of clinical intestinal transplantation. Hum Immunol. 2024;85(3):110788. https://doi.org/10.1016/j.humimm.2024.110788. Epub 2024 Mar 22. PMID: 38519405
162. Deltz E, Schroeder P, Gundlach M, Hansmann ML, Leimenstoll G. Successful clinical small-bowel transplantation. Transplant Proc. 1990;22(6):2501. PMID: 2264126
163. Veith FJ, Marin ML, Cynamon J, Schonholz C, Parodi J. 1992: Parodi, Montefiore, and the first abdominal aortic aneurysm stent graft in the United States. ;19(5):749-51. doi: 10.1007/s10016-005-6858-9. PMID: 16052384. https://doi.org/10.1007/s10016-005-6858-9. Ann Vasc Surg. 2005 Sep. PMID: 16052384.
164. J Vasc Bras. 2021 Mar 24;20:e20200192. PMID: 34093692; PMCID: PMC8147878 https://doi.org/10.1590/1677-5449.200192. J Vasc Bras. 2021 Mar 24;20:e20200192. PMID: 34093692; PMCID: PMC8147878

Chapter 11
Evidence, Surgical Research, Informed Consent

Archie Cochrane's account of a dying man at Elsterhorst, a World War 2 prisoner of war camp, first appeared in his memoir *One Man's Medicine*, 1989 (Fig. 11.1).

> *The Germans dumped a young Soviet prisoner in my ward late one night. The ward was full, so I put him in my room as he was moribund and screaming as I did not want to wake the ward. I examined him. He had obvious gross bilateral cavitation and a severe pleural rub. I thought the latter was the cause of the pain and the screaming. I had no morphia, just aspirin, which had no effect. I felt desperate. I knew very little Russian then and there was no one in the ward who did. I finally instinctively sat down on the bed and took him in my arms, and the screaming stopped almost at once. He died peacefully in my arms a few hours later. It was not the pleurisy that caused the screaming but loneliness. It was a wonderful education about the care of the dying. I was ashamed of my misdiagnosis and kept the story secret.* [1]

11.1 Development of Evidence-Based Practice

A poll conducted by the British Medical Journal (BMJ) ranked evidence-based medicine (EBM) as the seventh most influential milestone in shaping modern medicine out of a list of 15. EBM is a medical practice approach that relies on the best available scientific evidence to guide clinical decision-making. It involves systematically searching for and critically evaluating relevant scientific literature before applying this evidence to clinical practice [2]. Dr Archibald Cochrane, an epidemiologist, was a strong advocate for systematic reviews which was rewarded by the establishment of the Cochrane Collaboration by Iain Chalmers in 1993, five years after Cochrane's death.

The BMJ poll milestones also included the introduction of antibiotics, immunization, sanitation, and radiology. Before the advent of evidence-based medicine (EBM), medical practice was primarily based on expert opinions and observations, an approach known as "expert-based medicine."

S. Abbas, D. Watters, *The Road to Modern Surgery*,
https://doi.org/10.1007/978-981-96-4337-0_11

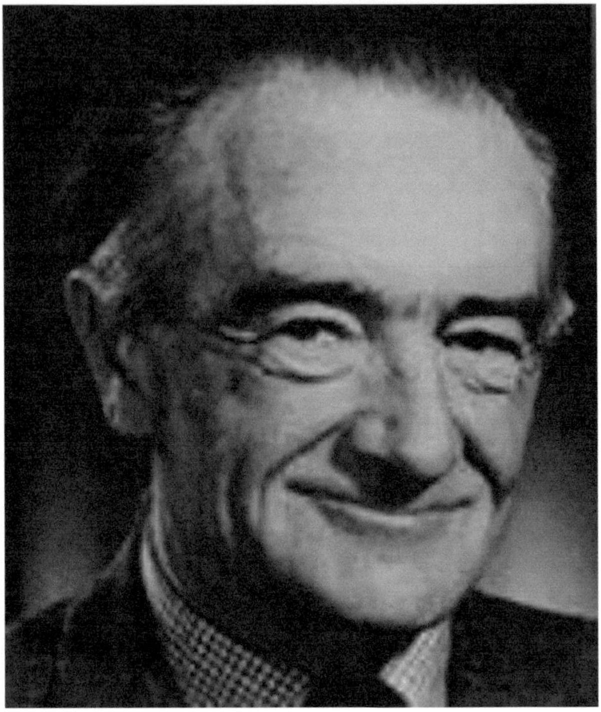

Fig. 11.1 Archibald Cochrane (1909–1988), Wikimedia, public domain. http://www.cochrane.org.au/libraryguide/pop_guide_archie.php

The evidence-based medicine (EBM) movement emerged in the early 1980s, led by a group of epidemiologists at McMaster University in Hamilton, Ontario, Canada, including David Sackett (1934–2015) (Fig. 11.2).

Sackett and his colleagues were concerned that medical decision-making often relied on tradition, authority, or anecdotal evidence rather than scientific evidence. They believed a more rigorous and systematic approach was necessary, one that utilized the best available scientific evidence to inform clinical decision-making [3].

To achieve this, Sackett and his colleagues developed a framework for evidence-based medicine involving five steps:

1. Formulating a clinical question
2. Searching for and critically appraising the relevant scientific literature
3. Applying the evidence to the individual patient
4. Evaluating the outcome
5. Reflecting on the process

Driven by a profound concern, Sackett and his erudite colleagues decried the prevailing reliance on tradition, authority, and anecdotal evidence in medical decision-making, advocating instead for a more rigorous and systematic approach. They envisioned a paradigm shift, one that would elevate the best available scientific evidence to the pinnacle of clinical decision-making [3–5].

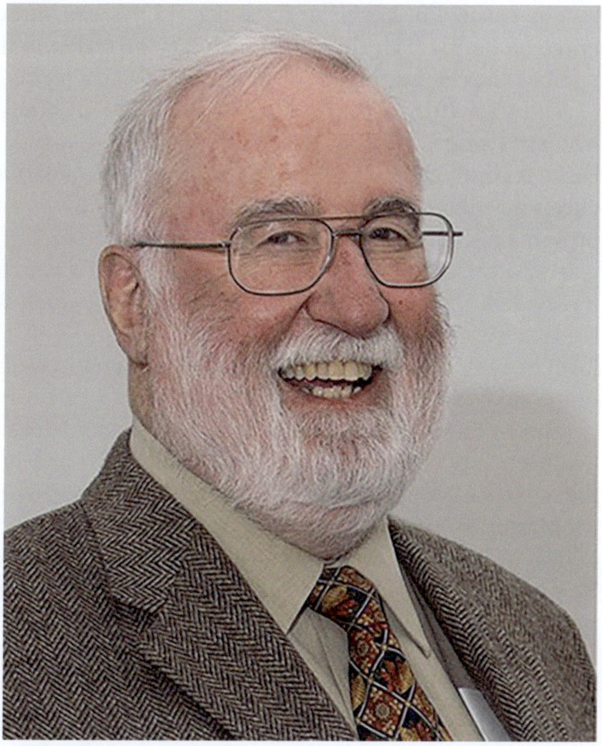

Fig. 11.2 David Sackett, from Canadian medical hall of Fame with permission

To realize this transformative vision, Sackett and his esteemed collaborators crafted a comprehensive framework for evidence-based medicine, structured around five pivotal steps: meticulously formulating a clinically relevant question, diligently searching for and critically evaluating the pertinent scientific literature, judiciously applying the evidence to the individual patient's unique circumstances, objectively evaluating the outcome, and thoughtfully reflecting on the entire process to refine and enhance future practice [2, 3].

The EBM movement has since grown and evolved, with the development of new tools and resources to support evidence-based practice, such as systematic reviews and clinical practice guidelines. Today, evidence-based medicine is a widely accepted and critical component of modern medical practice, helping to ensure that patients receive the best possible care based on the most up-to-date scientific evidence.

The term "evidence-based medicine" was first coined by Gordon Guyatt (b1953), a Canadian physician and clinical epidemiologist who was the Program Director of Internal Medicine at McMaster University in the early 1990s. Guyatt was a member of the same group of clinical epidemiologists at McMaster University who developed the framework for evidence-based medicine in the early 1980s, led by David Sackett. But it was Guyatt who first used the term "evidence-based medicine" in a paper published in the Journal of the American Medical Association in 1992 [3, 5].

The concept of Levels of Evidence (LOE) was introduced by the Canadian Task Force on Periodic Health Examination (CTF-PHE) in the 1970s, prior to the development of evidence-based medicine (EBM) as a formalized framework.

The CTF-PHE was established in 1976 as a joint effort of the Deputy Health Ministers across the ten Canadian provinces. Its mandate was to develop evidence-based recommendations for periodic health examinations, which are routine health check-ups that are intended to identify health problems and promote disease prevention.

As part of its work, the CTF-PHE developed a system for ranking the strength of the evidence supporting its recommendations, which was based on a hierarchy of study designs. This system, known as the Levels of Evidence (LOE), assigned a level of evidence to each study design based on its potential for bias and the strength of the study's internal validity.

The LOE system proved to be a valuable tool for assessing the strength of the evidence supporting clinical recommendations, and it was later incorporated into the evidence-based medicine framework developed by Sackett and his colleagues at McMaster University.

David Sackett (Fig. 11.2), the physician who is considered the father of evidence-based medicine (EBM), was born in Chicago in 1934, but he was a Canadian by choice.

Sackett obtained his medical degree at the University of Illinois in 1957 and then moved to Canada to pursue a residency in internal medicine at Toronto General Hospital. He subsequently completed a fellowship in nephrology at the Royal Victoria Hospital in Montreal before joining the faculty at McMaster University in 1967.

It was at McMaster University that Sackett became a leading figure in the development of evidence-based medicine, working alongside colleagues such as Gordon Guyatt and Brian Haynes to develop the framework for EBM and to promote its adoption within the medical community [5–7].

Looking back, Archie Cochrane is considered a forerunner of evidence-based medicine (EBM) due to his advocacy for the use of randomized controlled trials (RCTs) in the evaluation of medical interventions.

Cochrane was a British physician and epidemiologist who is best known for his influential book, *Effectiveness and Efficiency: Random Reflections on Health Services*, published in 1972. In this book, Cochrane argued that medical treatments should be evaluated using rigorous scientific methods, particularly RCTs, which he saw as the gold standard for assessing the effectiveness of medical interventions.

Cochrane was particularly concerned about the widespread use of medical interventions that had never been properly evaluated, leading to unnecessary harm and expense for patients. He argued that the medical profession needed to take a more scientific approach to the evaluation of treatments and that RCTs were the best way to do this.

Cochrane's advocacy for RCTs paved the way for the development of evidence-based medicine as a formalized framework, and his legacy is celebrated through the Cochrane Collaboration, established in 1993, an international network of researchers and healthcare professionals dedicated to promoting evidence-based healthcare [3, 6].

Sackett writes that the movement had its "philosophical origins" in the mid-nineteenth century, by Florence Nightingale (1820–1910) as the one who started it. Some now call this the "fourth revolution" in American medicine. Florence Nightingale, a British nurse and social reformer, is often credited with laying the groundwork for the modern nursing profession and for the development of evidence-based medicine. Nightingale emphasized the importance of collecting and analyzing data to inform medical decision-making, and her work in the Crimean War helped to establish nursing as a profession.

Florence Nightingale is famous for her work during the Crimean War, where she and her team of nurses used evidence to reveal the nature of infection in hospitals and on the battlefield. Through careful data collection and analysis, Nightingale was able to show that poor sanitation and overcrowding were contributing to high rates of infection and mortality among wounded soldier.

Florence Nightingale was a pioneer in the use of statistical evidence in healthcare decision-making. In the mid-nineteenth century, she was asked to advise on the renovation of St. Thomas' Hospital in London, England. To inform her recommendations, Nightingale collected extensive data on the hospital's mortality rates and causes of death.

Through her analysis, Nightingale was able to demonstrate that the hospital's mortality rates were significantly higher than those of other hospitals in England and that many of these deaths were preventable through improvements in sanitation and hygiene. She used this statistical evidence to develop a set of recommendations for the hospital, including the installation of proper ventilation and sewage systems, the use of clean linens and clothing, and the establishment of a trained nursing staff [5].

Nightingale's recommendations were controversial at the time, as they challenged conventional medical wisdom and required significant changes in hospital practices.

Nightingale was a highly respected figure in her lifetime, and her contributions to nursing and public health were widely recognized. In 1883, she was awarded the Royal Red Cross by Queen Victoria in recognition of her work during the Crimean War. The Royal Red Cross is a military decoration awarded to members of the armed forces and civilians who have shown exceptional devotion to duty in a medical capacity. In 1907, King Edward VII personally urged Nightingale to accept the newly created Order of Merit, which is one of the highest honours that can be bestowed upon a British citizen. Nightingale was the first woman to receive the honour.

Archie Cochrane, published his seminal book *Effectiveness and Efficiency: Random Reflections on Health Services* in 1972. His work was the inspiration for the Cochrane Collaboration, which has played a central role in promoting EBM.

Brian Haynes, a prominent figure in the development of evidence-based medicine, has spoken about his early experiences with critical thinking and evidence-based practice. Haynes has stated that he first became interested in the idea of evidence-based medicine during his medical training in the late 1960s, when he questioned the validity of the theories of Sigmund Freud.

During a lecture on psychoanalytic theory, Haynes asked the lecturer for evidence to support the claims being made. When the lecturer was unable to provide satisfactory evidence, Haynes became interested in the idea of evaluating medical practices and treatments based on empirical evidence. This experience helped to shape Haynes' approach to medicine and eventually led him to become a leading advocate for evidence-based practice.

Haynes went on to become a professor of clinical epidemiology and biostatistics at McMaster University in Canada, where he played a key role in the development of the evidence-based medicine movement.

Sir Iain Chalmers is a British medical researcher and health services expert who is best known as one of the co-founders of the Cochrane Collaboration, a global network of healthcare professionals and researchers who work together to promote evidence-based healthcare.

Chalmers began his career as a physician in the UK's National Health Service but became increasingly interested in the use of evidence to inform healthcare decision-making. In the early 1990s, he helped to establish the Cochrane Collaboration, which was named after the British epidemiologist Archie Cochrane [2–5, 7].

The Cochrane Collaboration is dedicated to producing high-quality, independent reviews of healthcare interventions and treatments, with the goal of promoting evidence-based practice and improving patient outcomes. The organisation has been highly influential in the development of evidence-based medicine and has helped to promote the use of systematic reviews and meta-analyses as key tools for evaluating healthcare interventions.

Evidence-based medicine (EBM) quickly gained popularity in the medical community for a number of reasons, including the support of senior clinicians who were open to new ideas and willing to challenge traditional medical practices, as well as the empowerment of young physicians and other healthcare professionals [3, 8].

David Sackett, one of the founders of EBM, emphasized the importance of engaging senior clinicians in the movement. He believed that EBM was more likely to be accepted and adopted if it was championed by respected and influential figures within the medical community. Senior clinicians who were confident in their own practice and open to need new ideas were often willing to challenge traditional medical practices and embrace new approaches to healthcare.

At the same time, EBM also empowered young physicians and other healthcare professionals by giving them the tools and resources to critically evaluate medical practices and treatments. By emphasizing the importance of evidence and data in healthcare decision-making, EBM helped to promote a culture of critical thinking and inquiry within the medical community. This, in turn, helped to create a more collaborative and interdisciplinary approach to healthcare, with physicians, nurses, and other healthcare professionals working together to provide the best possible care for their patients [8, 9].

Evidence-based medicine (EBM) has faced criticism and backlash from some quarters, particularly among those who were accustomed to more traditional approaches to medical practice and decision-making.

David Sackett acknowledged that the movement faced resistance from some physicians who were used to making authoritative pronouncements based on their own clinical experience and intuition. These "middle-level guys," as Sackett referred to them, may have felt threatened by the emphasis on empirical evidence and data-driven decision-making that characterized EBM.

One particularly notable example of this backlash was an unsigned editorial that appeared in The Lancet in 1995, which was titled "*Evidence-based medicine, in its place*." The editorial criticized what it saw as the excessive emphasis on evidence-based practice at the expense of other forms of clinical expertise and judgment. The authors argued that EBM needed to be seen as just one part of a broader approach to healthcare that took into account a range of different factors, including patient preferences, clinical experience, and intuition. EBM was described as "*it is impossible to practice, cookbook medicine, the creature of managers and purchasers.*"

Despite these criticisms, however, EBM has continued to gain traction and influence in the medical community. Today, EBM is widely recognized as an important tool for improving the quality of healthcare and promoting patient-centered, evidence-based decision-making [9, 10].

11.2 Randomized Controlled Trials

The journey of clinical trials starts with dietary therapy—legumes and lemons. Then we move to drugs. In the eighteenth century, the basic approach to clinical trials was established.

The world's first clinical trial is recorded in the Babylonian times. This experiment resembling a clinical trial was conducted by King Nebuchadnezzar a military leader. Nebuchadnezzar ordered his people to eat only meat and drink only wine during his rule in Babylon. He believed this diet would keep them in good physical shape. But several young men who preferred to eat vegetables, objected. The king allowed them to follow a diet of legumes and water for 10 days. When Nebuchadnezzar's experiment ended, the vegetarians appeared better nourished than the meat-eaters [11, 12].

Avicenna, a renowned Persian physician and philosopher who lived in the tenth and eleventh centuries, made important contributions to the field of medicine, including in the area of drug testing. In his encyclopedic work "*The Canon of Medicine*," he outlined some rules for testing drugs that are still relevant today.

One of the key principles that Avicenna emphasized was the importance of testing drugs on both healthy individuals and patients with the condition being treated. He recognized that the effects of a drug could differ depending on the health status of the individual taking it and that testing on healthy individuals could help establish a baseline for evaluating the drug's effects [12, 13].

Ambroise Paré (1510–1590), a famous French surgeon who lived in the sixteenth century, accidentally conducted what is considered to be one of the first clinical trials of a novel therapy by accident.

In 1537, Paré was treating soldiers who had been injured in battle using a traditional treatment of boiling oil to cauterize their wounds. However, when he ran out of oil during a battle, he turned to a mixture of egg yolks, rose oil, and turpentine as a substitute. To his surprise, he found that this mixture was just as effective as the boiling oil but caused less pain and scarring [14].

The Scottish physician, James Lind (1716–1794), is often credited with conducting one of the earliest recorded controlled clinical trials of the modern era.

In 1747, Lind conducted a trial to test the efficacy of different treatments for scurvy, a disease that was common among sailors at the time. He selected 12 sailors with scurvy and divided them into 6 groups, each of which received a different treatment, including citrus fruits, vinegar, seawater, and a purgative.

Lind observed that the sailors who received citrus fruits, particularly lemons and oranges, showed significant improvement in their symptoms, while the other treatments had little effect. This led him to conclude that scurvy was caused by a deficiency of "vitamin C," which is found in citrus fruits, and that these fruits could be used to prevent and treat the disease. It took 50 years for the British Navy to make lemon juice a compulsory part of the seafarer's diet. Soon, they replaced it with lime juice because it was cheaper.

While Lind's trial did not meet the rigorous standards of modern clinical trials, it is considered to be an important early example of controlled experimentation in medicine [15].

A century later the invention of placebo took place; "placebo" comes from the Latin word "placere," which means "to please." Hooper's Medical Dictionary of 1811 defined it as "*an epithet given to any medicine more to please than benefit the patient*." In medical terms, a placebo is a treatment or substance that has no therapeutic effect but is given to a patient as if it were a real treatment, typically in the form of a pill, injection, or other medical intervention. Sometimes the patient will respond to a *placebo,* a treatment which produces no known physiologic effects at all [16, 17].

The use of placebos in clinical trials began in the mid-nineteenth century, when doctors and researchers started to recognize the need for a control group in their studies. Placebos were used as a way to control for the "placebo effect," which is the phenomenon where patients experience an improvement in their symptoms simply because they believe they are receiving a real treatment.

The use of placebos has become an essential part of modern clinical trials, allowing researchers to test the effectiveness of new treatments against a control group. Today, all clinical trials are required to include a placebo control group unless there is a strong ethical or medical reason not to do so.

In the early 1940s, the Medical Research Council (MRC) in the UK conducted a clinical trial to investigate the use of patulin, an extract of *Penicillium patulinum*, as a treatment for the common cold.

The trial was conducted during the winter of 1943–1944 and involved over 1000 participants. The participants were divided into two groups, one receiving patulin and the other receiving a placebo. The results of the trial showed that there was no significant difference in the number of colds or the severity of symptoms between the two groups, indicating that patulin was not an effective treatment for the common cold, a condition caused by a virus, not a bacterium [16, 17].

The ethical framework for human subject protection has its roots in the ancient Hippocratic Oath, which emphasized the importance of doing no harm to patients. However, this principle was not always respected in human experimentation, particularly during periods of war and other crises when researchers felt pressure to quickly develop new treatments. The atrocities committed during World War II, particularly the medical experiments conducted by Nazi doctors, led to a renewed focus on protecting human subjects in medical research. In response to these abuses, the Nuremberg Code was developed in 1947, which laid out ten principles for the ethical conduct of medical research involving human subjects. Subsequently, a number of other ethical guidelines and regulations have been developed to protect the rights and welfare of human subjects in research, including the Declaration of Helsinki, the Belmont Report, and various national and international regulations. These guidelines emphasize the importance of informed consent, minimizing harm, and ensuring that the benefits of research outweigh any potential risks [16–18].

The first randomized controlled trial of streptomycin was conducted in 1946, by a team of researchers led by Dr. Albert Schatz and Dr. Selman Waksman at Rutgers University in the United States. The trial involved 15 patients with tuberculosis who were randomly assigned to receive either streptomycin or a placebo. The researchers found that those who received streptomycin had significantly improved outcomes compared to those who received the placebo. This landmark study demonstrated the effectiveness of streptomycin in treating tuberculosis and paved the way for the development of other antibiotics.

This trial was meticulous in design and implementation, with systematic enrolment criteria and data collection. It is worth noting that there were ethical issues with the study, as some patients who received the placebo ended up dying from their disease while an effective treatment was available. However, the trial was important in establishing the use of randomized controlled trials as a gold standard for evaluating the efficacy of medical intervention [15, 17].

The streptomycin trial helped to establish the importance of randomization and blinding in clinical trials, which are now widely used to reduce bias and ensure the reliability of study results. The trial also highlighted the need for careful planning and execution of clinical trials, including appropriate sample size calculations and data analysis methods.

The thalidomide tragedy, which occurred in the late 1950s and early 1960s, had a significant impact on the regulation of pharmaceuticals in the USA and the world. Thalidomide was a drug that was widely prescribed in Europe to treat morning sickness in pregnant women, but it was later found to cause severe birth defects in thousands of children. In the USA in response to the thalidomide tragedy, Congress passed the Kefauver-Harris amendments to the Federal Food, Drug, and Cosmetic

Act in 1962. These amendments strengthened federal oversight of drug testing and approval, requiring drug companies to provide more extensive testing and data on the safety and efficacy of their products. The amendments also included a requirement for informed consent, ensuring that patients are fully informed about the risks and benefits of participating in clinical trials [15, 17].

In 1964, the World Medical Association outlined the research guideline in the "The Helsinki Declaration" which is a set of guidelines for the ethical conduct of medical research involving human subjects.

The Helsinki Declaration sets out a number of general principles and specific guidelines for the conduct of medical research, with a focus on protecting the rights and welfare of human subjects. The principles include requirements for informed consent, minimizing risks to subjects, and ensuring that the benefits of research outweigh any potential harms.

Over the years, the Helsinki Declaration has been revised several times to reflect changes in medical research and evolving ethical standards. For example, the most recent revision in 2013, includes new provisions on the use of placebos in clinical trials and the protection of vulnerable populations [18–20].

While the science of medicine has advanced rapidly over the last two centuries, with many breakthroughs in understanding the body and developing new treatments, the practice of medicine remains an art because it involves a complex interaction between scientific knowledge, clinical experience, and individual patient factors.

Each patient is unique, and the way they respond to treatment may be influenced by a variety of factors, including their genetics, lifestyle, social environment, and psychological state. Therefore, the practice of medicine often requires a great deal of judgment and interpretation, as physicians must weigh the available evidence and consider the specific needs and preferences of each individual patient.

While scientific knowledge can certainly inform clinical decision-making, it is not always sufficient to predict how a patient will respond to treatment. Physicians must often use their intuition and clinical experience to adjust treatment plans and make decisions in real time based on the unique circumstances of each patient.

In this way, the practice of medicine remains an art, as it requires a great deal of skill, creativity, and empathy in addition to scientific knowledge [19, 20].

The randomized controlled trial (RCT) is the gold standard for clinical research, particularly for evaluating new drugs and other medical interventions. The RCT compares random-assigned groups that receive an experimental treatment and a control treatment (which may be a placebo, a traditional treatment, or no treatment). The study is double-blind, meaning researchers and participants don't know which group they're in. Comparing treatment groups, researchers can determine if the experimental treatment is more effective (or less harmful) and estimate the chance that any differences are due to chance. This helps clinicians to measure the effect and harm of any treatment which requires mathematical formulae and modules of statistics [15, 18, 20].

11.3 Statistics

The history of statistics can be traced back to ancient civilizations, such as the Babylonians and Egyptians, who used data to track economic activities, population numbers, and other important metrics.

Athenians in the fifth century B.C. used a method to estimate the height of ladders necessary to scale the walls of Platea by having multiple soldiers count the bricks. However, it is not clear if they specifically used the mode to determine the most frequent count.

Abu Yusuf Ya'qub ibn Ishaq al-Kindi was a Muslim philosopher, mathematician, and scientist who lived in the ninth century. He made significant contributions to various fields of knowledge, including cryptography.

Al-Kindi's *Manuscript on Deciphering Cryptographic Messages*, which he wrote around 850 A.D., is considered one of the earliest works on cryptography. In the manuscript, Al-Kindi explained how to use frequency analysis to decipher encrypted messages [20, 21].

The modern science of statistics started in the seventeenth and eighteenth centuries. The development of probability theory and statistical methods was largely driven by the needs of astronomers and navigators to quantify and make sense of large amounts of data. The scientific revolution was inaugurated by Newtonian mathematics, but biology and life science proved to be too complex to explain by math equations, because there are so many unknowns.

Francis Bacon (1561–1626) is often credited as being one of the earliest proponents of the scientific method, which emphasizes the importance of empirical evidence and systematic observation in the pursuit of truth. While he did not develop statistical methods, his approach to scientific inquiry influenced the development of statistics as a field of study.

Bacon emphasized the importance of induction, or the process of generalizing from specific observations. He advocated for the use of systematic data collection and experimentation in order to establish causal relationships between variables. This approach laid the foundation for statistical inference [13, 20, 21].

One of the key figures in the development of modern statistics was the Englishman John Graunt (1620–1674), who in the seventeenth century studied mortality data in London and developed the concept of life tables, which are still used today to analyze survival data. In the eighteenth century, methods were developed for measuring variability and correlation, laying the foundation for the field of biostatistics [21, 23, 24].

The term "statistics" was first used in 1749 by Swiss mathematician Daniel Bernoulli.

John Arbuthnot's work in 1710 is often credited as the first use of significance tests in statistics. In his work, Arbuthnot (1677–1735) analyzed data on the number of male and female births in London over a period of several years, and he used statistical methods to test whether the observed differences between male and female births were statistically significant or simply due to chance. He used a form of the chi-squared test, which is still widely used in statistical analysis today.

Arbuthnot's work is considered a landmark in the development of statistical theory, and it laid the foundation for the use of statistical significance tests in hypothesis testing and Decision-making [16, 22].

Napoleon Bonaparte (1769–1821) in France, as did other States, recognized the potential of statistics in improving governance and controlling empires. In 1800, he established the Imperial Academy of Political and Moral Sciences, which was responsible for collecting data on population, agriculture, industry, and commerce. Under Napoleon's leadership, statisticians were tasked with standardizing data collection methods and developing statistical techniques to analyze the data. This allowed Napoleon to make informed decisions about resource allocation, taxation, and other policies.

While the use of statistics in this context can be seen as a tool for improving governance, it is also true that statisticians were often at the service of powerful rulers and governments, and their work could be used to justify policies that oppressed and marginalized certain populations [14].

In the nineteenth century, statistics became a better established academic discipline, with statistical methods being used increasingly in many fields, including medicine, economics, sociology, and political science. In the 1840s and 1850s, the emerging field of medical meteorology gained attention as physicians and scientists sought to understand the relationship between weather and disease. One prominent figure in this field was William Farr (1807–1883), who became the first Medical Statistician to the General Register Office in England in 1839. Farr was responsible for analyzing and interpreting data on births, deaths, and diseases, and he used this data to investigate the impact of meteorological conditions on public health [14].

Karl Pearson (1857–1936) was a British mathematician and statistician who played a crucial role in the development of modern statistics. He is best known for his contributions to the field of correlation and regression analysis, which have become fundamental tools in many areas of science and social science. He founded the first University statistics department at University College, London in 1911.

Pearson's work was based on the idea that statistical analysis could be used to study biological and social phenomena in a more objective and rigorous way. He believed that statistical methods could help researchers to identify patterns and relationships that might be obscured by subjective observation or anecdotal evidence.

One of Pearson's most important contributions was the development of the correlation coefficient, which is a measure of the strength and direction of the relationship between two variables. Pearson also developed a number of other statistical techniques, such as curve-fitting and goodness-of-fit tests, that are widely used in modern research. Another physician embraced Pearson ideas, Major Greenwood (1880–1949) was a British epidemiologist and statistician who was heavily influenced by the work of Karl Pearson. Greenwood was one of the first medical researchers to recognize the potential of statistical methods for studying disease patterns and risk factors, and he was a vocal advocate for the use of quantitative data in medical research [24].

One of the first figures who advocated using numbers to analyze medical ads was Alexandre Louis (1787–1882) in 1830s. Louis was an early pioneer in the use of statistical analysis in medical research, and his work laid the foundation for evidence-based medicine.

Louis believed that medical decisions should be based on objective, quantitative data rather than subjective observations or traditional medical practices. He stressed the importance of collecting data systematically and analyzing it rigorously in order to draw meaningful conclusions. He collected data on patients. Louis argued that bloodletting was doing more harm than good.

Louis's approach was controversial at the time, as many of his colleagues were skeptical of the idea that medicine could be reduced to a set of mathematical formulas. The term "statistical evidence" remained controversial throughout the nineteenth century [25, 26].

In the twentieth century, the development of modern computing technology and the widespread availability of computers allowed for more sophisticated and efficient statistical analysis. This, in turn, led to the rapid expansion of the field of statistics and its application in a wide range of industries, including finance, marketing, and biology. Today, statistics is a vital tool for making sense of complex data and for testing hypotheses about the relationships between variables.

Ronald A. Fisher (1890–1962) was a British statistician and geneticist who made significant contributions to the fields of statistics, genetics, and experimental design. In 1926, Fisher introduced the concept of randomization tests, which involve randomly assigning subjects to treatment groups in order to reduce the effects of bias and confounding variables in experiments. This approach has become a standard method for analyzing data in many fields.

Fisher also developed the analysis of variance (ANOVA) method, which is used to determine whether differences between groups in an experiment are statistically significant. He also promoted the design of experiments, emphasizing the importance of careful planning and randomization in order to minimize errors and increase the validity of results [27].

William Allen Wallace (1906–1979) was an American statistician who made significant contributions to the theory of sequential analysis, which is a statistical method for analyzing data that arrive over time. His work laid the foundation for the development of optimal stopping theory and decision theory, which have important applications in fields such as engineering, economics, and finance. Wallace also worked on statistical inference, estimation theory, and nonparametric statistics [18, 21].

Sir David Roxbee Cox (1924–2022) is another prominent British statistician who has made important contributions to the field of statistics. He is known for his work on survival analysis, where he developed the proportional hazards model, which is widely used to model time-to-event data in medical research. Cox also made contributions to the theory of regression analysis, experimental design, and Bayesian inference. The profound influence of Cox on the field of medicine is vividly illustrated upon examining his seminal contributions. His enduring legacy in medical research is undeniable, as it is exceedingly rare to find an issue of any esteemed journal for that matter devoid of articles meticulously crafted using Cox's groundbreaking methodologies. Indeed, the very fabric of medical research methodology can be distinctly categorized into two distinct eras: the period preceding Cox's revolutionary work and the era that has flourished in its wake [18, 20, 21, 28].

Andrey Kolmogorov's book, *Foundations of the Theory of Probability*, published in 1933, is considered a seminal work in the field of probability theory. In the book, Kolmogorov (1903–1987) presented his axiomatic approach to probability theory, which is still widely used today. He also introduced the concept of a probability space, which is a mathematical framework for studying probability that includes a set of possible outcomes and a probability measure that assigns a probability to each outcome.

Kolmogorov's contributions to probability theory went beyond his book. In 1935, he became the first chairman of the department of probability theory at Moscow State University, which became a leading center for research in probability theory.

Today the practice of medicine is guided by evidence, which itself is supported by the statistics that enables researchers to compare data and interpret its meaning [29, 30].

11.4 Medical Ethics, Informed Consent and Shared Decision-Making

11.4.1 Informed Consent

In the past, it was not uncommon for surgery to be performed without the explicit consent of the patient. In ancient times, surgical procedures were often performed on unconscious patients or those who were restrained, such as prisoners, slaves, or soldiers.

During the medieval period, consent was not always sought or given, particularly in cases where the patient was considered unable to make decisions for themselves. In some cases, patients were operated on without their consent, either for religious or superstitious reasons or to satisfy the curiosity of medical practitioners.

Medical ethics developed predominantly within the profession of medicine until the early modern period. With few exceptions, patients and research subjects were not given consent or self-determination. The perspective on truthfulness and inclusivity in disclosure was mostly one of maximizing medical benefits through careful management of medical information. There was inherent fear that full disclosure could be harmful or distressing, particularly if it was conveyed abruptly and starkly. Withholding information on many occasions led to clear deception on the premise of trying to prevent such harm and spare the patient from the painful truth.

However, as medical ethics developed and patient autonomy was promoted as a key principle of healthcare, the concept of informed consent became more established. Today, surgical procedures cannot be performed without the patient's informed written consent, which requires the surgeon to explain the risks, benefits, and alternatives before the surgery is scheduled. The patient must also be informed of the potential outcomes and given the opportunity to ask questions and provide their consent before the procedure is carried out.

The idea of informed consent hinges on the ethical principles of justice invoked by Immanuel Kant (1724–1804) which stated that a patient's autonomy cannot be violated physically without consent given by a well-informed patient without duress or coercion.

Ethics is a broad term that covers the study of the nature of morals and the specific moral choices to be made. Normative ethics attempts to answer the question, *"Which general moral norms for the guidance and evaluation of conduct should we accept, and why?". Some moral norms for right conduct are common to all human kind: they transcend cultures, regions, religions, or other group identities, and constitute a set of values and principles by which people ought to live (not to kill, nor harm, nor cause suffering to others, not to steal, not to punish the innocent, to be truthful, to obey the law, to nurture the young and dependent, to help the suffering, and to rescue those in danger). A good example is the physician's "accepted role" to provide competent and trustworthy service to their patients. However, complying with the standards of professional organizations may not always fulfill the moral obligations as the codes developed have "often appeared to protect the profession's interests more than to offer a broad and impartial moral viewpoint or to address issues of importance to patients and society" due to the vagueness of the terms "accepted role" and "professional institution*" [31–33].

The four pillars of medical ethics are indeed beneficence, non-maleficence, autonomy, and justice.

Beneficence refers to the principle of doing good, and it requires healthcare professionals to act in the best interests of their patients and to promote their well-being. In addition to that, the moral principle needs to protect and defend the right of others, prevent harm, remove conditions that will cause harm, help persons with disabilities, and rescue persons in danger.

Non-maleficence is a simply stated principle that supports several moral rules—do not kill, do not cause pain or suffering, do not incapacitate, do not cause offence, and do not deprive others of the goods of life; on the other hand, it also refers to the principle of avoiding harm, and it requires healthcare professionals to avoid actions that may cause harm to their patients. Practically this puts the physician under obligation to weigh the benefits against burdens (risks) of all interventions, to eschew those that are inappropriately burdensome, and to choose the best course of action and minimize suffering [31, 33].

Autonomy refers to the principle of respecting patients' right to make their own decisions, and it requires healthcare professionals to provide patients with the information they need to make informed decisions about their healthcare. The underpinning principle of autonomy is what Immanuel Kant and John Stuart Mill (1806–1873) stated that everyone has intrinsic and unconditional worth. This means they should be able to make rational decisions and moral choices and should be allowed to exercise their capacity for self-determination.

Today, the principle of autonomy remains a fundamental principle of medical ethics, and informed consent is required before any medical procedure or treatment can be performed. The principle of autonomy recognizes and upholds the individual's right to make decisions about their own body and healthcare, and it ensures that patients are treated with respect, dignity, and compassion.

Justice refers to the principle of fairness, and it requires healthcare professionals to treat all patients equally and to allocate healthcare resources in a fair and equitable way.

These four principles are the foundation of medical ethics and guide healthcare professionals in their decision-making and interactions with patients. They are meant to ensure that patients receive the highest standard of care and that their rights and well-being are respected and protected.

Among these four pillars of medical ethics, autonomy is the basis for informed consent, truth-telling, and confidentiality. Informed consent requires that the patient or subject (1) is competent to understand and decide, (2) receives a full disclosure, (3) comprehends the disclosure, (4) acts voluntarily, and (5) consents to the proposed action.

The principle of informed consent requires that healthcare professionals provide patients with clear and accurate information about their condition, treatment options, and potential risks and benefits. Patients must be allowed to make their own decisions without undue coercion about their healthcare, and healthcare professionals must respect those decisions. In a previously autonomous, but presently incompetent patient, his/her previously expressed preferences are to be respected. Incompetent patients and previously competent (autonomous), but presently incompetent patients would need a surrogate decision-maker (i.e., a next of kin or legal representative).

Informed consent is a modern idea; it appeared first in 1957, and has been increasingly implemented since 1972. Prior to that there was no such commitment to obtain a formal informed consent, although the majority of practising surgeons would have obtained some form of consent, at least verbally. Many important figures in medicine through ancient, medieval, and early modern times wrote about openness in medical practice. These writings are a treasure trove of information about doctors' commitment to disclosure and discussion. But there was little formal requirement to implement any document covering informed consent.

In the Hippocratic Corpus, medical ethics centered on physicians' obligations to provide benefits and protect patients from harm. The purpose of medicine, (in the Hippocratic oath) was to benefit the sick and keep them from harm. Managing information with patients was portrayed as prudence and discretion in Hippocratic writings.

Benjamin Rush (1745–1813) and John Gregory are both known for their contributions to the field of medical ethics in the eighteenth century.

Rush was an early advocate for greater transparency and honesty in medical practice, and he believed that physicians had a moral obligation to fully disclose information to their patients. He argued that patients had a right to know the risks and benefits of medical treatments and that physicians should be honest about their own limitations and uncertainties. Rush also believed in the importance of public education about health [32–34].

John Gregory (1724–1773), a Scottish physician and professor of medicine, was also a proponent of medical ethics and professionalism. He believed that physicians had a duty to act in the best interests of their patients, and that they should avoid conflicts of interest and maintain high standards of professional conduct. Gregory emphasized the importance of patient confidentiality, and he argued that physicians should avoid unnecessary treatments and focus on providing compassionate care.

Both Rush and Gregory were influential in shaping the early development of medical ethics as a field of study, and their ideas continue to inform modern discussions about ethical principles in healthcare. Neither of them had the concept of informed consent. For example, Rush told physicians to give patients "relatively unimportant" choices but keep authoritarian control over "important" decisions and choices. Gregory and Rush valued patient input and dialogue, but they did not write about informed consent and self-determination was nonessential [33, 34].

Thomas Percival's historic Medical Ethics (1803) was of the same opinion. It's similar to previous codes and treatises on consent solicitation and respect for decision making. Percival (1740–1804) recommended benevolent deception, citing the patient's right to the truth against the obligation to benefit the patient in cases of conflict. He said: "*a patient … who makes inquiries which, if faithfully answered, might prove fatal to him, it would be a gross and unfeeling wrong to reveal the truth. His right to it is suspended, and even annihilated; because its beneficial nature being reversed, it would be deeply injurious to himself, to his family, and to the public.*" [34, 35]

In 1847 the Code of Medical Ethics was issued by the American Medical Association (AMA). Many of the above passages cited verbatim, in this code the AMA position on the obligations of physicians in regard to truth-telling. There was no recommendation to obtain the patients' consent or to respect their autonomy for the sake of autonomy. Worthington Hooker was the first to champion patient rights to information in the mid–nineteenth century. Hooker was unusual in opposing the medical tradition and swimming against the tide in regard to truth-telling. Despite his ingenious argument, it did not amount to the recommendation of informed consent in the way it is known today. It was more about truth telling than decision-making.

Prior to the 1950s, obtaining consent in surgery was not as standardized as it is today. There were several factors that influenced the practices of obtaining consent during this time, including concerns about medical reputation, malpractice suits, and practicality in medical institutions.

In terms of medical reputation, physicians were often concerned about being seen as competent and trustworthy. Patients were often viewed as passive recipients of medical care, and there was little emphasis placed on obtaining their consent for surgical procedures. Physicians were often expected to make decisions on behalf of their patients, without consulting them first.

Malpractice suits also played a role in the development of consent practices. As medical malpractice became more common, physicians and hospitals became more concerned about protecting themselves from lawsuits. Obtaining written consent from patients was seen as a way to protect against malpractice claims, as it provided evidence that the patient had been informed of the risks and benefits of the procedure.

Practicality in medical institutions was another factor that influenced the practices of obtaining consent during this time. Hospitals and medical facilities were often overcrowded and understaffed, making it difficult to obtain consent from patients. In some cases, consent forms were signed by patients shortly before surgery, or not at all.

The same applies in research involving human subjects. In the nineteenth century, for example, it was not uncommon for research to be conducted on slaves and servants without their consent or knowledge [35, 36].

During this time period, there was a belief among some researchers that they had the right to use vulnerable populations for their experiments without any regard for their well-being or autonomy. Slaves and servants, in particular, were seen as property rather than individuals with rights and, as such, were often used in medical experiments without their consent.

However, it is important to note that over time, attitudes toward informed consent in research have evolved. In the twentieth century, several high-profile cases, such as the Tuskegee Syphilis Study, helped to bring attention to the need for ethical guidelines in research involving human subjects.

American army surgeon Walter Reed's (1851–1902) yellow fever experiments at the turn of the century involved formal procedures for obtaining the consent of potential subjects.

In 1900, the US Army Surgeon General appointed a commission, led by Reed, to study yellow fever in Cuba. The commission was tasked with determining whether the disease was transmitted by mosquitoes and if so, how to prevent its spread [37].

As part of the study, Reed and his team recruited volunteers to participate in experiments to test their hypothesis that yellow fever was transmitted by mosquito bites. The volunteers were informed of the risks and benefits of the study and were given the option to decline participation.

Reed's team also established a medical board to review the consent process and ensure that the volunteers understood the nature of the experiments and their right to withdraw at any time.

These formal procedures for obtaining consent were groundbreaking at the time, as they represented a significant departure from the prevailing attitudes toward human subjects in medical research. Reed's experiments helped to establish the importance of informed consent in medical research and set the stage for future ethical guidelines in human subjects research.

In the early twentieth century, the behaviour of physicians as well as health institutions was often considered egregious, particularly with regard to patient autonomy and informed consent. In response to these issues, courts began to use strong language and sweeping principles to denounce these practices and establish legal precedents that protected patients' rights.

Schloendorff v. New York Hospital (1914) was a landmark case in the field of medical ethics and patient autonomy. The case involved a woman named Mary Schloendorff, who was admitted to New York Hospital for surgery where the surgeon removed her uterus without her informed consent. Schloendorff argued that her rights to bodily integrity and self-determination had been violated by the hospital. Schloendorff v. New York Hospital has been cited in numerous legal cases and has had a significant impact on medical ethics and patient rights. It is often cited as a landmark case in the development of the legal doctrine of informed consent.

The court stated that "no right is more sacred than the right of every individual to the control of his own person, free from all restraint or interference of others, unless by clear and unquestionable authority of law."

Justice Cardozo's ruling in this case affirmed the principle of autonomy, stating that "*every human being of adult years and sound mind has a right to determine what shall be done with his own body.*" This decision had a significant impact on medical ethics and established the principle of informed consent as a cornerstone of medical practice [36, 38–40].

Another example of strong language can be found in the case of Pratt v. Davis (1923). The court stated "the physician is not a god, and the law does not require us to put our lives and our health in his hands without recourse or protection." This statement emphasized the importance of informed consent and the right of patients to be fully informed about the risks and benefits of medical procedures. During the 1950s and 1960s, there was a significant evolution in the legal and ethical principles surrounding informed consent in the USA. Prior to this time, the duty to obtain consent was largely based on the physician's professional judgment, and the standard of disclosure varied widely [40, 41].

There was a growing recognition that patients had a right to know about the risks and benefits of medical procedures and that physicians had a duty to disclose certain types of information to patients. This led to the development of an explicit duty to disclose certain types of information and then to obtain consent.

One of the key factors that contributed to this evolution was the Nuremberg Code, a set of ethical guidelines that emerged from the Nuremberg trials in the aftermath of World War II. The Nuremberg Code emphasized the importance of informed consent and established the principle that research involving human subjects must be conducted with the voluntary informed consent of the participants.

In Salgo v. Leland Stanford Jr. University Board of Trustees (1957), Martin Salgo underwent a translumbar aortography procedure to evaluate the extent of his arteriosclerosis. The procedure involved injecting a contrast medium into his aorta through a needle inserted through his back. Unfortunately, Salgo suffered severe complications from the procedure, including paralysis of his lower body. He filed a lawsuit against the physician and hospital, alleging that he had not been adequately informed of the risks of the procedure. The Salgo case was a significant milestone in the development of informed consent law in the USA. It helped to establish the legal standard for informed consent that is still used today, emphasizing the importance of patient autonomy and the right of patients to be fully informed about the risks and alternatives of medical procedures [36, 42, 43].

The case of Natanson v. Kline (1960) was another landmark case in the development of informed consent law in the USA. The Kansas Supreme Court pioneered the use of the legal charge of negligence in informed-consent cases, rather than that of battery. The court established the duty of disclosure as the obligation "to disclose and explain to the patient in language as simple as necessary the nature of the ailment, the nature of the proposed treatment, the probability of success or of alternatives, and perhaps the risks of unfortunate results and unforeseen conditions within the body."

The Judicial Council of the American Medical Association made a statement in 1981 about consent. For the first time, the AMA recognized that informed consent is "*a basic social policy.*" The history of informed consent shows that the provision medical service has changed under legal and moral requirements for informed consent and autonomy but also that informed consent is a process that changes over time [36, 44].

11.5 Shared Decision-Making

Shared decision-making (SDM) describes the process of coming to a decision about treatment that involves the healthcare team, patient and their family or carers. In terms of perioperative care and the decision to undergo surgery, it involves understanding the patient's values, goals, and preferences, ensuring their expectations of what surgery can achieve are realistic, and the risks and benefits are considered. There should be consideration of the options available for treatment including non-surgical interventions (e.g., physiotherapy, hand therapy, pain management) and not undertaking any treatment at all. Shared decision-making requires good communication between the perioperative team and patient and thus depends upon listening as well as imparting information as to what surgery and recovery involves. Good shared decision-making, particularly for a complex or comorbid patient, requires multidisciplinary input involving expertise in the disease, expertise in the options for care, and expertise on the individual patient, the last being most likely provided by the patient, their family, or carers. The options considered and decisions made should be documented as should the patient's goals of care. Some patients will decide with their perioperative teams to undergo surgery but may not wish to be treated in an intensive care unit or have mechanical ventilation or failing organs supported in the event they develop complications. Limits of care (and limits of suffering from interventions) may be set prior to surgery to guide the postoperative care provided. Effective, documented SDM results in less decision regret both for patients and clinicians. When postoperative complications occur, the patient suffers, but there is also considerable emotional impact on the surgeon, or at least on surgeons who care.

Informed consent is particularly focused on professional and legal issues, ensuring the patient is aware of the significant and relevant (to them) risks of surgery, with the patient (or delegated carer) providing written consent for the procedure.

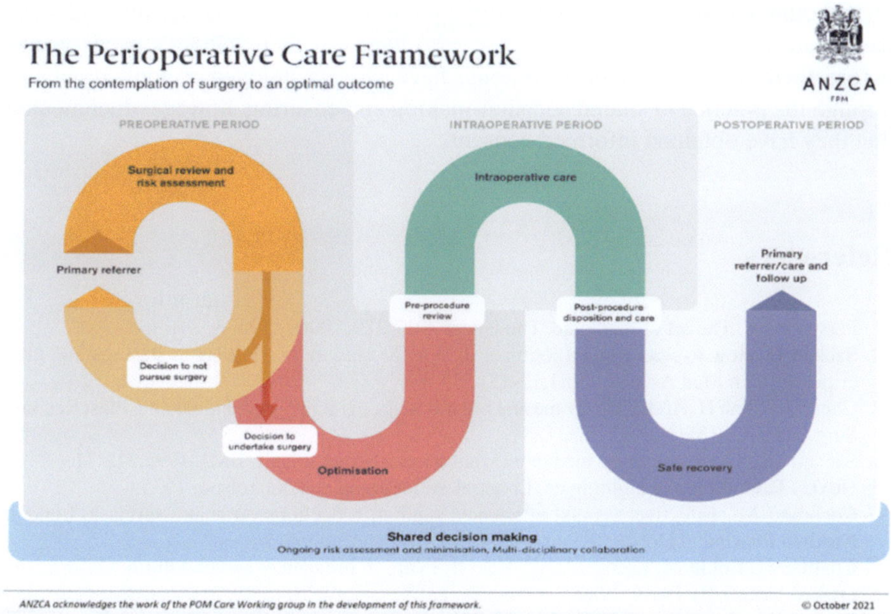

Fig. 11.3 ANZCA's perioperative care framework [47]

The information provided needs to be accurate, given in a language the patient or carer can understand and at a level appropriate to their health literacy. However, SDM involves much more than informed consent, because it includes expectations, values, preferences, and goals of care. It requires listening to the patient, not just informing the patient. It aligns decisions with the patient's values, underpinned by shared understanding and collaboration. Although informed consent can be given or withdrawn at any point along the preoperative journey, it is targeted at one particular intervention (the operation). SDM engages the patient all along the journey, defining the limits of care and all the options chosen before, during and after surgery (Fig. 11.3).

Throughout history patients have always had some say in whether they underwent surgery, though the more hierarchical the society and health system, the less likely were the wishes of the patient adhered to. The term shared decision-making (SDM) was only introduced in the early 1980s, challenging the mid-twentieth century more hierarchical style of decision-making in which doctors and surgeons often told patients what treatment they should have [45]. Prior to that the term had been used in writings on ethics in medicine [46]. However, it wasn't until 2001 that the first international conference on SDM was held in Oxford (UK). Over the next two decades of the twenty-first century, with the development of perioperative medicine, SDM has come to become a part of modern surgical, anesthetic and perioperative practice. In addition, lived experience, consumer voice, and input have been introduced to inform more patient-focused delivery of care at the health service level and how health systems are designed to meet the needs of the community.

It should also be recognized that throughout history, the majority of good, compassionate doctors of every age, those who have put their patient's needs wishes before their own benefit or ambitions, have always enjoyed a good reputation through the practice of shared decision-making and ensuring, however documented, that they have obtained informed consent.

References

1. Perspectives. The art of medicine. The lancet 2017;389(10069):594–5.
2. Sackett D. How to read clinical journals: I. Why to read them and how to start reading them critically. Can Med Assoc J. 1981;124(5):555–8.
3. Chung K, Shah H. Archie Cochrane and his vision for evidence-based medicine. Plast Reconstr Surg. 2009;124(3):982–8.
4. Sackett DL. Evidence based medicine: what it is and what it isn't. BMJ. 1996;312:71.
5. Huxley EJG. Florence nightingale. London: Weidenfield and Nicholson; 1975.
6. Cochrane AL. Effectiveness and efficiency: random reflections on health services. London: Nuffield Provincial Hospitals Trust; 1972.
7. Chalmers I, Enkin M, Keirse MJNC. Effective care in pregnancy and childbirth. Oxford, UK: Oxford University Press; 1989.
8. Sackett DL, Rosenberg WMC, Gray JA, Haynes RB, Richardson WS. Evidence based medicine: what it is and what it isn't. BMJ. 1996;312(7023):71–2.
9. Evidence-based medicine, in its place. Lancet. 1995;346(8978):785.
10. Smith R, Rennie D. Evidence-based medicine—an oral history. JAMA. 2014;311(4):365–7. https://doi.org/10.1001/jama.2013.286182.
11. Bull JP. A study of the history and principles of clinical therapeutic trials. MD Thesis: University of Cambridge; 1951.
12. Twyman RA. A brief history of clinical trials. The Human Genome. 2004. Accessed 5 Oct 2009.
13. Bacon F. The advancement of learning. Paperback edition, Dent & Sons; 1973.
14. Rusnock AA. Vital accounts: quantifying health and population in eighteenth-century England and France. Cambridge: Cambridge University Press; 2002.
15. Collier R. Legumes, lemons and streptomycin: a short history of the clinical trial. CMAJ. 2009;180:23–4.
16. Graunt J. Natural and political observations upon the bill of mortality; 1662.
17. Sparks J. Timeline of laws related to the protection of human subjects Office of History National Institutes of Health. html. Accessed 20 Sep 09.
18. Dodgson SJ. The evolution of clinical trials. J Eur Med Writers Assoc. 2006;15:20–1.
19. Farr W. Report on the mortality from cholera in England, 1848--1849. London: Her Majesty's Stationery Office; 1852 [Also published as Farr W. Registrar General's report on cholera in England 1849--1850. London: W. Clowes & Son; 1852].
20. Hart PD. A change in scientific approach: from alternation to randomised allocation in clinical trials in the 1940s. BMJ. 1999;319(7209):572–3.
21. Hardy A, Magnello ME. Statistical methods in epidemiology: Karl Pearson, Ronald Ross, Major Greenwood and Austin Bradford Hill, 1900-1945. Soz Praventivmed. 2002;47(2):80–9.
22. Matthews JR. Almroth Wright, vaccine therapy, and British biometrics: disciplinary expertise versus statistical objectivity. In: Magnello E, Hardy A, editors. The road to medical statistics. Amsterdam-New York: Rodopi; 2002. p. 125–47.
23. John CH, Graunt FRS. (1620-74): The founding father of human demography, epidemiology and vital statistics. J Med Biogr. 2024;32(1):57–69.
24. Shannon H. A statistical note on Karl Pearson's 1904 meta-analysis. J R Soc Med. 2016; 109(8):310–1.

25. Morabia A. Pierre-Charles-Alexandre Louis and the evaluation of bloodletting. J R Soc Med. 2006;99(3):158–60.
26. Louis PCA. Researchers on the effects of bloodletting in some inflammatory diseases, and on the influence of tartarized antimony and vesication in pneumonitis (trans: Putnam CG). Boston: Hilliard, Gray; 1836.
27. Thompson EA. R.A. Fisher's contributions to genetical statistics. Biometrics. 1990;46(4): 905–14.
28. Pavlos, et al. Medicine before and after David Cox. Msaouel. Eur J Internal Med. 98:1–3.
29. Dudley RM, Cook SL, Llopis J, Peng NP. A. N. Kolmogorov and statistics: a citation bibliography. Ann Stat. 1990;18(3):1017–31.
30. Marks HM. The progress of experiment science and therapeutic reform in the United States, 1900–1980. Cambridge: Cambridge University Press; 1997.
31. Beauchamp TL, Childress JF. Principles of bioethics. 7th ed. Oxford University Press; 2013.
32. Berkman ND, Wynia MK, Churchill LR. Gaps, conflicts, and consensus in the ethics statements of professional associations, medical groups, and health plans. J Med Ethics. 2004;30(4):395–401.
33. Guyer P. Kant on the theory and practice of autonomy. Soc Philos Policy. 2003;20(2):70–98.
34. Gregory J. Lectures on the duties and qualifications of a physician, New edition. London: Strahan & Cadell; 1772.
35. Bazzano LA, Durant J, Brantley PR. A modern history of informed consent and the role of key information. Ochsner J. 2021;21(1):81–5. https://doi.org/10.31486/toj.19.0105. PMID: 33828429; PMCID: PMC7993430.
36. Faden RR, Beauchamp TL. A history and theory of informed consent. Oxford: Oxford University Press; 1986.
37. Tobin MJ. Fiftieth anniversary of uncovering the Tuskegee Syphilis Study: the story and timeless lessons. Am J Respir Crit Care Med. 2022;205(10):1145–58.
38. Cardozo B. Basic right to consent to medical care—Schlendorff vs the Society of the New York Hospital, 211 NY 125 105 NE 92 1914 LEXUS 1028. (1914).
39. Angell M. Ethical imperialism? Ethics in international collaborative clinical research. N Engl J Med. 1988;319(16):1081–3.
40. Katz J. The silent world of doctor and patient. Baltimore: JHU Press; 2002.
41. Schloendorff v. Society of New York Hospital. 211 N.Y. 125, 129, 105 N.E. 92 (1914).
42. Salgo v Leland Stanford, Jr University Board of Trustees 154 Cal App 2d 560, 317 P2d 170 (1957). Accessed 5 Feb 2021.
43. Permissible medical experiments. In: Trials of war criminals before the Nuremberg military tribunals under control council law No. 10, vol. 2. Washington, D.C.: US Government Printing Office; 1949. p. 181–2.
44. Natanson V (1960) Kline, 186 Kan 393, 411, 350 P. 2d 1093.
45. President's Commission for the Study of Ethical Problems in Medicine and Biomedical and Behavioral Research. Making health care decisions. The ethical and legal implications of informed consent in the patient-practitioner relationship. Washington; 1982. p. 33.
46. Veatch RM. Models for ethical medicine in a revolutionary age. What physician-patient roles foster the most ethical relationship? Hast Cent Rep. 1972;2(3):5–7. https://doi.org/10.2307/3560825. JSTOR 3560825. PMID 4679693.
47. Australian and New Zealand College of Anaesthetists (ANZCA). The perioperative care framework. https://www.anzca.edu.au/safety-and-advocacy/standards-of-practice/our-perioperative-care-framework.

MIX
Papier aus verantwortungsvollen Quellen
Paper from responsible sources
FSC® C105338

If you have any concerns about our products,
you can contact us on
ProductSafety@springernature.com

In case Publisher is established outside the EU,
the EU authorized representative is:
Springer Nature Customer Service Center GmbH
Europaplatz 3, 69115 Heidelberg, Germany

Printed by Libri Plureos GmbH
in Hamburg, Germany